CRANIOSACRAL
BIODYNAMICS

CRANIOSACRAL BIODYNAMICS

VOLUME ONE

The Breath of Life, Biodynamics, and Fundamental Skills

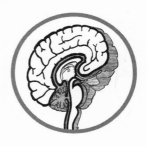

FRANKLYN SILLS

Illustrations by Dominique Degrangés

North Atlantic Books
Berkeley, California
and
UI Enterprises
Palm Beach Gardens, Florida

Craniosacral Biodynamics

Published by   and
North Atlantic Books   UI Enterprises
P.O. Box 12327   11211 Prosperity Farms Road
Berkeley, California 94712   Palm Beach Gardens, FL 33410

Printed in the United States of America

Illustrations by Dominique Degrangés
Cover design by Paula Morrison
Book design by Jan Camp

Craniosacral Biodynamics is sponsored by the Society for the Study of Native Arts and Sciences, a nonprofit educational corporation whose goals are to develop an educational and crosscultural perspective linking various scientific, social, and artistic fields; to nurture a holistic view of arts, sciences, humanities, and healing; and to publish and distribute literature on the relationship of mind, body, and nature.

North Atlantic Books' publications are available through most bookstores. For further information, call 800-337-2665 or visit our website at www.northatlanticbooks.com.

Substantial discounts on bulk quantities are available to corporations, professional associations, and other organizations. For details and discount information, contact our special sales department.

Library of Congress Cataloging-in-Publication Data

Sills, Franklyn, 1947–
    Craniosacral biodynamics: the breath of life, biodynamics, and fundamental skills / by Franklyn Sills.
        p. cm.
    Includes bibliographical references and index.
        V. 1.—V. 2.
    ISBN 1-55643-354-9 (alk. paper)
    1. Craniosacral therapy. I. Title.
    RZ399.C73 S57 2001
    651.8'9—dc21

                                                                                00-067885
                                                                                        CIP

                    1 2 3 4 5 6 7 8 9 / 06 05 04 03 02 01

Contents

Preface

In sitting down to write this preface, I was overwhelmed by the acknowledgment of the journey it took to get to this point. I started to write this book fifteen years ago. My understanding of work within this field was dramatically different then. Each time I attempted to complete the writing work, my understanding and perspectives changed. This book has gone through at least ten drafts. I drove my colleagues, students, and family to distraction with my constant rewritings. Each time a piece was completed, my perception of things had changed. Most of this arose from my clinical practice. As my clinical understanding of what I was encountering and doing changed, so did my conceptual framework. The training course also continually underwent changes in an attempt to align it with clinical practice. This has been a real negotiation and mutual learning process for me and all of the teaching staff here at the Karuna Institute, and also at the Craniosacral Therapy Educational Trust in London. Each year training approaches changed here at Karuna and somehow had to be conveyed to colleagues not directly associated with us. Then the validity of these changes had to be experienced and challenged within the teaching format and within clinical practice. A truly humbling process!

There have been many influences on my clinical work, on my understanding of the nature of healing processes, and on the teaching processes derived from these. The first and foremost teachers have been my patients. Clinical work is the true ground of learning. My first entrée into the world of complementary medicine was through the work of Dr. Randolph Stone, D.O. I first encountered his work in 1975, and it was a powerful introduction into the realm of energy medicine. His work was, and still is, a huge contribution to the field of energy medicine. I also want to thank and give appreciation to Dr. James Said, who brought a semblance of real order to the polarity therapy field after Dr. Stone's retirement. I am forever indebted to his clarity. My first introduction to the cranial field was through Dr. Stone's work. He considered it part of a wider energy medicine. I became entranced by the nature of what he called the neuter essence and understanding its unfoldment within the human system became a calling. It led me directly to the work of Dr. W. G. Sutherland and to the field of clinical work he founded. Dr. Stone had studied with Dr. Sutherland and his influence on Dr. Stone's work is clear. My clinical focus very early became the neuter essence of Dr. Stone's work and the potency of the Breath of Life, which Dr. Sutherland discussed.

This set me off on what has become a lifetime journey into what might be called energy medicine, and an attempt to listen to the human system in such a way that I could hopefully be led into its mysteries. I attended osteopathic college and underwent an apprenticeship in the field. This was a wonderful addition and ground to my understanding of both structure and function and of work in the cranial field. The contacts and friends I made in osteopathic college have been an ongoing blessing.

I am deeply grateful to the teaching staff here at Karuna. They brought their own massive clinical experience to the training course. Our ongoing conversations about the nature of work within the cranial field and how to teach it at a foundation level were the ground for the current training format. I have been deeply influenced by the writings of Dr. Rollin Becker, D.O. I first came across his four articles on palpation while in osteopathic college. Although they touched me, I could not make heads or tails of them then. Rereading them ten years later was an eye opener. Not only did it resonate, but much of it made total sense to me. I have incorporated some of Dr. Becker's terminology into the training course and into the writing of this volume. I find his concepts extremely helpful in framing the work. *Craniosacral biodynamics,* the term I now use for the work, originates from his use of the term *biodynamic* to indicate the action of the potency of the Breath of Life within the human system. I have also deeply appreciated the writings of Dr. James Jealous, D.O., on work in this field. I first came across his writings in 1995; they were a real gift at a time when I was attempting to reframe the course and its language. His words resonated with our clinical experience and were inspiring. Although Dr. Jealous also uses the word *biodynamics* to describe his work, our work here is not derived from his, but a deep resonance and respect for his clarity and insight is felt by all the staff here at Karuna. Quotes from some of his articles are used in this volume with his kind permission.

These two volumes are geared to be textbooks for students and practitioners. They outline a particular biodynamic outlook in the cranial field. The work within this volume is different from most foundation coursebooks currently available. Dr. Sutherland, the founder of this work, emphasized that the human system is not just a mechanism, but is ordered by the deepest spiritual sources. He called the Creative Intelligence in action within the universe the *Breath of Life*. It is this Breath of Life that is the focus for a clinical understanding, even if we only perceive the forces it generates. This book focuses on the Breath of Life as the ordering and organizing principle, not just of the human system, but within the world at large. Craniosacral biodynamics is an energy medicine, which attempts to align us to the deepest wellspring of life. It takes a *biodynamic* approach in that the intentions are to clarify our relationship to the Breath of Life and its ordering processes, and to function clinically as a servant to the healing processes it unfolds. Our work is clearly seen to be one of supporting these intentions. We do not "do" the healing; we listen to and support its unfoldment. I also have strongly deemphasized the CRI level of action. This book and the course we teach focus much more on the deeper tidal rhythms within the human system. It is within these rhythms that the resources of the system are found and within which our unresolved experience, be it traumatic or pathological, is centered. Our focus is squarely on the action of what Dr. Sutherland called the potency of the Breath of Life as it unfolds within our human condition.

I use words in particular ways in this volume. Readers may be unfamiliar with many of the terms I use. Please bear with it and, as you work with the concepts via clinical applications, the usage will, I hope, become clearer. I have also coined a number of terms, such as *mid-tide, primal midline, bioelectric matrix, dynamic equilibrium,* and others. Their use has an internal consistency, so please read them within the context of the whole presentation.

I find that I am finally relatively happy to put this text out into the world. I am sure that it will be received in different ways by different people. Its intention is to delineate one approach to work within this field. I do not claim to have the ultimate truth here, nor do I deny other equally valid beliefs and approaches. The intention is simply to share discoveries and hopefully help in the alleviation of suffering, even to a small measure. It is time that people within this and other fields stopped taking positions and began to share insights. We are all in this together. We are not things, nor are we the forms we generate. We must not be narrowly defined by the professions we create. These are hopefully all skillful means to alleviate suffering. We are a living unfoldment of life itself. No one owns or can control this unfoldment. It is beyond our machinations. There is the possibility of paying attention, of truly being present, and of listening to our human condition. Can we share our learning for the betterment of all? There is suffering. How can we help in its alleviation? For me it is as simple as that. In this process we must not fool ourselves, but must continue to develop both clinically and spiritually. Trainings must reflect this and must be geared to produce safe and efficient practitioners. This has been an ongoing process here at Karuna. So my intentions here are simply to share what I and close colleagues have discovered and developed over the years. I hope that this volume will be read by students and practitioners of the work with an open mind, and that it will be of some use to many of you. Colleagues and students have been asking me to complete this work for many years now. So here it is, in a two-volume format.

In the words of my own spiritual tradition:

May all beings be peaceful!

May all beings be happy!

May all beings be liberated!

May this book be of some value in the alleviation of suffering.

Acknowledgements

First, I wish to acknowledge the colleagues with whom I have worked closely over the years. They have all had their part to play in the unfolding of the training program here at the Karuna Institute. I wish to thank Claire Dolby, D.O., for pushing me to develop a training program geared for practitioners in the health and helping professions. Until then this work was largely taught only in the osteopathic world. It was felt that it was important at that time, especially here in Britain, to train practitioners who might be able to take the work into the National Health Service. We also felt that it was important to redefine the work in terms of a field of practice in its own right. I know that this is controversial in some quarters. I want to thank Michael Kern, D.O., for pushing me to develop a training program in London. The CTET has developed from those roots and is continuing to provide an excellent foundation in this work. Michael is the current coordinator of training there and continues to contribute to the field. I would like to thank Paul Vick for his tenacity in sticking with this work and helping to develop the CTET course. Paul has developed a unique teaching style and is organizing a new training program in London. I wish him well. I would like to thank Katherine Ukleja, D.O., for her ongoing contributions to the Karuna course as a senior lecturer and for her clarity and frankness. Katherine has always managed to ground me when my musings went beyond my clinical experience. She still does this,

and for this I am eternally grateful. I would like to thank both Colin Perrow and Mij Ferrett for their contributions to the course at Karuna, and for the great dialogues we have had about the work. I want to deeply acknowledge the work of Mike Boxhall in postgraduate courses for cranial practitioners. Mike is one of the old men of the work. He admirably brings practitioners to the Stillness and to a deeper trust in the nature of our human condition. We have had very important dialogues over the years and much thanks to him for that.

I would like to acknowledge the practitioners who brought me to Switzerland many years ago, and who now have founded their own training program with integrity and heart. They include Peter Wydler, Dominque Degrangés, Marcell Bryner, Alex Huberthur, and Heidi Baumann. I would also like to acknowledge Susi Iff for her kindness in setting up my original seminars in Switzerland and for introducing me to Switzerland and to the Swiss people. I want to thank Christopher and Mary Louise Muller for organizing my first American training and for their ongoing commitment to the work. I think of their kindness to me over the years with much appreciation. Likewise, I want to thank Doug Janssen for his role in setting up the Boston training and for his continuity in offering trainings on the east coast of America and in other places. He took such good care of me in Boston. I am always appreciative of his generosity and the laughs we had together. I also want to thank John and Anna Chitty for introducing me to the Boulder crowd, and for setting up an excellent training program there. John, Anna, and Scott Zamurut have heart-fully developed a full cranial program in Boulder with the facilities to back it up. I would also like to thank Scott for his stepwise, gradual approach to learning and teaching this work.

I would also like to thank Tanmayo Krebber-Woehrle for twisting my arm to come to Germany and for setting up a program there. All have greatly contributed to the development of this form of the work. Finally, I would like to appreciate the work of Dr. Michael Shea, Ph.D., in developing and teaching a biodynamic approach to work in the cranial field. Michael has been a student and colleague of mine for a number of years now and the gradual development of his approach to work in this field has shown integrity and clarity at all levels.

I would like to acknowledge with much respect the pioneering work of Dr. John Upledger, D.O. It was because of Dr. Upledger's single mindedness in offering his work to the world that the consciousness of the cranial field has been hugely raised among a suffering population. The Upledger Institute continues this important work.

Most emphatically, I wish to acknowledge my wife and family. My wife Maura Sills, is the founder of Core Process Psychotherapy, a Buddhist-influenced therapy form. It is an elegant therapeutic form, which reflects the deep truths of relationship, suffering, and the potential to heal, and I am greatly indebted to Maura for sharing her journey with me all of these years. She has put up with my endless writing and sometimes babbling and incoherent statements about the nature of life. I love her deeply. In all honesty, I have learned my deepest lessons in my role as father. My two children, Laurel and Ella, are the joy of my life and my greatest teachers. I wish to joyfully thank them and wish them both well in their respective journeys.

I would like to thank Dr. Jim Jealous for permission to use quotes from his writings and for the dialogue we have had over the last few years. I would also like to acknowledge and thank the American Academy of Osteopathy for permission to use quotes from Dr. Becker as they appeared in the Academy of Applied Osteopathy Yearbooks. Their website can be found at:

www.academyofosteopathy.org.

Finally, to Dominique Degrangés, another emphatic thank you for the wonderful illustrations in this work. Dominique is an excellent teacher and practitioner of the work, and is also an excellent illustrator. I would also like to thank Michael Kern, D.O., for his early feedback on the text. I would also like to thank Paul Vick and Mike Boxhall for feedback on the text and also the staff here at Karuna for their on-going feedback on the written chapters. I know that I may have inadvertently omitted various colleagues and staff in these acknowledgments. If this is the case, please let me know.

Thank you.

SECTION ONE
Fundamental Principles

1

In the first few chapters of this book, I will introduce a particular understanding and approach to work within the cranial field. The way I describe this perspective is based largely on my own perceptual understandings and clinical experience. It is a perspective that has been influenced by many sources, by deep discussions over many years with colleagues, students, and friends, and, most of all, by my clinical practice. This viewpoint entails a paradigm shift from a mechanistic orientation to work within this field to a truly dynamic one. In this perceptual shift, there is an appreciation of life as it unfolds its intentions within the creation of a human being. With this awareness, there is a recognition that the organizing forces at work within the developing embryo are still at work in the eighty-year-old. It is seen that these forces are *epigenetic*, that is, they underlie and precede genetic expression. It is a viewpoint which acknowledges that life originates in the infinite present and that healing can only occur in the present time-ness of life. Healing is thus about present process and organization, not about past or future experience.

In this chapter we will:

- *Introduce some basic concepts.*
- *Outline some of the history of the work.*
- *Give some of the basic premises and intentions of the work.*

Inquiry

Work in the cranial field is largely perceptual. The heart of clinical practice is listening. This demands both stillness and humility on the part of the practitioner. In this inquiry all one can do is to enter into a stillness and see what our journey brings. The foundation of this endeavor is the experience of our own perceptual and inner processes. An appreciation of our inner world is crucial for efficient clinical practice. This awareness of our own interior world is critical in the creation of a safe and efficient healing relationship. In this process, we will come directly into relationship to our own human condition and our own suffering. This is a huge undertaking. It means truly inquiring into who we are. The ground of this exploration is a commitment to learn about ourselves. It is about inquiry and awareness.

In this context we can develop a relationship to our unfolding process as a sentient human being. From this ground, it is possible to form clear and healing relationships with others. Work in the cranial field is very intimate. It entails an intimacy of contact and communication. Within the context of a clinical relationship, you explore what it means to be a human being. In this process, the practitioner must truly learn what it means to have a depth of contact with another person. However, this process has vast implications for everyday life. Our relationships are the ground of our experience. It is from our relationships that we mold our sense of the world and our place within it. Thus the work, in a powerful way, can only bring us back to ourselves.

Suffering

As we pay attention to our lives, questions will naturally arise. The most pressing of these for me are about the nature of the suffering that I feel within me and see in the world around me. In the work I do, I constantly meet suffering and its personal manifestations. There is a whole spectrum of suffering ranging from an inherent sense of dissatisfaction, to physical, emotional, and spiritual torment. From my experience, I have seen that suffering is truly a relational process. That is, suffering arises within the context of relationship. The nature of our experience is that it happens within relationship. Whether it is the relationship we have to our inner life, to our particular experiences, or to the people within our life, traumatization and suffering are seen to be relational processes. The ground of this is our relationship to our inner world and to our experience of the outer world we inhabit. Suffering may even arise due to our relationship to the universe we inhabit and our sense of selfhood within its vastness. Existential crises are not unusual and play a large part in the suffering I see around me. A sense of meaninglessness can be overwhelming. Who am I in this seemingly vast and impersonal universe? Even more so, if there is a sense of "something other," a greater power, something that underlies the seeming arbitrariness of things, another kind of self-crisis can ensue. A painful experience of emptiness can grip us as a sense of separation from the divine, or from the deeper creative forces within our human condition.

Perhaps the deepest suffering that we hold is the suffering which arises due to the loss of trust in relationship itself and to the subsequent pain of intimacy. In this, we lose trust in the safety and potential of relationship, and intimacy itself is experienced as painful. Intimacy, the experience of a depth of contact with self and other, becomes painful and threatening. People end up both deeply yearning for intimacy and deeply afraid of it. For some, the closer a relationship becomes, the more threatening it becomes. Because of this, it seems that the deepest healing processes are those that occur within the context of relationship. In the cranial field we consciously create a relationship that holds open the possibility that trust in intimate contact can be renegotiated. This must occur within a nonjudgmental field of presence and respectful listening. There must be a fundamental intention to create a safe and meaningful relational field within the context of clinical exploration.

The Buddha taught extensively and deeply about the nature of suffering, and his teachings have been of great personal benefit to me. The first noble truth of the Buddha is about suffering, or *dukkha*. *Dukkha* is a basic sense of unease, a state of anxiety, which arises as we experience life. It is inherent within the conditions of life. The Buddha, in this, did not say that everything is suffering, or *dukkha,* as is sometimes said. He simply and profoundly stated that *there is suffering and it must be understood*. This simple statement is the ground of therapeutic inquiry. The understanding of *dukkha* is not just a mental understanding, but an embodied, almost visceral insight into the nature of impermanence and self-construct. Suffering is seen to be a relational process. If we are in the world in a certain way, then there will be suffering. If that way of being is relinquished, then suffering is also relinquished. Simply put, if we hold onto things, onto fixed positions, onto self-construct, self-view, and past history, then there will be suffering. If we relate to the world within the context of attachment and aversion, and if we are confused about the nature of present reality, then there will be suffering. If we are ignorant about the present nature of things, then we suffer. Most of us, most of the time, tend to see the present through the filters of the past. But if we can find a way to truly live in the present, in the present time-ness of things, then there is the possibility of not suffering. There may be pain, but there needn't be suffering. Within the

Xerox

Netter Figure

Palette 1
2
3
6

cranial context, it is seen that suffering is relinquished when the system truly aligns with the present time-ness of things. It is an alignment to something else beyond the fear that seems to hold our sense of selfhood together. It is a realignment to a universal, an Intelligence much greater than our human mentality. To something still, yet potently present. This occurs when the oppositional forces of our past experience are reconciled within us, in states of balance and stillness. Within the Stillness, known only in this present moment, something else can occur beyond the suffering held. It is as simple as that.

Questions

Over the years I have been privileged to be able to engage in an exploration into the human condition, and into the nature of suffering and healing, with many people, in many contexts. It has been a journey that has not only encompassed the cranial concept, but has embraced many avenues of inquiry. These included journeys into many healing arts and spiritual traditions. As one engages in this process of inquiry, some deeper questions about the work we do and about life itself begin to unfold. Some of these are:

Questions about suffering, health, and disease, like:

- *What is the nature of suffering and dissatisfaction?*
- *What generates suffering, and can one be free from it?*
- *What is health?*
- *Can health be accessed even in the midst of the greatest suffering?*
- *What processes and forces express and maintain health?*
- *Can healing be facilitated from within?*
- *What is healing and what heals?*

Questions about meaning, like:

- *What are the deeper roots of my existence?*
- *Does my life have meaning?*
- *What is the spiritual ground of my life?*
- *What is my relationship to spirit and the source of existence itself?*
- *What centers my existence?*
- *Who dies?*
- *What is really going on here?*

I believe that questions like these will naturally arise as one listens to the human condition and explores suffering, health, healing, and life and death issues. The more we are with suffering and the healing processes we are privileged to witness, the more questions of meaning and truth will arise. The questions that arise will be personal ones. They will be expressions of our own unique journey and need. They are, however, essential to allow and to meet, even within a clinical context. Indeed, one might say they are the very heart of clinical understanding. In this endeavor, we must allow ourselves to observe and listen to our human condition without preconceptions, expectations, judgments, or fear. Can we, as practitioners, truly listen to suffering, pain, hope, joy, and the deeper forces at work within our lives, without fear? Can we leave all agendas behind and be open to the forces of life itself? This is our challenge and the heart of the healing journey.

Beginnings

Let's start our journey in this book with a look at the beginnings of work in the cranial field. Something remarkable happened at the turn of the twentieth century. A young osteopathy student sat musing over the nature of the human skull. As he was viewing a disarticulated temporal bone, an extraordinary thought struck him: *"Bevelled like the gills of a fish and indicating a primary respiratory mechanism!"* This seemingly bizarre thought started William Garner Sutherland on a lifelong exploration into the roots and depths of the human system and led to a deep appreciation of what is called *primary respiration.* By all accounts, William Garner Sutherland was an extremely gentle and spiritual man and felt that this thought was given to him as a pointer to his life's direction and work. In his ongoing research, he used his keen palpation skills and his knowledge of anatomy and physiology to uncover the workings of a primary life force within the human body. During his career he developed concepts and treatment approaches based upon his discoveries, which were revolutionary and profound. His discoveries have huge repercussions for all of the healing arts.

As a student, in his anatomy classes, he was taught that the cranium is fused in the adult and that cranial bones do not move. When he closely inspected the nature of the human skull, he could not understand why, if it was fused, it was designed with sutures that seemed to allow movement. He then set out to investigate whether or not cranial bones move. To do this, he set up a number of experiments. He decided to experiment on himself first, with the insight that if he could sense the repercussions of the process within himself, then he would have real knowledge, not just information. I have always appreciated his clear understanding of the difference between information and knowledge. He reasoned that if the cranial bones move, then, if movement was restricted, some sort of pathological state would result. He designed a helmet to place on his head, which could be adjusted to restrict different cranial bones. As he experimented on himself, he noticed various responses in his body and mind, from gastric responses to mental confusion. He began his quest in order to prove, as he was taught, that the cranial bones don't move. Instead, he proved to himself that they do move and that they have physiological importance. This spurred him on to explore the physiological aspects of this movement and then to discover its deeper implications.

Dr. Sutherland's Discoveries

When Dr. Sutherland began his exploration, being an osteopath, he was initially interested in the physical manifestations of cranial bone motion. When he began to relate to the movement dynamics of the whole body, he discovered not just bony movement, but a whole series of interrelated pulsations. In his explorations, he discovered that he was sensing the dynamics of a powerful yet subtle physiological force within the human system. He realized that this force is the most fundamental ordering and healing principle within the human body-mind. He believed that this ordering principle was generated by the action of what he called the *Breath of Life.*[1] The Breath of Life is a concept that is difficult to define. The best I can do is to call it the action of a divine intention. This divine wind expresses and orchestrates the intention to create. I will discuss this in much more detail in later chapters. The Tibetans call a similar concept *rigpa,* the pure and divine state of *pristine awareness,* or pure consciousness, which is the ground of all phenomena. Dr. Sutherland realized that the Breath of Life generates a primary life force which is expressed within the human system. This life force is a bioelectric principle, which has physiologically integrative and healing functions in the human system.

In his palpation studies, he also realized that he was exploring a subtle physiological system that is critical in the maintenance of health and vitality in the mind-body system. He called this system the *Primary Respiratory Mechanism,* or the *Involuntary Mechanism.* He discovered some amazing things about its functioning and expression. He noticed a subtle rhythmic impulse that is palpable to sensitive hands throughout the body. As he explored this impulse, he realized that he was palpating a basic motility, or inherent motion, which was driven by what he termed the *potency* of the Breath of Life. This potency was sensed to permeate the cells and tissues of the body, maintaining its order and healing processes. As we shall see, this potency is an expression of a subtle bioelectric ordering field, which orders and enlivens the human body. It is its most essential life force and is an expression of a deep Intelligence at work within the human condition. In accord with this view, some researchers in biophysiology are beginning to view the organization of the human system as a dynamic and coherent *quantum bioelectric* field phenomenon. This has huge implications for healing work of any kind.[2]

By the end of his career, Dr. Sutherland believed that the potency of the Breath of Life is an expression of the Intelligence of life itself and is fundamental to the proper functioning of both mind and body. He also perceived that the cerebrospinal fluid that surrounds the brain and spinal cord becomes potentized with this life principle. He described the process of potentization as one of *transmutation.* Transmutation means a *change in state.* In other words, there is a change in the state of the bioelectric potency within the fluids, which allows it to act as a direct physiological ordering force within the body. This transmission of the potency of the Breath of Life into the cerebrospinal fluid became the most fundamental concept in his treatment modality.[3]

As potency is received by the cerebrospinal fluid, a tide-like motion, or fluctuation, is generated within the fluids of the body. Dr. Sutherland learned that it is this fluctuation of fluid that conveys and transports the potency of the Breath of Life to all of the cells and tissues within the body. So here we have the makings of a concept of the human system based on an understanding of the dynamics of an inherent life force. We also have the revolutionary concept that it is the fluid systems of the body that convey this ordering principle to all of its parts. Thus the fluid dynamics of the body are essential to its expression of health.

As we shall see, the potency of the Breath of Life conveys the *Original blueprint* or *matrix* of a human being to every cell and tissue via the body's fluid systems. The Original matrix[4] is a bioelectric form expressed at the moment of conception and is the organizing matrix of the human system until the moment of death. The Original matrix is a direct expression of the creative intentions of the Breath of Life. As we shall see, the Breath of Life, and its potency within the system, is the inherent ordering principle around which the cellular and tissue world organizes. It arises at the time of conception, drives the initial phases of embryological development, and is with us until the day we die. This seems, at first, an incredible concept, but the amazing clinical results that Dr. Sutherland and other practitioners obtained were based directly on this very understanding.

There are similar concepts in many forms of traditional medicine that place the main healing focus on life energy or life force. In Chinese medicine, for instance, the emphasis is on the balance of *qi* and the potency of *jing* in the body. Interestingly, *jing,* or essence, is similarly sensed to be an inherent ordering principle in the human body that is intimately related to its fluid systems. In Ayurvedic medicine, there is also a similar concept in which *ojas* is seen to be an essential ordering energy which again manifests in the fluid systems of the body at a cellular level. Finally, in Tibetan medicine, the most primary life force is called the *wind of the vital forces* and is considered to be the inherent ordering principle of the body. In the Tibetan system of medicine it is traditionally experienced as being located along the central axis of the body and within the cerebrospinal fluid and central nervous system. From here, let's get started on some basic concepts.

A Unit of Function

The human system is a *unit of function;* it is an integrated whole. It is only our minds that fragment that whole. This truth can be perceived both within our immediate experience of suffering and within the experience of the underlying Health which centers that suffering. Within the cranial concept, it is seen that Health is never lost. Health is a principle; it is not dependent on particular mind-body states. Even in the most desperate health situations, this inherent principle is never lost. In our work we learn to palpate and to be in direct relationship to the expressions of this inherent Health within human form. This Health has been with us from the moment of conception and will be with us until the day we die. It never becomes diseased. It is a function of the *universal* within us. It is the true *neutral* that centers our existence. *Neutral* is a term that is commonly used within the cranial concept. It encompasses a number of concepts. Here I mean that there is a still center, or a depth of Stillness, around which our whole being is organized. It is the most essential and fundamental ground of our being.

We are whole from the moment we are conceived and, in this wholeness, we discover that our human system is unified and it is never fragmented. Fragmentation is an illusion, which the mind generates due to its tendency to focus on the results and affects of experience, rather than on the inherent forces that organize our mind-body process within this present moment. If Health is truly perceived, we discover that it is never lost. We discover that structure and function are mutually interdependent, that the body is self-healing, self-regulating, and self-integrating. The key to this process of discovery lies in our God-given abilities to be aware, to be present, to be able to deepen and widen our fields of awareness and simply listen. It is in the ability to be still and listen that the truth of the human system unfolds its mysteries. As we listen, a true humbleness arises as we meet the awesome Intelligence within the human system.

Basic Premises

Let's discuss the nature of the therapeutic work involved in the cranial concept. Dr. Sutherland evolved his work in the context of his osteopathic profession. He considered the therapeutic aspects of the work to be an extension of the osteopathic concept. There are a few important premises of osteopathic practice that are crucial to understand. One important concept is that form and function are interdependent. In this it is seen that function, whether it is the functioning of a joint or of an organ system, is dependent on the relationships of the form, or structure, of the body. Form is precise; liver cells are liver cells, neural tissue is neural tissue.

Another aspect of this is that all form is seen to be in motion, and the movement dynamics of form are of crucial importance in the functional health of the system.

Thus the structural relationships of the system are considered to be of extreme importance in the functioning of the human body. Another way of saying this is that the anatomy of the body is of crucial importance in relationship to its functioning. This may seem obvious, but it is not emphasized in orthodox medicine to the degree seen in osteopathic practice. Again, this is especially seen to be crucial in motion dynamics. Life is expressed via motion. Whether this is seen in the voluntary motions of the musculoskeletal system or the involuntary motions of the cells, fluids, and tissues of the body, life is in motion. Resistances and congestion within the tissue and fluid relationships of the body are seen to be precursors of pathology, and early pathology can be perceived as subtle resistances within fluid, cellular, and tissue motion.

A further belief is that the body is a self-healing and self-regulating entity. It already has all the information it needs to heal and maintain a balanced state. This is critical. There is an Intelligence at work within the mind-body process. This Intelligence knows what to do. The practitioner, within this context, does not have to work out what to do. He or she has to find a way to access this knowledge. In this work it is seen that the treatment plan, the exact sequence of what needs to happen within a treatment context, is *inherent* within the disturbances found in the system. The role of the practitioner is seen as assisting and facilitating this inherent healing intelligence. In this book, we will explore this natural intelligence and suggest ways to relate to it. It is of crucial importance that practitioners learn to relate to the inherent health of the system and not just to its patterns of resistance.

A last important aspect to appreciate is that the human being functions as a *whole*. The human dynamic is a unit of function, a unified dynamic that cannot be reduced down to a conglomerate of its parts. Hence, inertia found in any part of the system has repercussions for the whole system. For instance, a sacroiliac disturbance may be due to a process located in another part of the body or even in another system of the body. Any discussion of the premises of craniosacral biodynamics must be seen in the light of these basic premises.

To summarize these basic concepts :

- *Structure and function are interdependent.*
- *The body is self-healing, self-regulating, and self-integrating.*
- *The human system is a unified entity and should function as such. It is a unit of function, a whole.*

Essential Intentions

Essentially, work within the cranial field is the art of intelligent and intuitive listening. Practitioners learn to perceive the body's intrinsic movement dynamics, rhythms, and pulsations. Within this context, they are able to appreciate the inherent Health within the system *and* its historical patterns of trauma, pathology, and inertia. Through this perceptual process, practitioners can assist both the expression of the inherent Health of the system and the resolution of its inertial forces and patterns.

In relationship to the basic osteopathic principles outlined above, practitioners learn to deeply appreciate the nature of the structure-form of the human body and its subtle motion dynamics. One basic intention is to be able to palpate and hear the Health within the system and to respond to the inertia within its fluids, cells, and tissues. Practitioners learn to comprehend the nature of the self-healing process and the role of primary respiration in these healing processes. They learn to deeply appreciate the arising of what Dr. Sutherland called the Breath of Life and the manifestations of its inherent healing potency. They develop the ability to sense this most fundamental resource within the human system and to facilitate its expression.

Finally, practitioners learn to sense the human body as a unified field whose inherent life process is an expression of the Breath of Life itself. They learn to perceive and receive the whole of a person. They discover the dynamic forces at work within the organization of the human system, and a reverence for life ensues. As you study the material in these volumes, do not forget, in the midst of all the technical and specific theory and clinical work presented, that it is the magnificent human system that does the healing. Most importantly, you can have a direct relationship to this most essential healing and organizing principle. As you will discover, the heart of the work rests in stillness, and stillness is the ground of our human condition. There is a saying from the Bible: *Be still and know me.* Perhaps that is the most important thing we can do. Let's all renew our journey and inquiry into life with an open mind and warm heart. As you will see, life continuously unfolds itself to the still and respectful observer.

1. See W. G. Sutherland, *Teachings in the Science of Osteopathy,* ed. Ann Wales (Rudra Press).

2. See Mae-Wan Ho, *The Rainbow and the Worm, the Physics of Organisms,* (World Scientific).

3. See W. G. Sutherland, *Teachings in the Science of Osteopathy,* ed. Ann Wales (Rudra Press).

4. *Original matrix* is a term coined by Dr. James Jealous, D.O.

2 Introduction to the Cranial Concept and the Primary Respiratory Mechanism

Dr. Sutherland explored the nature of the human system and its healing processes. In this journey, he made some extraordinary discoveries. These discoveries became known as the cranial concept. This concept grew out of Dr. Sutherland's inquiries and explorations into the human system and the forces that organize its expression in both health and disease. This exploration was a clinical one, yet in such an inquiry, wider questions about the human condition are bound to arise. The more one delves into the human condition, the more its mystery begins to call to you. It was these kinds of questions which, over many years, led the team at the Karuna Institute to develop a unique form of work called craniosacral biodynamics. We will unfold the nature of that approach later in this book. In this chapter we will look at the classic primary respiratory mechanism which Dr. Sutherland discussed in his work and then outline an important paradigm shift in subsequent chapters.

In this chapter we will:

- *Introduce the primary respiratory mechanism.*
- *Discuss its classical dynamics.*
- *Discuss the paradigm shift from a primary respiratory mechanism to a primary respiratory system, where the focus is on the biodynamic forces generated by the Breath of Life.*

Introduction to the Cranial Concept

When Dr. Sutherland began his exploration, being an osteopath, he was initially interested in the physical manifestations of osseous motion. When he subsequently explored the inherent motion dynamics of the human system, he discovered not just bony movement, but a whole series of rhythmic tissue and fluid pulsations. He believed that these pulsations were manifestations of a deeper principle at work within the human body. As we have seen, Dr. Sutherland called this life principle the Breath of Life. As he continued his researches into the inherent motions within the human body, he realized that he was exploring a subtle physiological system that had vast clinical implications. He discovered some amazing things about its functioning and expression in the body.

He noticed a subtle rhythmic motion that is palpable to sensitive hands throughout the body. As he explored this motion, he realized that he was palpating a basic motility, or inherent motion, which was driven by what he termed the potency of the Breath of Life. This potency was sensed to permeate the cells and tissues of the body, maintaining its order and healing processes. Dr. Sutherland believed that the potency of the Breath of Life is an expression of the Intelligence of life itself and is fundamental to the proper functioning of the body. He further perceived that this Intelligence was taken up by the cerebrospinal fluid which surrounds the brain and spinal cord.

This transmission of the potency of the Breath of Life to the cerebrospinal fluid became the fundamental concept in his treatment modality. As the potency is received by the cerebrospinal fluid, a tide-like fluid motion, or fluctuation, is generated in the body. Dr. Sutherland learned that the fluid systems of the body convey the potency of the Breath of Life to all of the cells and tissues in the body. So here we have the makings of a concept of the human system based on an understanding of the dynamics of an inherent life principle. This echoes the teachings of Dr. Andrew Taylor Still that the fluid systems of the body convey this ordering principle to all of its parts. Thus the fluid dynamics of the body are essential to its expression of health. In this concept, it is perceived that it is the *fluids* that convey a potency, an ordering matrix, to every cell and tissue. This may at first seem an incredible concept, but the amazing clinical results that Dr. Sutherland obtained was based directly on this very understanding.

This principle is seen in every level of body functioning. It is the fluids that allow the exchange of information throughout the body via messenger molecules. Even more deeply, the fluids have been seen to convey bioelectric or biomagnetic information throughout the body at lightning speeds. It has been found that fluid molecules are unified throughout the body via discrete hydrogen bonding. There is literally a unified fluid matrix within the body. It has also been discovered that this fluid field conveys discrete and ordered bioelectric wave forms throughout its matrix.[1] Dr. Sutherland called the action of potency within the cerebrospinal fluid *liquid light*. The potency within the fluids was perceived to convey an Intelligence which ordered the fluid and tissue world. Recently Russian scientists have discovered a high concentration of light photons within cerebrospinal fluid. This all points to an intelligent bioelectric field of action underpinning the organization of form. Indeed, it may even be a universal quantum field of Intelligence that organizes a particular human being. We will look at the action of the potency of the Breath of Life as such a field. More on all of this later.

The Breath of Life and Its Potency

Dr. Sutherland pointed to the deep spiritual roots found within the human condition. He stressed that there is an invisible and intelligent potency at work within the human system. This potency is a force generated by the intentions of a higher Intelligence, which he called the Breath of Life. What can one say about the Breath of Life? Perhaps it is best to simply say that it is the divine or universal intention in action. This intention is really unfathomable, but its ordering principles and the forces it generates are palpable and have vast clinical significance. The Breath of Life is the unseen Presence that orchestrates the unfoldment of the form and function of the universe. It is the Tao in action; the *Tai Ji;* the Great Breath that enlivens all living things. From the New Testament:

> *God is breath.*
> *All that resides in the Only Being*
> *From my breath*
> *To the air we share to the wind that blows*
> *   around the planet:*
> *Sacred Unity inspires all.*[2]

And:

> *Ripe are those who reside in breath;*
> *To them belongs the reign of unity.*
> *Blessed are those who realize that breath is*
> *Their first and last possession;*
> *Theirs is the "I can" of the cosmos.*[3]

Perhaps this is close to what is called the Holy Spirit within the Christian tradition. There is an awareness of Great Presence when one senses its contiguity. I once had a dialogue with a Buddhist abbot who became a great spiritual friend. He shared a meeting he had with an orthodox Russian priest. The priest shared his understanding of the Trinity. Very elegantly, he said that the Father was the potential in all things; the Son, that potential manifest; and the Holy Spirit, that which unifies. Yes, perhaps that is it. The Breath of Life is that which unifies and holds all things together.

Dr. Sutherland said that the Breath of Life generates a potency, a force within the living system. It is this potency that enlivens and maintains that unity in form. Potency can be considered to be the most fundamental life force found within the human system. Dr. Sutherland stated that there is a transmutation of this most essential life force within the cerebrospinal fluid. The potency that manifests within the cerebrospinal fluid and, indeed, within all the fluids of the body can be thought of as a fundamental bioenergy, a biodynamic life force, which manifests at conception and whose expression within the system is essential for its proper functioning throughout life.

Transmutation means a change in state. There is a change in state within the cerebrospinal fluid that allows the potency of the Breath of Life to be expressed as an ordering principle within the fluid, cellular, and tissue world. Cerebrospinal fluid was thus perceived to be potentized with the Breath of Life. Dr. Sutherland likened cerebrospinal fluid to the sap in a tree. He stressed that there is an invisible element within the cerebrospinal fluid, which is an expression of a universal Intelligence at work. He conceived of this invisible breath as the basic biodynamic life force within the human system. This invisible element is seen to have ordering and healing functions and is considered to convey a basic Intelligence to all the cells and tissues of the human body.[4] Indeed, it is perceived to be an inherent blueprint or bioelectric matrix around which they are organized. As we shall see, as one comes into relationship to its biodynamics, the three functions of potency, fluids, and tissues are seen to be a unified field of action. In osteopathic language, potency, fluids, and tissues are a unit of function. This unity allows the body-mind to maintain its dynamic homeostasis and respond to the various forces of life.

Fluctuant Phenomena

This understanding is based on the experience and belief that the body is not just a mechanical system, but a dynamic process of Intelligence manifesting within physical form. Dr. Sutherland found that the action of the potency of the Breath of Life generates rhythms within the fluids and tissues of the body. He called these phenomena *tides*. These rhythms are expressed as tidal fluctuations palpable throughout the body. Thus, the subtle dynamics of the human system are available to human perception. For instance, in palpating the deeper fluctuant motions of cerebrospinal fluid, a practitioner can tune into its qualities, its strength, its tendencies, and its patterns. He or she can even sense the potency, or the life force, which is driving it. This can communicate information to the practitioner as to how the body can express this most inherent resource, the potency of the Breath of Life. Practitioners can sense this fluctuation and also allow it to communicate to them. When respectfully listened to, the dynamics of this most inherent life force will communicate to the practitioner the totality of the person's life story. In the cranial field, this quality of attention is sometimes called *reading the nuances of the tide*.

Dr. A. T. Still, the founder of osteopathy said that the cerebrospinal fluid is the *highest known element* in the human body. This concept acknowledges the role of cerebrospinal fluid as an essential element of the human body. Cerebrospinal fluid was thought to be essential in the body's homeostatic and self-healing mechanisms. Dr. Sutherland believed that the potency of the Breath of Life is an invisible element found within the cerebrospinal fluid. This element does not actually mix with the cerebrospinal fluid, but has potency that drives its fluctuation.

The potency of the Breath of Life was thus experienced to manifest as a biodynamic ordering force within the fluids of the body. Dr. Sutherland considered the fluctuation of cerebrospinal fluid to be a key factor of his concept. Cerebrospinal fluid was considered to be the initial recipient of the

Breath of Life. This occurs via a transmutation process whereby the cerebrospinal fluid becomes potentized with this ordering principle. The potency within the fluid can be perceived to have an electromagnetic quality. An electromagnetic field of action is generated, and the fluid and tissue world organize around it. The natural tidal fluctuation of cerebrospinal fluid has been called its *longitudinal fluctuation*. The strength of its longitudinal fluctuation is sometimes called its *fluid drive*. This drive is an expression of the action of the potency of the Breath of Life. The stronger the fluid drive, the more potency is available for ordering and healing functions. A potent system will strongly manifest its fluid drive and its healing resources.

As we shall later see, the action of the Breath of Life generates different tidal phenomena and rhythms within the human system. These have been called the *CRI* (cranial rhythmic impulse of 8–14 cycles per minute), the tidal potencies, or *mid-tide* (tidal rhythm of 2.5 cycles per minute), and the *Long Tide* (the most formative tide of the Breath of Life, 100-second cycles). Each has different qualities and functions. As we shall see, it is possible for the practitioner to synchronize his or her awareness to these various tidal phenomena. Each rhythmic manifestation is holographically enfolded in the other. Clinical work in relationship to each rhythmic unfoldment calls for different skills and intentions. We will be exploring all of this as the work in these volumes unfolds.

The Primary Respiratory Mechanism

Dr. Sutherland, in his researches into the human system, discovered that certain core anatomical and physiological relationships are key elements in the expression of primary respiration and in the dissemination of the potency of the Breath of Life throughout the body. He called these relationships the *primary respiratory mechanism*. On a tissue and fluid level, the primary respiratory mechanism is defined by the boundaries of the dura mater, which surrounds the brain and spinal cord. The dural membrane system is the outermost membrane surrounding the central nervous system and is relatively tough and inelastic. (See Figure 2.1.) The primary respiratory mechanism includes all of the fluids and structures found within it and all of the structures directly attached to it. The primary respiratory mechanism became one of the early principles of the Cranial Concept. The primary respiratory mechanism is also commonly called the *in-*

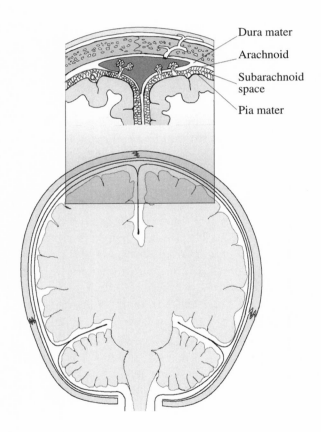

Dura mater

Arachnoid

Subarachnoid space

Pia mater

2.1 Dural membrane system

voluntary mechanism. This term has also been used in a wider sense to indicate the whole involuntary unfoldment of primary respiration within the human body-mind system.

The term *involuntary mechanism* expresses the understanding that the subtle fluid and tissue motions palpable within the human system are driven by an inherent life force and not by voluntary processes or outer agencies. These involuntary forces underlie and organize form in order to express the original intention, or blueprint, of a human being. As we shall see, this blueprint is a bioelectric matrix that is epigenetic, that is, it precedes genetics and underlies embryological formation and differentiation. It is with us from the moment of conception until the day we die. The primary respiratory mechanism is the system of anatomical and physiological relationships that express this primary potency as motion and motility within the core of the human system. It is composed of the anatomical and physiological relationships that express the potency of the Breath of Life as motility within the core of the human body. This motility is expressed like an inner breath in two respiratory phases, which Dr. Sutherland called primary *inhalation and exhalation.* Thus every cell and tissue expresses an inner respiratory motion, or motility, which manifests in reciprocal phases of inhalation and exhalation. These inner respiratory motions were sensed to be very stable and were found to yield important diagnostic and clinical information.

The primary respiratory mechanism is classically composed of five interrelated aspects. These five relationships make up the tissues and fluids within the core of the human body. They are perceived to express an inherent rhythmic motion called motility, which can be palpated and sensed by the aware practitioner. Motility is a direct expression of the potency, or biodynamic forces, of the human system and is considered to be an expression of its deepest resources. Figure 2.2 summarizes these anatomical and physiological relationships and a lengthier discussion follows.

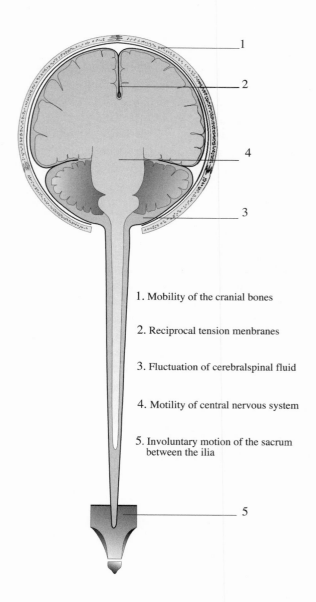

1. Mobility of the cranial bones

2. Reciprocal tension menbranes

3. Fluctuation of cerebralspinal fluid

4. Motility of central nervous system

5. Involuntary motion of the sacrum between the ilia

2.2 Primary respiratory mechanism

The Primary Respiratory Mechanism

- *The Inherent Fluctuation
of Cerebrospinal Fluid*

  This is the tide-like motion of the cerebrospinal fluid driven by the potency of the Breath of Life. It manifests as longitudinal fluctuations within the core of the body. It manifests in the inhalation phase of primary respiration as a general fluctuant rising of fluid and potency in the body as a whole and, in the exhalation phase, as a general sinking or receding. This is sensed to be a tide-like fluctuation, not a linear current of fluid.

- *The Inherent Motility of the Brain
and Spinal Cord*

  As the cells of the brain and spinal cord express the potency of the Breath of Life, a rhythmic motility within the central nervous system is generated. This occurs as the long axis of the nervous system shortens towards the lamina terminalis in inhalation. Its motility manifests as a inherent respiratory motion, or pulsation. These subtle reciprocal respiratory motions can be palpated by sensitive hands.

- *The Reciprocal Tension Membranes*

  The dural membrane system also expresses a rhythmic motility and motion. This is expressed as a bipolar reciprocal motion in the two phases of primary respiration. The dural membranes are always under a reciprocal tension in these phases. They always hold a natural tension in their rhythmic motion and motility. This motion is naturally organized around the anterior aspect of the straight sinus, Sutherland's fulcrum. It must be emphasized, however, that all respiratory motion in the human system is expressed as reciprocal tension motion driven by the Breath of Life.

- *The Articular Mobility of the Cranial Bones*

  This was the first aspect of the system that attracted Dr. Sutherland's interest. He was taught that the cranium is fused in the adult and discovered that this is not the case. The cranial sutures have mobility and allow the various cranial bones to also express primary respiration in rhythmic, reciprocal cycles of motility and mobility.

- *The Involuntary Motion of the Sacrum
Between the Ilia of the Pelvis*

  The sacrum is firmly attached to the dural membrane system and is thus an integral part of the primary respiratory mechanism. It too expresses an involuntary or inherent motility and mobility as the inferior pole of the primary respiratory mechanism.

The Five Aspects of the Primary Respiratory Mechanism

Classically, the primary respiratory mechanism is considered to be the physiological heart of the human system. As you palpate its tissues and fluids, you will discover that the potency of the Breath of Life manifests as a dynamic force that organizes all inherent motion. As you listen, you will discover very subtle rhythmic fluid and tissue motions and an underlying potency or force driving them. As the Breath of Life unfolds within tissues and fluids, there is a synchronous unfolding of inherent motions called motility. All cells and tissues express motility as an inner breath. This inner breath is, in turn, an expression of the respiratory cycles generated by the intentions of the Breath of Life. The individual aspects of the primary respiratory mechanism are introduced here in more depth.

1. The Inherent Fluctuation of Cerebrospinal Fluid

Dr. Sutherland considered the fluctuation of cerebrospinal fluid to be the fundamental principle in his concept.[5] Cerebrospinal fluid is a highly filtered fluid. According to orthodox physiology it has a number of vital functions. It bathes the structures of the brain and spinal cord and functions as a fluid shock absorber. It acts as a nutrient fluid and fulfills the role that lymphatic fluids play in the rest of the body. It is the fluid medium for exchange of messenger molecules, neuroactive polypeptides, throughout the central nervous system. The cerebrospinal fluid is an important medium which carries neuroactive molecules from the central nervous system, the endocrine system, and the immune system as they communicate with each other. It helps to maintain a stable electrolytic, neurohormonal, and chemical balance around the central nervous system. It also acts to dampen down the arterial pulse so that rapid changes in pressures do not effect the central nervous system. It thus helps maintain a relatively stable pressure dynamic around the central nervous system.

Practitioners of the cranial concept, however, have seen that it has other vital functions. Cerebrospinal fluid was called by Dr. Andrew Taylor Still, the founder of osteopathy, "the highest known element in the human body." Dr. Sutherland experienced and described a pulsatory, tide-like motion of cerebrospinal fluid, which he called its *inherent fluctuation*. He meant that the cerebrospinal fluid fluctuates by a power found within itself and that it is not moved by structures or mechanisms found outside of itself. Its rhythmic motion was called the *cerebrospinal fluid tide*.

Dr. Sutherland pointed to the primary role of the potency of the Breath of Life within the human system and its action within the fluids of the body.

Cerebrospinal fluid is thought to be an essential fluid mediator between potency and the cells and tissues of the body. It is thought to convey potency to every cell and tissue within the body as a physiological ordering principle. It is, in turn, moved by the action of the potency it carries in a tide-like manner. This potency is considered to carry the universal blueprint or the Original matrix[6] of a human being. It is an expression of the universal within each of us and is precisely expressed from the moment of conception to the moment of death. This is important. The matrix that the Breath of Life lays down is precise. There are no deviations. It is the universal, the Original Intention, made manifest. Deviations from this universal only occur when our genetics and the further experiences of our lives are encountered. This Original matrix is carried by the potency of the Breath of Life through the fluids to each and every cell in the human body. Most importantly, this inherent biodynamic force was considered to be an expression of the Intelligence of life itself and to be the fundamental ordering principle of the human system. Thus in Dr. Sutherland's concept, cerebrospinal fluid was considered to be the initial recipient and conveyor of the Breath of Life.

Dr. Sutherland maintained that the cerebrospinal fluid is the initial recipient of the potency of the Breath of Life. This life force was considered to be the spark that is the life principle in the human body.[7] As we have seen, the cerebrospinal fluid is considered to be the agent by which this spark was conveyed to all cells and tissues. One of the chief aims of cranial work, as we shall see, is to assist the system in expressing this healing and ordering principle and to help whatever has become inertial and chaotic to reconnect with this potency. It is believed that if the potency of the Breath of Life cannot be expressed, then chaos and pathology will result.

Dr. Sutherland also stated that the Breath of Life is an expression of a higher Intelligence at work in the human system. The cerebrospinal fluid is seen to convey this intelligent ordering principle and its inherent healing potency to all parts of the body. Thus, in the cranial concept, the essential ordering principle of the body, the potency of the Breath of Life, is conveyed to all cells and tissues via the body's fluid systems. Only the fluids of the body literally touch and are in physiological relationship to all of its tissues and cells. It could only be via the fluid system that this potency can be conveyed physiologically to all body areas.

I would like to quote from the work of another osteopath, Dr. Randolph Stone, D.O. Dr. Stone was the founder of another healing art, polarity therapy. He studied with Dr. Sutherland and was very interested in the energetics of the human body. Like Dr. Sutherland, Dr. Stone spent his life seeking to understand the human condition. He wrote:

> The cerebrospinal fluid seems to act as a storage field and conveyer for the ultrasonic and light energies (e.g., the Breath of Life as a "neuter essence"). It bathes the spinal cord and is a reservoir for these finer energies, conducted by this fluidic media through all the fine nerve fibers as the first airy mind and life principle in the human body. Through this essence mind functions in and through matter as the light of intelligence.[8]

Here, Dr. Stone is echoing the ideas of Dr. Sutherland. He is saying that cerebrospinal fluid stores and conveys the life principle throughout the body. He also states that cerebrospinal fluid acts as a reservoir for these finer energies and that these are conducted via nerve roots to all parts of the human body. This at first seems to be a fantastic claim, but recent research has shown that small quantities of cerebrospinal fluid do indeed leave the core of the body via the dural sleeves, which cover the nerves as they leave the spinal canal. This is an accepted fact in German anatomy texts. He then states that it carries the life principle with it and that through this essence the "light of intelligence" functions. Indeed, he is saying, as did Dr. Sutherland, that the intelligence of life itself is conveyed through it. In other words, he is claiming that the cerebrospinal fluid carries the ordering and integrating principle of the human body to all of its cells and tissues. Dr. Stone further states,

> The cerebrospinal fluid is the liquid medium for this life energy radiation. . . . Where this is present, there is life and healing with normal function. Where this primary and essential life force is not acting in the body, there is obstruction, spasm, or stagnation and pain, like gears which clash instead of meshing in their operation.

This statement is the corollary to the above understanding. If cerebrospinal fluid is fluctuating without impediment, then the potency of the Breath of Life is available as the "light of intelligence," and normal functioning is possible. Indeed, Dr. Sutherland called the potency within the cerebrospinal fluid *liquid light.* But if this fluctuation is restricted or has broken down in some way, then this "primary and essential life force" cannot act and chaos will result. The fluid systems of the body thus maintain its functioning integrity and bring healing resources to all cells and tissues. This is true both energetically and physiologically. It is an intelligent process in which order is maintained and chaos held at bay. It is no wonder that Dr. Still, the founder of osteopathy, focused on the fluid systems of the body in his work. He stated, "The rule of the artery is supreme." Dr. Sutherland expanded this and said, "And the cerebrospinal fluid is in command."

Cerebrospinal fluid (CSF) can be perceived to fluctuate like the ocean tide. This is not a current or wave flow, but a pulsation, which can be sensed as a simultaneous tide throughout the whole body. This fluid tide is an expression of the action of the potency of the Breath of Life within the human body. In its inhalation phase CSF can be sensed to generally rise in a cephalad direction and in the exhalation phase, it can be sensed to descend in a caudal direction. Upon palpation, the practitioner will sense a cephalad surge in the inhalation phase and a caudad settling in the exhalation phase. In this tide-like motion all of the fluid is moving at once. It is not a current flow of fluid. Within the dura, there are also the physiological currents of CSF, which flow around the structures of the brain and spinal cord like the currents that flow in the ocean within the movement of the tide. The fluctuation of cerebrospinal fluid is palpable by sensitive hands. (See Figure 2.3.)

2. The Motility of the Brain and Spinal Cord

Because the central nervous system is located within the boundaries of the dural membranes, it is an integral part of the primary respiratory mechanism. All the tissues of the human body are enlivened, organized, and moved by the Breath of Life. This is expressed as an inherent pulsatory tissue motion. The central nervous system is no exception. It expresses a clear and palpable motility and primary respiratory motion. As the principle organizing system of the human body, the central nervous system is intimately related to the homeostatic action of the Breath of Life. To understand the motion of the central nervous system as it expresses primary respiration, we must grasp two concepts.

One is the simple fact of cellular motility as pulsation, and the other comes from an understanding of the embryological formation of the nervous system. First of all, it has been experimentally noted that the oligodendroglial cells of the neuroglia undulate in a pulsatory, rhythmical fashion, and that continuous pulsations occur in the finer structures of the brain and spinal cord, independent of respiratory or cardiac rhythms. This is an expression of cellular motility or inner breath. The second aspect is a unified motility, which can be perceived throughout the central nervous system. The brain and spinal cord rhythmically express a pulsatory movement that follows its embryological axis of development. The central nervous system develops embryologically as the cephalad aspect of the neural tube curls up like a ram's horn. This movement occurs around the lamina terminalis, the end point of the neural tube in the embryo, which becomes

the anterior wall of the third ventricle in the fully developed nervous system.

In the inhalation phase of primary respiration, the neural axis shortens towards the lamina termi-

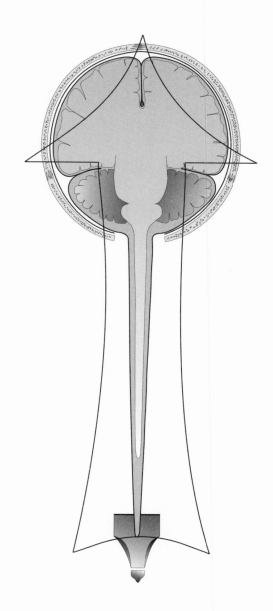

2.3 Longitudinal fluctuation of cerebrospinal fluid in inhalation

nalis. Dr. Sutherland likened this to a tadpole pulling up its tail. (See Figure 2.4.) This caudad to cephalad shortening occurs through the spinal canal and the ventricles of the brain. As this occurs, the ventricles also rotate around a transverse axis through the foramen of Monro. Dr. Sutherland also likened the overall motion of the ventricles in inhalation to a bird taking flight. (See Figure 2.5.) As this occurs, the brain becomes more compact in its longitudinal dimension. This motion is expressed by the ventricles and was likened to the tightening of a ram's horn. During inhalation, the ventricles and waterbeds of the cranium also widen transversely.

There is thus a general cephalad shortening through the neural axis towards the lamina terminalis of the third ventricle. During this time, the brain compacts anterior to posterior and widens side to side, while the spinal cord rises as it follows the shortening of the neural axis towards the lamina terminalis. This action occurs through the spinal canal and the ventricles of the brain. The cortex is like a dense sponge, which follows this action by

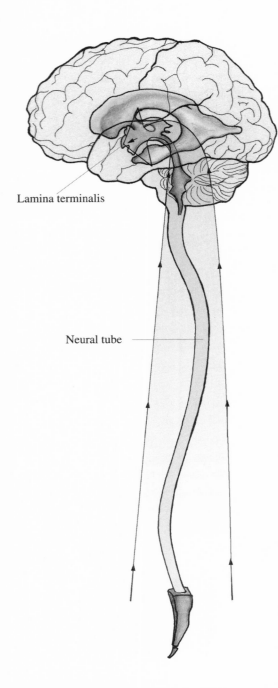

Lamina terminalis

Neural tube

2.4 Shortening of the neural tube in inhalation towards lamina terminalis

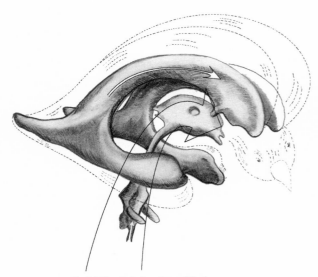

2.5 The bird takes flight
The ventricles like a bird

reciprocal cycles of compaction and expansion, first in one direction during inhalation and then in the other during exhalation. The basic motility of the system in the inhalation phase is expressed as a widening side to side, a shortening front to back, and a shortening top to bottom. (See Figure 2.6.)

3. The Reciprocal Tension Membrane

The dural membranes form the boundaries of the primary respiratory mechanism. The dura mater in the cranium is a tough, relatively inelastic tissue with a double layered structure. It forms the natural boundary for the central nervous system and cerebrospinal fluid. In the cranium, its outer layer is continuous with the periosteum of the cranial bones. Its inner layer forms the membranous compartments of the cranium. These are created by the vertical and horizontal invaginations called the falx cerebri and cerebelli and the tentorium cerebelli. These inner membranes peel off from the cranial walls and form the partitions that compartmentalize the cranium. Where they peel off from the cranium, spaces are formed that are part of the cranial venous sinus system. (See Figure 2.7.)

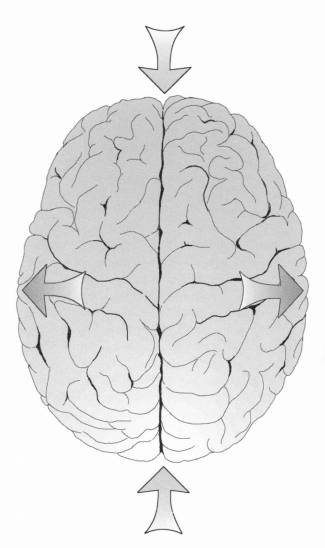

2.6 Motility of the cortex in inhalation

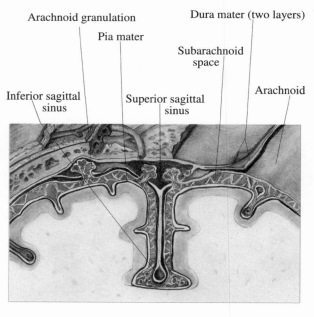

2.7 Double layer of the dura and venous sinus

21

In orthodox physiology the dural membranes create partitions and are a support for the cerebellum and cerebral hemispheres. They also have shock-absorbing functions like the inner straps of a motorcycle helmet. As the dura leaves the cranium at the foramen magnum to become the dural tube and enclose the spinal cord, it is formed of only one layer of membrane. The dural tube can be thought of as an integral part of the reciprocal tension membrane (RTM) and its dynamics. (See Figure 2.8.)

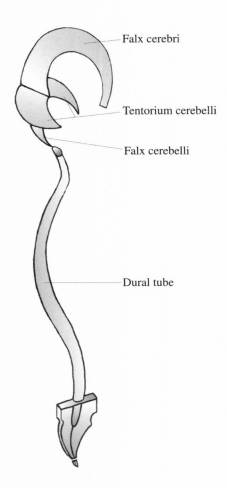

Falx cerebri

Tentorium cerebelli

Falx cerebelli

Dural tube

2.8 Reciprocal tension membranes
and dural tube

The dural membrane system was called the reciprocal tension membrane by Dr. Sutherland. This term denotes the nature of the membranes' tension and motion dynamic. They function as a singular, unified movement structure that is always under tension. The RTM thus expresses the two phases of primary respiration, inhalation and exhalation, like a reciprocal tension structure. The membranes are always under tension as they express motility and motion, first in one direction and then in the other. In their expression of motility and motion, they cannot be separated from the cranial bones. The motion dynamics of membranes and bone are a unit of function.

The movement of the membranes has a natural point of balance, or a fulcrum, within the straight sinus where the leaves of the falx cerebri and tentorium cerebelli meet. This natural fulcrum was considered so important by cranial practitioners that it became known as Sutherland's fulcrum. Sutherland's fulcrum is a point of potency ideally located within the anterior aspect of the straight sinus where the falx and tentorium meet the great vein of Galen. (See Figure 2.9.) It is a moving point of balance that shifts with the respiratory cycles of the Breath of Life. Dr. Sutherland called it a *suspended automatically shifting fulcrum*.[9] It is suspended within the field it operates and automatically shifts with the phases of primary respiration. The natural tensile motion of the reciprocal tension membrane is organized around it. It is thus the main organizing fulcrum for the dural membrane and is the point of balance for all of its natural tensions.

As the membranes express their reciprocal tension motion, all of the tensions held within are naturally resolved and balanced around Sutherland's fulcrum. As dural membrane and cranial bone express motility and motion as a unit of function, Sutherland's fulcrum can be thought of as the organizing point of balance for their unified motion dynamic. The leaves of dural membrane in the cranium can be thought of as being suspended from this fulcrum within the straight sinus. No matter what orientation the head assumes, there is always

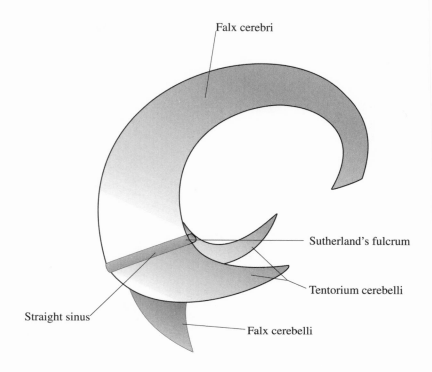

2.9 Sutherland's fulcrum

a reciprocal tension balance around Sutherland's fulcrum throughout the membrane system. Seeing the membranes as suspended from the straight sinus in this way, will give you a better sense of their movement when we learn to palpate membranous motion. We will discuss its origins and function in much more detail in later chapters.

Motion of the Reciprocal Tension Membranes

The poles of attachment of the reciprocal tension membranes in the cranium are important to understand as you follow their motion dynamics. The falx and tentorium can be thought of as arising from the straight sinus. The falx cerebri has its anterior pole of attachment at the crista galli of the ethmoid bone, and its posterior pole of attachment at the occipital squama and internal occipital protuberance (inion).

(See Figure 2.10.) In the inhalation phase the falx cerebri shifts anteriorly towards its anterior pole, the crista galli of the ethmoid bone. As it does this, it follows the arc of its sickle shape, and the aspect of it that is curled under, attached to the crista galli, moves posteriorly. During these motions, the falx cerebri also generally deepens caudad. At its posterior pole, it moves anteriorly as a unit of function with the occiput and the sphenobasilar junction. In summary, in inhalation, the falx generally shortens front to back and lowers.

The tentorium has its anterior poles of attachment at the clinoid processes of the sphenoid bone, its lateral poles at the petrous ridges of the temporal bones and its posterior pole at inion and the occipital squama. (See Figure 2.11.) In inhalation, the tentorium cerebelli widens and flattens. Its anterior poles at the clinoid processes of the sphenoid move posteriorly and superiorly. At its lateral poles, the

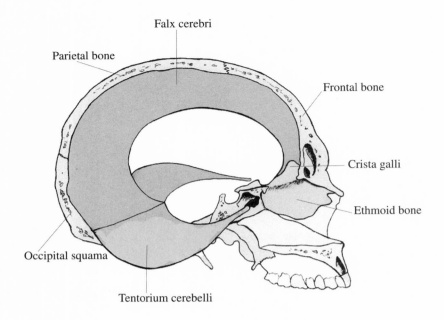

2.10 Poles of attachment of falx cerebri

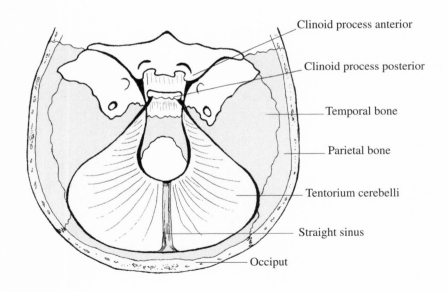

2.11 Poles of attachment of tentorium

petrous portion of the temporal bones, the tentorium shifts superiorly and anterio-laterally. In summary, in the inhalation phase the tentorium flattens and widens side to side and narrows front to back, and its anterior aspects at the clinoid processes move posterior and superior. (See Figure 2.12.)

4. The Articular Mobility of the Cranial Bones

Orthodox Western anatomy has frequently taught that the cranial sutures fuse and that there is no allowable movement in the adult skull. Middle Eastern and Eastern European anatomy, however, always taught that the cranial sutures allow movement and that fusion of sutures was pathological. It was the insight that the cranial sutures have mobility that led Dr. Sutherland to his exploration of the

primary respiratory mechanism. If you remember, as a student, he was looking at the sutures of the temporal bones when the thought struck him, "bevelled like the gills of a fish for Primary Respiration!" This seeming bizarre thought started Dr. Sutherland on his lifelong journey of exploration into the human condition.

In studies with high-powered microscopes, connective tissue, blood supply, and nerve endings have been found within cranial sutures. There is now enough anatomical evidence for orthodox anatomists to accept the reality of sutural motion. Cranial bone movement is easily palpable. As the phases of primary respiration are expressed within the system, the central nervous system, cerebrospinal fluid, and membranes are all in motion. The most important point here is that mobility is allowed within the sutural relationships of the cranial

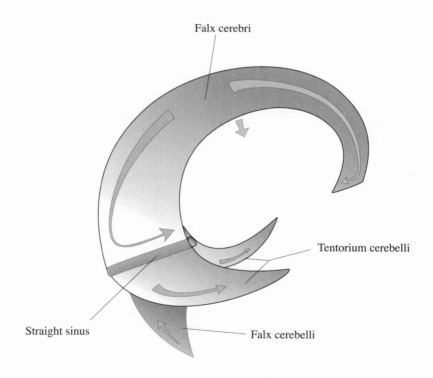

Falx cerebri

Tentorium cerebelli

Straight sinus

Falx cerebelli

2.12 Motion of reciprocal tension menbrane in inhalation

bones. Furthermore, these bones express an inherent motion driven by the potency of the Breath of Life, commonly called craniosacral motion.

As we shall later see, the Breath of Life generates different tidal phenomena and rhythms within the human body. Cranial bones express this as both mobility and motility. Mobility is based upon the ability of sutures to express motion. Motility is an expression of the action of potency in cranial bones and membranes. This is what truly enlivens and orders their function. Cranial bones, like any other tissue, express their motility as an inner intraosseous breath. The practitioner can perceive this as a welling up and receding within bony tissue. It is thus the most important dynamic palpable within bony motion. As we shall see, this inner breath is most easily perceived within the deeper tidal rhythms of the body.

One can perceive a rhythmic motion dynamic between bones and all tissue structures called *craniosacral motion*. Craniosacral motion arises as the individual structures of the body develop and begin to come into relationship. The craniosacral motion of structures is a factor of the deeper inherent forces at work within the system. Dr. Sutherland called this inner force the *inherent potency* of the system.[10] This inner force generates tissue motility and motion. As we shall see, with a perception of the deeper tidal forces within the system, a practitioner can be aware of the fact that all tissue motility and craniosacral motion within the human body is truly whole. The motion of individual structures are seen to be part of a unified motion dynamic. The practitioner can even begin to sense that the tissues of the body form a *unified* tensile field, which expresses a *unified* reciprocal tension motion. This will be described in much greater detail in later chapters. How our bones and tissue structures express their motility and craniosacral motion is conditioned by our experiences of life. Inherent motions become conditioned by our genetics, by our developmental issues, by nervous system activity, and by the unresolved forces of our experience. These motions also express our individualization.

Again, we will discuss this in much more detail in later chapters.

As introduced above, the action of the tide generates various rhythms within the human system. Tissues can be perceived to move at different rates of expression depending on the level of action we are listening to. It is a matter of synchronizing our perceptual fields with the different levels of action within the system. As we shall see, in the CRI level of perception, craniosacral motion is sensed to be a motion between individual tissue structures expressed at a rate of 8–14 cycles per minute. At the mid-tide level of perception, the motion of individual structures is perceived to be part of a greater whole. The tissues of the body can be perceived to be moved by the potency of the Breath of Life as a whole. Here the craniosacral motion of individual tissue structures are sensed to be part of a unified dynamic. A unified tensile tissue field can be experienced by the still observer. At the mid-tide level of perception, tissue motility and craniosacral motion is perceived at a slower rate of 2.5 cycles per minute. If there were no inertial factors within the system, the motion of the cranial bones would ideally be balanced and oriented to the midline. As we build up life experience, tissue motion becomes very individualized.

Introduction to Craniosacral Motion

Cranial bones are perceived to move in very particular ways. These movements were named by Dr. Sutherland according to their anatomical relationships. The movements of the cranial bones and, indeed of all body structures, were named in relationship to the motion between the sphenoid bone and the occiput. This relationship is traditionally considered very important in the cranial concept. The sphenoid is classically considered to be the major gear of cranial bony motion. As the sphenoid bone rotates one way, the other midline bones in the cranium rotate in the opposite direction. These midline movements are called *flexion* and *extension*. Hence flexion and extension, which are descriptions of bony motion in general, are used to describe craniosacral motion.

In the inhalation phase, the midline bones of the cranium rotate in flexion (sphenoid, occiput, vomer, and ethmoid). The anterior aspect of the body of the sphenoid bone rotates anterior and caudad (footward) around a transverse axis. As this occurs, its greater wing complexes subtly widen. In relationship to this, the occiput also rotates around a transverse axis, but in the opposite direction. As this is occurring, the junction between them, the sphenobasilar junction, moves cephalad. (See Figure 2.13.) Meanwhile, the other midline bones

also rotate in the opposite direction to the sphenoid. In this inhalation phase, the inferior aspect of the sphenoid and occiput move closer together and this movement is called flexion. In the exhalation phase their inferior aspects move apart and this is called extension. (See Figure 2.14.)

Simultaneously, in the inhalation phase, the paired bones of the cranium express a movement called *external rotation*. These include the frontal bone, parietals, temporals, maxillae, lacrimals, nasal bones, palatines, and zygomas. In external rotation each bone has its unique motion. Basically all of these movements tend to express a widening of the

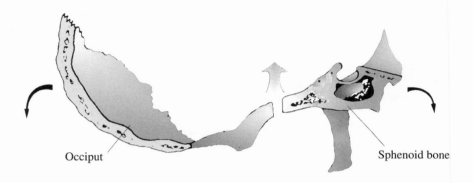

2.13 Motion of the sphenoid and occiput in flexion

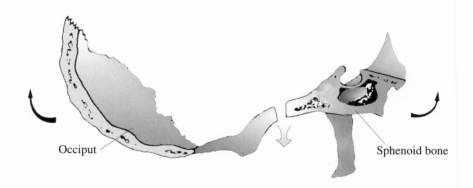

2.14 Motion of sphenoid and occiput in extension

skull side to side while it narrows front to back. Most paired bones exhibit a flaring out or opening out movement. For instance, the lateral aspects of

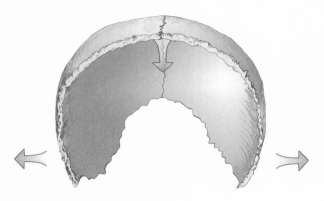

2.15 External rotation of the parietal bones

the parietal bones widen apart in the inhalation phase. (See Figure 2. 15.)

In the exhalation phase, the movements of the paired bones occur in the opposite direction and are called *internal rotation*. Thus, in the inhalation phase of primary respiration, the bony relationships exhibit flexion-external rotation and in the exhalation phase, they exhibit extension-internal rotation. A subtle change in cranial shape occurs during this process. In inhalation, the cranium shortens front to back, widens side to side, and becomes shallower from its vertex to its base. (See Figure 2.16.)

5. The Involuntary Movement of the Sacrum between the Ilia

The final aspect of the primary respiratory mechanism is the involuntary movement of the sacrum between the ilia. It is called the *involuntary movement* of the sacrum to differentiate it from the voluntary movements of postural mobility. The sacrum is an integral part of the primary respiratory system because it is directly and strongly attached to the dural

membrane system via the dural tube. Because of this, the dural tube has also been called the *core link*. The dural tube is a single layer of dura mater that is continuous with the dura of the cranium and hence continuous with the reciprocal tension membrane. There is a firm attachment of dura at the foramen magnum of the occiput, which forms a ring of tissue sometimes called the dural ring. From here the dural tube has attachments within the vertebral column to the bodies of C2 and C3. The dural tube then descends through the vertebral canal and firmly attaches to the second sacral segment in the sacral canal. There are also attachments to the bodies of the lower lumbar area. The firm attachment at the second sacral segment becomes the axis of ro-

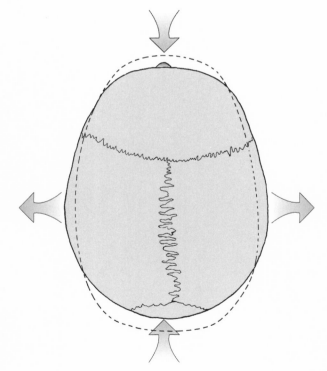

2.16 Change of shape in cranium in inhalation

tation for the craniosacral movement of the sacrum. (See Figure 2.17.)

The dural tube should be relatively free to glide within the vertebral canal as it expresses respiratory motion. During the movement of the reciprocal tension membranes, the craniosacral motion of the sacrum is synchronous with the movement of the dural membranes. In the inhalation phase, the dural tube rises superiorly towards the cranial base. The dural tube follows the foramen magnum and sphenobasilar junction generally superior in this phase. There is also a subtle rising of the sacrum as it follows the rising of the central nervous system cephalad. This is an involuntary motion because it is driven by the potency of the Breath of Life and its respiratory phases. In fact, all tissue motion in the body occurs simultaneously as a unified tissue response to the action of the potency of the Breath of Life. (See Figure 2.18.)

In the inhalation phase of primary respiration, the sacral base subtly rises cephalad and rotates posterior and superior in flexion. The central nerv-

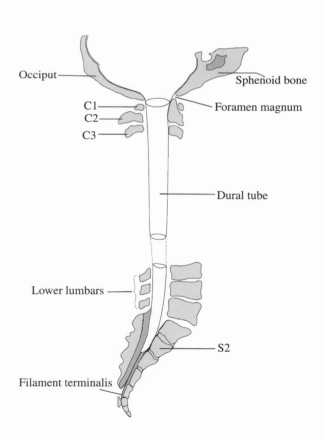

2.17 The attachments of the core link

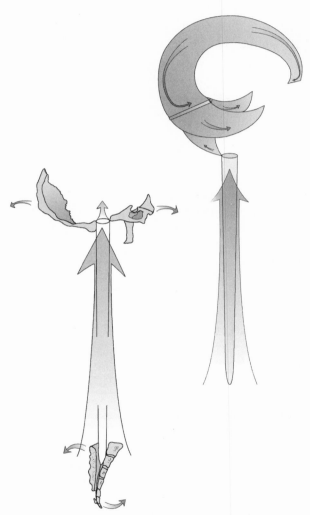

2.18 Rising of the dural tube in inhalation

ous system is attached to the sacrum and coccyx via the filament terminale. As the nervous system shortens towards the lamina terminalis, the sacrum also moves cephalad. (See Figure 2.19.) The sacrum expresses both an intraosseous motility and craniosacral motion, which is an expression of its involuntary movement between the ilia. As you palpate the sacrum, you may sense a subtle inner breath being expressed. You may sense this as a welling up and receding within its tissues. You may also sense a subtle intraosseous widening and uncurling in the inhalation phase and the opposite in exhalation.

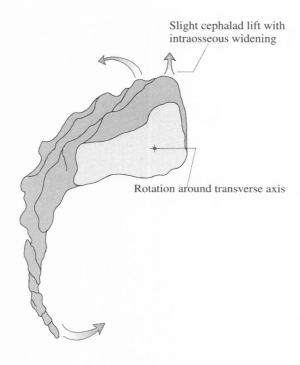

Slight cephalad lift with intraosseous widening

Rotation around transverse axis

2.19 The motion of the sacrum in inhalation

A Paradigm Shift

From my understanding, Dr. Sutherland's later emphasis clearly shifted to the primacy of the Breath of Life as the system's motivating and organizing factor. This is the foundation of a biodynamic understanding of the human system. From a biodynamic viewpoint, the fluids and tissues of the human system are seen to organize as a unified tensile field around the bioelectric matrix of the potency of the Breath of Life. The deepest tide, called the Long Tide, is perceived to be expressed from the "outside in" as it generates an ordering midline around which the cellular and tissue world organizes. This is initially expressed as the notochord within the embryonic disc and is the subtle midline around which the vertebral bodies and cranial base form. Its action will be described in later chapters.

The concept of the primary respiratory mechanism composed of tissue and fluid elements is superseded by that of the primary respiratory function of the Breath of Life. Hence the primary respiratory mechanism truly becomes the *primary respiratory system* (PRS). As we shall see, this primary respiratory function is expressed as a series of unfolding tidal forces and rhythms. These generate the motility and motion of the potency, fluids, and tissues that comprise the human system. This unfolding process maintains its integrity and wholeness. The primary respiratory system is dynamic and nonlinear and is an unfoldment of the intentions of the Breath of Life. We will discuss the basis for all of this in the next few chapters. A perceptual experience of this unfolding process is the ground for clinical practice from a craniosacral biodynamic viewpoint of the human system.

1. See Mae-Wan Ho and David P. Knight, "Liquid Crystalline Meridians," *American Journal of Complementary Medicine*.

2. John 4:24, trans. Neil Douglas-Klotz, *The Hidden Gospel* (Quest Books).

3. Matthew 5:3, trans. Neil Douglas-Klotz, *The Hidden Gospel* (Quest Books).

4. See W. G. Sutherland, *Teachings in the Science of Osteopathy* (Rudra Press).

5. Ibid.

6. *Original matrix* is a term coined by Dr. James Jealous, D.O.

7. See W. G. Sutherland, *Teachings in the Science of Osteopathy* (Rudra Press).

8. Randolph Stone, *Polarity Therapy,* vol. 1 (CRCS Press).

9. See Chapter Twelve for a more detailed discussion of suspended automatically shifting fulcrums.

10. See W. G. Sutherland, *Teachings in the Science of Osteopathy* (Rudra Press).

3 Introduction to a Biodynamic Viewpoint

This chapter introduces some of the concepts that underpin a craniosacral biodynamic approach to work in the cranial field. This approach entails a major shift in perceptual understanding, clinical subtlety and efficiency, and, indeed, in our state of consciousness. In following chapters we will enlarge upon these ideas via discussion and clinical explorations.

In this chapter we will:

- *Introduce the concept of the primary respiratory system.*
- *Introduce concepts about the Breath of Life and its potency within the human system.*
- *Discuss the spiritual roots of the work.*
- *Introduce the groundswell of the Breath of Life, its midline expression, and the tidal phenomena.*
- *Introduce the three functions.*

A Paradigm Shift: A Biodynamic Viewpoint

The last chapter introduced the primary respiratory mechanism and its five aspects. This chapter introduces a *craniosacral biodynamic* viewpoint to work in the cranial field. This viewpoint represents a paradigm shift from the concept of a primary respiratory mechanism, which expresses a mechanistic cranial rhythmic impulse, to a dynamic system of tidal unfoldments that express the ordering imperatives of the Breath of Life. A biodynamic perspective is one in which the primacy of the Breath of Life is perceived and understood. It is one in which the Breath of Life and its transmutations are the focus of the work. In the original concept, the primary respiratory mechanism was a grouping of anatomical and physiological functions and parts, which were originally believed to be an expression of, and responsible for, a primary physiological respiration. As we have seen, the primary respiratory mechanism is composed of:

1. The inherent fluctuation of cerebrospinal fluid
2. The inherent motility of the brain and spinal cord
3. The reciprocal tension membranes
4. The articular mobility of the cranial bones
5. The involuntary mobility of the sacrum between the ilea

The perceptual shift to the primacy of the Breath of Life as the system's motivating and organizing factor is the foundation of a biodynamic understanding of the human system. Within a biodynamic viewpoint, the human system is seen to organize as a unified field around the imperative of the Breath of Life. The concept of the primary respiratory mechanism composed of tissue and fluid elements is superseded by that of the primary respiratory function of the Breath of Life. Hence the primary respiratory mechanism (PRM) becomes the *primary respiratory system* (PRS). The primary respiratory system includes:

- *the Dynamic Stillness*

- *the potency of the Breath of Life, the Long Tide, also called the Tide, the bioelectric matrix, and the primal midline*

- *the organizing and integrating function of the potency of the Breath of Life within the fluids; the mid-tide*

- *the organization of the fluid and tissue world to the imperative of the Breath of Life and its blueprint*

- *the manifestation of these as a unit of function in primary respiratory cycles of inhalation and exhalation*

In the next few chapters, we will unfold these concepts and begin our exploration into this important perceptual shift within the context of clinical work. We will begin with a discussion of the Breath of Life as a fundamental life principle at work within the human system.

A Fundamental Life Principle

The heart of clinical work rests in our awareness of the Intelligence found within the human system. As we shall see, this occurs as the practitioner holds a particular kind of *field of presence* in relationship to the patient's unfolding process. The Breath of Life is considered to be the fundamental ordering principle of the human system. It is mysterious. The Breath of Life is the Creative Intelligence in action. It is the divine intention in action. Its presence is humbling. The Breath of Life generates an organizing force, which is expressed as respiratory motion called the Tide. It, in turn, generates and maintains the universal blueprint, or matrix, of a human being around which the cellular and tissue world constantly organizes. This matrix is a bioelectric form around which the fluid, cellular, and tissue world organize. Within this concept, the Breath of Life manifests its function as an *unerring potency* within mind and body. This occurs via a process that Dr. Sutherland called transmutation. Transmutation means a *change in state*. In transmutation, the potency of the Breath of Life manifests within the human system via changes in state. In this process, a transmutation occurs within the cerebrospinal fluid, and fluids of the body generally, in which the Breath of Life generates a life force called *potency*. In this process, the fluid systems of the body become potentized with the intention of the Breath of Life.

Potency is perceived to be a living biodynamic ordering force active within the body-mind. It is expressed as a bioelectric or biomagnetic force within the fluids of the body. Within the human system, the potency of the Breath of Life maintains the *blueprint principle* of a human being. Cerebrospinal fluid was considered to be the initial recipient of this principle. In this process, a bioelectric matrix or blueprint manifests a physiological ordering principle. This principle becomes the organizing matrix for structure and function within the human being. This organizing principle manifests like a subtle breath within the human system. This invisible breath is the basic biodynamic[1] principle within the body-mind, having potency and healing functions. The Breath of Life was considered to be the primary agency that maintains the body-mind's order and integrity. Furthermore, it was considered to convey a basic Intelligence to all the cells and tissues of the human body and to express an inherent blueprint around which they are organized. It can be thought of as the inherent health of the system. As we shall see, this Health is never lost.

Creativity and Biodynamic Potency

Health is a universal. It is an expression of universal creativity. We live in a constantly creative universe. Each moment is a moment of creation. The human system is an expression of this constant, moment to moment creation. Creation unfolds its intentions via the Breath of Life. The unfolding of the human system is a living biodynamic process in which the Breath of Life is constantly manifesting its creative intentions. The Breath of Life generates a biodynamic potency within the fluids of the body. It is this *biodynamic potency* that maintains the original intention of a human being as an inherent blueprint within the system and that has an active physiological functioning. It maintains this original intention in every cell and tissue, and allows them to manifest in specific ways. This is true Health manifesting in the human system. Dr. Randolph Stone, D.O., called it the *pattern energy* around which all cells express their intention. Genetics unfold secondarily and in relationship to its imperative. Think of the Breath of Life as generating the basic blueprint or Original matrix of a human being and then think of genetics as being overlaid upon that original form. The Breath of Life is the universal that maintains the Original intention, and genetics is the conditional force that allows for individualization and particularization.

The potency of the Breath of Life carries the fundamental blueprint of the human form and is continuously expressed as an inherent ordering principle throughout our life. The primal intention of the Breath of Life is maintained through our life as a living biodynamic, physiological potency in the fluids, cells, and tissues of the body. As the Breath of Life unfolds within the human system, the cellular and tissue world organizes around its expression. The expression and maintenance of this inherent blueprint, or matrix, occurs via transmutation. This transmutation process begins at the time of conception, is expressed as the Original matrix of a human being throughout life, and continues until the day we die.

A Universal Principle Unfolds

The Breath of Life is an expression of a universal creative principle. It may be considered the divine intention in action. It is a manifestation of the Creative Intelligence, which infuses the universe and is its organizing principle. Its action is ever present within our mind-body system. Its potency manifests as an ordering matrix around which the human system is constantly organizing. This potency is taken up by the cerebrospinal fluid. This blueprint principle is then carried within the fluid system as the inherent organizing principle of the mind-body complex. The potency is received by the fluids and, in turn, the fluids convey this neuter essence[2] to every cell in the human body. This neutral is the Original matrix around which the cellular and tissue world organizes and which underpins genetics. The potency of the Breath of Life is an expression of this universal within a particular form. This type of understanding is seen throughout classical forms of medicine and spiritual understanding. It is an expression of an ancient wisdom in modern clinical practice. In the Chinese Daoist tradition, the Dao *(Tao)* is the true essence of reality. It is perceived to be the essence of the natural state. In the ancient text, the *Dao De Jing,* Laozi states,

> *Great De and its features*
> *Flow entirely from Dao*
> *Dao objectified*
> *is only intangible and illusive.*
> *Intangible and illusive,*
> *yet within it are images.*
> *Illusive and intangible,*
> *yet in it are forms.*
> *Shadowy and obscure,*
> *yet within it is essence.*
> *Essence so real,*
> *that within it is true potency.*[3]

In this extraordinarily poetic classic, all of manifestation is seen to be an expression or outflow of Dao. Dao is *essence*, the absolute that is empty and still, yet dynamic and potent. Dao is the Emptiness inherent within all form. Emptiness unifies. Dao and all manifestation is seen to be whole. The universe is one thing. Dao is the essence of this reality. The first unfoldment from Dao is a universal ground of Stillness. Stillness is "Dao objectified." As such, it is the ground of emergence for all form. Within a biodynamic context, this ground of emergence is called the *Dynamic Stillness*. As we shall see in later chapters, the intentions of the Breath of Life arise from such a depth of Stillness. This ground of Stillness is implicate within all form. It underlies the whole. It is what connects and allows everything to be in relationship. Within this Stillness, all potential form, that is, all the images inherent in Dao, are enfolded. From this stillness, all form arises. Within this arising, the empowerment to be here is enfolded. This is Great De.

Great De can be thought of as the empowerment of Dao within each of us. De, as our discrete empowerment, is far deeper than our sense of separate self or personality. It is an expression of the *Great Ultimate*, the *Tai Ji*. It is a universal, the Original matrix or blueprint of life. This universal is expressed and unfolded from Dao as De, the true potency within our human form. This potency is this universal at work within each of us. It precedes and underlies genetics and maintains order. Potency maintains the organization of life. In the Chinese medical tradition the function of potency is sometimes called jing *(ching)*. In the Chinese system, this essence is also perceived to be concentrated within the cerebrospinal fluid and fluids of the body generally. As we begin to relate to the power of the potency within the fluid system, we are learning to relate to this universal. It is the neutral within us and is expressed as the great Tide of life.

Each of us is thus empowered to be here, to incarnate as a manifest human being, as a direct function of Dao and De. In the terms of the cranial concept, the potency of the Breath of Life is an expression of this universal. This inherent principle within our system must be a direct perceptual experience. Once this is a direct experience, clinical intentions can be grounded in its expression. Dr. Sutherland's journey was a perceptual journey. This is how it must be. All of this work has been developed through direct perception and observation of the human condition. As Dr. Sutherland listened to the human system, he discovered subtle forces, and related tidal phenomena unfolding under his intelligent touch. As he learned to listen and respond to these inherent forces, he realized that he had come into direct palpatory relationship with the universal forces of life. This is the great gift that he has given to us all.

A Biodynamic Viewpoint

In a biodynamic viewpoint of work in the cranial field, the Breath of Life is seen to be the primary mover and organizer of the human system. Awareness and appreciation of its manifestation become the heart of clinical work. In this understanding, the unfoldment of the human system is perceived to be holistic and dynamic. Dr. Jim Jealous, D.O., states,

> The breath of life comes into the body. We can sense various rhythms that are created from it, and we can perceive that process taking place.... We can actually perceive the breath of life come into the body, come into the midline, and from the midline, generate different forms of rhythms in the bioelectric field, fluids, and tissue. Essentially, what's happening is genesis. It never stops. Moment to moment we are building new form and function.[4]

In this elegant statement, Dr. Jealous is restating an ancient truth. Our embryological arising, our creation, is a constant and ever-present process. We are continually being created and that is one of the great gifts of life. For in that continual creation there is the continual and immediate potential for health, order, and change. In the next section, we will introduce some of the phenomena that are generated by the action of the Breath of Life within the human system. These phenomena include the Dynamic Stillness, the Long Tide, the mid-tide, and the cranial rhythmic impulse. I will introduce these below and we will discuss them in much more detail in later chapters.

The Dynamic Stillness

As we listen to the human system in silence, sometimes a mysterious gateway seems to open. We enter a state that is hard to describe in words. There is a deep sense of presence, yet I am not separate from that presence. There is a depth of stillness, yet it is not a blank or void stillness. It is alive and dynamic. It is not empty, but vibrant and full of potential creativity. In this state, there is perception, but no independent perceiver; there is keen awareness, but no subject-object relationship; there is unity, yet no merging. As this gateway opens, a deep clarity arises, yet it is not "me" being clear, it is clarity itself. This state is beyond words; it seems to be beyond phenomenology. I again turn to the *Dao De Jing:*

> *Attain complete emptiness*
> *Hold fast to stillness*
> *The ten thousand things stir about*
> *I only watch for their return*
> *Things grow and grow*
> *But each returns to its root*
> *Returning to its root is Stillness*
> *This means returning to what is.*

Stillness is the root of our being, and it is also the root of creativity. It is the silence from which the "ten thousand things" arise. It is a stillness that is alive and pregnant with potential manifestation. Stillness expresses the potential for creativity, and through stillness one can begin to come into relationship to the deeper manifestations of Health within the human system. In a clinical context, when what is called the "mysterious gateway" in Daoism

opens for both practitioner and patient, both enter a formative state of primordial organization. It is potential organization in its most primal form. In this state, healing can be instantaneous, and if physical healing does not occur, a much deeper state of the human condition is experienced. I have had patients who, even in the midst of great pain from intractable clinical conditions, have found a gateway into profound peace and reassurance.

The Long Tide

The intentions of the Breath of Life seem to arise out of this great Stillness. As this occurs a tidal phenomenon is generated, which carries the Intelligence and organizing intentions of the Breath of Life into form. This original tidal phenomenon is called the Tide and the Long Tide.[5] The Long Tide seems to act like a great wind which seemingly arises out of nowhere. It is the *Original motion,*[6] which is an expression of the creative intentions of the Breath of Life. The Tibetans call this Original motion the "winds of the vital forces." It has a vast field of action and manifests locally as the organizing wind of the human bioelectric field. This can be perceived as centrifugal and centripetal spiral-like motions within a large field of action around the human body. These motions express a *dynamic equilibrium* in space, and a stable bioelectric form is generated. The action of the Long Tide generates this bioelectric field, which grounds the creative intention in form. This is an expression of the creative intentions of the Breath of Life in which its potency is expressed as a local field phenomenon. This is literally a coherent quantum-level field of light.[7] It can be perceived as an energetic field around and within the body. The Breath of Life organizes space in order to organize form.

The clear expression of the Tide is commonly considered to be an important landmark in the healing process. When the Long Tide manifests clearly, it is there to be deeply appreciated. If you allow your mind to be settled and fully widen your perceptual field, you may sense a slow rhythm or Tide that manifests in about 100-second cycles (e.g., one phase about every 50 seconds). It is a field phenomenon; you may sense it all around you. The key to perceiving the Long Tide is to allow the mind to be in its natural state: a mind that is still and neither coming nor going. The sensory and motor functions of awareness itself are in total balance. This quality of mind holds a very wide perceptual field and can appreciate the Long Tide and its direct expression of the potency of the Breath of Life. When you perceive it, you will be surprised by its power. The Long Tide is the underlying tidal form generated by the Breath of Life and is the basic resource of the human system. When you perceive the Long Tide, it will seem to permeate everything. It may even seem that you are within the Tide itself, a living experience of being in the waters of life. It surrounds and permeates everything and is a direct expression of the mutually arising nature of all phenomena.

The clear expression of the Long Tide indicates that Breath of Life is manifesting its healing resources at a very deep level. When a patient naturally expresses this, simply appreciate how the system is reconnecting to its Original matrix. In a clinical experience of this Tide, there is nothing to be done except to maintain a keen awareness within a wide perceptual field and to deeply appreciate whatever unfolds. Healing occurs through resonance and humility. Patients commonly note a depth of stillness and a deep sense of well-being when their perceptual field shifts to this level of unfoldment. The initial perceptual discovery of the Long Tide can be a very special experience. This direct perception and experience of the potency of the Breath of Life can have deep healing and even spiritual repercussions. When you are in relationship to the Long Tide, you are at a very formative level of organization within the system. The Original matrix is becoming an emergent reality and the universal within the human system is clearly evident. At this level, the potency of the Breath of Life is more directly sensed to do the healing, and this does not depend on practitioner intervention.

The Mid-Tide

Once the bioelectric matrix is established, another tidal phenomenon is generated. Potency from this field steps down in intensity and undergoes a transmutation within the fluids of the body. It is via this transmutation process that potency becomes an embodied reality in the human form. Dr. Sutherland considered the cerebrospinal fluid to be the initial recipient of this transmutation of potency. It is this transmutation and ignition of potency within the fluids that allows it to be a physiological ordering principle in the body. As potency manifests within the fluids, the cellular and tissue world organizes around its blueprint imperative.

As this occurs, another tidal phenomenon is generated, the mid-tide. This tide can be perceived to express inhalation and exhalation cycles of 2.5 cycles a minute. Within this unfoldment, *potency, fluids, and tissues* can be clearly perceived to be a unity, or a unit of function. These three functions are perceived by the practitioner as a unified field of action. Potency is the organizing factor, fluid is the medium of exchange and cells and tissues organize around its action. The mid-tide is thus a level of unfoldment in which the organizing forces of the human system manifest as a direct physiological ordering principle. Cellular and tissue motility are generated as fluids and tissues are moved by the deeper action of the potency within the fluids field of the body. Within the mid-tide the practitioner can perceive all three functions of potency, fluids, and tissues to be moving at the 2.5 cycles a minute rate. The fluid motion within this is called the *fluid tide*. An awareness of the fluid tide will give the practitioner information about how the system can manifest its potency as a driving and organizing force within the body.

The Cranial Rhythmic Impulse

Another rhythm can be perceived by the receptive listener. This is the cranial rhythmic impulse (CRI), the rhythm upon which most basic cranial courses focus. The CRI represents the conditioned nature of the human system. It is a rhythm that is conditioned by genetics and experiential processes. It is the wave form of our experience, it is not a direct expression of the Tide, yet is driven by these deeper forces. It is like the wave forms that ride on the deeper tides. This rhythm expresses the patterns of our unresolved experience. The quality and rate of this rhythm is an expression of the action of genes as they unfold, of the state of the central nervous system and its autonomic functions, and is further conditioned by the various experiences and forces we meet in life. It manifests as the result of genetics, personal history and experience, and the suffering we encounter in life. The quality and state of the CRI is directly effected by the state of the autonomic nervous system. Autonomic set points will affect CRI expression. It is also strongly affected by unresolved shock states held in the system. The CRI has a variable rate of 8–14 cycles a minute, which is an expression of conditioned processes. Its rate of expression will change due to the forces of unresolved trauma and the nature of the unresolved experiences held in the system.

At a CRI level of perception, the deeper forces generated by the Breath of Life generally are not directly perceived by the practitioner. Within the CRI one tends to focus on the results and affects of experience, commonly perceived as tissue compression, adhesion, changes in quality of tissues, strains, and fluid fluctuations. The practitioner's perception is drawn to form and resistance; it is about how and where we hold unresolved trauma and resistance. These are seen as CNS hyper- and hypo- states, as tissue and fluid inertia, as resistance between parts, as emotional affects, as psychological positions, and as pathological processes.

Summing Up

A biodynamic viewpoint is one in which the primacy of the Breath of Life, and of the forces it generates, is acknowledged as the prime focus of clinical work. The intentions of the Breath of Life generate tidal phenomena. These phenomena are expressions of organizing forces, which are in turn expressions of the intention to create. They are manifestations of creativity in action. The organizing Tide of life is thus a manifestation of a universal intention to create. As I unfold the concepts in the book, this will be my emphasis. The primary respiratory system (a term that allows us a "shorthand" to denote this grand process of creation) is an expression of a biodynamic unfoldment that can be appreciated and tracked by the still observer. This understanding has vast clinical repercussions.

Some Terms within a Biodynamic Framework

- *The Breath of Life*

  The Creative Intelligence in action. Its Presence is humbling. It is the divine intention in action. It arises from a profound and Dynamic Stillness.

- *The Dynamic Stillness*

  An intrinsic and alive Stillness, the ground of emergence for all form.

- *The Tide, the Long Tide*

  The great organizing wind generated by the Breath of Life. The Long Tide functions within a huge field of action. It seems to arise from, and to return to, "somewhere else." When its centrifugal and centripetal motions are in a dynamic equilibrium, a stable bioelectric field, or matrix, is generated.

- *The bioelectric matrix*

  The Long Tide acts to generate a stable bioelectric matrix, which is the organizing field for the human system. This seems to be a quantum-level coherent field of organization, literally an organizing field of light energy.

- *Potency*

  The intrinsic ordering force generated by the Breath of Life within the human system. It is expressed as a field phenomenon and is embodied within the fluids of the body as a direct organizing force with physiological function.

- *The mid-tide and the fluid motion called the fluid tide*

  The mid-tide is the tidal phenomenon generated by the action of the potency of the fluids of the system. Potency, fluids, and tissues are the three functions within this tidal phenomenon. Each function can be perceived to express a primary respiratory rhythm of 2.5 cycles a minute. Tissues express this as motility, an inner breath-like motion in all the tissues of the body. The fluid component of this tidal motion is called the fluid tide.

- *The CRI, the cranial rhythmic impulse*

  The outer manifestation of motion generated by the interface of the Breath of Life with all of the conditions of our life. It is variable and conditional. It is the wave form that rides the deeper tidal forces.

- *Primary respiration*

  The Breath of Life generates various tidal rhythms that manifest in two cycles of inner breath called inhalation and exhalation.

In the following chapters we will start much the way I begin foundation course work. We will look at contact and relationship, at the creation of a safe clinical space, and will slowly begin to unfold clinical skills. Much of the concepts and information are unfolded in a different time space and order than in an ongoing course. I do, however, discuss the clinical skills and the relationships of the body in a similar way as in the ongoing course at the Karuna Institute. This book can be used as a reference that tracks the unfolding of skills in a logical and hopefully dynamic way.

1. Dr. Rollin Becker, D.O., introduced the word biodynamic to the cranial concept. It was synonymous with the potency of the Breath of Life The term had also been used by Dr. Alexander Lowen in the creation of his therapy form, Bioenergetics, and by Dr. Wilhelm Reich in his explorations into psychology, psychotherapy and life force.

2. Neuter essence is a term coined by Dr. Randolph Stone, D.O.

3. Laozi, *Dao De Jing,* Chapter Twenty-one, translation from personal notes of Franklyn Sills during studies with Daoist master Hsi Chi Liu. All subsequent quotes from the *Dao De Jing* are from these studies.

4. Jim Jealous, "Healing and the Natural World," interview in *Alternative Therapies* 3, no. 1 (January, 1997).

5. *Long Tide* is a term coined by Dr. Rollin Becker, D.O.

6. The term *Original motion* was coined by Victor Schauberger, an Austrian scientist who focused on the dynamics of water within the natural environment. See Chapter Five.

7. We will discuss this idea in Chapter Five via the work of Dr. Mae-Wan Ho and her extraordinary book, *The Rainbow and the Worm, the Physics of Organisms.*

4

The Holographic Paradigm

In this chapter, we will begin to explore an understanding of primary respiration, which is based on universal holographic principles. The hologram is a wonderful analogy of the human system and its unfoldment. In a hologram, every part is an expression of the whole and has the whole enfolded within it. In the new physics, some physicists consider the universe to be a super-hologram in which every part of the universe has the whole enfolded within it. This idea is seen over and over again in traditional spiritual and medical traditions. Hence the Chinese sage Laozi can say that is possible to perceive the whole universe without leaving your room!

As we shall see, the human system unfolds holographically in each moment of life. The Breath of Life holographically unfolds a blueprint principle, or Original matrix,[1] at the moment of conception. This matrix is a universal principle around which the cellular and tissue world organizes. This process is at work in every moment of our lives, from conception until death. We will see that as the Breath of Life unfolds, various rhythms, or tides, are generated, which underpin and support our experience of life.

In this chapter we will:

- *Introduce the concept of a hologram.*
- *Introduce the holographic paradigm.*

A Holographic Understanding

One way to appreciate the expression of the Breath of Life within the body is to understand how a hologram works. A hologram is a very useful concept and understanding the holographic process has repercussions for all the healing arts. Every part of a hologram has the information of the whole enfolded within it, yet the whole is greater than the sum of its parts. Information about any aspect of the whole is reflected within its parts, and every part has the image of the whole enfolded within it. This is one of the most important concepts to understand in our experience of life. Understanding the hologram can help us understand the unfoldment of life as a whole. Life is whole, and the human system is an expression of that wholeness. Furthermore, life is nonlinear; everything is enfolded within everything else. One of the easiest ways to begin to grasp the concept of the hologram is to discuss how a laser hologram is made.

The Photographic Hologram

A photographic hologram is a three-dimensional projected image created by using a laser beam in a special way. A laser gun produces a beam of pure laser light. This beam captures an image on a photographic plate and represents it holographically.

The photographic plate encodes the whole of that experience.

A laser beam is a very intense and pure light source. To create a photographic hologram, a laser beam is projected from a laser gun and passed through a prism, where it is split into two beams. It is as if one river has been split into two streams, or forks. It is, however, still the same river. One fork in the river is called the *reference beam;* the other fork is called the *working beam.* The working beam goes out into the world and has experience and is effected by that experience. The working beam is directed to an object. It meets the object and, in a way, experiences that object. A pattern of laser light results, which is an expression of that experience. The reference beam, in the meantime, remains in its pure state. The recombination of the two beams on a photographic plate encodes and captures the experience. This pattern is then used to create a three-dimensional image, which exactly describes the whole of what has been experienced and encoded. Let's describe this in a simple example.

Creating a Photographic Hologram

A pure beam of light is passed through a prism and is separated into two beams, the reference beam and working beam. The working beam is directed towards some object. Let's say that it meets an apple. As the working beam meets the apple, it is broken up into specific wave forms that are called *interference patterns.* Interference patterns are really patterns of experience. It is like a stream of water that meets a rock, and then very specific ripples arise directly from that experience. This interference pattern is directed onto a transparent photographic plate. In the meantime, the reference beam has maintained its purity. It has not been effected by experience. It is also directed onto the same photographic plate. So both the interference wave *and* the pure beam of light (the reference beam) meet the plate. As this happens, the whole of the experience is encoded on the photographic plate. Once this is completed, a beam of pure laser light is shot through

the plate to produce a three-dimensional image in space. It is an exact representation of the encoded experience. It has captured the "all about appleness" of the experience. (See Figure 4.1.)

Let's take this a step further. There are some important aspects of holographic functioning that are useful to understand. Let's say that, after I made the hologram, I went out walking and I dropped the glass photographic plate. It shatters into pieces. You might think all is lost. However, if I take a piece of the plate, no matter how small, and then shine the pure laser light through it, I find to my astonishment that the *whole* image is still intact and is projected. It may lose clarity, but it is all there. This is one of the most important principles of the hologram. The whole is found within each of its parts, no matter how small the part is. I could break the pieces into smaller and smaller parts, and still the whole image would be contained and projected! (See Figure 4.2.) In healing work, this is a principle that is critical to understand. No matter how desperate the situation, the information of the whole, the inherent ordering principle, or Original matrix, is still found within each part. The blueprint of health is thus present in each part and is still available if it can be accessed.

Let's explore another scenario. If, for some reason, the reference beam is blocked and only the working beam, with its pattern of experience, meets the plate, important consequences arise. Let's say that in the above example, only the working beam meets the photographic plate. I then shoot a beam of pure laser light through it. In the absence of the reference beam, an astounding thing occurs. What comes out the other side is chaos. There is no clarity, no coherent image, no order, no integration. The reference beam, that pure source of light, is *essential* to maintain order and cohesion. This analogy has vast repercussions in the understanding of all healing work. It is the reference beam that maintains order and allows coherency and integration of function. In Dr. Sutherland's terms, the reference beam of the human body *is* the Breath of Life and its Intelligence is required to maintain order and proper functioning. (See Figure 4.3.)

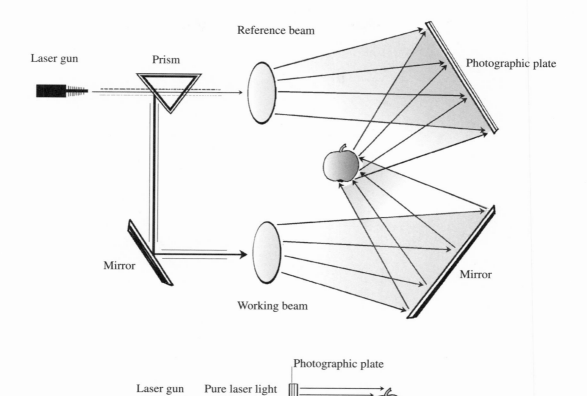

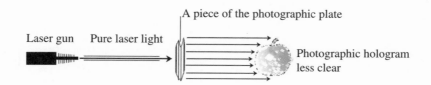

4.1 The photographic hologram

4.2 Less clarity of photographic hologram

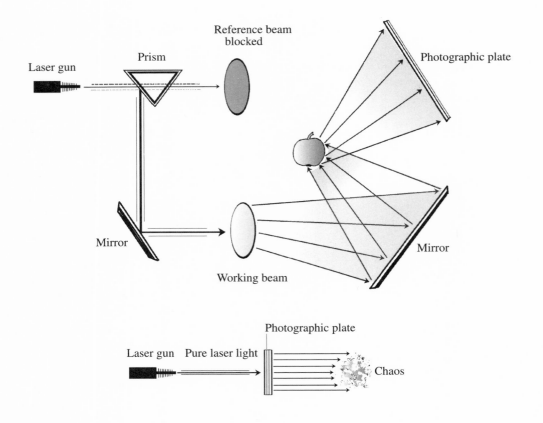

4.3 Reference beam blocked; chaos results

The Breath of Life is thus analogous to the reference beam of a hologram. All must refer back to it for order to be maintained. This intention holographically unfolds within the human system and is expressed as a bioelectric, or biomagnetic, potency that organizes each and every cell of the human body. This intention must be maintained throughout life. It is what maintains order and integration as the cells and tissues of the body have experience. If it is blocked or impeded in any way, chaos and disorder result. We will later see that the potency of the Breath of Life becomes inertial in order to center and compensate for disturbances in the system. This is a corollary to the reference beam becoming blocked. Fluidity and connection to the intentions of the Breath of Life is lost. Tissues and fluids respond to inertial potencies by also becoming inertial.

As we saw earlier, the cerebrospinal fluid is considered to be the initial recipient of the Breath of Life and its potency is thought to be conveyed throughout the body by it. The cerebrospinal fluid is thus considered to be a fluid medium for its expression. Hence, in traditional cranial work, great importance was placed on cerebrospinal fluid and fluid dynamics generally. In this framework, the Breath of Life can be likened to the reference beam of a hologram whose medium of physiological expression is found within the fluid systems of the body.

Research Highlight

In the 1970s, Dr. Karl Pribram proposed a holographic model of the brain to explain brain functioning generally and memory specifically. Recently, Dr. Ray Gottlieb has extended this idea by proposing how this may actually function. He proposes a *phase conjugate holographic brain model*. Phase conjugate mirrors use two crossed lasers in a reactive medium to create a light structure, which can, in turn, reflect and interact with other lasers. This creates what is sometimes called a super-hologram. A super-hologram can hypothetically store an infinite amount of information, which can be retrieved extremely precisely without any loss of detail.

A source of laser light in the brain may have been discovered by German scientists. They have found evidence that brain cells emit coherent light in the form of photons, which travel in organized wave fronts. They suggest that the DNA molecule may have the ability to emit these photons. Gottlieb proposes that phase conjugate mirrors are located in the ventricles of the brain where photons are organized into coherent wave fronts within the cerebrospinal fluid. He postulates that the cerebrospinal fluid is the reactive medium in which the photons are organized.

Are we again seeing Dr. Sutherland's perceptual insight being explored in a different context? Dr. Sutherland described the potency within the CSF as liquid light. Perhaps the cerebrospinal fluid, and the fluid systems of the body generally, function as the reactive medium for the conveyance of the Breath of Life, like the reference beam of a superhologram, to all of the cells and tissues of the human body. Nature never misses a trick, and it would be narrow indeed to assume that the only method of sending, receiving, and storing information in the brain would be a linear system of wired brain and nervous system cells.[2]

The Holographic Paradigm

Let's take the holographic concept outlined above a huge step forward. In this section we will explore the *holographic paradigm* of Dr. David Bohm. Understanding the holographic paradigm can give us great insight into the unfoldments of the various rhythms and tides attributed to the Breath of Life. David Bohm has used the holographic concept to describe the nature of the universe. He envisioned the universe to be, in a sense, a vast hologram with two aspects. One is called the *implicate* or *enfolded* aspect and the other is called the *explicate* or *unfolded* aspect. The explicate or unfolded realm is the realm of the measurable, touchable world. It is the world that is available to the five senses. What we see, hear, feel, smell, taste, and even think is in this explicate realm. The tangible explicate world is governed by its own laws, which Bohm calls the laws of *heteronomy*. These are the physical laws of our observable universe. In a sense, they are the laws of the parts and their interrelationships. Newtonian physics, anatomy and physiology, the senses, the sun, moon, and stars all are governed by these laws. In Bohm's model even the subtleties of the quantum realm[3] are seen to be just a subtler expression of the explicate. Scientific and medical research is carried out at this explicate level. It is the level of the material world with its measurable quantities and physical processes.

There is, however, something beneath, or within, this tangible world, a whole other realm that Bohm calls the *implicate order*. Bohm postulated that enfolded within our explicate universe of time, space, and matter is a subtler reality, the implicate order. The universe is likened to a vast hologram in which every part of the hologram has all the information of the whole enfolded within it. Within the observable is a whole implicate realm which ties every seemingly separate thing, being and experience into one universal whole. The implicate realm is a holographic realm literally enfolded within the more obvious explicate world. It is a realm of holographic wholeness that underlies explicate processes and binds things together as a whole. This inner, implicate order underlies our physical "real" world. Due to this holographic reality, every part of the explicate has the information of the whole enfolded within it. In this deeper sense, the universe is literally whole and undivided. The implicate can also be thought of as a realm of potential. The Original matrix of everything is enfolded within it and the blueprint of any form is implicit within it. Once a form is made explicit, this Original matrix is always inherently present within the unfoldment. It is like the reference beam of a photographic hologram, which is always present in order to maintain the integrity of form.

Figure 4.4 is a simplified two-dimensional drawing to try to show some of Bohm's ideas. Here we

have the whole unfolding of information into an explicate expression of itself. When one is observing from the viewpoint of the explicate, the implicate order is generally not perceived. It is like being on the surface of the earth, seeing the mountains, and not being able to perceive the core of the earth within. Or it is like being a wave on the surface of the ocean, seeing other waves as separate. It is easy to identify with the wave, to become the wave, and to forget that we are really the water. As we do this, we lose touch with the wholeness of the life that we are part of.

In the diagram, each bump is an unfolded aspect of reality, which, in turn, may have further inherent implicate and explicate relationships. Each unfolding will have within it further enfolded information and thus further potential for unfoldment and exfoliation. Each unfoldment is thus an aspect of a universal fractal design in which each piece is an expression of the whole. Here we see the seeming paradox of the implicate being within the explicate

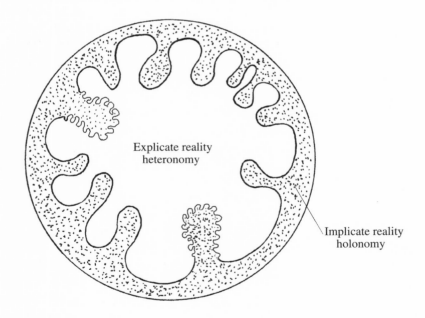

4.4 The implicate and explicate order

and yet the explicate being a local expression of a greater whole. Thus what may at first appear to be unrelated random occurrences may actually be completely interrelated at an implicate level. As seen in traditional spiritual and medical systems, the "whole is contained within every part and the part is an expression of the whole." This simple schema can be carried to any level of complexity with various expressions contingent on each other; worlds within worlds, and universes within universes. Worlds literally enfolded and contingent on each other.

Consciousness Unfolds

This enfolded order becomes unfolded, or explicit, due to implicit laws of the whole, or of *holonomy*. As we shall see, what is unfolded from the implicate depends on an interplay of consciousness and perception. Bohm has postulated that the interplay of implicate and explicate realities, is an interplay of consciousness. In other words, all unfoldments of implicate order into an explicate expression are, at their root, an unfoldment of consciousness. Thus consciousness and explicate form are a unified whole. Here it is important to understand that it is the play of consciousness that determines the nature and quality of what unfolds from the implicate. Every physical event may thus be an expression of consciousness unfolding. This notion also concurs with traditional philosophies, which see no creation possible without the play of consciousness involved. Here, in Bohm's work, we have a new expression of traditional cosmology, where everything is seen as a whole and, depending on one's perceptual viewpoint, one can perceive the implicate whole or its explicate expressions. Furthermore, depending on the quality and state of one's perception at any time, one may become aware of different unfoldments of the implicate into explicate expression. Thus as you shift your perceptual field, a different unfoldment becomes apparent. As we shall see, this understanding has important clinical implications. The continuity of consciousness and perception with the

implicate and explicate orders has important consequences in the practice of cranial work.

In the next chapters, we will explore these concepts of holographic unfoldment within the human system. We will see that the Breath of Life unfolds within it as an *emergent reality*. In this process of unfoldment from the implicate to the explicate, the Breath of Life unfolds the basic blueprint or matrix of a human being. It is a holographic process in which each unfoldment contains all others and every part has the information of the whole enfolded within it.

The Breath of Life and the Holographic Paradigm

In Bohm's terms, the Breath of Life can be seen as a fundamental unfoldment of implicate order into an explicate reality. This is a process of consciousness unfolding. In the human realm, it is the unfolding of the intention to incarnate. It is the implicate manifesting, or unfolding, an intention into the explicate. The implicate unfolds an inherent blueprint or Original matrix within the human system. This Original matrix is the root of our embryological unfolding and maintains the integrity of our form throughout life. The process of the intention of a human being unfolding into form is expressed in the unfolding of the tides generated by the Breath of Life. These manifestations of the Breath of Life order the cellular and tissue world and maintain their integrity. It is an inherent, implicit ordering principle, which is an expression of the Intelligence of life itself.

As we have seen, the Breath of Life arises from Dynamic Stillness as an intention to incarnate. In the embryo, its intention is expressed as a midline phenomenon within the embryonic disc. This midline is expressed as the primitive streak and notochord within the embryo, and as the midline around which the vertebrae and cranial base organize in the adult. From this midline, different rhythms, or tides, unfold. These unfoldments allow the Breath of Life to express a physiologically functioning potency within the system. This potency conveys the Original matrix, or intention, to every cell and tissue within the body. The various unfoldments of the Breath of Life allow the Original matrix to be expressed as a biodynamic potency within the fluids and tissues of the human body. In this process, the groundswell of the Breath of Life generates a number of "tides within tides." It is the holographic unfolding of these tides that is at the heart of the primary respiratory cycles within the body and is the underpinning of our experience of life. In the next chapter, we will discuss these concepts within a holographic context.

1. See James Jealous, "Around The Edges," quoted with permission of author.

2. See *Brain/Mind Bulletin 21,* no. 6 (March 1996).

3. The quantum realm is the realm of the very small, i.e., that of subatomic particles.

5

The Holographic Human System

In the last chapter, we discussed the concept of the hologram and the holographic paradigm. In this chapter, we will explore the holographic unfolding of the Breath of Life within the human system in more detail. We will see that the human system is a particular unfoldment within a greater whole and is totally interconnected with all of life. Some of these concepts were introduced in Chapter Three and will now be developed further.

In the following paragraphs, I will attempt to discuss concepts and perceptual experiences that are hard to describe. In an ongoing course these ideas are slowly introduced over time and are discussed according to each person's own perceptual experience. I have to admit to my own limitations here in using terms clearly and precisely. Words are always difficult. What resonates and has meaning for one person, does not for another. For instance, I commonly talk about the Breath of Life as a palpable experience, yet what we commonly sense is its potency and the results of its actions, rather than its purity or essence. Somehow, we must all find our own words to describe our unique perceptual experiences as the action of the Breath of Life unfolds within our field of awareness. My words have arisen from my particular experience of the human condition and the Health that centers that condition. The following words are simply mine; I encourage all of you to find words that have meaning for you. This is all part of an active experiential journey. It

is a journey based on our perceptual processes. It is about awareness and observation. It is not an intellectual exercise. Listen for your own truth in this inquiry. I believe that the only way to do this is to enter into the Stillness and to listen deeply to our human condition. As you read this chapter, you may have reactions and judgments. Listen to all of that too. Hold what arises as you read this in a state of balance in your inquiring mind.

In an ongoing training, the information in this chapter normally unfolds over time within the context of a group of fellow travelers inquiring into the nature of the human condition. What is written here is meant for reference purposes on this kind of journey.

In this chapter we will:

- *Discuss the holographic unfolding of the human system.*
- *Explore the concept of transmutation in more detail.*
- *Explore the basic embryological unfolding of the system and the midlines.*
- *Explore the unfolding of the tides and rhythms of primary respiration.*

Creativity

We live in an incredibly creative universe. Each and every moment is a moment of creation. We are constantly being created in every moment. From the moment of conception to the moment of death there is creation. At the time of conception, the potency of the Breath of Life manifests as an organizing intention within the fluid and cellular world. It is a "neutral" around which development occurs. This neutral is the universal blueprint of a human being. It is constantly being expressed in each and every moment of our lives. Our embryological organization is not just happening in the first few months of life; it is constantly expressed every moment of life. One can truly say, "as in the embryo, so in the adult." In this grand process of creation, we are the surfers on the tide of life. Our human unfoldment is a universal within the greater context of life and is constantly being renewed. In the following sections, we will explore the Breath of Life in its holographic unfoldment and attempt to create a blueprint for our explorations in the rest of this book. In this process, Stillness is seen to be the ground of emergence for all reality. From this ground, the emergent reality of a human being takes shape. This process is a holographic one. Each holographic unfoldment manifests as a change in state. Each level of expression is holographically enfolded in the next. At each level of unfoldment, a new state emerges. Within each emerging state, all others are enfolded. We will begin this journey by discussing the relationship between emptiness and Stillness. This is not an easy thing to conceptualize or describe, but I will do my best.

Emptiness

Emptiness is a mysterious ground of potential. It is implicit in all form. Stillness is that implicate realm expressed as a manifest potential. Stillness is the creative ground of the universe. In the holographic paradigm, explicate reality unfolds from the implicate realm. In many Eastern spiritual traditions, such as Buddhism and Daoism, this implicate realm is called emptiness *(shunyata)* and is understood as the inherent ground for all of manifestation. In the Christian tradition, this understanding of the divine was beautifully expressed in "The Cloud of Unknowing," a medieval spiritual text.[1] One can only know God through *unknowing* all created things in love. God is the ground of unknowable emptiness from which all creation arises. Also in medieval times, the godhead as the unknowable emptiness was beautifully described by Meister Eckhart, a Dominican friar. This understanding is not based on beliefs or religious forms, but on direct contemplative and meditative experience. From this ground, all of the universe is said to emerge. Whether this *ground of emergence* is talked about in terms of the Godhead, God, the Dao, emptiness, or the Master Mechanic, this idea is an expression of a depth experience of life. In Buddhism the essence of reality is said to be *shunyata,* emptiness. This emptiness is not a vacuum, but is the essence that allows all form to manifest. It is said that all forms are inherently empty and that emptiness is the ground of existence. In David Bohm's terms, emptiness is implicit in all form.

The Heart Sutra is one of the shortest spiritual treatises in the Buddhist tradition. It is said that it was given by the bodhisattva Avalokitesvara. A bodhisattva is a manifestation of archetypal, universal energies. These archetypal forms are in potential and inherent within all of us. Avalokitesvara is the bodhisattva of compassion and is said to be the root energy of the universe. In other words, compassion is at the heart of the unfoldment of the universe and is inherent within our human condition. The Daoists call the unfoldment of life the Primal Sympathy. Life unfolds life in compassion. This discourse was said to be given by Avalokitesvara out of universal compassion for the suffering of sentient beings. In the Heart Sutra, Avalokitesvara tells Shariputra, a great disciple of the Buddha, the following:

Listen, Shariputra,
form is emptiness, emptiness is form;

*form does not differ from emptiness,
emptiness does not differ from form . . .
all dharmas are marked with emptiness; they
are neither produced nor destroyed . . . neither
increasing nor decreasing.*[2]

This seemingly enigmatic statement is considered by many scholars to be one of the clearest and most profound descriptions of our human condition found in world religion. In this understanding, emptiness is not void. It is not a vacuum. It is the inherent ground from which all form unfolds. All *dharmas*, that is, all things and all truths, are marked by emptiness. All things have emptiness as their root. Furthermore, all things are neither "produced nor destroyed." As modern physics claims, in the universe as a whole, energy is neither destroyed nor created; it is simply transformed. In this sense, all creation is about transformation. In these transformations, nothing new is created. Things simply undergo change. As we shall see, the Health in our system is also "neither produced nor destroyed" and neither increases nor decreases. Health is never lost and is ever present and available. The great Buddhist master Thich Nhat Hanh explains these ideas:

> Form is the wave and emptiness is the water. . . .
> So "form is emptiness, emptiness is form" is like wave is water, water is wave. . . . A wave on the ocean has a beginning and an end, a birth and a death. But Avalokitesvara tells us that the wave is empty. The wave is full of water, but it is empty of a separate self. A wave is a form which has been made possible thanks to the existence of wind and water. If a wave sees only its form, with its beginning and end, it will be afraid of birth and death. But if the wave sees that it is water, identifies itself with the water, then it will be emancipated from birth and death. Each wave is born and is going to die, but the water is free from birth and death.

The Breath of Life is like the water and our separate existences are like the waves. Our separateness is an illusion and our sense of selfhood will die, but the Breath of Life is like the water, which is free from birth and death. It is neither produced nor destroyed. It is a universal, which upholds the unfolding of life in this human form. It maintains the blueprint and is the inherent Health within the system. Dr. James Jealous, D.O., writes,

> The health that we speak about in Osteopathy is at the core of our being and cannot be increased nor decreased to a greater or lesser degree. In other words, the health in our body cannot become diseased. The health in the body actually transcends death. The health in our body is one hundred percent available 24 hours a day from conception until death, then it transpires, it does not expire.[3]

Like Avalokitesvara says above, "all dharmas are marked with emptiness; they are neither produced nor destroyed. . . neither increasing nor decreasing." Health cannot be increased or decreased. It is a constant. This understanding of health is so important to us all. Health is ever present, is never diseased, and does not die; "it transpires, it does not expire." The Tide of life is greater than the concept of "myself" and the passing of the body is not to be feared. As Laozi says in the *Dao De Jing,* "Dao endures, your body dies, there is no danger."

Emptiness and Stillness

The relationship between emptiness and stillness is important to understand. They are not the same, yet they are not different. Emptiness is the inherent ground and stillness is this ground made manifest. One tradition that describes this interplay is the Chinese Daoist tradition. In Daoism there is the concept of Dao. The Dao is the essence of reality. It is eternally silent and empty, yet within this emptiness is the potential for the unfoldment of all things. The emptiness of Dao is sometimes called *Wu Ji.* Wu Ji is the great primordial emptiness which underlies and unifies all of existence. Dao is the absolute which has the potential enfolded within it for all forms of being. In essence the whole universe is enfolded in potential in Dao.

From this emptiness emerges *Tai Ji,* the *Great Ultimate* from which the *great breath* unfolds. Tai Ji is the primal unfoldment from emptiness. Tai Ji is the being-ness that unfolds from the unchanging nonbeing. It is vibrant and alive with potential. It is potential made manifest. Its function is at the heart of all creation. In the *Dao De Jing* Laozi says, "All things originate from being, being originates from non-being." Tai Ji is intrinsically still. Yet within it are the potentials and images of *all* forms and, depending on the play of consciousness, polarities will arise and specific forms will unfold.[4] In Chinese philosophy these polarities are called the *yin* and *yang* forces active within the universe. In David Bohm's holographic principles, depending on states of consciousness, specific implicit forms unfold and become explicit. Tai Ji is the Stillness enfolded within all form. In the cranial concept this stillness has been called the Dynamic Stillness. Dynamic Stillness arises from the emptiness of Dao. Dynamic Stillness is emptiness unfolded as potential form and being-ness. Stillness is, in turn, enfolded in all manifest things. The Stillness is a ground of emergence from which all forms arise. Within its nature are enfolded all potential manifestations.

The Tibetans call the Dynamic Stillness *Kun Zhi,* the "ground of emergence." It is considered to be an everyday awareness. It is the ground of the manifest world. It is usually in the background of things, but can be brought to the foreground via stillness and contemplative practices. When you are in the natural world, a forest glen or high up on a mountain, as you settle into listening and your field of perception widens to include all of the natural world, the Dynamic Stillness naturally unfolds its presence to you. In many ways it is not "special." It is simply an expression of the whole. It is the natural ground of emergence for form within this world. It is an experience of the holographic nature of reality. It is an expression of oneness. Life is whole and will forever be whole. The Dynamic Stillness can also be like a mysterious gateway into deeper spiritual awareness and process. In many spiritual traditions the first thing you are asked to do is to settle into a wide listening within this Stillness. Deeper spiritual realms may then unfold. This kind of journey needs a spiritual teacher or tradition, because journeying in these deeper realms has many pitfalls. In clinical work we are simply accessing a subtle level of the emergence of interrelationship and wholeness within the natural world

It is thus possible, as a practitioner, to perceive this Dynamic Stillness as an inherent ground of emergence. As we saw, Stillness is not separate from the forms of the world; it is its foundation. This Stillness is not void; it is dynamic and alive. From this, the intentions of the Breath of Life, like great winds, arise. An appreciation of this, and the unfoldment of the natural world from it, has important clinical implications. It allows a direct appreciation of the emergence of the Original or primal matrix. This matrix is the inherent bioelectric ground of organization of human form. Within this process of deepening awareness, there is a reverence for life that naturally arises the deeper one perceives. The stiller one becomes, the more one experiences awe and humility in the presence of life's unfoldment.

An Emergent Reality

This non-linear, holographic process orients the human system to Health and its Original matrix, an original, or primal organizational form. From the Dynamic Stillness, intention arises. This is the intention of creation itself. This intention is mediated by the Breath of Life as it orchestrates and organizes the formative forces of creation. This is the emergence of Originality. The true Health of the human system is seen in this emergence. Again, Dr. Jim Jealous DO elegantly writes,

Health can be defined as the emergence of Originality. The Originality expresses a complete balance of both structure and function as intentionalised in the creation of a human being . . .

Our existence is totally dependent upon this Original matrix expressing its intention. . . .The Original matrix is a form that is carried through the potency of the breath of life around which the molecular and cellular world will organize itself into the Original pattern set forth by the Master Mechanic.[5]

Originality is an expression of divine intention. It is the intention to create. Originality is creativity made manifest. Originality is a direct expression of the intentions of the Breath of Life in the creation of a human being. As it emerges, a divine intention to create emerges. The Original matrix is a direct expression of Originality. It is a precise bioelectric form that defines the geometry and the structure-function of a human being. It unfolds at conception and is continuously expressed until the day we die. This matrix is a universal and is precise in its expression. It is through the expression of the Original matrix that our human life is continuously being created and renewed. This bioelectric matrix is expressed as force, or potency, within the fluids of the body. As we have seen, there is a transmutation, or change in state, of potency within the fluids of the body. It is this potency expressed within the fluids around which the cellular and tissue world continuously organizes. In the cranial field it is possible to sense these formative forces at work and to support this most primal level of organization within the human system.

The Groundswell and the Three Rhythms

As we have seen, in the biodynamic concept, as I am describing it, the Breath of Life is perceived to manifest its intentions via a series of holographic unfoldments. This is expressed as a fundamental biodynamic ordering process within the human system. It is by the action of the Breath of Life that the Original matrix is laid down as a precise bioelectric form. It is through this process that the Original intention and plan of a human being is maintained. As the Breath of life manifests its intentions, a tidal phenomenon is generated, which Dr. Sutherland called the Tide. This Tide brings the creative intentions of the Breath of Life into manifestation. As the Tide manifests, the bioelectric matrix is generated and a series of enfolded tidal phenomena arises. Dr. Sutherland called these tidal phenomena the *groundswell* of the Tide. The groundswell of the Tide is the inherent tidal swell generated within human form by the action of the Tide. Like a great tidal force, the groundswell generates the cyclical motions of primary respiration. These tidal forces allow the Breath of Life to be expressed as a physiologically functioning potency within the system. This potency conveys the intention of the Original matrix to every cell and tissue. Thus, the various unfoldments of the Breath of Life, like the various tides within the body, allow the Original matrix to be expressed as a living biodynamic potency within its fluids and tissues.

The generation of tidal phenomena echoes the holographic paradigm of David Bohm. Each intention of the Breath of Life manifests as an unfoldment from implicate realms of potential to their explicate expressions. In this process, the Breath of Life generates a number of "tides within tides." The unfolding of these tides is at the heart of the primary respiratory cycles in the body. Later, we will also see that each unfoldment has enfolded within it various states of mind and consciousness. This again echoes Dr. Bohm's work, in which consciousness is seen to be implicit within the unfoldment of the whole universe. There are three rhythms, or tides, which are directly attributed to the action of the Breath of Life in the human system. In this book I am calling them the Long Tide, the mid-tide, and the cranial rhythmic impulse (CRI). These particular rhythms relate to the unfolding groundswell of the Breath of Life within our human experience.

The Long Tide is also called the Tide. The Long Tide (a term coined by Dr. Rollin Becker, D.O.) is the potency of the Breath of Life per se, expressed as a radiant field of action and as a slow and deep tidal phenomenon. It can be perceived to permeate everything. It is commonly experienced within the human biosphere at a rate of one cycle every 100 seconds. It is the most inherent resource of the system and is a direct expression of the potency of the Breath of Life and the Originality it manifests. It is a very stable rhythm, which is an expression of the organizing intentions of the Breath of Life within the human form. The Long Tide, as we shall see, is like a great wind which, when perceived within and around human form, expresses an ordering intention as a local field of action. This local phenomenon occurs within a huge field, which may actually be the whole universe. Like a whirlwind, it can seem to arise out of "nothing" and return to "nothing." The Long Tide generates a bioelectric field of potency, which is the most fundamental organizing matrix of the human system. This field phenomenon is sometimes called the Original matrix.

The mid-tide is an expression of the transmutation of potency from the Original matrix into a physiologically functioning principle within the fluids of the body. Transmutation is a change, or shift in state. Via the process of transmutation, bioelectric potency is expressed as an ordering force within the fluids of the system. The mid-tide is the embodied expression of the organizing potency at work. It is the force generated by the Breath of Life manifesting within cerebrospinal fluid and all of the fluids of the body generally. This force carries the intention of the Original matrix to each cell and tissue. Its action generates a rhythm within the fluids and tissues of the body, which is commonly perceived at a rate of 2.5 cycles a minute. The cerebrospinal fluid tide, or *fluid tide*, which is moved by the potency of the Breath of Life, can be perceived to fluctuate at this rate. The mid-tide is thus an expression of the ordering matrix as a force within the fluids and is a stable rhythm.

Finally, the cranial rhythmic impulse (CRI) can be perceived at variable rates from 8 to 14 cycles a minute. It has also been called the *cranial rhythm*. Dr. Rollin Becker, D.O., called it the "fast tide."[6] The CRI is the rhythm that is most commonly explored

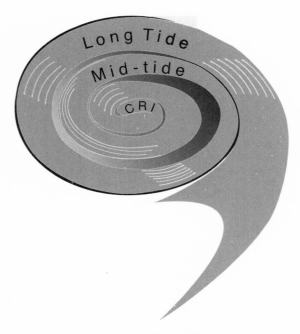

5.1 The tidal rhythms

in basic cranial courses. The CRI is generated as the potency of the Breath of Life acts to center the conditions of our life. The CRI manifests as an expression of the conditioned relationships of the individual parts of the body, the inertial forces at work within them, and their unresolved history. The CRI is like the wave form riding on deeper tidal forces. The cranial rhythmic impulse is thus not really a tidal phenomenon per se, but is generated as potency acts to center and contain the unresolved forces of our experience. These experiential forces even include genetic processes. The CRI will express all of our history in its shape and rate. It is a conditional rhythm which expresses historical forms and autonomic nervous system activation. It is unstable and variable in its expression.

Each rhythm is an expression of the groundswell generated by the Breath of Life and each tide is holographically enfolded in the other. Each tidal unfoldment is thus implicate in the other. Each rhythm is a holographic shift in state from an implicit Stillness into explicate form. They are the unfoldments that manifest via transmutation from one state to another. Each tide is enfolded within the other, like spirals within spirals, as the groundswell manifests itself in the human system. (See Figure 5.1.) It is this groundswell that creates the reciprocal or cyclical expressions of primary respiration. This is an inherent biodynamic process, in which the Breath of Life is manifesting its unerring potency as the creative intention is grounded in form. Let's spend more time discussing each of these rhythmic unfoldments in more detail.

The Long Tide

Remember Chapter Four on the holographic paradigm and our discussion of the work of David Bohm. In this concept, the universe is seen to be a conscious, unified holographic form. All of the information within the universe is seen to be held as a whole, and every part has this information enfolded within it. All discrete phenomena are seen to be local unfoldments of information held within the universe as a whole. Form unfolds from an implicate order into explicate reality. Furthermore, all of the unfoldment of form within the universe is seen to be a function of consciousness itself. Local phenomena are seen to be expressions of creative intentions within a grand holographic play of consciousness. All of this arises from what David Bohm called the implicate realm. In work in the cranial field a deep appreciation of this implicate realm has also arisen. Stillness is perceived to be the implicate ground from which all phenomena arise. With this awareness, the intentions of the Breath of Life seem to arise out of a Dynamic Stillness and to return to it. This Stillness can be thought of as a universal ground of implicate potential. From this ground, specific forces arise. Within the cranial concept, a phenomenon known as the Long Tide has been perceived by many clinicians. This deepest tidal phenomenon was named by Dr. Rollin Becker, D.O.

Think of the Long Tide as an expression of an intention generated by the Breath of Life as a discrete organizing force, or form, within the wider play of the universe. An *intention to create* generates motion and force. These arise out of Stillness and act to organize the nature of the form being created. This is expressed as a tidal phenomenon that carries the Intelligence and organizing intentions of the Breath of Life into form. The Tibetans call this level of unfoldment the "wind of the vital forces," a primal organizing wind, which is a universal within the mind-body complex. The Long Tide seems to come from "somewhere else" as it manifests within the human system. Like a tornado, it seems to arise out of "nowhere" and return to "nowhere." This is really an expression of wholeness, or the unity of all phenomena. It is an expression of the totally interdependent nature of all things. As the Long Tide manifests, a local phenomenon is generated within a huge field of action. Consider the whole universe as the field of action and the generation of a human form a local manifestation of creativity within this huge field. The Long Tide manifests, and a local phenomenon is orchestrated. This local phenomenon is expressed as a bioelectric or biomagnetic form, which arises in a way similar to how a cyclone forms within the atmosphere as a whole.

Thus the Long Tide manifests like a great wind that allows potency to coalesce in order to form the organizing matrix of a human being. To help describe this, I'd like to use images from the work of a scientist who I feel thought deeply about the nature of the natural world. I was very struck by the work of an Austrian scientist from the first half of the twentieth century. His name was Victor Schauberger and his work is described by Callum Coates in a book called *Living Energies*.[7] Victor Schauberger was a very original thinker and had amazing insights into the nature of the most formative forces of life. He gained his insights as he observed the actions of these forces within the natural world. He stated that all organizing forces in nature come from the "outside in." Form is organized by forces that cycle and spiral inward in order to form cohesive living structures. Furthermore, like Dr. Sutherland in the medical field, he had the insight that water becomes potentized with these energies and conveys their organizing intentions to enliven all living form in the natural world.

Schauberger perceived that living form is organized via cycles of centrifugal and centripetal motion generated by the formative forces of the universe. These forces are generated by the Creative Intelligence at the heart of all manifestation. Call this Intelligence God, Dao, Atman, Buddha, Nature; names are but symbols, which can only point to the essence of this truth. Centrifugal expansive energies flow out from a universal source, the "big bang" of physics, and centripetal motions and forces coalesce within this huge outflowing field to generate form. This is not an arbitrary process: it is an expression of the deepest Creative Intelligence at work. This process is seen in the creation of stars and galaxies. It is a universal principle of creation. Schauberger called these centrifugal and centripetal creative forces within the universe the "Original motion" that generates all living form. In his therapeutic discussions Dr. Randolph Stone, D.O., also emphasized the centrifugal and centripetal nature of the most formative forces within the human system.

Think of the Long Tide as a direct expression of these Original centrifugal and centripetal motions. The Long Tide moves from a ground of Stillness in a centrifugal outpouring of creativity. You might call this the emerging reality of a human being. Like a great wind, the intention to generate specific forms within this centrifugal outpouring occurs via a centripetal inward spiraling of forces. Victor Schauberger claimed that *all* form within the natural world is generated this way. The Original matrix of a human being is an expression of these centripetal inflowing energies. As mentioned above, the Tibetans call these motions the *wind of the vital forces*, an unconditioned emergence of Originality. The Long Tide is the grand organizing wind of the human system. In its centripetal and centrifugal expression, it lays down a stable bioelectric matrix, the ordering field for the human body. This matrix represents a *dynamic equilibrium* within the centripetal and centrifugal action of the Long Tide. Dynamic

equilibrium is a state in which all forces involved in the generation of a form are in balance. It is a dynamic state in which there is a rhythmic balanced interchange[8] between all of the forces present. It is not static, but an alive and dynamic state of interchange and balance. As the forces in play come to a state of dynamic equilibrium, potency is concentrated and a form is generated. We will see that this concept of dynamic equilibrium is a key to the healing processes in this field of work. The classic state of balanced tension, discussed later in this volume, is a state of dynamic equilibrium in which healing potencies come into play and inertial forces are processed.[9]

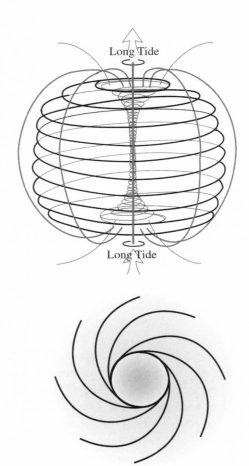

5.2 The spiral forces of

Within the state of dynamic equilibrium, potency is concentrated in order to organize form. As the Long Tide concentrates potency in order to organize form, a stable quantum-level bioelectric matrix coalesces. This matrix is not a mechanical or purely physical form. It is imbued with Intelligence. Indeed, it is an expression of the Creative Intelligence at work. Within this matrix a midline axis also forms. This axis is like the vortex that forms within the spiraling forces of a tornado. This axial vortex within the bioelectric field generates uplifting or uprising forces along the midline of the field. It becomes the ordering axis for the differentiation and motion of cells within the embryo. Victor Schauberger stressed that it is this uprising force that becomes the axis of organization for all living form. I call this axis the *pri-mal midline*. The primitive streak and notochord within the embryo form in relationship to it, and it remains the organizing axis throughout life. We will discuss the primal midline in more detail below. In his work, Dr. Sutherland also talked about spiraling forces. He talked about the Tide as a reciprocal spiraling outward and inward from a point source. He called this reciprocal spiraling action of the Tide the *groundswell*. It is the groundswell of the Tide that generates the cycles of primary respiration within our human form. The unfoldment of the Tide is likened to a pulsation, which arises from a point source and which returns to it via centrifugal and centripetal spirals.[10] This is a direct perceptual experience of the tidal forces that Victor Schauberger called the "Original motion." (See Figure 5.2.).

Clinical Highlight

As the practitioner settles into a perceptual stillness and holds a wider perceptual field, the Long Tide may become evident. Perception of the Long Tide allows the practitioner to have a direct experience of the potency of the Breath of Life and the inherent treatment plan as initiated by the Intelligence within the system. From here, the practitioner may perceive the potency of the Breath of Life arising within the primal midline and condensing, or coalescing, within sites of inertia as the inherent treatment plan is expressed. There is a shimmering within the system, and inertial issues are attended to. At this level of work, healing is perceived to be a factor of the Breath of Life and the healing priorities of its potency are more directly perceived. This level of work is based upon presence, upon a clarity of awareness, upon resonance with the function of the potency within the system, and upon the maintenance of a very wide and still perceptual field.

The Human Bioelectric Matrix

The Original matrix is a manifestation of an Intelligent life force in action. The human system is organized as a whole by extremely subtle and intelligent bioelectric interactions. An understanding of bioenergy, or life force, was an integral part of almost all traditional medical systems. The concept of life force, or bioenergy, was always an essential aspect of treatment processes. In essence, most classical systems of medicine were energy medicine. In recent years the wisdom of this understanding has been described in modern terms by researchers in biology and biophysics. For an excellent overview of these concepts and research I can refer you to the book, *The Rainbow and the Worm, The Physics of Organisms,* by Mae-Wan Ho.[11] The development and organization of the human system is seen to rely on a level of order which Mae-Wan Ho calls the "coherent quantum electrodynamical field." The organization of living organisms is seen to be based on coherent, dynamic, and unified quantum field phenomena. This organizing field manifests as a unified electrodynamic field at a quantum level of interaction. In terms relevant to body-oriented therapies, it means that there is a level of organization within the human system which is always coherent and whole, which is based on a quantum interplay of bioelectric phenomena and which is perceived in the living system as an interplay of bioelectric potencies within a unified field of action. The question arises, how can one clinically interface with this most subtle level of organization? I believe that the work of Dr. Sutherland and the extension of his work by later practitioners speaks directly to this question.

In classic yogic teaching this level of organization is described in terms of the chakra system and its field pulsations. Life force, called *prana,* is organized in very discrete ways. Again, in this tradition, the chakra system is seen to be a local phenomenon within a universal field of action. (See Figure 5.3.) It is this bioenergy field that is first laid down at conception and that forms the organizing principle for human form. The Chinese speak of organizing centers called Dan Tian *(Tan T'ien)* and of *ji,* or life force, which manifests in various ways within the human body. I believe that all of these ways of describing reality, whether in terms of quantum mechanics and field phenomena, in terms of holographic principles, of potency and the Breath of Life, of bioenergy and the chakras, of prana and jing, all point to the same truth. The human system is whole and can never not be whole. It is organized via subtle bioelectric/biomagnetic fields, which are expressions of a deeper Creative Intention at work. When practitioners hold a relatively wide perceptual field and allow their minds to become still within this field of listening, these phenomena can actually become discernible. Awareness of this level of organization has very important clinical implications. A practitioner's consciousness can resonate with this level of unfoldment. Healing processes can be initiated from the depths of the creative principle, which underpins all of the biodynamic interchanges within the human system.

The bioelectric matrix can be thought of as a local phenomenon not separate from the universe it is part of. In terms of the Long Tide, motion can be perceived to arise within a much wider field of action than the human system being palpated. The practitioner can literally perceive a tidal phenomenon that seems to come from "somewhere else" and that expresses its intentions within the local field of the human system. The Long Tide seems to unfold out of a Stillness and to return to that Stillness. Within this dynamic, the organization of a living system is generated. This is literally a holographic, universal field of interplay. The Long Tide can be thought of as an organizing force that coalesces and generates a local, quantum-level bioelectric organizing field. This field, or bioelectric matrix, is what organizes the development of the embryo and is a constant throughout life.[12] As we have discussed above, this bioelectric form can be considered to be the "Original matrix," a subtle quantum-level template of "light" for the human system. Its ordering energies are carried within the fluids of the body via transmutation and the cellular and tissue world organizes around its action. Remember Dr. Sutherland's description of liquid light. This concept is not just a metaphor; it is based on direct perceptual experience. Recently light photons have been found to be present within the cerebrospinal fluid and throughout the fluids of the body.[13] From this most primal ordering field, potency undergoes a transmutation within the fluids of the body. The organization of the bioelectric matrix is then directly expressed as an organizing force within the fluids. In essence, potency becomes embodied in form via the medium of the fluids. This force can be thought of as expressing quantum levels of organization within the fluid-tissue matrix of the body. This is the realm of the mid-tide, the tidal expression of embodied biodynamic organizing forces. Here the practitioner can literally sense the nature of potency, fluids, and tissues as a unified field of motion and organization.

One of my colleagues, a very experienced osteopathic practitioner, considers this level of clinical

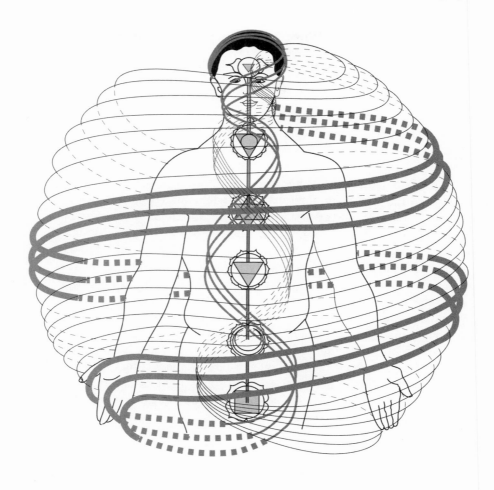

5.3 The chakra system

work as an interface with a realm of "quantum interplay." A realm where all phenomena and their inter-relationships, are perceived as one. It "hums" with quantum shifts, biophoton interplay and coherent information exchange. Dr. Rollin Becker D.O. described what he called a *quantum touch,* a quality of perception and palpation which opens to this subtle world of quantum organization.[14] Many modern researchers into biophysics consider the human system to be organized by discrete and coherent bioelectric quantum fields of action, that manifest a unified and fluid wholeness. Here the unity and coherence of the human bioelectric field at a quantum level of manifestation can be appreciated. All of these concepts and perceptual experiences have vast clinical importance. Many will be outlined in following chapters.

Ignition and Incarnation

In our discussion of the Long Tide, we reviewed some concepts which come from the work of Victor

Schauberger. In his concept, there is a Creative Intelligence that imbues the universe. This is similar in some ways to David Bohm's concept that the universe is a conscious holographic whole. In many spiritual traditions the roots of this interplay are seen to be a function of divine creativity. This Creative Intelligence is seen to organize form via the centripetal, spiraling motion of subtle forces. Nature, in his concept, organizes form via implosive, centripetal action. Form is organized from the outside in. The formation of the bioelectric field with its quantum effects can be thought of as arising from such action. The Long Tide generates organizing forces like great winds, which spiral in centripetal and centrifugal action to coalesce the Original matrix. These organizing forces manifest as an ordering principle within the conceptus. This ordering principle literally ignites within the fluids of the embryo. At the time of conception, there is an *ignition* of the intention to incarnate as a human being. Dr. Randolph Stone, D.O., talks about the moment of conception as being an extremely fiery process in which the bioelectric field ignites as an organizing form within the single cell of the conceptus.[15] This ignition process is the initial embodiment of Originality within the world of form. This is the original primal ignition at the moment of conception.

At conception, as these forces manifest, the bioelectric matrix of a human being ignites within the fluids of the conceptus as an ordering principle for the creation of the form of the human body. The potency of the Breath of Life manifests within the fluids of the conceptus, the Original matrix is embodied, and cellular division and differentiation are literally ignited. It is the forces within the fluids of the embryo that convey this principle. These potencies drive the initial development of the human system. Throughout life it is the fluid systems of the body that serve to embody the ordering intentions of the Breath of Life within human form. The human bioelectric matrix is with us from the moment of conception until the day we die. Once the blueprint is laid down, the cellular world organizes to its imperative. Dr. Jim Jealous writes,

The Original design and function is in the fluids of the embryo. . . . The Original matrix is a form that is carried through the potency of the breath of life around which the molecular and cellular world will organise itself into the Original pattern set forth by the Master Mechanic.[16]

The "Original design and function" of a human being ignites within the fluids of the conceptus and the Original matrix is embodied within form. The Original matrix is a bioelectric form embodied within the fluids as an expression of the "Original pattern set forth by the Master Mechanic." Thus life is organized at its earliest and deepest roots by this Original intention being made manifest, not just by genetic drive. The Long Tide is not bound by the limits of the physical body. It is what originally generates its organization. It connects the individual to the whole and is an expression of the unified biosphere of life. There is a later ignition process at birth where potency literally ignites within the cerebrospinal fluid as the infant leaves the womb and enters the outside world. We will describe this process in later chapters.

The Primal Midline

As we have seen, Victor Schauberger wrote of the uprising midline forces that arise within the center of all organizing matrices. As the centripetal and centrifugal forces of the Tide generate an ordering matrix, a midline axis within the field is expressed. The spiraling forces coalesce a bioelectric field of potency, and uprising forces are generated within its core. The organizing matrix of human form is no exception to this rule. Victor Schauberger likened this midline to the vast vortex-like uprising force generated within the center of a tornado. Within the human bioelectric matrix, these uplifting forces generate a midline organizing axis for the cellular and tissue world to orient to. It is around and within this most primal midline that the primitive streak and notochord of the embryo forms. (See Figure 5.4.) The vertebral bodies, in turn, form around the no-

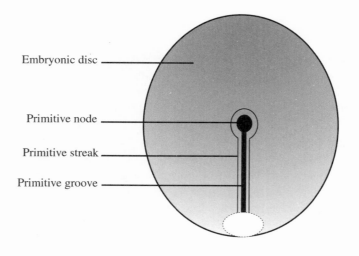

Embryonic disc

Primitive node

Primitive streak

Primitive groove

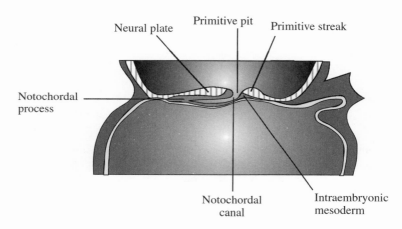

Neural plate Primitive pit Primitive streak

Notochordal process

Notochordal canal Intraembryonic mesoderm

5.4 Primitive streak and notochord

tochord as does the heart of the cranial base. The primal midline can be sensed as an uprising force ascending from the coccyx, through the vertebral bodies and cranial base, to the ethmoid bone from where it seems to disappear in space. Dr. Randolph Stone D.O. called it the "fountain spray of life." The primal midline is discussed in detail in Volume Two. This midline phenomena is a *primal midline* around which we continually orient. Its uprising force, and the bioelectric field it is part of, are expressions of a precise intention to create. The primal midline constantly orients us to the precision of this creative impulse within us. We are continually

being created and that is one of the great gifts of life. For in that continual creation there is the continual potential for health, order, and change. Again Dr. Jim Jealous, D.O., states,

The breath of life comes into the body. We can sense various rhythms that are created from it, and we can perceive that process taking place.... We can actually perceive the breath of life come into the body, come into the midline, and from the midline, generate different forms of rhythms in the bioelectric field, fluids, and tissue. Essentially, what's happening is genesis. It never stops. Moment to moment we are building new form and function.[17]

This elegant statement points to the roots of our human existence. The action of the Breath of Life is expressed within the midline of the embryo. This primal midline is maintained as the primary organizing axis of the human system throughout life. From it, the tidal groundswell is generated as the fluid and tissue world constantly organize around the creative impulse. Hence, there is continual genesis, continual creation, and continual orientation to the Original intention to create a human being. From this midline, different tidal phenomena are generated within the potencies, fluids, and tissues of the human body. These three, the potency, the fluids, and the tissues, become a unified biodynamic field of action.

Dr. Randolph Stone, D.O., called the primal midline the *fountain spray of life*. He called its uplifting force the *neuter essence*. He also called it the "ultrasonic core" of a human being. He likened it to the midline of the caduceus and chakra system, the core of the organization of a human being. (See Figure 5.3.) The midline of the caduceus is called *sushumna*, the neuter essence at the heart of the bioelectric matrix. He wrote,

> The center line through the body is the location of the path of the ultrasonic energy substance as the primary life current and the core of being . . . the central core is the ultrasonic energy current of the soul. It is the primary energy which builds and sustains all others. . . . This core is the center of attraction and emanation of all currents from the brain to the extremities. It is the internal gravity of the individual energy and lines of forces, distinct from the gravity lines of the earth.[18]

Here Dr. Stone is using his own terminology to describe the nature of the primal midline. He likens it to an "ultrasonic energy current," a wave form of extremely high vibration. This is the uplifting force

which Victor Schauberger stresses is at the heart of every organizing field in the natural world. From this vibration emanates the classical chakra system and its bioelectric field. These emanations and vibrating fields organize the form of the body. The fluids are the media for that organization. Victor Schauberger stressed that it is water which conveys the life principle and allows forms to be organized within the natural world. Picture a glass of water. As you vibrate the glass, the water takes various shapes and motions in response. As the fluids are "vibrated" by the potency of the Breath of Life, the cellular and tissue world take on specific form and motion. This process is precise. From this core, all other manifestations of potency are generated: "It is the internal gravity of the individual energy and lines of forces. . . ." In other words, it sets up a precise internal matrix of forces and potencies which maintains the universal design of a human being. In the body, this neuter essence is expressed along the midline from the coccyx through the cranial base to the ethmoid bone. This is the axis of the uplifting forces within the human form. It rises up this midline and disappears into space at the ethmoid bone like a fountain spray of life. Most importantly, it is possible to perceive this midline function. It can be a direct perceptual experience for the practitioner, which, as we shall see, has important clinical significance.

Transmutation and Precision

As we have discussed, there is a *transmutation* of potency into a biodynamic ordering force within the fluids of the system. This shift in state within the fluids allows the bioelectric matrix to become an embodied force within the living system. The anatomy and physiology of the system must refer back to this most primal force. The transmutation process is naturally precise. Every cell is aligned to its function. Dr. Randolph Stone, D.O., used to say, "Man cognises, God geometrises." The laying down of the bioelectric matrix is a precise process that is never wrong. It is the universal principle that maintains the intention of incarnation and form. It is the "Original pattern set forth by the Master Mechanic" and is precise and ever present. As the bioelectric field is generated, and a midline function forms within it, a series of tidal phenomena unfold via a process of transmutation. Remember from earlier discussions that transmutation is a change in state. It is a transformation from one state into another. In this unfolding holographic process, each transmutation is enfolded within the other and each emerges from the other.

The organizing winds of the Breath of Life arise from the Dynamic Stillness. As the Long Tide is generated, the Original matrix is expressed as a dynamic bioelectric matrix. The potency within this field steps down in intensity as it transmutes within the fluids of the body. The fluids become potentized with its force. The cellular and tissue world then organizes around the Original matrix like the waves riding the Tide. Embryonic differentiation and cellular migration unfold in response to this pattern energy. Later, this potency is received by the cerebrospinal fluid and ignites within the fluid system of the body as a physiologically active, biodynamic ordering force. This ordering principle is with us from the moment of conception until the day we die.

How we organize around this universal principle is modified by our genetics and our life experience. Yet it is always possible to reorient to its potency and to its Original intention. In clinical process, tissues, fluids, and potency will naturally align to the intention of the Breath of Life. This is the heart of our work in the cranial field. As you listen to a person's system, you can actually perceive this process happening. This process of transmutation is whole: it unfolds in unity. It is a holographic, biodynamic process. Within each unfoldment, the whole is ever present. Reconnecting to the Original matrix is a reconnection to Health and wholeness. Health is an expression of Originality made manifest. This is the transmutation process. It is palpable and perceptible by the still observer. This idea of transmutation is important to understand. If you truly understand transmutation as a perceptual reality, then you understand how potency unfolds, and you understand healing processes.

Basic Biodynamic Unfoldments

- *Dynamic Stillness*

  The ground of emergence, an inherent aliveness. The whole that has implicate within it all of potential manifestation. We are always and forever part of this whole: it is implicate in our very existence.

- *The Breath of Life*

  An expression of the divine creative intention, which generates the Long Tide, the organizing Tide of life. It generates the ordering principles to which all form is inherently oriented.

- *The Bioelectric Matrix/Original Matrix*

  A bioelectric field of potency is generated and organized by the Long Tide. A precise matrix is laid down around which the fluid and cellular world will organize.

- *The Primal Midline*

  Within the bioelectric matrix an organizing and orienting midline is generated. Fluids, cells, and tissues naturally align to this midline as the main orienting axis of the body. The structural axis of the body is a derivative of this midline function. Structure and function naturally orient to the primal midline.

- *The Potency*

  The potency within the bioelectric matrix is expressed as an organizing force within the fluids of the body. This process occurs via transmutation, or change in state. The potency within the fluids becomes the inherent biodynamic ordering force within the body.

Basic Biodynamic Unfoldments *continued*

- *The Potency*

  The intention of the Breath of Life is made manifest. It is the neutral around which the cellular and tissue world naturally organize.

- *The Fluids*

  There is a transmutation, or shift in state, of potency within the fluids. Potency becomes an embodied force within the fluids. This process brings this neuter essence into rela-

tionship to every cell and tissue within the body. This is a fundamental biodynamic principle. This generates the fluid tide, an expression of the available resources within the system.

- *The Tissues*

  The cellular and tissue world organizes around the precision of the Original matrix carried within the fluid systems of the body. The tissue world expresses this imperative as an inner motion called motility.

The Mid-Tide

Once the bioelectric matrix is established as a function of the Long Tide, another tidal phenomenon s then generated. As seen above, potency from this field steps down in intensity and undergoes a transmutation within the fluids of the body. It is via this transmutation process that potency becomes an embodied reality within the human form. This change in state allows the potency of the Breath of Life to fulfill its function as the ordering principle of form. Dr. Sutherland considered the cerebrospinal fluid to be the initial recipient of this transmutation of potency. It is this transmutation and ignition of potency within the fluids that allows it to be a physiological ordering principle within the body. As potency manifests within the fluids, the cellular and tissue world will organize around its blueprint imperative.

As this occurs, another tidal phenomenon is generated, the mid-tide. This tide can be perceived to express inhalation and exhalation at 2.5 cycles a minute. Within this unfoldment, potency, fluids, and tissues can be perceived to be a unity, or a unit of function. These three functions are perceived by the practitioner as a unified field of action. Potency is the organizing factor, fluid is the medium of exchange, and cells and tissues organize around its action. The mid-tide is thus a level of unfoldment in which the organizing forces of the human system

manifest as a direct physiological ordering principle. This biodynamic potency within the body physiology maintains the Original intention and plan of the human being from the time of conception to the moment of death.

Within the mid-tide the three functions of potency, fluids, and tissues are thus perceived to express a unified dynamic. The skilled practitioner can also sense each function as a *tensile field of action*. Thus potency, fluids, and tissue can each be sensed to express reciprocal tension motion as whole tensile fields. The craniosacral motions of individual structures are discernible, but are experienced to be part of a larger tensile field. We will discuss and explore this in much greater detail later. As we have seen, Dr. Sutherland considered the cerebrospinal fluid to be the initial recipient of potency as an organizing force within the body. It is through the fluid systems of the body that the Original matrix constantly manifests within its cells and tissues. We have also seen that Victor Schauberger considered water to be the medium for the life force throughout the natural world. As potency is expressed within the fluids, a tidal phenomenon is generated. This tidal phenomenon is the motion of the fluid function within the mid-tide. This was originally called the *cerebrospinal fluid tide* by Dr. Sutherland. Cerebrospinal fluid is moved by the action of the potency within it and the fluid tide is generated.

However, it is important to think of the fluids and tissues of the body as a unified field of action. This idea has physiological reality. Recently it has been found that the water molecules within all connective tissues form discrete hydrogen bonds. These bonds literally create a unified fluid matrix throughout the body. Furthermore, the connective tissues of the body have peptide side chains that bond with these water molecules. A unified fluid-tissue matrix results. This unified fluid-tissue field exhibits phenomena that Mae-Wan Ho likens to liquid crystalline structures.[19] The body is literally a unified fluid-tissue crystalline matrix. It is literally a liquid crystalline whole. As noted above, researchers have discovered discrete quantum effects and wave forms within this fluid-tissue matrix. The presence of bio-photons, light photons within living cells and fluids, has also been clearly documented.[20] The nature of liquid light, as Dr. Sutherland called this level of reality, is being scientifically unfolded. Tissues, fluids, and bioenergy phenomena are literally a unified dynamic. This reality is palpable and perceptible by the still observer.

As we have seen, within this fluid-tissue matrix, there is a transmutation of potency, or bioenergy, which is directly expressed within the body's cells and tissues. As this occurs, cells and tissues express primary respiratory cycles of inhalation and exhalation as an inner motion called motility. Motility is a function of the relationship of fluids, cells, and tissues to the potency of the Breath of Life. As potency moves, fluids and tissues move. It is one unified dynamic. Potency permeates the fluids and fluids permeate the tissues. In the Venerable Thich Nhat Hanh's words, they *interbe*. At this level of perception, the human system is experienced to be whole. Thus, when the practitioner's perceptual field is resonant with the mid-tide, he or she will perceive a unified field of action. Potency, fluids and tissues will be perceived to express motility at a rate of 2.5 cycles a minute as a unified tensile field. The unity of things become more obvious and the wholeness of the system becomes apparent. Tissues, as a particular field of action, are experienced to be a unified tensile field that expresses motility as a whole, rather than simply as separate parts in motion. Within the mid-tide, inertia and resistance within the system is experienced as an interplay of forces at work. Patterns of unresolved trauma and past experience are seen to be a function of universal and conditional forces at work. These inertial patterns may be perceived as distortions within whole tensile fields of action, rather than as resistance between separate structures. We will explore all of these concepts in much more detail in later chapters.

Clinical Highlight

Perception within the mid-tide is precise. The human system is perceived to be whole. At this level of perception, the practitioner experiences tissues as a unified field of action. What is sensed to be resistance and pathology at the CRI level (see below) is here perceived to be a function of forces at work. The biodynamic potencies of the Breath of Life and their expression of the inherent Health of the system are more obvious here. Tissues are sensed to be a unified tensile field. This tensile tissue field is sensed to express motility as a whole around the natural fulcrums of the system.

The whole tensile tissue field will be perceived to distort precisely around any inertial force held within the system. The precision is an inherent factor of the centering function of the bioelectric matrix. Moreover, in treatment sessions, this unified tensile field will express its distortions according to an *inherent treatment plan*, which is a function of the intentions of the Breath of Life. Motion testing and analysis are not necessary here. The system directly unfolds its story and its healing intentions to you. The answer is inherent within the enquiry. Within the mid-tide level of perception, the practitioner also has direct access to the cerebrospinal fluid tide. Via awareness of the quality of this tide, the available resources within the patient's system can be assessed.

Cranial Rhythmic Impulse

Finally, the most superficial rhythm is expressed at rates of 8–14 cycles a minute. This is the cranial rhythmic impulse (CRI). This term was later shortened by some to the cranial rhythm. According to Dr. Rollin Becker, Dr. Sutherland did not coin this term.[21] It was created by others for the purpose of counting phases of motion. The CRI is the most common rhythm discussed in basic cranial courses. In common usage, the terms *cranial rhythmic impulse* and *cranial rhythm* can be misleading. As we have seen, there is not one cranial impulse or rhythm. There is a series of enfolded rhythms, which can all be perceived. Whereas the Long Tide and the mid-tide are stable rhythms, the CRI is not stable. The rate of the CRI is variable depending on the particular tissues and fluids being palpated, upon the level and nature of the autonomic activation, and upon the nature of the suffering and inertia held within the system.

I believe that the CRI is generated as early as genetic differentiation. As individual tissue structures develop and genetic forces come into play, these genetic forces are directed and centered by the action of the Breath of Life. The CRI is first and foremost an expression of the conditions of our lives as these conditions must be met and centered in some way. Any unresolved force held within the system, such as unresolved trauma or toxins, will affect the expression of the CRI in some way. The CRI is the wave form that arises in relationship to these forces. The CRI is thus not a direct expression of the Tide, but is a rhythm generated as the Breath of Life interfaces with the conditions of our life. It is about individualization and particularization. Its rate of expression is effected by the level of autonomic activation present within the system. The CRI changes in rhythm, tone, and tempo as the autonomic nervous system changes. It is a composite rhythm, which manifests in relationship to all of these factors. As the system experiences inertial forces of various kinds, and as it holds the effects of these as tissue resistance and fluid congestion, the rate of the CRI is affected.

Within the CRI one becomes aware of the results and affects of past traumatization and suffering. The underlying forces and bioelectric phenomena are not easily perceived here, but the results of these forces are. Thus the results of unresolved experience are seen as tissue resistance, fluid congestion, emotional charge, and psychological form.

In a Buddhist context, the potency of the Breath of Life must interface with our individual *karma*, the energies of our past actions and tendencies. The affects of our experience, such as tissue changes, psychological patterning and the maintenance of emotional affects in the body-mind, are all expressions of karmic processes. These karmic tendencies, or predispositions, must also be centered by the Breath of Life in some way. This interplay of universal and conditional forces will also greatly effect the expression of the CRI. Health is expressed within the CRI as the Breath of Life moves to center the conditions of our life. When you are in relationship to the CRI, you are in direct relationship to the suffering of a person within this human form. This must be appreciated and respected. Within the CRI level of perception, the practitioner has a direct relationship to the results and affects of suffering. Witnessing and acknowledging suffering at this level *can* have a profound effect. It can allow the person to be heard within his or her experience of suffering and can facilitate a reconnection to the deeper tides and the inherent healing forces at work within the system.

The CRI has become associated with what is known as *craniosacral motion*. Within the CRI, tissue structures, such as bones, are perceived to express separate motions usually called craniosacral motion. These externalized motions are commonly termed *flexion/external rotation* and *extension/internal rotation*. When your perceptual field is resonant with the CRI, bones, membranes, connective tissues, and organs may be perceived to express separate and individualized motions. Tissue structures may seem to be separate in their expression of motion and motility. These same motions are perceptible within the mid-tide, but are perceived at a much slower rate and as part of a unified tensile dynamic.

Within the mid-tide, individual structures are directly sensed to be part of a greater whole. At the level of the CRI, inertia within the system will be perceived as fluid and tissue resistance within and between the separate structures. Information at this level is commonly gained via motion testing and by the application of palpation methods such as fluid direction and tractioning or compression of tissues and tissue structures.

Clinical awareness of the CRI can indicate how tissue structures are holding the shape of our experience. The overall detail of this is, however, clearer when viewed through the mid-tide. As tissue and fluid inertia is resolved, the craniosacral motion of tissue structures will reorient to the natural fulcrums and midlines within the system. They will then become more balanced in their motions and the amplitude of the CRI will be perceived to be stronger. This is a function of the lowered inertia within the system. It must be understood, however, that healing forces are perceived within the deeper tidal phenomena. Awareness of the Long Tide and the mid-tide allows a more direct appreciation of the forces at work within the human system. It then becomes possible to have a direct therapeutic relationship to these organizing forces. Clinical work becomes more dynamic and less tiring.

Clinical Highlight

As the practitioner becomes aware of the various unfoldments of the Breath of Life, different perceptual and clinical skills are appropriate for each different unfoldment. The introduction below may not make much sense at this point, but will become obvious as we unfold the concepts and perceptual exercises in this book. Here we will discuss the relationship of the practitioner to resistance within the system.

CRI: 8–14 cycles/minute

At the level of the CRI the individual motions of tissues, structures, and fluids are most apparent. The practitioner sees the individual wave forms of structures as discrete entities that express individual motion. At this level, inertia within these relationships is experienced as resistance between tissues and structures and as fluid fluctuations. Resistances are perceived through tissue and fluid dynamics. The CRI level of awareness is one of results and affects. The practitioner perceives the results of suffering. Clinical skills tend to revolve around engagement of the tissues and fluids in various ways in order to release resistance. There may be a tendency for the practitioner to relate to resistance, inertia, and emotional cycling as problems to solve or processes to release.

Healing then tends to be a function of practitioner intervention. *Therapeutic work tends to be resistance- and affect-based.*

Mid-Tide: 2.5 cycles/minute

At the level of the mid-tide, potency, fluids, and tissues are perceived as a unified field phenomenon. The practitioner perceives the wholeness and unity of the system. The unit of function of tissue, fluid, and potency is clearly apparent. The practitioner perceives tissue motility as a whole tensile field of action. Although individual tissue structures and their relationships are clearly available to awareness, tissue motility is perceived to be part of a greater whole. The overall organization of tissue motility around inertial fulcrums becomes obvious. Inertia within the system is perceived through the inherent forces at work, and a precise awareness of the details of this becomes possible. Clinically, the practitioner facilitates states of balanced tension and relates to inertial potencies rather than to tissue resistance per se. Space, rather than form, is more to the forefront. The unit of function of tissue, fluid, and potency, accessed via states of balance and stillness, is the "agent" of healing. *The therapeutic work is potency and transmutation based.*

Clinical highlight *continued*

Long Tide: Field phenomena perceived within the biosphere as cycles of 50-second inhalation and 50-second exhalation

At the level of the Long Tide healing is perceived to occur from the "without to the within" and the "within to the without."[22] In other words, healing forces are perceived to arise within huge fields of action and move right into the center of an individual's healing process. The field of action may indeed be the whole universe as a unified holographic entity. The winds that organize the bioelectric field become discernible. They may be discernible within and around the biosphere of the person being palpated. Epigenetic, biodynamic forces may become discernible. The practitioner may have the direct experience of being in the Tide. Potency is perceived to be a field phenomenon and seems to permeate everything. A radiance may be sensed moving through all things. The practitioner's mind is neither coming nor going and resonates with the emerging reality of the Long Tide. The potency of the Breath of Life is more directly perceived as it establishes the Original matrix within and around the body space. Healing processes occur through clarity of practitioner awareness, the ability to maintain a wide perceptual field, and via a resonance with the deeper epigenetic, biodynamic forces at work. *Therapeutic work is resonance based.*

Mental Unfoldments

At the CRI level of manifestation, you are experiencing the conditioned mind. At this level the mind is busy. The practitioner's mind may be analyzing and seeking solutions. Therapeutic work revolves around a linear, rational approach. There is a problem, here is a solution. The work is goal oriented and can be based on fixing whatever is found to be inertial and holding resistance. There is little sense that within the heart of this resistance there is health at work. Therapeutic interventions tend to be based on techniques and methods applied to release resistance and fix problems.

At the level of the mid-tide, the mind is quieter. The practitioner's mind is still but may wander. The mind is taking in the whole and the details within the whole become clear. The practitioner learns to trust the inherent treatment plan and does not have to analyze or motion test to understand the dynamics at work. The practitioner can access and rely on his or her intuitive mind, and therapeutics are therefore less linear and more holistic. The practitioner appreciates the forces at work. Therapeutic interventions are perceived to truly be conversations with the three functions of potency, fluids, and tissue. In these therapeutic conversations the healing and inertial forces are more directly perceived. Work at this level is much less tiring and more clinically efficient.

At the level of the Long Tide, the practitioner's mind is truly neither coming nor going. The mind literally breathes with the Breath of Life. The mind is still and holds a very wide perceptual field. The practitioner is aware of the breathing of the bioelectric field, and its organizing matrix is appreciated. The practitioner has the experience of being in the Tide, and the mind is still and acutely aware. Potency seems to permeate everything. Healing is resonance-based, and the practitioner is simply open to the inherent healing process as a function of the Breath of Life.

Emotional Unfoldments

Each unfolding tide has enfolded within it the potential for the expression of various feeling tones and states. At the level of the CRI, emotional affects may arise in relationship to our particular conditioned state (e.g., our particular life experience). They are thus conditioned and conditioning. At CRI level, the activation of fight or flight emotions during treatment is more likely. Hyperarousal and hypoarousal states may manifest. These processes are the affects left over from unresolved past trauma. These may include a spectrum of emotion from fear to terror and from anger to rage. During a session, they may be expressed in a overwhelming and dissociated way. Emotions may flood, or the patient may experience freezing states. Then the person may reexperience overwhelm, dissociation, and traumatization. This is not necessarily therapeutic. The system may experience this as a reinforcement of the original traumatization. As these traumatic emotional states become inertial within the system, they will effect the expression of the CRI in some way.

Emotions at the mid-tide level of expression are more about present time. Emotions will arise appropriate to the circumstances being experienced and will then pass. Our emotional life is lived within the immediacy of our experience and is a direct expression of the quality of the relationships within our life. The fluidity of our emotional life is appreciated here. During treatment, emotional affects of past trauma may also be activated, but they tend to be expressed in much milder forms within the resources of the person. Emotional processes are experienced as a completion of past experience and do not continue to cycle. Emotional affects complete; they are not reinforced. Emotional resolution may occur very quietly here and be experienced as a streaming of energy, warmth, and feeling. Within the Long Tide are enfolded expansive feeling tones relating to safety, joy, warmth, and contact. These expansive feeling tones are about the actualization of compassion, love, and the movement towards contact. These are less about protection and more about connection and loving contact. They tend to allow the person the felt sense of inter-connection with others. Empathy with another is more possible as our mutual interconnection is more obvious here. This can be a truly healing experience. Below some terms are defined; some were highlighted in Chapter Three.

Some Terms within a Biodynamic Framework

- *The Breath of Life*

  The Creative Intelligence in action. Its Presence is humbling. It is the divine intention in action. It arises from a profound and Dynamic Stillness.

- *The Dynamic Stillness*

  An intrinsic and alive stillness, the ground of emergence for all form.

- *The Tide, the Long Tide*

  The great organizing wind generated by the Breath of Life. The Long Tide functions within a huge field of action. It seems to arise from, and to return to, "somewhere else." When its centrifugal and centripetal motions are in a *dynamic equilibrium*, a stable bio-electric field, or matrix, is generated.

- *The Groundswell*

  The tidal swell generated within human form by the action of the Tide. Like a great tidal force, the groundswell generates the cyclical motions of primary respiration.

- *Dynamic Equilibrium*

  A state in which all forces involved in the creation of a form are in balance. It is a dynamic state in which there is a rhythmic balanced interchange between all of the forces present. It is not static, but an alive and dynamic state of interchange and balance.

Terms *continued*

- *Ignition*

  A process by which the intentions of the Breath of Life literally ignite within the human experience. The first ignition occurs at conception, when the Breath of Life literally ignites within the conceptus and the human bioelectric matrix is generated. The second ignition process occurs at birth, when the potency of the Breath of Life fully ignites within the cerebrospinal fluid as a final empowerment to take form within the human realm.

- *The bioelectric matrix*

  The Long Tide acts to generate a stable bioelectric matrix, which is the organizing field for the human system. This is a quantum-level coherent field of organization, literally an organizing field of light energy.

- *The Midlines*

  The Breath of Life establishes two ordering axes around which the fluid, cellular, and tissue worlds orient. The first is the *primal midline*, an uprising force generated within the embryonic disc of the embryo around which the notochord and spinal axis form. This force is part of the wider bioelectric matrix, the Original template of human form. This orienting axis is with us until the day we die. The second midline relates to the ignition of the potency within the cerebrospinal fluid. A *fluid midline* arises within the neural axis as the groundswell surges within the fluids as an embodied force.

- *Potency*

  The intrinsic ordering force generated by the Breath of Life within the human system. It is initially expressed as a field phenomenon, and is embodied within the fluids of the body as a direct organizing force with physiological function.

- *Transmutation*

  The process by which the potency of the Breath of Life undergoes a change in state within the fluids of the body to become an embodied ordering force within the human system.

- *The mid-tide and the fluid motion called the fluid tide*

  The mid-tide is the tidal phenomenon generated by the action of the potency within the fluids of the system. Potency, fluids, and tissues are the three functions of this tidal phenomenon. Each function can be perceived to express a primary respiratory rhythm of 2.5 cycles a minute. Tissues express this as *motility,* an inner breath-like motion within all of the tissues of the body. The fluid component of this tidal motion is called the *fluid tide.*

- *The CRI, the cranial rhythmic impulse*

  The outer manifestation of motion between structural parts generated by the interface of the Breath of Life with all of the conditions of our life. It is variable and conditional. It is the wave form that rides the deeper tidal forces.

- *Primary respiration*

  The Breath of Life generates various tidal rhythms, which manifest in two cycles of inner breath called inhalation and exhalation.

- *Phases of the Tide*

  The action of the Tide is perceived to generate two primary respiratory phases of motion within the human system, called inhalation and exhalation. In the inhalation phase, there is a welling up of potency and fluid within the system. Cellular and tissue motion is also generated. These motions are called motility, the inner inherent motion of tissues driven by the potency of the Breath of Life.

In this chapter, I attempted to introduce some concepts which at first may seem, to some, to be a nice fairy tale, or a conceptual model. Please understand that this is an attempt to discuss direct perceptual and clinical experience. Awareness of these phenomena depends on a deepening ability to listen with a perceptual field that is whole and still. Within the context of an ongoing training course, these concepts are unfolded in relationship to perceptual experience and to the student's deepening appreciation of the system. Students are encouraged to find their own words for their experience and to trust their own perceptual processes. The reality of the Breath of Life and its dynamics unfolds itself in its own way, according to our perceptual ability to hear its constant call. The work then begins to teach itself. The next chapters introduce perceptual exercises to encourage this self-taught process to occur. We will slowly introduce clinical concepts and practices related to these unfoldments as the book progresses.

1. *The Cloud of Unknowing,* trans. by Robert Way (Anthony Clarke).

2. *The Heart of Understanding,* trans. Ven. Thich Nhat Hanh (Parallax Press, 1988).

3. James Jealous, *Around the Edges,* quoted with permission of author.

4. In some Daoist traditions, the first unfoldment from *Wu Ji* is called *Wang Ji,* the Dynamic Stillness and the *Tai Ji* is the motion which arises from it. From Stillness, yin and yang arise and the ten thousand things are born.

5. Jim Jealous, "Around the Edges" ; quoted with permission of author. The term "Master Mechanic" is a term that Dr. Still coined to indicate God and His organizing and creative action within the world of form. Dr. Randolph Stone, D.O., used to say, "Man cognises, God geometises."

6. See Rollin Becker, *Life in Motion* (Rudra Press).

7. Callum Coates, *Living Energies* (Gateway Books, 1996).

8. See Chapter Twenty-four for a discussion of *rhythmic balanced interchange*, a concept originally developed by Dr. Rollin Becker, D.O.

9. See Chapter Fifteen for a discussion of this concept.

10. See W. G. Sutherland, *Teachings in the Science of Osteopathy* (Rudra Press).

11. Mae-Wan Ho, *The Rainbow and the Worm, the Physics of Organisms* (World Scientific).

12. For interesting aspects and research into embryological development in morphogenic fields, see *The Rainbow and the Worm,* and also the work of the great embryologist Erich Blechschmidt, *Biokinetics and Biodynamics of Human Differentiation* (Charles C. Thomas).

13. See Mae-Wan Ho, *The Rainbow and the Worm, the Physics of Organisms* (World Scientific).

14. See R.E. Becker, *Life in Motion* (Rudra Press).

15. See R. Stone, D.O., *Polarity Therapy* (CRCS Press).

16. See, Around The Edges; Dr, James Jealous; quoted with permission of author.

17. Jim Jealous, "Healing and the Natural World," interview in *Alternative Therapies* 3, no. 1 (January, 1997).

18. R. Stone, *Polarity Therapy* (CRCS Press).

19. Mae-Wan Ho, *The Rainbow and the Worm, the Physics of Organisms* (World Scientific).

20. Ibid.

21. See Rollin Becker, *Life in Motion* (Rudra Press).

22. A saying of Dr. Randolph Stone, D.O.

SECTION TWO
Palpation Skills and Tissue Motility

6

Presence, Negotiation, and Palpation

In this chapter we will explore some of the fundamental ground necessary for competent clinical practice. It is of critical importance that the practitioner have the ability to be present for the patient's arising process. The work we do is largely perceptual, and our listening skills are the heart of the clinical process. The ability to be fully present and to consciously work with perceptual processes is of tantamount importance.

In this chapter we will:

- *Discuss and explore presence.*

- *Inquire into relationship, contact, and touch.*

- *Discuss and explore stillness and palpation.*

- *Discuss and explore issues of contact and boundaries.*

- *Learn to access the practitioner neutral.*

- *Establish practitioner fulcrums and learn to negotiate contact.*

- *Learn to establish a wide perceptual field.*

Presence and Perception

Presence is natural and inherent within our human condition. Presence is an expression of the Intelligence of life itself. It is a manifestation of the *whole* and is not bound by our limited and conditioned ego constructions. Presence manifests as we allow our mind to still and rest wholly in present time. Presence is the miracle by which we master and restore ourselves to ourselves. In the end that is all we can do. If we restore ourselves to ourselves, we restore ourselves to life itself. It is a restoration to Wholeness so that we can live fully each moment of our life. In stillness, it is possible to sense the presence of a deeper Intelligence at work within our human system. It is the expression of the Health that is never lost within all of our experience. Presence is the foundation of our clinical practice. Our work is to perceive the inherent Health within our conditions; to recognize the innate Intelligence at work no matter how extreme these conditions may seem to be.

From this ground, the work that we do in the cranial field is largely perceptual; it is about *presence in relationship*; it is about the refinement of our perceptual skills. In this endeavor, the practitioner deepens his or her ability to be wholly in the present with full awareness. This awareness is whole; it is not fragmented. The ability to perceive Health is based on maintaining an open and wide field of awareness in which conditioned thoughts, imagination, opinions, judgments and beliefs simply do not arise. The practitioner is not reflecting on the past or projecting into the future. In this, our mind is not moving in its conditioned state, but is resting in the eternal present. Dr. James Jealous, D.O., states in an interview:

> The core of this work is perceptual; the work grew out of repeated observation until the laws of nature became more clear. We learn to sense the whole. When one meets a patient one sees the Whole—a very unique and rare event in our modern world. One does not divide life into soma/psyche/ visceral etc. This is an event contained only in the moment one is in. It's extra-ordinary. Patients are very much aware that a different attention is present. They comment on it. It's not intellectual or intuitive. It's aboriginal, instinctive. The moment is filled with the effort to be present with the Health in the patient and the story as it unfolds into its own answer. [1]

In this work, the quality of presence and perception that we bring to the session is the fulcrum for the unfolding of the therapeutic relationship. This attention is whole. It must be. We can only perceive the whole of the human condition, and its unique expression within the patient, if we ourselves are resting in this state of unified awareness. Another way to say this is that our perceptual field is not fragmented. We bring a still and wide field of awareness to the relationship and from that we learn. As Dr. Jealous states above, this kind of attention is instinctual, aboriginal. Although we must initially make an effort to be present, this state is natural and the key to its attainment is to simply notice what is in the way of it, that is, to notice whatever arises in me that is in the way. Presence allows our perceptual field to be clear and allows us to really listen to the patient's unique story. Thus, in order to appreciate the Intelligence at work, my perceptual field must be whole. In our culture we are not encouraged to maintain a perceptual field that takes in the whole. We are taught to narrow our perceptions, our outlook, our listening. We reduce experience to its parts and lose the wider awareness of the whole. It can be a real challenge to make a shift from this way of perceiving to a more

holistic perceptual process. This is always the challenge in training courses and is an ongoing process of continual learning for us all.

Thus, the work we do is largely perceptual. It is based on an appreciation of the Intelligence within the system and the healing intentions it unfolds. One of the most important skills within this context is the ability to be present. By this I mean the ability to deeply and widely listen to the human condition without fear. In this listening there is no judgment, no preconception, no shoulds. Simply have the courage to listen, and truth makes itself known. The heart of this is the ability to be still, to listen in the silence, and to trust the wisdom of the very system you are listening to. This wisdom is the inherent Health of the system. Our most important clinical skill is the ability to hear this Health and its expressions in another person. In this listening there will be communication. Both the Health and the history will be communicated. Health is a universal and is always present. History is relative and particular. As we listen through palpation and perceptual process to a person's history, expressions of suffering will be heard. These also must be acknowledged and understood. I believe that our task in this life is one of acknowledgement. It is an acknowledgement and deep appreciation of our present condition. That is the starting point. Can we, in the present, be a witness to the conditions of our lives? Can we, within that present condition, reconnect to a deeper Intelligence at work and to the inherent Health it manifests?

In essence, as you shall see, we are present for the health in the patient's system, and we learn to perceive, appreciate, and facilitate it. Indeed, the state of presence and the attainment of a unified perceptual field allow us to resonate with the expressions of this Health as it unfolds in the human system. Within this field of awareness, the story of the patient, his or her patterns of experience, disturbance and dis-ease, have within them all the answers that are necessary for the healing riddle to be answered. Thus, inherent within the disease process is the state of Health itself. The treatment plan is inherent within the disturbance or obstruction perceived in the system. In essence, as Dr. Jealous states above, "The moment is filled with the effort to be present with the Health in the patient and the story as it unfolds into its own answer." This is our greatest challenge. It is the heart of healing practice and of the clinical intentions within the cranial concept.

The Practice of Presence

In the following sections, you will explore some ways of maintaining attention and awareness in the therapeutic relationship and of creating clear boundaries between practitioner and patient. Presence is at the heart of our work. It is through presence that compassion and clarity will flow. On a deep level, presence cannot be created. It is part of our birthright. On another level, our ability to be present becomes clouded. Our minds become conditioned and habitual and we get caught up in repetitive patterns, repetitive thinking, and narrowed perception. In order to work in any depth within the cranial concept, it is necessary to wake up. It is essential to be present in order to simply listen. The conditioned mind is really very ephemeral and transitory. Once awake, our former life may seem like a dream. In our work we learn to listen deeply to the human condition, its inherent Health, and the very personal story that it has to tell.

I use a number of processes in teaching to help encourage practitioner presence and also to help anchor or ground the student. I find this necessary because it is not enough to tell someone to be present. Our ability to be present must be constantly developed and refined. Presence has a soft quality to it. Yet it also has a fire to it, a clarity. In our work, attention is not narrowed or forced. It takes in the whole and notices the particular. It is as if you are in the presence of a newborn baby and softly meet the whole of the baby with care and compassion. Yet you also notice the particular, the movements, the expressions, the sounds.

The first step in the practice of presence is to become aware of ourselves. This may seem obvious, but how many of us really take the time to become aware of our innermost processes and their outer manifestations? The development of presence is really a development of the ability to know oneself. It is largely about learning what gets in the way of just simply being here, just simply being still. This perception of our sense of self must be rooted in the body and its sensations, otherwise contact with our own state and the state of others would be impossible. The following simple process may help you with this.

Clinical Application:
Breath and Sensation

In this process, you will use the natural motion of your breath to help settle your attention. The breath is always present and is a useful reference point from which to explore your ability to simply be present. In the tradition of Tibetan Buddhism, there is a saying that if one really "lives in the breath," insight and a serene life will ensue.

1. As you sit comfortably erect, simply become aware of your breathing. Follow your breath into your body as you inhale and out of your body as you exhale. Be aware of the sensation of breathing and simply follow this sense in and out. This first step helps direct attention into the body and its sensations. It also helps to initially create an anchor for your awareness. As you do this, notice the quality of your breath. Is it easier to inhale or exhale? Is one phase fuller than the other? As you inhale, how far into your body can your attention go? Can you inhale and allow your attention to follow the movement of your breath right down into your pelvis? Are there areas of your body that are not available to your attention?

2. Now follow your breath in one more time, and then just keep your attention within your body without following your breath. Let your breath

go on in its natural expression and shift your attention to the quality of *sensation* in your body. Are there any areas of pain or distress? Are there any emotional tones or feelings?

3. After holding this awareness of sensation, let that go too. Now see if you can simply sit with yourself, noticing anything that arises. You may notice feeling tones, thoughts, images, sounds, and so on. Can you have an open relationship to them? Can you notice whatever arises and let it pass away? Can you not get caught up in it? Can you be like a vast sky of awareness? Can you let whatever arises within your field of perception pass like clouds moving through it? Is there the space to simply listen and notice what arises within the field of your presence?

4. As you listen, hold the *whole* of yourself within your field of awareness. Extend your perceptual field to include your body and the field around it. Soften your attention and see if your mind settles into a simple space of listening. There is nothing you can *do* to make this happen. It is about allowing and letting go. What do you notice? Does your mind still? Is there more clarity?

5. If you find that your mind becomes caught up in thinking, or images, or feelings, simply notice that and return to the breath to settle your awareness. Then once again see if you can simply be aware first of sensation and then of whatever arises within your larger field of perception. Once again soften and widen your listening and see if your mind settles naturally into a still yet aware state. Do this exercise a number of times a day. Let the potential for inner awareness and space become part of your life.

Later, once you learn palpation listening skills, as outlined in the next few chapters, you can do this exercise in threes. One person takes the practitioner position, one the client position, and one that of a neutral observer. The practitioner, while she is palpating the client's system, keeps fifty percent of her attention inward. The practitioner then continually describes her inner experience to the observer while the client also gives feedback.

Relationship, Contact, and Palpation

Relationship is at the heart of our journey on this earth. Through relationship we can see the reflection of who we are. Presence is the foundation for exploring relationship. A clinical relationship, in turn, demands more than the mere passive presence of the practitioner. Presence, in this sense, is not passive. Therapeutic presence is about *contact*, which is *presence in relationship*. It requires a keen and precise quality of attention. It implies the ability to be in a direct and appropriate relationship to the patient's arising process. In this context, the clinical relationship can be a mirror of truth. As we shall see, one of the practitioner's roles is to clearly reflect the patient's arising process through palpation and touch. In this reflection, something can be rediscovered that was forgotten, something can be reclaimed that was seemingly lost.

In the cranial concept, the perceptual art of palpation is at the center of our work. Palpation is about touching, and touch generates a powerful relationship. In our culture touch means so many things; the touch of a friend, of a loved one; sexual touch; touch in anger, or touch in need. Touch takes on so many shades of psychological and emotional quality and tone. In our context, there is the therapeutic touch of the practitioner. This is ideally a touch that is still and neutral, that has the intention to actively listen and to relate to the inherent forces at work. Even here, practitioners can be caught up in need. This may include the need to heal, to change things. Personal issues will also cloud the quality of contact and relationship. The practitioner's need to be okay, to be accepted, to be a great healer, his anxieties and fears: all can get in the way of the healing relationship. Practitioners' unfinished business, their personality constructs, will get in the way of a clear therapeutic relationship. These must be dealt with in an ongoing manner, with a developing awareness and a growing insight into the nature of self-view, defensive strategies, and self-organization.

Touch and the Inherent Treatment Plan

The Alexander Technique has a useful concept about touch. Tutors ask the student teachers to touch the patient without "wanting." Can you make contact from a deep place of not wanting or needing anything from the patient? Our needs will dramatically get in the way of the healing process. Furthermore, can you access a truly neutral place that is open to learning, that does not assume that you know best? This is not the neutral of the disengaged observer; it is an engaged, interested neutral. It is alive. It is in relationship, yet it does not arise out of need, even the need to know. Can you touch from a place within yourself that does not know, a place of *unknowing*? For it is only from this that we can truly be open to, and learn from, the patient's unique process. Can we allow patients to access their own inherent intelligence and deeply heal themselves? Can we trust this? In the interview mentioned above, Dr. Jealous continues,

> We use our hands diagnostically, perceptually, and therapeutically—that's how simple and profound this is. We are not listening for symptoms but for a pre-established priority set in motion by the Health in the patient." [2]

This is fundamental to understand. In a state of presence, using our perceptual skills, we do not do the healing, nor do we have to figure out what to do. The program for healing, its treatment priorities and mechanisms, is already inherent within. We listen for the "pre-established priority set in motion by the Health in the patient." All we have to do is hear it, appreciate it, and facilitate it. In essence, the treat-

ment plan is already inherent within the disturbance. We can never know what needs to happen in another's healing process. It is up to us to be able to hear and to be in an intelligent relationship to what is heard. In the cranial concept, palpation is the heart of this process.

In this work we must develop a touch that is open to perception on all levels. As we learn to touch and palpate the human system, our touch must be one that truly listens. I find that many students and practitioners attempt to develop a listening touch, but in their listening they tend to grasp the system and its tissues. This occurs either through a touch that subtly grabs on to the forms and motions perceived, or through a quality of attention that is too close and too grasping. In this work it is important to develop a quality of palpation which does not generate defensive reactions. It is a quality of touch that does not limit, lock up, or restrict the motility and mobility of the tissues being palpated. It does not limit or restrict the structure and function of the tissues being palpated. Likewise, it does not limit their field of action, nor effect their motion. In essence, it is a touch that allows the tissues to be who they are and to tell their story without coercion or constraint. In this depth of contact, the practitioner is in direct relationship to the living history of the patient. As this relationship unfolds, you will discover that the treatment plan is inherent within the disorder, and naturally unfolds itself. Again, as Dr Jealous states, "The moment is filled with the effort to be present with the Health in the patient." Within this wide-ranging perceptual field, the tissues and the forces that organize them will directly communicate the "story as it unfolds into its own answer." Our challenge is to listen, to hear the Intelligence as it unfolds itself, and to respond appropriately.

Contact and Boundaries

Stillness lies at the heart of perception. As we listen in stillness the patient's system will start to speak to us. In stillness, the story and its answers will unfold themselves. Even deeper, stillness is intrinsic to our human experience. This stillness is alive and dynamic. Stillness is not a dead or vacant emptiness; it is the basic aliveness of our human condition. Stillness is the essence of the contact we make in the cranial field. This Stillness is the ground of palpation. It is the key to accessing the "story as it unfolds into its own answer."[3] The challenge we face is to access a quality of mind that has perceived its basic ground of Stillness. From here we can perceive the Health that is never lost and truly be of service to ourselves and our patients.

Work in the cranial field is the art of doing-not-doing. It is about working with a deep appreciation of the inherent Intelligence and Health of the system. In this process there is no judgment about the patient's condition or state. It begins with an acceptance of how things are as a mutual starting point and ends with a recognition that the answers were already present within the conditions presented. In this, we recognize that we are all in this human condition together and that we are fellow travelers in this journey of life. There are, however, pitfalls in this journeying.

It is important for practitioners to have a sense of boundary and personal process within the work. It is very easy for boundaries between what we are sensing and the patient's own process to become blurred. Is what I am feeling mine or hers? Is that my pain or his? Is that my intention or hers? It is also easy to project personal process onto the patient. Ultimately these are all issues of boundary and interface. For instance, personal needs and desires projected into the therapeutic relationship will get in the way of the healing process. These must be attended to. We must all work on our personality constructs, our needs, our desires, and our interior shadow world, in order to be clear and skillful helpers.

It is important for the practitioner to approach the patient from a *neutral*; not wanting, needing, or expecting anything. Just listening to, appreciating, and facilitating Health. In this we help the system to do what it already knows and wants to do, not what I, as practitioner, need or want. It is very easy to fall into the trap of doing, wanting or needing change. Perhaps the pitfall lies in needing to be the great practitioner, or seeking approval, or needing to be successful. It may lie in a real intention to alleviate suffering, but even that may get in the way of the healing process.

Contact is the ability of the practitioner to reach out to patients and meet them where they are, not where we would like them to be. The intention in the work as practitioner is to be fully engaged in the healing process. Yet for a depth of healing to occur, you must also maintain a clear sense of space and boundary between yourself and the patient's process. The obvious ethical boundaries must be maintained. You must internalize a clear code of ethics for your work. Beyond this, there are vital issues of boundary that will arise through the depth of palpation and contact demanded in the cranial field.

Due to the intimacy of contact that arises in the work, subtle boundaries between practitioner and patient can become blurred. If you don't understand these issues, you will find yourself getting lost in your patient's system and will end up in confusion and/or in a mentally foggy state. You may get lost in the doing and not respect the boundaries of the system. You may fall into the trap of making things happen and lose the possibility of truly listening to what wants to happen. You may even subtly invade the patient's system with your intentions and end up unknowingly re-traumatizing him or her. Even your attention, if not negotiated, can be invasive. You may find yourself chasing fulcrums or patterns that are really the system's defensive responses to your invasion. If you do this, you will end up chasing shadows. This can all be very tricky and confusing. Furthermore, if your boundaries are not clear, the patient's system will not be able to trust your contact and will not allow you to touch the depth of his process. You will become an obstacle to his healing process, rather than an intelligent facilitator. You may not even be aware of this and carry on in your invasive intentions. Things will appear to happen, but you have missed a real opportunity for a deep healing relationship. This is the greatest tragedy of all and it need not occur.

Let's explore some of these concepts in a perceptual exercise. Listen to your own system and note what gets in the way of your listening to the patient's system. This is something that you will come back to again and again.

Clinical Application:
Presence and Patient Contact

You will make a physical contact with another person. In this process you will sit at the foot of a treatment table and simply make contact with the person's feet. The intention will be to center yourself on your breath and sensations and to see what arises within yourself that gets between you and your listening.

1. Sitting at the foot of the table, simply make a light contact with the dorsal aspect of the other person's feet. Remember the discussion above about your quality of touch. *Let your hands float on the person's tissues* and allow them to show you their motions, pulsations, and patterns. Do not be in a hurry. Do not expect to sense anything. Let yourself listen for a while without any preconceived concept of what you should be sensing.

2. When practicing palpation, as you sit or stand by your patient, is there any sense of anxiety or other feelings that color the relationship? As you bring awareness to yourself, do you notice any thoughts that arise? Judgments, opinions, fantasies, memories? Are there feelings or emotions? Fear, anxiety? Senses or thoughts of insecurity?

3. Now, see if you can create some space between yourself and anything that may arise within you

which may come between you and your patient. Thoughts, needs, anxiety, fear, insecurity, pride, judgments, beliefs will all close down your receptivity to the patient's process. The first step is to simply become aware of these. Try to have no judgments about your judgments or feelings. Simply become aware of them.

4. See if you can sit in a space of open awareness. Try to maintain a gentle, light, open awareness as you notice your breath and sensations. In clinical work, it is this quality of nonjudgmental presence that allows you to sense the inherent Health of the system. In this state of present open awareness, your hands will be your perceptual antennae and your patient will be within your soft and open perceptual field. It comes back to whether you can be in the present without a preconception of how things should be.

This exercise can be a very important meditation. What keeps me from being present? What challenges or threatens this sense of "me"? What gets between me and the present moment? What gets between this me and a simple listening to my patient's system?

Accessing a Practitioner Neutral

I would like to take our exploration a step further. The concept of the neutral, and of states of balance, are central themes in the cranial concept, and you will gradually grow to appreciate their importance. In the following process, you will be accessing a *neutral* within yourself, which will be used as a reference point for your relationship to the patient. This neutral is not that of a dissociated or disengaged observer. It is rather one that is fully engaged in listening and can have a direct yet respectful relationship to the patient's system. It is one from which compassion can flow as a natural consequence of a deep and appropriate contact. Accessing a neutral within yourself is the first step in establishing a clear practitioner-patient relationship.

Let's begin to explore establishing this neutral ground within yourself. We will start with an internal process, which you will later learn to apply to your palpation sessions.

1. Once again, simply become aware of your breathing. Follow the inhalation and exhalation of your breath. Follow it into your body as you inhale and out as you exhale. Stay with this simple process for a while.

2. As you do this, notice what takes you away from awareness of your breath. It may be thoughts, imagery, fantasy, feelings, sound, sensations, and so forth. As you notice this movement away from your breath, gently acknowledge it and return to your awareness of breath. Again stay with this process for a while. See if you can bring equal attention to both (i.e., equal attention to the breath and on what takes you away from the breath).

3. Now I will ask you to explore a possibility. Notice the *coming back to your breath* and the *being taken away from your breath*. Notice what takes you away and the intention to return. You may notice thoughts taking you away from the breath, or images, or sensations, or external input such as sounds. Notice this and then notice your intention to return to the breath. As you move towards your breath again, see if you can find a neutral between the two, a place of balance. As you sense this polarity of staying with your breath and being drawn away from it, notice a neutral point between the two states. It is a point or state of balance between the coming and going of your attention and intention. It is a place of balance between the two. As you experiment with this, you may notice that this point of balance has a sense of *place* within your mind and body. See if you can rest in this place of relative balance and ease within yourself.

This will be a still center. Your mind will be in a state of balance between its coming and going. Accessing this state where the mind is neither coming nor going is an important clinical skill.

When you begin to palpate a patient's system, establishing your practitioner neutral will aid in establishing a clear and negotiated contact. From this inner neutral, your perceptual field can hold the patient's system within a sense of presence that is grounded in the stillness within. It can become a refuge where presence and present time-ness can be accessed on an everyday basis. Before actually touching a patient, access your neutral and only make contact when this is achieved. This neutral will come and go. The most important thing initially is to maintain your intention to rest in it. When you establish an inner neutral, a clear relational field is also established. It gives the patient's system a new fulcrum and a clear relationship from which to explore its process. The fulcrum you create is essential. It is an anchor around which the whole healing process can unfold. It grounds you as practitioner and generates a still and safe listening space. In the following sections, you will learn further processes to help clarify boundaries and relationships. These are called establishing practitioner fulcrums. The process is meant to help you understand the subtleties of negotiating contact with a patient's system.

Clinical Application:
The Negotiation of Contact

There are many ways to initiate a healing relationship. The intention is to initiate and develop a safe and trustworthy clinical space. One might even call it a sacred space. I would like to present some useful ideas, which are best practiced and internalized in your own way. These ideas are guidelines that you can work with. In the end each of us must find our own way back into conscious relationship. In the following exercise, decide on where you will touch the patient's system and go through the following steps in a conscious and gradual way. All of this becomes second nature and intuitive. If you are negotiating a contact from the head, don't worry about your exact hand position for now; it is the quality of the contact that we are focusing on here.

Step One: Checking In

The first step is to sense your own internal space. The important thing is to begin to appreciate your own inner state. It is imperative that you have a clear sense about where you are starting off as you enter the therapeutic relationship. It is a checking-in process. The simplest way is to enter your inner *body space*. The intention is to be inside your body with awareness from the top of your neck to your pelvic floor. *This is an embodied realm of feeling tone.* Try following your breath into your body and its sensations. As you inhale, follow the feeling sense of your breathing into your body space. An alternative is to "inhale" your way into your body from the bottom up. To do this, imagine that you have nostrils on the soles of your feet and as you inhale, imagine/sense that you are drawing your breath from the soles of your feet up your legs into your abdomen. The intention is to have a sense that you are listening within your body space and allowing the "all about-ness" of your present state to speak to you. What is the sense of yourself now? What may get in the way of your relationship with the client? See the Clinical Application above, "Presence and Patient Contact." See what you need to acknowledge. Can you hold this with space?

Step Two: Moving Towards

Once you have a sense of your inner state, the next step is to make contact with your patient. This must be a negotiated process. It is about establishing a conscious relationship and a negotiated contact with your patient. Slowness helps. As you sit or stand by the patient, first bring an intention to move towards her. Verbally let her know that you are moving towards physical contact and will be contacting her body. Let your hands move slowly with a listening intention. Listen for the response to your intention even before you actually make physical contact. See how this is communicated within the field between you and the patient.

Step Three: Negotiating Physical Contact

Once you are in a physical contact, no matter where on the body, the next step is to negotiate that contact. Let the patient lead you here. In class situations, students learn to give each other clear verbal feedback. Am I too close? Is the contact okay? Is it too heavy, too light? Over time you begin to read the negotiation of contact via the nature of the communications from the system picked up by your sensing and listening hands.

Step Four: Negotiating Attention

Once physical contact is negotiated, also negotiate the quality of your attention. This really occurs simultaneously with the physical contact, but for learning purposes I am breaking it down into two movements: physical touch and the touch that your attention brings to the system. If your attention is too close or too distant, the quality of contact may not feel safe or contained. Many practitioners subtly invade the patient's system with their attention without realizing it. It is common to unknowingly grab onto the tissues with your attention. All that you will be following then is the system's response to your attention, not its inherent motions. Practice moving your attention towards the patient's system and away from it. See if both you and the patient can sense a contact that feels right. There may be a sense of meeting and contact within your perceptual field. Play with this. I will go into more detail on this issue below.

Step Five: Establishing a Field of Listening

The final step in this process is to establish a dynamically still listening field. By this I mean a field of awareness that has a still quality to it, yet which is deeply engaged in listening. To do this I will introduce the idea of the *biosphere,* a term used by Dr. Rollin Becker, D.O. Dr. Becker used this term to indicate the nature of the practitioner's field of awareness, or perceptual field. In this idea, the practitioner holds an awareness of the whole of the person, his body, and the field of environmental exchange around them. This is a wide field of listening, which places you in a relationship to the whole of a person. After establishing your contact as described above, establish this wide field of listening and see what kinds of communications arise form the patient's system within this field. The challenge, as we shall see, is to not narrow your perceptual field down as you listen to these communications. Sense them within the context of the whole. See if the nature of the space you are providing creates a context for communication and a deepening into a healing relationship. We will develop these concepts in great detail later in this volume. For now, simply let yourself explore these ideas.

In the following sections, I am introducing processes that give more structure to the ideas explored above. This process is called establishing practitioner fulcrums. We will work with some structured approaches to the issues explored above. Again, in the end, you must find your own way here. See what works and develop your own approaches if necessary. All of this becomes natural and intuitive as you continually intend a conscious relationship to the patient's system.

Practitioner Fulcrums

In the next sections, you will explore a further process that helps practitioners clarify their relationship to their patients: *establishing practitioner fulcrums.* The intention of this process will be to establish and maintain your own boundaries and to respect the boundaries of the patient's system. As you will see, all motion is organized around *fulcrums.* A fulcrum is simply a still place that organ-izes motion. Motility and motion are always organized around fulcrums. For instance, a site of inertial forces, and any related tissue and fluid resistance, may become a still or inert place around which motility and motion will have to organize. There are also *natural fulcrums* within the system which develop embryologically. These naturally organize the intrinsic motions of the body's fluids and tissues. In the following exercise, you will use this concept of fulcrums creatively by establishing fulcrums, or anchors, from which your presence can move. If you can do this, you will have a clear sense of ground within yourself, and your boundaries in relationship to the patient will become clearer. You will also learn to use these fulcrums in order to negotiate your contact and distance to the patient's system.

Establishing Practitioner Fulcrums

Let's try a simple procedure. We will again approach this first as an inner exercise. Establish a comfortable sitting position. Keep your feet flat on the floor and your back comfortably erect. First establish your ground of presence. From here, you will establish three basic *practitioner fulcrum,* which can help to organize your relationship to your patients.

First Fulcrum

1. Place your attention inwardly within your back and spine. See if you can visualize your spinal cord as you feel yourself in that part of your body. If you haven't a clear image of this, look up this area in your anatomy atlas. Feel/sense/see the cauda equina of the spinal cord, and see the filament terminalis as it descends through the sacral canal to your coccyx. Now imagine your filament terminalis extending downward from the coccyx, through your chair, into the earth. Allow your visualization of this to extend as deeply into the earth as you feel appropriate. This point in the earth will be one of the fulcrums you are establishing. Sense how

far into the earth this fulcrum needs to project for you to feel grounded.

2. In this process, you are establishing your relationship to the earth as you work and relate to the patient. This is not a fixed place. It is an *automatically shifting fulcrum* at the end of the imaginary straight line that extends inferior from your spine. After you establish this fulcrum, notice that it is a point in the earth under you at the end of the extended straight line from your spine. You can experiment with this earth fulcrum. Slowly lean forward and backward. As you lean forward, your spinal axis changes and your earth fulcrum will move with it. As you lean backward, it will move anterior. It is an automatically shifting fulcrum point of reference, not a fixed, rigid place. (See Figure 6.1.)

Second Fulcrum

Now you will establish a second posterior fulcrum. The first related you to the earth; the second relates to the physical relationship between yourself and your patient.

1. First place your attention at your external occipital protuberance (inion). See/sense the internal and external occipital protuberance. This is located on your occipital squama above the hollow at the top of your spine. You will feel a bump centrally located about an inch above this hollow. Internally this is where the straight sinus meets the confluence of sinuses. The straight sinus is the natural fulcrum for reciprocal tension membranes and of osseous-membranous

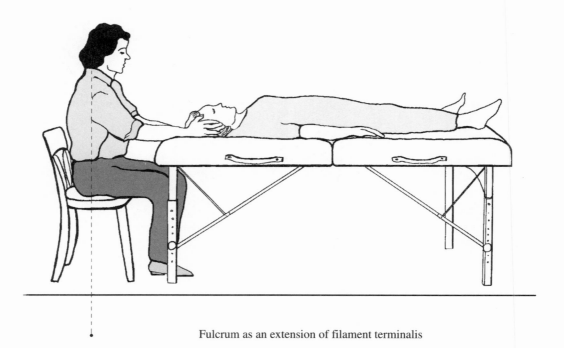

Fulcrum as an extension of filament terminalis

6.1 First fulcrum to earth

motility generally. This fulcrum has been called Sutherland's fulcrum.

2. Imagine that you project a line outward from the straight sinus and inion to a place on the floor behind you, at about a 30-degree angle to the ground. See if you can have a felt sense of this axis meeting the ground behind you.

3. You will discover that this will eventually help define your spatial relationship to the patient. The fulcrum behind you will actually help you

establish a clear sense of the space in front of you. It will be a reference point to return to when you discover that you've lost this sense. This line that you project just touches the ground somewhere behind you. It is *not* a fixed point attached to the ground. You can experiment with this. As you lean forward, notice that this straight line projected from the straight sinus lifts off the ground. When you settle back into your upright position, your posterior fulcrum also settles back onto the ground. (See Figure 6.2.)

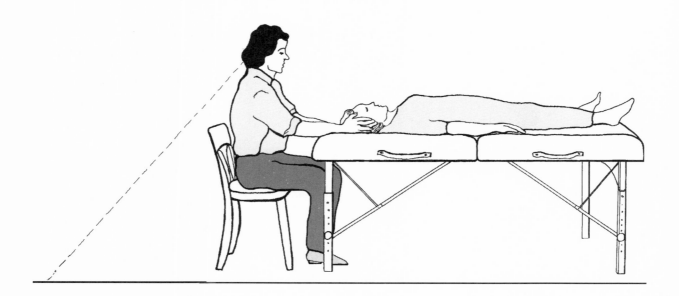

Fulcrum as posterior extension of straight sinus

6.2 Second fulcrum to earth

Sensing Both Fulcrums

Spend some time visualizing/sensing both of these fulcrums. As you do this, notice what happens to them as you move. These aren't meant to be fixed places, but moving fulcrums that help you define your relationship to the patient. Experiment with them again. When you lean forward, the fulcrum projected from the filament terminalis under you will shift posterior, while the one projected from the straight sinus behind you will lift off the ground. These are straight lines whose end points are your reference points, or fulcrums. If, while palpating the patient's system, you lose the sense of the space in front of you and collapse into it, you will notice that you lose your fulcrums. They move with the motion of your spine and your straight sinus. You now have these reference points to reestablish the sense of groundedness and the sense of the space in front of you. Recenter yourself and reestablish the two fulcrums under you and behind you. You will find that this visualization will help you maintain a sense of the boundaries and space between you and the patient. This is of critical importance in a field where the contact is so intimate and boundaries are so subtle between patient and practitioner.

These two fulcrums establish your physical relationship both to the earth and to the patient. Although they are imaginary, they are very practical. Many students and practitioners do not appreciate the subtlety of the patient's boundaries, physically, psychologically, and energetically. I have witnessed many students and practitioners intensively concentrating on what they were perceiving in the patient's body. They may move too close to the patient's system, not be aware of the patient's subtle boundaries, and even subtly grab onto the tissues that they are palpating. They may go beyond the safe energetic boundaries that the patient's system has set up for herself. If you do this, you will not get clear information and communication from the patient's system. The patient's system will either close you out, shut down, or may seem to go along with your in-tention, but will return to its own needs and patterns soon after the session is over.

If you get too close to a patient's system or have no sense of the patient's energetic boundaries, you may lose sense of both your own boundaries and those of your patient. This can be a very subtle process. The practitioner may sense that he is in a deep relationship to the patient's system, yet is really invading it and not respecting its boundaries. You may even lose yourself in the patient's system. Commonly, if you lose yourself in your patient's system, you may feel mentally foggy and unclear. It is also common, as the practitioner gets lost in the patient's system, for his or her body to slump and lose a sense of place in relationship to the patient's system. I've even seen sessions in which the practitioner becomes so physically and mentally lost and disoriented that her forehead ends up touching or even banging the patient's head. We would say that the practitioner has lost the sense of her own fulcrums! When this happens, the practitioner can reestablish a clear relationship to the patient by imagining these two fulcrums. First, return to the spine, the filament terminalis, and your projection into the earth. Then establish the fulcrum from inion to the earth behind you. This reestablishes your upright position and a sense of physical place. Once again you can reestablish your sense of space and boundary in relationship to your patient.

Inner Fulcrum

The final fulcrum that I will ask you to establish is an *inner fulcrum*. This fulcrum establishes an inner anchor for your awareness to rest in. You have already worked with this idea when you established a practitioner neutral. In one classic version of this process, the practitioner simply becomes aware of, and anchors his attention in, the straight sinus. The straight sinus is an important internal fulcrum of the primary respiratory system. In this version of accessing an inner neutral, the practitioner learns to rest in the straight sinus and to look at the patient's system from there. You might want to try this. In a more open version, the practitioner finds the most focal point within herself to rest in. This might be within the straight sinus, the third ventricle, the "third eye," the "heart center," the abdomen, and so on. The practitioner looks within and finds his own still center from which to sense the patient's process. Try this. Seek a neutral within yourself and try to rest there as you look/listen outwardly. Try to maintain this place of watching as an inner anchor for your attention. Allow your attention to arise from here and direct your sense of presence towards the patient. This anchors your awareness and helps maintain clarity. It also creates space between your system and that of the patient's. (See Figure 6.3.)

Although this is a practice commonly taught in foundation cranial courses, I recommend that you use the process earlier described, that of accessing a practitioner neutral. If you do this, you will honor your own state of balance and will relate to the patient in a more natural way. It also allows you to more easily establish a wide perceptual field, which we will work with below. Reread the section above on establishing a practitioner neutral.

Let's summarize these sections on practitioner fulcrums. The main thrust was to clearly establish your therapeutic relationship with the patient. To do this you set up a number of fulcrums from which you could relate to the patient. You set up two fulcrums that established your physical relationship to

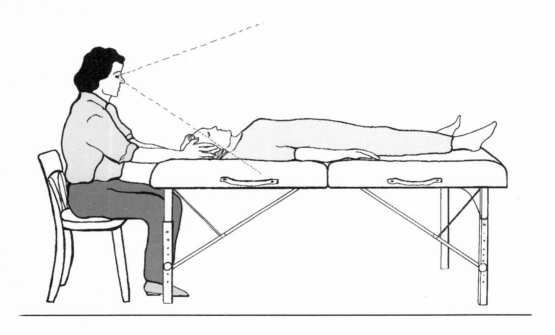

Listening from your inner fulcrum

6.3 Inner fulcrum

the patient, one was to the earth below and the other, to earth behind. The two together should give you an immediate sense of place and distance in relationship to the patient. Finally, you also established an inner fulcrum, a neutral, which anchored your sense of presence. These concepts may at first seem strange to you, but please work with them, and I believe you will discover their value. Now that you have established these fulcrums, we will use them to help negotiate our relationship to the patient and his or her system.

Negotiating Distance and Boundary

We talked earlier about the subtlety of palpation and contact in cranial work. When you establish your fulcrums and a sense of boundary and space between you and your patient, you can also establish the appropriate sense of *distance*. I will try to clarify this by using a common practical example. The quality of touch in cranial work is usually very, very light. It is a contact that uses no physical pressure; it uses intention and suggestion rather than pressure or force. The sense of the quality of touch is that of lightly palpating a cork floating on water. You want to sense how it is moving on the tide. You do not want to place any pressure on it, as it will then have to respond to your pressure. You will then lose a sense of what it is doing *as though you are not there*.

However, even with the lightest of physical touches, a patient may still experience your touch as heavy-handed or pressured. I have noted this many times in supervising student and practitioner work. The patient here is perceiving not a heaviness of physical touch, but a heaviness of concentration and attention, and a loss of clarity of boundary. In moving your attention to the patient's system, your concentrated awareness can be perceived by the patient as very heavy, pressured and invasive. You may not be sensitive enough to the patient's boundaries and move past what the patient senses to be safe. Although this is of critical importance in cases where there has been abuse, it is equally important

in your relationship to every patient.

If your intention is too heavy, or if you inadvertently cross a patient's energetic boundaries without negotiation, the patient's system isn't given enough space to show you how it has become structured. It will have to react to or resist your presence. Your contact isn't experienced as safe enough. It will be sensed as intrusive or invasive. You may subtly invade the patient's system without realizing it. This obviously will not be experienced by the patient as safe. You may be invasive with your attention and intention. What also happens many times is that the practitioner is trying too hard, concentrating too hard, and, although being gentle with touch, is not being gentle with attention. Because of this, it is important to establish a sense of appropriate distance in relationship to the patient's system.

Clinical Applications:
Negotiation of Boundary and Distance

It is clinically important to establish an appropriate contact and listening distance to the patient's system. In this section, you will explore some processes that will clarify your relationship to touch and contact with the patient's system. The focus will be on the negotiation of boundary and distance to the patient's system. In this section, you will imagine that you are doing this, and in the section that follows, you will set up an actual palpation session.

1. Sitting comfortably, imagine that you are at the head of a treatment table, then bring your attention to your own body. Establish your neutral and your practitioner fulcrums as described above. Then place your hands in front of you. Imagine that you are gently holding your patient's head with your fingers spread. Imagine that your touch has the quality of meeting a cork floating on water. You do not want to place any pressure on the cork because this would stop its own inherent motion. After establishing

89

your gentle and light contact, reestablish your practitioner fulcrums as above.

2. Now imagine that you are sitting behind your-self, maybe ten or fifteen feet (three meters or so) back from where you are physically sitting, and imagine that you are sensing the person's system from a distance. Some practitioners imagine that their arms are growing longer and that they are moving further away from the pa-tient's system. As you move behind yourself to a distant vantage point, be sure your practi-tioner fulcrums are established, because these will ground you in your body and in physical space. They will also give you a clear sense of the physical distance between you and the pa-tient. Some practitioners imagine that they are outside the room, or even outside the building.

3. After creating this sense of space, you will ne-gotiate the distance between yourself and your imaginary patient. The intention is to find the appropriate sense of space and distance from which the patient's system can accept your con-tact. It will help you to sense the energetic boundaries of a patient's system. Experiment with this by projecting your fulcrums several feet behind yourself as described above. Start at least ten feet (three meters) behind where you are sitting and slowly draw your intention and attention closer to the patient's system. Re-member, you are still in physical contact with the patient's body. You are simply trying to ad-just the quality and distance of your attention. The intention here is not to "leave your body," but to create space and to negotiate contact and distance.

4. In a real situation, as you draw closer to the pa-tient, his or her system will give you clues as to the appropriate viewing distance. This may be quite far away from the patient's physical sys-tem, or may be quite close or deeply inside. The

distance will depend on the relationship you have with your patient, the appropriateness of the contact, and the sense of safety felt by the patient. This will change during a session and over a period of time. Each patient will be unique and, indeed, each body part and each session will be different. Thus negotiating dis-tance and boundaries is an ongoing process. This process gives the person's system a sense of space and, I believe, a feeling of being re-spected and not manipulated or controlled. You may sense the patient's system opening to you, showing you its inherent Health, or a clear sense of its life shapes and patterns.

This may all sound a bit esoteric, but these are use-ful and important skills, which help maintain and clarify the therapeutic relationship. Try it and you will notice that a greater depth of perception be-comes available to you and a greater sense of clar-ity arises. After you experiment with this, you may find your own ways of negotiating space and clari-fying boundaries. Let's take this the next step and move into an actual palpation session with a real person.

Clinical Application:
Negotiating Distance in a Session

Let's now spend some time using these principles in a real situation and work to negotiate space and dis-tance with a person's system.

1. With a person in the supine position on a treat-ment table, set up your practitioner fulcrums as described above. Establish your neutral, then slowly move to a contact in which you place your hands on either side of the patient's head. Let your index finger touch the greater wing of the sphenoid and your ring finger touch the squama of the occiput. Spread the rest of your fingers comfortably on the patient's cranium. I am not concerned here with the exact place-

ment of your fingers; this will be stressed in later sections. This hold will later be developed into a *vault hold*. (See Figure 6.4.)

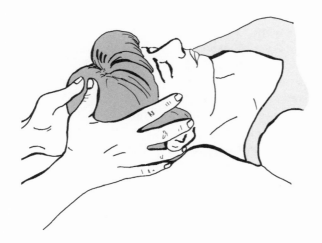

6.4 Vault hold

2. Once you make physical contact, be sure that you are holding the person's head with a very light contact. Imagine that your touch has the quality of meeting a cork floating on water. Again, you do not want to place any pressure on the cork that would stop its own inherent motion. Ask your patient for feedback on the quality of your touch. Is it too heavy? Is it not firm enough? Is it pressured?

3. Now, as described above, after you have established your fulcrums, project/imagine that you are sitting ten or fifteen feet behind the person. From that position, slowly move towards the person's system. Notice how the person's system responds to this. See if you can sense where the person's system begins to resist your presence. See if you can sense the edge of the boundary; the edge just before you sense resistance to your presence. You may sense that

the patient's system is pushing you away, or that it is shutting you out. You may even sense that it withdraws from you. See if you can sense the boundary where you meet the patient's system, where there is communication between you rather than reaction. This distance might be ten or more feet behind yourself, or it may be very close to the person. You may find that the person's system allows you to be anywhere from very far away to right inside its dynamics. I have had many patients for whom, initially, I had to set my fulcrums very far away; outside the room, or in the next county, or on the other side of the world, or even in outer space! This distance will change as the therapeutic relationship deepens, as you approach different parts of the body and different issues. Many practitioners initially relate to their patients from far away, perhaps outside the building, and then negotiate the viewing distance.

4. Ask your practice patient for feedback about the quality of your touch, sense of pressure, and distance. Note the response of the person's system as you do this. Ask your patient how he or she perceives your touch, as to its heaviness, closeness, and quality. In a classroom situation you can give each other very precise feedback. Take advantage of each other's sensitivity. See if you can both sense the appropriate listening distance. Work fifteen minutes or so each way, and then spend some time sharing your experience of the process.

In the next sections, you will explore a further essential skill, that of establishing a wide perceptual field. The usefulness of this will become clear as we introduce more clinical concepts and applications.

A Wide Perceptual Field

In previous sections, you worked to establish your practitioner neutral, worked with practitioner fulcrums, and worked with the negotiation of contact and distance. The next step is to establish a wide perceptual field. The intention here will be to learn to listen to the *whole* of a patient, even when focusing on a particular relationship or part. The ability to perceive the whole and to note the particular within that whole may have vast repercussions for your understanding of life and of perception itself. It may effect your everyday sense of who you are and what the world is about. It is based on a still and naturally balanced mind and the establishment of a wide perceptual field.

I once undertook a perceptual training in the Nyingmapa tradition of Tibetan Buddhism. Day after day, I had to visually trace the Tibetan letter "ah" while sitting with its image on the wall in front of me. I endlessly traced it over and over again, letting my eyes follow its contours for hour upon hour. At first I had to struggle with the sheer boredom and seeming absurdity of the practice. Then I struggled with my emotional responses and anger. Then with fear and even terror. I can't tell you why all of these emotions came up, but they did, and they all became part of the practice. We carried this on for weeks until the letter was totally incorporated into our consciousness. I could see it in front of me at will. We were then taught to project it in front of us and to make it three-dimensional. I learned to turn it upside down, around and around, and even to flip it over and see its opposite side, projected in space in front of me. Finally, once a day, for a number of weeks, we hiked to the top of a high hill. From here we could see the expanse of the world around us. Then we practiced something that literally changed my perception of my world and of the perceptual process itself. We learned to project and extend this letter "ah" into the environment. Further and further we projected it, until it even projected beyond the horizon. Finally, after some practice, within this wide perceptual field, I learned to project it behind particular things. I could project it behind the building or the forest far away. I learned, in essence, to extend my consciousness to see behind things and

to see what was there. I would see a car before it emerged from behind a building, a person before he stepped out from behind a tree. These were not considered to be "psychic" powers, but very mundane, everyday perceptual processes. In other words, the ability to take in a wider perceptual field and to gain information from a more holistic relationship to the world was considered by the Tibetans to be our birthright and part of our natural abilities. The letter "ah" was simply the vehicle that broke down my fixed view of the world and concepts of my perceptual capabilities. It had a lasting effect.

Holding a wide perceptual field is an essential skill within this work. As we said above, the heart of the work in the cranial field is perceptual. It is about an attunement to the whole unfoldment of a human being. Indeed, it leads to a deeper resonance with the universal nature of the healing forces at work within the human system. This is critical to understand. As you palpate a patient's system, you are meeting a living reality, which is Intelligent and conscious. It is important to hold this interface with lightness and respect. It is important to establish a wide perceptual field so that you are not limiting the potential of the therapeutic encounter. You must meet the patient's system without judgment and as a fellow traveler. At any time your perception will be attuned to particular layers of experience. It is possible to widen and deepen your field of perception to take in more and more of the human condition. In the next chapter we will introduce perceptual exercises that help you to shift your perceptual field to the different unfoldments of the Breath of Life within the human system. As you will see, there is very clear clinical value in the ability to shift your perceptual fields to different layers of the system and to different unfoldments of the Breath of Life in the human system. Perception is multidimensional. In experience, perceptual processes should not be fragmented. Thus, in setting up a wide perceptual field, you have the opportunity to be in relationship to the whole of the human system and the possibility of shifting your perceptual processes to appropriate relationships and un-foldments. Later on you will also learn to appreciate that it is in this state of unified awareness that, in stillness, you can listen to the unfolding of the Breath of Life and perceive its healing priorities. Sensing the *Whole* is wider and deeper than you may first imagine. Let's take some steps to open to this possibility.

Clinical Application:
Establishing a Wide Field of Perception without Patient Contact

The next clinical application is about the generation of a wide perceptual field within the therapeutic context. It may, however, have wider repercussions for you. It is really about how you relate to the world and how you perceive that world. This process may become a way of being in the world. It will challenge your fixed views about perception and how you gain information. It is about everyday awareness. Can you hold a wide perception that takes in the whole while you walk down the street? Can you notice the particulars within that whole as you walk down that street? Can you hold a wide perceptual field while sitting in a coffee bar? While talking to another? While in a confrontational situation? Can you gain information about the particular from the whole? These are very real and challenging questions for us all.

Let's explore the possibility of establishing a wide perceptual field that will help you sense the *whole* of a patient and maintain the integrity of your attention. The establishment of a wide perceptual field is a useful starting point in your perceptual exploration of the system. It will allow you to start from a wide perspective before learning to consciously shift to the different tidal unfoldments. We will begin to explore this conscious shift in the next chapter. You will practice this exercise internally before actually palpating a patient's system. Start from a comfortable sitting position and first work with this exercise on your own, rather than in a clinical setting.

1. Settle into your sitting position and relax as best as you can. First access the neutral as described above. Again use your breath to help access the state of balance, or the practitioner neutral within. Again notice what takes you away from your breath. It may be thoughts, fantasies, memories, feelings, sound. As you notice that you have lost your awareness of the breath, gently return your attention to it. Find the neutral point of balance between bringing your attention to your breath and being taken away from it. This neutral may have a sense of place within yourself. See if you can rest in this still center.

2. From this sense of neutral, the intention will be to create a wide perceptual field within which to hold the patient. From the neutral that you have just established, gently and slowly extend your attention out to the horizon, with your patient within that field. Widen your perceptual field only to where it still feels safe and you do not experience dissociation or spaciness. If possible, let your attention move past the horizon, even if it is just in your imagination. Now, within this wide perceptual field, notice what information comes back. Simply be attentive and receptive and notice what sensory information returns within your field of perception. This is an active process. You are a neutral yet engaged listener. As you explore this field of listening, you may notice that there is a point, or state of balance, between the extension of your attention as it moves out and the sensory information that returns. You may sense this to be another neutral, a state where your attention moving out into the world is at balance with the perceptual information that is returning. In other words, your sensory and motor fields are in balance. This is a state where you have let go of controlling your attention and field of aware-

ness and have settled into a still yet engaged state of perceptual balance. It is a true state of listening with need or direction. In this state of balance, simply be open to whatever sensory information enters your field of awareness.

3. Spend a few minutes listening to your world this way. You may be surprised what is communicated to you. Then gently and slowly again narrow your perceptual field to your immediate environment and to your body, and stretch and make contact with your surroundings.

Clinical Application: Establishing a Wide Perceptual Field with Patient Contact

In this application, you will work with the same concepts as above while in contact with another's system. As you continue in your course of study, this exercise will take on more and more meaning and clinical relevance.

1. Sit at the head of the treatment table with your patient in the supine position. From this position, again access your neutral and extend a wide perceptual field. Let this field extend to the horizon, or as far outward as feels safe and contained for you.

2. Now slowly move to holding the patient's head in the vault hold as already practiced. Let your hands float on the tissues as though they are in fluid. See if you can maintain your practitioner neutral and a wide perceptual field. While holding this wide field, include the person you are in contact with as the center of that field. Be aware of the particulars within that field, that is, the particulars which include that person. Listen into it. It demands a keen and sharp quality of awareness. The field is wide and soft, the quality of attention is sharp and incisive.

See what information comes to you. Again let your hands simply float on the tissues and listen to whatever information is given. Do you sense tissues breathing? Do you sense tissue motion? Do you sense fluid fluctuations? Do you sense rhythmic motions? Listen and note what you become aware of.

3. Stay with this exercise for fifteen minutes or so and then exchange places. Come together in small groups and in the larger class context to see what you have all discovered. Once you are familiar with this exercise, practice it in threes with two people in the practitioner position holding different body parts of a fellow student. Each person can give the others feedback. The intention is to discover what is happening for yourselves.

Sacred Space, Summary of Process

In this chapter you learned to meet your patient's system with respect and spaciousness. If you followed my suggestions, you may have realized that the whole process has a ritual quality to it. This process can be an entrée into the creation of a *sacred space*. This term has many connotations. It is, for me, about creating a space that can hold something larger than conditioned reality. It holds more than just the suffering of the person. It is about generating a space that can hold a relationship to the *Health*, which is always centering the personal suffering of a person. This relationship is a gateway to the deeper forces and intentions that center the human experience as a whole. It is about a space that invokes a relationship to something deeper than personal experience, something that may be called the divine.

These sections were meant to introduce some concepts of presence, contact, palpation, and relationship. The key to all of this is the practitioner neutral and your wide perceptual field. In this book, and in a compatible training course, you will come back to these ideas over and over again. In the next chapter we will continue with this exploration and begin perceptual exercises which will include a more defined process to help you gain entry into an awareness of the different unfoldments of the Tide.

1. James Jealous, "Healing and the Natural World," interview, *Alternative Therapies* 3, no. 1 (January 1997).

2. Ibid.

3. Ibid.

7 Palpation and the Tidal Unfoldments

In the previous chapter, we began to explore a particular kind of presence and field of awareness. You learned to access a neutral within yourself and to listen within a wide perceptual field. The next step is to explore what there is to perceive. Dr. Sutherland talked about the Breath of Life, the Tide it generates, and its manifestations within the human body. The intention of this chapter is to work with some perceptual exercises geared to open your perceptual fields to these phenomena. This will be an ongoing process of deepening awareness over many months and years. These are our first tentative steps in this direction. In an ongoing training course, these exercises may be spread over a number of seminars and returned to often as the particulars of the system are explored.

As we began to describe in earlier chapters, the Breath of Life generates various tidal rhythms, which can be perceived as an inherent *primary respiration*. Primary respiration manifests in subtle rhythmic cycles of inhalation and exhalation within the mind and body. These arise as the Breath of Life generates the energetic blueprint, or the Original matrix, of a human being. They are an expression of an intention to incarnate, and the subsequent unfoldment of our lives. As we have previously outlined, the potency of the Breath of Life is expressed as a midline phenomenon within the human bioelectric field. We called this midline the *primal mid-*line. From this midline various tidal phenomena are in turn generated within the body-mind. These unfoldments manifest via *longitudinal fluctuations*, the tidal fluctuations of potency and fluid within the human system. Longitudinal fluctuations are expressions of the midline action of potency as it expresses respiratory cycles. We will slowly begin to unfold the possibility of perceiving these various phenomena via perception and palpation.

In this chapter we will:

- *Begin to come into relationship to the Health of the system and its tidal unfoldments.*

- *Introduce and explore the concept of transmutation.*

- *Learn perceptual exercises to help access different tidal unfoldments.*

- *Learn to palpate the fluid tide from a number of vantage points.*

First we will discuss the concept of health in a biodynamic context. This is a different view of health than is common in our culture. You will then enter an open listening session in which you will simply listen for *expressions of Health* within the human system. After this perceptual exercise, you will begin to form a relationship with the different expressions of Health within the system. You will start this exploration with an open listening process. The intention will be to simply listen and to note what phenomena you perceive. You will then work with an exercise that initiates an inquiry into transmutation and the shifts in state of the Breath of Life. From here you will explore an important perceptual exercise which we will use in various ways throughout the book. This specific exercise is geared to help you gain perceptual access to the different tidal phenomena and rhythms generated by the action of the Breath of Life. These are the CRI, the mid-tide, and the Long Tide. Lastly, you will explore a specific tidal phenomenon, *the fluid tide,* and we will begin a discussion about resources and the Breath of Life. All of the work in this chapter is introductory. All of the processes are worked with in an ongoing fashion in biodynamically oriented courses. These particular perceptual skills take time to practice and explore. It may take months and years of listening before the phenomena become more obvious. I always tell students to have patience; be gentle with yourself in your work. Remember that self-judgments and self-doubt will get in the way of your learning.

Health

In learning to relate to the human system, it is important that you begin to gain an appreciation of the Health that is its essence. Dr. Jim Jealous, D.O., eloquently writes in his paper "Around the Edges,"

> The health that we speak about in osteopathy is at the core of our being and cannot be increased or decreased to a greater or lesser degree. In other words, the health in our body cannot become diseased. The health in our body is one hundred percent available 24 hours a day from conception until death, then it transpires. It does not expire.[1]

It is important to open our perceptual processes to this principle. It is extremely important to grasp this truth. Health is never lost, nor is it increased or decreased. It is a universal, a constant. Health, in this concept, is not just about an absence of symptoms or even about a sense of well-being, although that may all be a part of its free expression. It is about a universal intention making itself known. It is about a *universal* interfacing with the conditions of our lives. This interface is an expression of the *Whole,* which we are part of. The Original matrix is an expression of this Health as it unfolds its intentions to organize the human system. In a craniosacral biodynamic context, we must be able to relate to this inherent Health, not just to patterns of resistance and fixation. Indeed, our primary role is to perceive this Health no matter what clinical circumstances we are faced with. It is really challenging for us all to shift to this way of perceiving.

Dr. Sutherland relates a story in which he describes what he considered to be one of his most successful treatments. He was called out to the house of a chronically ill man. The man was in great pain and his family were all despairing. Dr. Sutherland treated the man at his bedside. He passed away in great peace with the love of his family all around him. He died in love, not despair. The treatment was a success because the dying man was able to sense something greater beyond the pain and the immediacy of his illness. As Dr. Jealous stated above, the Breath of Life transpires, it does not expire. This is a radically different paradigm of health from that which is current in our orthodox medical system.

In our culture we are conditioned to see parts and local events. In perceiving the Whole, and the Health which is its expression, we must make a perceptual shift to a wider and deeper viewpoint. This is the essential task in our clinical work. As we shall see, even within the most seemingly disoriented and chaotic patterns and pathologies, this Health is never lost and is always in potential. It is the role of the practitioner to be able to hear and facilitate its expression. Dr. Jealous continues,

> This health, this Original matrix within the human body, interfaces with every physiological, structural and psychological stress that one contacts. This interface begins as early as our encounter with our genetics and ends at death with a shift in our perceptual field. . . . Regardless of the patient's state of disease it is possible for individuals to bring their own consciousness into direct contact with this health and experience through their entire sensory field the expression of the breath of life. [2]

This is a particular understanding of health. Again, in this perceptual shift, Health is seen to be all-pervasive and eternally present. It is not a function of the physiology of the body, or of any physiological system, but is its organizing essence. Nor is it a function of time or temporal processes. Health interfaces with every experiential process we encounter from the moment of conception until the day we die. This all occurs in the eternal present. All stresses, including the unfolding of our genetics, are centered in some way by its action. In this context, it is the role of the practitioner to perceive Health and to facilitate its perception by the patient, in even the most seemingly desperate situations.

Clinical Application:
The Perception of Health

In the following exploration, you will simply listen to the system. You will hold a wide perceptual field and simply listen for expressions of Health. This awareness is of critical importance when you, as practitioner, begin to relate to patterns of distress and dis-ease. As we unfold the work in this and following chapters, we are unfolding a relationship to the different expressions of Health within the system. Here, you will begin your explorations into the manifestations of Health by simply listening for

them. Please be open to *not knowing*. Don't look for anything. Simply inquire into how Health manifests its intentions within the human system. Float the question, "How does Health manifest here?" and see what is communicated to you.

1. With the patient in the supine position, place your hands in the vault hold. This time you will use a classic vault hold in which your index fingers are touching the greater wings of the sphenoid, your middle fingers are over the zygomatic process of the temporal bone (anterior to the ears), your ring fingers are over the mastoid portions of the temporal bone (behind the ears), and your little fingers are over the squama of the occiput. (See Figure 7.1.)

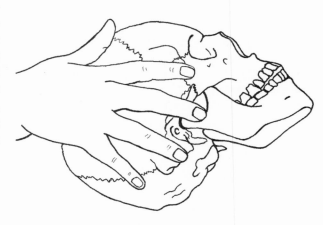

7.1 Vault hold

2. Establish your inner neutral, negotiate your contact, and extend a wide perceptual field. Gently and softly extend your field of awareness out towards the horizon to whatever distance feels safe, without spacing out or losing a sense of ground. As you do this, keep the patient within the center of that field.

3. Now simply listen and float the questions mentioned above. Do not narrow your perceptual field as you become aware of phenomena within the patient's system. Let them come to you; don't narrow your field of awareness and don't grasp what you perceive. This is a simple listening for expressions of Health. How is this communicated to you? What tells you that Health is at work? How does Health manifest here? Do not hold any expectations. Be in a state of unknowing and inquiry. Be open to any answer. Listen.

Clinical Application:
Perceiving Health—The Tidal Phenomena

Within the cranial concept, Health is an expression of the action of the Breath of Life in the human system. As we have seen, the Breath of Life generates tidal phenomena which are expressions of its intentions and ordering functions. In this section you will extend the exercise above and listen for these tidal expressions of Health in the system. You will again listen to the system with an open awareness without expectation. You can give yourself the luxury of not having to perceive any particular rhythm, pulsation, or phenomenon. You will simply be in a receptive space, actively listening to the system. In this space, you will initiate an inquiry into primary respiration. In his student days, Dr. Sutherland was sitting and musing over the structure of the temporal bone. He claimed that a thought then struck him: "Bevelled like the gills of a fish for primary respiration." As we have seen, this seemingly bizarre thought started him off on a lifetime journey. In this section we will start, or renew, our own journey.

In this palpation session I want you to establish your contact and relationship to the patient's system as previously learned. Then simply be open to any communication by the system as to how it expresses primary respiration. Can you perceive any kind of tidal phenomena? For instance, you may sense a phenomenon that seems like a welling up and receding. See if the concept of primary respiratory motion begins to clarify. What is communicated to you by the system? Do not *look* for any particular motions, rhythms, or rates. Let them come to you. If you were taught in previous courses to relate to a particular motions, rhythms or rates of expression, put these aside for now and simply be open to *anything*.

In this book, I will stress over and over again, do not look, but listen. *Looking* is very focused and intense. It may project you into the patient's system in ways that do not respect boundaries. It may not give the patient's system enough space to simply show you what is relevant to communicate. *Listening*, however, is softer and will allow a respectful relationship with the possibility of being truly responsive to the human condition. The intention to listen is through all of the senses. This includes the information you are receiving from your hands, information from all your senses, and all sensory phenomena that arise within your field of awareness. Listen with your ears, your eyes, your touch. Listening is a state of receptive yet active awareness. Listen with a gentle intention coupled with keen awareness and curiosity. Establish your neutral, create your relationship, and bring an open inquiry to the system. It will begin to speak to you and will unfold its story naturally.

1. With the patient in the supine position, gently establish a contact in the vault hold as above. Establish your practitioner fulcrums and negotiate your contact with the patient's system. Again extend a wide field of awareness with the patient at the center of that field.

2. The contact that you make should be as though your hands are floating on corks which are in turn floating on fluids. Your touch should be so light that you do not disturb the floating of the tissues within fluids. See if you can sense the underlying fluid and tidal motions that are moving the raft. Any pressure or resistance on your part will enlist the system's defensive responses. A

narrowed attention or a grasping attention will also do this. If you narrow your field of listening, you may be hearing the responses to your contact rather than the underlying tides, rhythms, and patterns of the system.

3. In this relationship, simply listen to whatever is expressed. See if you can sense any kind of tidal phenomena or primary respiration. Gently inquire into primary respiration. There is no right or wrong here. Simply listen. Relax, don't try to find anything, and listen to what comes your way. Note whatever is communicated to you. Work for fifteen minutes or so and then exchange with your partner.

In this exercise, you may have sensed subtle qualities of welling up and receding or tensile motions of tissues. You may have sensed reciprocal surges of fluid and/or potency (force) with a subsequent settling and receding. You may sense midline expressions of longitudinal fluctuations, the rising and sinking of the Breath of Life and its potency within the midlines of the body. You may also sense the rising and receding of the fluid tide, the cerebrospinal fluid fluctuation that is one of the classical aspects of the primary respiratory mechanism. You may sense a number of different rhythms and rates. You may have sensed various kinds of patterns of motion and qualities of expression. Don't worry about these right now; all of it will clarify over time.

There are a number of tidal rhythms generated by the intentions of the Breath of Life. Each has its own characteristic rate and qualities. Be open to any kind of tidal phenomenon that clarifies in your perception and palpation session. Later in this chapter, you will more directly learn to shift your perceptual fields to the various unfoldments of the Breath of Life. The next perceptual exercise continues with this concept of open listening and will focus on the awareness of transmutation, or the shifts in state of the Breath of Life. This is another exercise that you will come back to many times in your learning process.

Transmutation

In the unfolding of the human form, a process occurs which Dr. Sutherland called transmutation. *Transmutation* is a change, a shift in state. The inherent blueprint, or Original matrix[3] of a human being is expressed and maintained via transmutation. There is a transmutation or change in state as the Breath of Life generates potency. There is a transmutation of potency within the CSF and a further transmutation within all of the fluids of the body. This is, in turn, expressed in each and every cell and tissue as a living blueprint. This process allows the Original matrix to function as an ordering force within the human system. Each successive transmutation is a change in state. At each level of unfoldment, a new state emerges. Within each emerging state, all others are enfolded. As we have described earlier, the unfoldment of the Breath of Life, and the Original matrix it conveys, is a holographic process. Within each unfoldment the *Whole* is enfolded. In our work, the imperative is to listen to the Whole and to life as it unfolds.

In summary, it is via transmutation that the Breath of Life generates potency within fluids. This is a universal principle. It is the manifestation of life force within the waters of the world which allows life to manifest. Water is the universal media for the expression of creativity. Just as this occurs within the world as a whole, it occurs within the fluid systems of the human body. There is a transmutation of potency within the fluids of the body. Potency is the biodynamic ordering force within the mind-body system. This is initially expressed as a precise bioelectric ordering field, as the Original matrix is laid down within the system. This matrix manifests the forces around which fluids, cells, and tissues organize. This is naturally precise. Every cell is aligned to this. Dr. Randolph Stone, D.O., used to say, "Man cognises, God geometises." The expression of the bioelectric blueprint is a precise process that is never wrong. Its proportions are always precise. When a practitioner gains awareness of the transmutation process, he or she begins to understand the organization and healing principles of the human system. This is no small thing. It heralds a critical shift in the perceptual abilities of the practitioner.

Stillness To Form

Stillness–Motion–Force–Fluid and Form

In Ayurveda, the traditional form of medicine in India, they talk about the process of consciousness coming into form as a process of transmutation. In this process, "pristine consciousness" undergoes transformations in order to become embodied and expressed through form. In simple terms, without going into the traditional terms and cosmology, the process can be described as follows:

From Stillness arises motion,
from motion arises force,
from force arises cohesion and from cohesion,
form is organized and integration
is maintained.

In this simple framework, *stillness* is the ground from which all else arises. *Motion* emerges from it as an intention to become something. In our circumstances we may consider it to be an intention to incarnate as a human being. This then manifests as *force*, a drive to become, around which the natural world organizes to complete this intention. This is expressed as *cohesion*, a fluidic function that conveys the "intention to become" into form. *Form is then organized around the Original intention to become.* (See Figure 7.2.)

In Ayurveda this is commonly discussed in terms of the elements, the traditional way of describing the inherent forces at work in the world: ether—air—fire—water—earth. Ether is the stillness at the heart of all physical manifestation. It manifests as space. It holds all potential forms and processes within it. Air is the first transmutation, or change in state from stillness towards form. It is motion, literally the motion of the intention to become something. Fire is the force or drive that is generated from this in-

tention. Water conveys the quality of cohesion and integration that is maintained by these forces. Finally, earth is the expression of form that organizes around the Original intention, which moves the whole process. It can be thought of, and perceived as, deepening condensations, from stillness and motion to the seeming solidity of form.

Here we have a simple conceptual structure for the perception of some of the basic transmutations generated by the Breath of Life. Stillness is the deep intrinsic ground from which all of manifestation arises. It is the ground of potential from which the Breath of Life emerges. Stillness is inherent within our existence. Within it resides all potential for manifestation. It is both dynamic and alive. From Stillness arises motion, in our terms, the intentions of the Breath of Life. The Breath of Life expresses its intentions as motion. In the Daoist system of thought this is called the "primal intention." This primal intention generates polarities, yin and yang, which are polarized forces that allow intention to take form. In our incarnation, it is the intention to create a human being. It is a manifestation of the divine in action and is an expression of the intention to incarnate, to become.

The Breath of Life expresses its intentions from this ground of stillness as a great wind. The Long Tide can be perceived like a great wind of life. It seems to come from "somewhere else" and, via centripetal, vortex-like forces, generates the Original matrix, the bioelectric ground of the human system. The Chinese call this the Tai Ji, or the great breath. The Tibetans call it the *wind of the vital forces*. This great breath generates the bioelectric field, which allows precise forms to be organized. This maintains the order of the form, or substance, of the body-mind complex. This motion carries with it the blueprint or Original matrix of a human being. From this motion emerges force. Force in our terms is the potency of the Breath of Life. It is expressed within the fluids as a palpable and biodynamically alive force. Cohesion, or the fluidic nature, is the next unfoldment. It is about the power of fluids to maintain form and cohesion. It is about the maintenance of

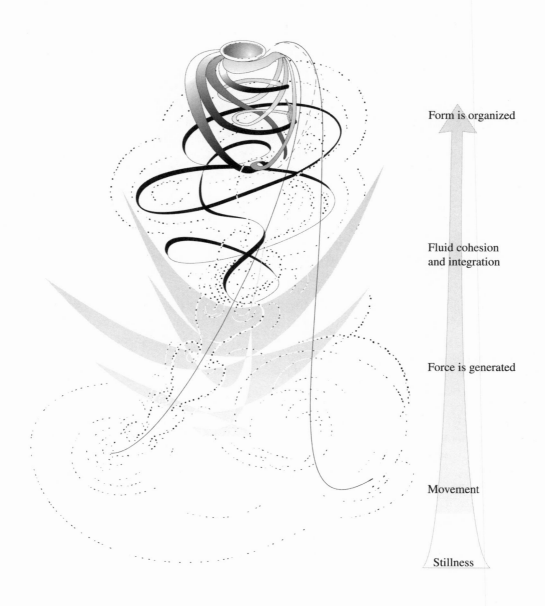

Form is organized

Fluid cohesion
and integration

Force is generated

Movement

Stillness

7.2 Transmutation

integrity. It maintains the expression of the whole within every part. Finally there is form. Form organizes around the Original matrix carried by the potency within the fluids of the body. Form, the cells and tissues of our body, are all moved and organized by this interplay. This interplay is an expression of the Whole within the particular. There are forces at work within the metabolic fields of the system and these forces organize and maintain the structure-function of the human body. Let's work with a simple perceptual exercise, which you will come back to many times within the framework of a training course.

Clinical Applications:
The Perception of Transmutation

Let's set up a palpation exercise to see if transmutation begins to have an experiential meaning for you.[4] This is an exercise that you will come back to many times. It is a perceptual process that will deepen as your experience deepens. If you understand transmutation, then you will understand the unfoldment of life in this human form and will have a perceptual access to its healing processes.

1. Again establish your inner neutral and wide perceptual field. Negotiate your contact with the patient's system. Hold the patient's system in the vault hold as established above. Again allow your hands to simply float and be moved. Listen; do not look.

2. Now bring the idea of transmutation into your awareness. Use the simple structure of *Stillness —motion—force—fluid and form (cells and tissues)* to inform your inquiry. Start from as still a place within yourself as possible. Remember our former exercise in generating a neutral. See if you can have a mind that is neither coming nor going, and listen within a wide perceptual field. See what information comes into this field. If all of these shifts in state are too much to hold

at the beginning, work more simply with an awareness of *Stillness—motion—force*.

3. Sense the Stillness. Sense the motion arising from it. Sense the force generated. Sense the fluids responding. Sense the tissues responding. See what rhythms and tides begin to speak to you. See if you sense the *transitions* between expressions of rhythms and tides. Simply be open to whatever information comes your way. What is important here? Do not worry about perceiving anything in this context. Let in whatever information comes.

4. Repeat this at the sacrum. Hold the sacrum from the side of the table. Place your chair near the patient's feet facing the opposite shoulder. Place your hand under the sacrum, fingers pointing cephalad. Do not bend your wrist too much. Place your elbow under/near the patient's knee. From here listen to the unfolding of *Stillness—motion—force—fluids and form.* (See Figure 7.3 and 7.7.)

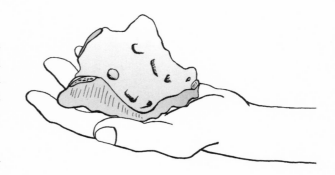

7.3 Sacral hold

The process of transmutation is a factor of the tidal unfoldments of the Breath of Life. As the intentions of the Breath of Life unfold via transmutation, the various tidal unfoldments are generated. In the next sections, we will again look at these unfoldments and work with a perceptual exercise that will help you begin to consciously gain access to them.

Synchronizing Perceptual Fields within the Tidal System

One of the most important skills within the cranial concept is the ability to consciously synchronize your perceptual field to the different tidal expressions of the Breath of Life. The human system is holographic—it is not linear. All of the unfoldments of the Breath of Life are expressions of the subtle physiological states of the human system. All tidal phenomena are expressions of the respiratory cycles generated by the Breath of Life. Each of the tides, or unfoldments, is enfolded in the others. It is possible for you, as practitioner, to shift your perceptual field in order to consciously perceive each of these tidal unfoldments. The deeper rhythms generated by the Breath of Life can become explicate and obvious to the still and perceptive observer. As mentioned above, all of these unfoldments have clinical significance and attunement to their expression is part of the palpation skills that the practitioner must learn. As the practitioner opens to the different tidal rhythms within the human system, different types and qualities of clinical skill come into play. Dr. James Jealous, D.O., writes:

> Our perceptual fields vary at different moments. However, it is possible to synchronise one's attention with the different expressions of health within the body. That is to synchronise one's attention with the movement of the cranial rhythmic impulse in the 8 to 14 range per minute. It is possible to synchronize one's perception with a rhythmic impulse that precedes at two and a half cycles per minute. It is also possible to synchronise one's perceptual field with a longer tidal movement that occurs six times in ten minutes

[about one cycle every 100 seconds—Ed.]. The shifting of the perceptual field to allow one to explore these different kinds of motion is a skill that all palpatory studies should address, otherwise only accidental contact with these "other" rhythms is possible. Accidental contact does not allow the physician therapeutic and diagnostic access to these other physiological states.[5]

You can think of these three rhythms as tides within tides. Each is an unfoldment of the implicate into the explicate, and each is implicit within the unfoldment of the others. Depending on the quality and nature of your perception, you can become aware of each of them. As you become aware of one unfoldment, the others tend to become more peripheral. It is a matter of sinking into deeper stillness and of holding a wider field of perception. As Dr. Jealous stresses, it is important to develop the skill to shift your perceptual fields in order to gain intelligent clinical information. Each unfoldment of the Breath of Life yields a different perceptual and clinical experience. Different kinds of perceptual phenomena arise within each unfoldment and different clinical skills are appropriate to each. Unless you become clear about the different qualities of each unfoldment, confusions can arise, both perceptually and clinically.

A number of years ago I was invited to teach a few seminars in an ongoing training. I came into the last seminar and asked the students how their skills were coming along. As I went around the classroom, I saw that some students were in tears. One student shared that she thought she was a fraud because she couldn't sense the tissue motions of flexion and extension. I asked her what she *could* perceive, and she explained that she sensed the tissues moving as one thing, that she sensed a surging and settling within the tissue field and that, rather than sensing places, or fulcrums of resistance, she perceived sites of condensation. I then asked her how her clinical skills were, given her experience. She answered that she worked through stillness, a settling of the whole system around that site of condensation, and then things happened. Well, I said, you're not a fraud, you are simply sensing through the mid-tide level of perception. That's wonderful! At that level, flexion and extension of structures are not sensed as independent phenomena: tissues are perceived as a unified tensile field, which expresses a unified tensile motion. I later helped her to upshift to the CRI level, and she felt greatly relieved. Clarity as to the perceptual possibilities within each tidal level is essential for a depth of clinical practice. This concept is an important thread of the work in this book and a keystone of a craniosacral biodynamic approach to work in this field.

Clinical Application:
Shifting Perceptual Fields

Let me introduce a perceptual exercise that will become the foundation for many future clinical explorations. We will return to it over and over again. In this process, you will use different modes of intention and a widening perceptual field to help gain access to the different tidal unfoldments. You will be establishing different fields of awareness in order to synchronize with the different tidal unfoldments. We will work within the three basic levels of the CRI, the mid-tide and the Long Tide. The CRI tends to express itself anywhere from 8 to 14 cycles a minute. The mid-tide expresses itself at a more stable 2.5 cycles a minute, and the Long Tide generates a 100-second respiratory cycle (50-second inhalation and 50-second exhalation). Refer back to Chapter Five for a more detailed discussion of each layer of unfoldment. Later, we will explore access to the Dynamic Stillness.

1. With the patient in the supine position, place your hands in the vault hold as described above. Access your inner neutral, negotiate your contact, and let your hands float on the tissues as though they are corks on the water. Do not place any pressure or force on the tissues.

Simply float and let yourself be moved by the tissues and fluids being palpated.

2. In the first perceptual process, you will shift, or synchronize, your attention to the *CRI level of perception*. To do this, maintain the image of your hands floating on the tissues like corks on the water. Narrow your perceptual field to tissues, bones, and membranes. Negotiate your contact and get interested in how these tissues are moving. Let your hands float on the tissues and let them show you their motions. Listen, don't look for anything, and don't expect anything. Let it come to you. See if the faster rhythm, the CRI, comes into your field of awareness. Stay with this for a number of minutes until you are clear about its expression. We will clarify the motions perceived within this rate of expression in later chapters.

3. Now shift your intentions to the *mid-tide level of perception*. To do this, you will shift your imagery and widen your perceptual field. In the CRI level of perception, your hands were floating on the tissues; in this shift, let your hands also float within fluids. Imagine/sense that your hands are floating in a wider field of fluid as they palpate the tissues. Your hands are immersed within this fluid field.

4. Now widen your perceptual field to hold the whole of the person and the field around him or her. Dr. Rollin Becker, D.O., called this the *biosphere*. The biosphere is a useful concept. It denotes the whole of the person, the body, and the field of potency and environmental exchange around the body. In this process, you widen your field of awareness from the individual tissues and structures palpated above to include the whole of the person and the wider field of potency around the person's body. Within this field you are sensing the fluids and tissues of the body *as a whole*.

5   As you do this, allow your mind to settle and be relatively still. Your quality of awareness is wide and soft, yet you also maintain a keen precision within your listening. You are now holding the *whole* of the person within your field of attention. You may sense a deepening and slowing of the rhythmic unfoldment. See if the slower rhythm of the mid-tide, 2.5 cycles a minute, begins to unfold its presence. Stay with this for a number of minutes.

6. Now shift your perceptual field to the Long Tide. To do this, you will again shift your intentions and widen your perceptual field. Above you imagined/sensed that your hands were immersed within fluid. Now see if you can imagine/sense that your hands are immersed within potency. Imagine a field of potency within which the patient is centered and within which your hands are immersed. It is like being within a subtle yet palpable bioelectric field.

7. With this sense, slowly widen your perceptual field towards the horizon. Move out towards the horizon while holding the patient within the center of your field of attention. Do not extend your awareness beyond what feels safe and contained for now. Simply let your mind hold a wider sense of the whole. Let your mind still, and see if you have the sense that your intention to move towards the horizon is at balance with the sensory information returning. It may seem as if your mind is literally being breathed by the Breath of Life in total balance. The patient is in the center of this widened field of perception.

8. See if the deeper, slower Long Tide unfolds within your perceptual field. It may seem as if the potency of the Breath of Life is radiating everywhere and permeates everything. It may also seem as if you are immersed within the ocean and the tidal forces are moving through you. Simply listen within this wider field. You may be surprised at the nature of communication within this widened field of attention. You may even have the experience of a vibrant field, or a bioelectric matrix, as you listen to the per-

Summary of Access to Perceptual Levels

CRI		
	•	HANDS float on tissues like corks on water.
8–14 Cycles a Minute	•	PERCEPTUAL FIELD narrows to tissue, bone, membrane.
	•	MIND is interested in individual structures and relationships of structures/parts.

Mid-tide		
	•	HANDS are immersed/float within fluid.
2.5 cycles a minute	•	PERCEPTUAL FIELD widens to hold the whole of the person and his or her biosphere. (The biosphere is the body and the field of potency and environmental exchange around it.)
	•	MIND is relatively quiet, holds a wider field, and is in relationship to the whole of the person.

Long Tide		
	•	HANDS are immersed/float within potency.
100–second cycles	•	PERCEPTUAL FIELD widens to the horizon.
	•	MIND is expansive and still: breathes with the Breath of Life.

son's system within this wide perceptual field. Stay with this awareness for a number of minutes, then gently and slowly shift your perceptual field back to the biosphere and the mid-tide level of perception. After anchoring your perceptual field within the mid-tide, slowly negotiate a disengagement of your physical contact.

Throughout this book you will repeat this process many times as you explore the different clinical intentions of the work. Once a practitioner has skill in this process, it occurs much more organically. It becomes possible to simply hold a wide perceptual field and to listen for the different tidal rhythms as they are expressed within the system. The exercise outlined above gives an entrée into the skills of synchronizing attention with these unfoldments. This perceptual practice is an ongoing learning process. A summary of this process is outlined above.

Listening to the Tidal Unfoldments

Do not worry if these rhythms were not clear to you in this first exercise. This will be an ongoing process. This exercise is commonly used throughout a training course over many seminars. It becomes a way to clearly invite students to work with different skills within different perceptual levels. Here we will summarize some of the salient features of each tidal unfoldment. See Chapter Five for a fuller description of the tidal unfoldments generated by the action of the Breath of Life. These concepts will be greatly expanded in later chapters. The most important thing to recognize is that you must listen and find out what is relevant and true for yourself. It is only by direct perceptual experience that any of this makes any clinical sense at all.

CRI Level

As you listen to one unfoldment, the whole system may be perceived to express it. For instance, if you are listening through the CRI, you will sense the faster, more discrete motions of structures and fluids. These are expressed at a rhythm of 8 to 14 cycles a minute. The CRI is a variable rhythm whose expression is influenced by past history, trauma, pathology, toxins, and genetics. These express the experience of the person, or the personal, rather than the universal. The state of the autonomic nervous system and of the neuroendocrine immune system also directly influences the CRI via trauma affects, hyper- and hypo-arousal states, and neuroendocrine set points.

The CRI will give information about the results and affects of experience and trauma within the system. You have a relationship to the results of suffering as they manifest within the person's system. This must be appreciated and acknowledged. It is also important to recognize that the inherent healing forces are at work within the deeper tides, and perceptual access to these deeper phenomena is essential for efficient clinical practice. Working through the CRI may touch off various trauma affects being centered within the system. These trauma affects are the result of overwhelming experiences. For instance, as you are tracking CRI level motion, shock and emotional affects may be activated and flood the system and dissociative states may arise. We will discuss these issues in more detail in later chapters. If trauma affects arise within a session, it is important to have the clinical skills to help moderate and process them.

Mid-Tide Level

As you shift to the mid-tide level of perception, you are shifting to an awareness of forces at work. This is the level of the transmutation of potency within the fluids of the body. If you are listening through the mid-tide, a 2.5 cycles a minute rhythm begins to clarify. As you listen through this unfoldment, the whole system may be perceived to express it. Fluids and tissues will be perceived to be a unitary experience in which this deeper rhythm is perceived. It will seem as if the system is moving within tidal potencies as a whole unified field of action. Here potency can be more directly perceived within the fluids, and tissue motility will be sensed to be a unified tensile field of action. Individual tissue structures and motions are still discernible, but their motions are more easily perceived to be part of the whole. Hence, tissues are sensed to be a true unit of function that expresses a unified dynamic. Within this unfoldment you have a direct perceptual entrée into the three functions of potency, fluids, and tissues. The action of potency, fluids, and tissues can be sensed to be a unified dynamic whose actions and motions are perceived to be a factor of the transmutation of potency within fluids. Thus the practitioner may have the experience of sensing the interplay of potency, fluids, and tissues as one functional reality.

Within the mid-tide level of perception, inertial potencies will also become clearer within your field of perception. As you will later discover, potency will become inertial in order to center and compensate for any unresolved issues within the system. We will discuss this in great detail in later chapters. At this level of perception, you can perceive and relate more directly to the inertial forces that organize and maintain tissue and fluid affects within the system. It is thus possible to sense the forces at work, not just the resultant fluid and tissue changes. It is much more clinically effective to relate to the forces at work, rather than to the affects or results of these forces.

Long Tide Level

As you widen your perceptual field, you may sense an even deeper, wider, and slower phenomenon, which seems to permeate everything. This is the Long Tide. The Breath of Life generates the Long Tide as the organizing "wind" of the human system. It is an expression of our unity with all of creation. The formation of the human organizing field, which is basically a bioelectric or biomagnetic field, is a local phenomenon within a huge field of action. The Long Tide may be sensed like a great wind that generates this organizing field. It may seem to pass through the body and through your hands. It is almost like the gathering of the winds of a tornado as

its organizing vortex is formed and a field is generated around it. As these winds gather in centripetal action, the bioelectric matrix of a human being is formed. You may sense this Original matrix as a perceptual reality. These are epigenetic, bioelectric potencies, which are with us from the day of conception until the day we die. In this Long Tide, you may perceive yourself to be surrounded by "tidal waters." It may seem as if you are sitting in the ocean and are even part of that ocean. Healing is perceived as the *shimmering* of potency within the bioelectric matrix as inertial issues are encountered. The practitioner's role is one of keen awareness and reflection as the Breath of Life is truly seen to be doing the healing work. Healing is perceived via resonance and reconnection. At this level of perception, one may sense the potency of Breath of Life moving into the midline and interfacing with sites of inertia and condensation. Healing is seen to be a factor of reconnection and realignment to the Original intention of life itself.

Dynamic Stillness

I haven't discussed the Dynamic Stillness in any detail so far. However, if you are resting in the Dynamic Stillness, self and other fade away and unity is directly experienced. Tidal rhythms are not obvious, but the unified nature of all phenomena is. The whole biosphere of life becomes more available within a still and open field of awareness. This can be a truly unitary experience; it is our nature to be whole. The practitioner's mind stills, settles, deepens, and expands, letting go of self-view. The practitioner's state of mind is unified, still, and expanded. There is no self, no self-constructs, no subject-object relationships, only Unity consciousness. It is, in essence, a unified field of compassion. The emotional qualities are nonpersonal and expansive. Equanimity and compassion are expressed as an illimitable and unified natural state of grace. There is great joy here, yet it is not a personal joy, it simply is. It is not personal, but is a universal. At this level of perception there is *perception without a perceiver*.

There are no tides, only an alive, Dynamic Stillness. Here vibrancy predominates and organization is perceived to be an expression of the intention of the divine. Entering the Dynamic Stillness is like entering a mysterious gateway. If you look for it, you won't find it, but if you settle into stillness and drop your self-view, it mysteriously presents itself. At this level of clinical work healing may be instantaneous. If healing does not occur, a much deeper perception of the nature of life can be experienced. A great peace arises. This has vast repercussions for intractable diseases and dying processes. The Dynamic Stillness is, in itself, a gateway into deeper spiritual realms. It is the realm of the implicate nature of subtle form. Within its vibrant field it holds the potential for all possible expressions of form and its organization. An awareness of the Dynamic Stillness and of the Long Tide allows one to appreciate that all individual forms, such as the human body, are an expression of discrete energetic phenomena within a huge field of action.

Attunement

In essence, you will perceive the unfoldment that you are attuned to. It is thus essential, as practitioner, to be able to attune to the different expressions of Health within the system. It's like tuning a radio to different frequencies or carrier waves. This attunement of your perceptual field is a *holographic* shift to another unfoldment of the Breath of Life. Remember that in a holography, all the information is enfolded throughout the hologram, and every part contains all the information of the whole and all of its possible unfoldments. Thus, as you shift your relationship to the hologram, the *whole* holo-

---

Summary of the Basic Tides of the Primary Respiratory Impulse

The Groundswell Expressed as the:

- Cranial Rhythmic Impulse

    CRI generated as the potency of the Breath of Life meets the genetics, experiences, and history of the person. The waves on the Tide; the interference pattern of the hologram. Information perceived via analysis and diagnosis.

    8–14 cycles/minute

- Mid-Tide

    Expression of the potency as a biodynamic force within the fluid system. Potency, fluids, and tissues perceived to be unified tensile fields. Information perceived directly through the whole.

    2.5 cycles/minute

- Long Tide

    Deeper expression of the potency of the Breath of Life per se, or the "such-ness" of its potency within the system. The Tide. The organizing "winds" of the human system. Information received through resonance.

    One cycle every 100 seconds

---

gram expresses the information of the new relationship. As in a hologram, the whole system expresses the tide of the unfoldment that you are attuned to. This process of attunement is a function of consciousness.

As discussed earlier, in David Bohm's concept, consciousness is enfolded in all phenomena. Depending on your state of consciousness, on where you are looking from or through, that is what will unfold and that is what you will perceive. The rate of rhythm that you will experience as a practitioner depends on what you are open to, the needs and capacity of the system, the level that you are tuning into, and the relationship you have with your patient. We are looking at a nonlinear system in which consciousness is seeing itself through itself, and rhythms are enfolded within rhythms. It is like a symphony made up of many notes, octaves and chords that all resonate to express the unified vibration of life. What you perceive within this symphony all depends on where you are looking from and what you are attuned to. This process of attunement to the different expressions of the Breath of Life must be addressed, at least in an introductory manner, within foundation courses in craniosacral biodynamics. It is my experience that this is possible to do, and greatly enhances the student's ability to be clinically effective.

The Fundamental Principle and the Fluid Tide

In the above sections, we introduced a perceptual exercise that may help you learn to synchronize your perceptual field to the different rhythms and tidal phenomena associated with the action of the Breath of Life. In this section, we will work to encourage an awareness of a particular tidal expression, the fluid tide. The *fluid tide* is the tidal expression of cerebrospinal fluid within the 2.5 cycles a minute mid-tide. Within the mid-tide there are three functions. They are (1) the potency of the Breath of Life, (2) the fluids, and (3) the tissues. The

potency is the organizing principle, fluids are the media of exchange, and tissues organize their form and motion around its action. In this sense, the fluids within the body are truly an expression of the waters of life. Within the natural world it is water that conveys the most primary and formative forces of life.

The three functions within the mid-tide

- *potency* is the organizing and driving force,
- *fluids* are the media of exchange, and
- *cells and tissues* organize their form and motion around the action of potency as conveyed to them via the fluid systems of the body.

The *fluid tide* is a term that describes the motion of the fluid function within the mid-tide. It is an expression of the action of potency within the fluids as it organizes and moves the cerebrospinal fluid fluctuation. Think of the potency as an invisible force that organizes and moves the fluids. Dr. Sutherland continually stressed this perceptual truth in his teachings and writings. Awareness of the fluid tide gives you direct information as to the quality and manifestation of the resources of the system. Dr. Sutherland considered the fluctuation of cerebrospinal fluid to be the most fundamental and essential principle within the cranial concept. Again, in this concept, it is seen that there is a transmutation of the Breath of Life into potency within the cerebrospinal fluid. Cerebrospinal fluid becomes potentised with this Breath of Life factor and acts to disseminate it throughout the body. Potency is an expression of the Breath of Life as a biodynamically active organizing force within the human system. It is perceived to be a fundamental and essential ordering principle active throughout the body-mind.

Potency is an expression of Intelligence itself. It manifests within the cerebrospinal fluid, yet its function is not diluted. Within the fluids of the system, the Breath of Life generates an organizing force, which is an expression of the intentions of life itself.

As potency is expressed within the fluid systems of the body, motion is generated. This motion is called the fluid tide. (See Figure 7.4.)

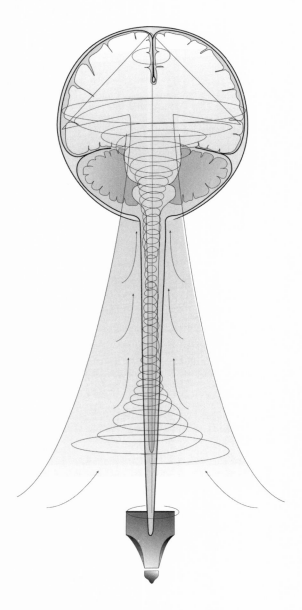

7.4 Potency: The organizing force within the system

The Generation of the Fluid Tide

Potency of the Breath of Life
is expressed as a most basic bioelectric matrix.

Cerebrospinal fluid
becomes imbued with potency
via transmutation or a change in state.

Cells and tissues
are organized around its imperative.

The Breath of Life generates potency, a biodynamically active force within the system. This potency is received by the CSF and is conveyed by it, and by all of the body's fluids, to every cell and tissue. Organization is a function of the potency of the Breath of Life and its transmutations within the human system. It expresses the Originality in form.

Longitudinal Fluctuation

When we talk about fluid fluctuation and the fluid tide, we are talking about a tidal pulsation, not a linear circulation. The natural motion of the fluid tide, driven by this primary breath, is called its *longitudinal fluctuation*. Longitudinal fluctuation occurs throughout the fluid system as a whole. It is perhaps clearest within the cerebrospinal fluid, as it is the initial recipient of the potency of the Breath of Life. The fluctuation of cerebrospinal fluid has also called the *cerebrospinal fluid tide,* or more simply, the *fluid tide*. The fluid tide naturally fluctuates in longitudinal tidal cycles. The longitudinal fluctuation of CSF is expressed along the dorsal, or neural, axis of the body. As this occurs, there are also *transverse fluctuations* of potency and fluids, most easily discernible within the ventricles of the brain. (See Figure 7.5.)

Thus, the dynamic of the fluid tide is expressed as longitudinal and transverse fluctuations along the axis of the neural tube. As the fluid tide rises, it rises along the longitudinal axis of the central nervous system and is also expressed transversely across its ventricles. In the sections below, you may palpate a longitudinal rising in the dorsal midline (e.g., the neural axis), and a transverse widening across the lateral ventricles, in the inhalation phase of the fluid tide. In the exhalation phase, the fluid tide recedes and is sensed to settle caudad.

There are expressions of longitudinal fluctuations within each tidal unfoldment.

- At the *CRI level* of rhythm, CSF can be sensed to fluctuate along the longitudinal axis of the body at a relatively fast rate of 8–14 cycles a minute.

- At the *mid-tide level*, longitudinal fluctuation is sensed as a more direct relationship between potency and fluid at the 2.5 cycles a minute rate within the dorsal or neural axis.

- At the *Long Tide level*, longitudinal fluctuation is sensed to be a direct expression of the potency of the Breath of Life as an uprising force within the ventral, or primal midline of the system. It can be sensed to be the "fountain spray of life."[6]

Dr. Sutherland perceived that cerebrospinal fluid is the initial physiological recipient of the Breath of Life. He likened it to an invisible force active within the fluids of the body.[7] He stated that it is this potency that generates and drives the motion of the fluid tide. The fluid tide, like all unfoldments of the Breath of Life, is an expression of the Health of the system. All tidal phenomena are expressions of the intentions of the Breath of Life. The cerebrospinal fluid is imbued, or becomes potentised,

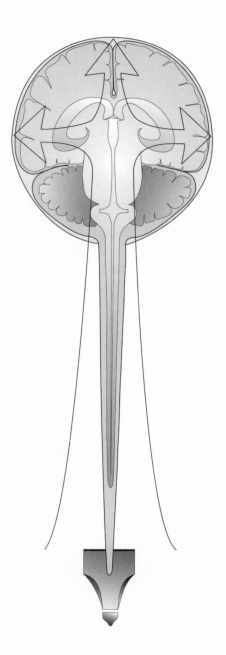

7.5 The longitudinal and transverse fluctuation of cerebrospinal fluid

with the potency of the Breath of Life. CSF conveys this ordering principle to every cell of the body. It is the potency of the Breath of Life that moves the fluids and creates the fluid tide.

Clinical Highlight: The Fluid Tide

Although there is longitudinal fluctuation within each tidal unfoldment, in this book, when I use the term "fluid tide." I am referring to the expression of fluid fluctuation within the tidal rhythm of 2.5 cycles per minute. It is within this particular unfoldment that the quality and availability of potency is most easily sensed. Listening through this unfoldment gives you a direct perception of the tidal potencies driving the fluid system. It allows you to perceive the patient's inherent resources and to sense how these can manifest within the system. Over time, after palpating many patients' systems, you will be able to establish clear baselines as to the availability of potency for the healing work undertaken. The building and liberation of potency is an integral part of work within the cranial concept. We will introduce these ideas more fully in later chapters.

Perceiving the Fluid Tide

The *fluid tide* and the *potency* that generates it are all expressions of Health. In the following sections, you will open to the possibility that you can directly perceive and palpate the longitudinal and transverse fluctuations of the fluid tide. You may have already had some perceptual experience of this from the exercises above. Remember that the potency of the Breath of Life is the driving force within the fluid tide. This is a direct expression of Health within the body-mind. This Health is never lost and always in potential. When palpating its expression within

the human system, you are perceiving an inherent biodynamic force, the ordering principle of human form. Let's see if we can begin to sense this dynamic. In the following section you will begin to palpate the Health within the system as it is expressed within its fluids. The intention in the following sections is to gain some experience in perceiving the vitality and potency of the system via the interchange between fluids and potency. This is an important first step in perceiving the Health of the system. To do this, you will see if you can begin to appreciate the nature, motion, and quality of the fluid tide as a sense of rhythmic force and tidal motion.

In the following, you will focus on sensitizing yourself to the quality of the potency and drive of the fluid tide. This *drive* is an expression of the healing resources of the system and is a manifestation of an inherent bioenergy, or biodynamic force, the potency of the Breath of Life itself. In this book, I am taking a biodynamic and biokinetic approach to work in the cranial field. This follows the languaging of Dr. Rollin Becker, D.O. The biodynamic force of the body is the potency of the Breath of Life expressed as a physiological ordering principle within its fluids and cells. This is maintained by the presence of potency within the fluid systems of the body. Let's see if you can begin to appreciate this groundswell via a perception of fluid fluctuation. You may even begin to get a sense of the potency of the Breath of Life, which drives the fluid tide and generates its motion.

Palpating the Fluid Tide

In the following exploration, you will use the cranium and sacrum as your vantage points. You will see if you can perceive the welling up and receding of the fluid tide as potency and fluid drive. If, in cranial courses, you have previously learned to specifically palpate craniosacral tissue motion as the *cranial rhythm*, please let this go for now. Start with a beginner's mind.[8] Simply listen. As you listen to the patient's system, wait for a perception of tide-like force and fluid fluctuation. This may be sensed as a welling up and receding of potency or force. It is like going under the waves and appreciating the welling up of the underlying force of the Tide within the ocean waters.

After having established a practitioner neutral and negotiated your contact, you will use the vault hold, the occipital hold, and the sacral hold as listening posts to sense the fluid tide. These will be used to encourage your palpation skills from different vantage points and to help you begin to relate to the fluid tide and the forces within it. The intention here will be to see if you can palpate the force or drive within the cerebrospinal fluid.

Clinical Applications: Perceiving the Fluid Tide

I. Palpation via the Vault Hold

1. To begin with, you will use the vault hold as your listening post. In this hold, you will be holding the patient's cranium in a specific way. Place your index fingers at the greater wings of the sphenoid, in the hollows just posterior to the corners of the eyes. Place your middle fingers in front of the temporal bones over the zygomatic processes. Place your ring fingers over the mastoid portions of the temporal bones posterior to the patient's ears. Place your little fingers over or as close as possible to the squama of the occiput. Let the palms of your hands and your thumbs rest comfortably and lightly on the parietals and superior aspect of their head. Do this in as fluid a manner as possible so that you are placing your fingers over these areas more or less simultaneously. (See Figure 7.1.)

2. Remember our previous discussions on palpation. It is important to allow your hands to float on the structures of the cranium and not to grab onto the motions and pulsations that you may be sensing. It is as if you are floating on a cork that is in turn floating on and being moved by

tidal water. If you place any pressure on the tissues whatsoever, you interfere with their natural motions as they are moved by this tide.

3. Establish your practitioner neutral. Now you will synchronize your perceptual field with the mid-tide level of perception. Imagine/sense that your hands are immersed within fluids. Let your hands float within fluids, yet do not lose contact with the tissues you are palpating. Now extend your perceptual field to include the whole biosphere as practiced above. Remember that the biosphere includes the whole body and the field of action around it. Hold the person's body and the field of potency and environmental exchange within your field of awareness. You are now holding the whole of the person within your perceptual field.

4. From this vantage point, see if you can perceive a sense of welling up and receding of a tide-like force under your hands. Keep your sense of distance and space and see if you can allow this awareness to come into your hands. It is important not to look for anything. Simply be present with a wide perceptual field and a gentle quality of palpation. Do not worry about rates or rhythms, but let the communications come to you. Don't seek or look for anything; simply listen with a side field of perception and genuine curiosity. Allow your hands to float within the fluid and notice how they are moved.

5. You may perceive a sense of force or power under your hands, which has a tidal, rhythmic nature to it. It is a very subtle sense of motion underneath your hands, like riding on a little boat that is being moved by the ocean tide. Look under the surface to the force that moves it. You may sense a subtle yet powerful welling up and receding of fluid and force under your hands. It has a tidal quality to its arising and receding. Let it take you. Do not interfere with it or try to grasp it in any way.

At some time, you may begin to differentiate the two phases of primary respiration, its inhalation and exhalation phases, as a welling up and settling. You may sense a rising and sinking of the cerebrospinal fluid in a tide-like manner. This is its longitudinal fluctuation and is considered to be the natural motion of the fluid system as it expresses the groundswell of the Breath of Life. You may also begin to sense simultaneously, in the inhalation phase, a transverse tide. As potency rises longitudinally in inhalation, you may sense a widening across the lateral ventricles. In exhalation, this transverse tide ebbs as it follows the general settling of potency and fluids. Basically, in inhalation the fluid tide rises and in exhalation it recedes and settles. You may sense the inhalation phase of the fluid tide the clearest. This is the cycle in which potency surges within the system. The inhalation phase of the fluid tide is generated by a cephalad surge of potency, while its exhalation phase is a settling after this surge. Thus primary respiration at this level of perception can be sensed to be expressed in rhythmic cycles of surge and settling.

Sensing the Fluid Tide

II. Palpation via the Occipital Cradle Hold

1. Once you have a sense of this dynamic, change your hand position to an *occipital cradle hold*. Be sure that you maintain or reestablish your practitioner fulcrums. In this hold, place your hands under the patient's head with your little fingers touching, fingers spread and pointing caudad. The fingers of your hands should be comfortably cradling the patient's head. Do not create any pressure against the person's occiput with the heels of your hands. (See Figure 7.6.)

2. In this position again see if you can sense the arising and receding of the fluid tide as described above. You may sense a force against

your palpating hands. You may sense the occiput expressing motion along with this force. Just simply notice the sense of a welling up and receding under your hands. You may sense a strong arising of fluids and a sense of receding. Again, listen with a gentle and wide perceptual field. Try to hold the *whole* of the person in that field and do not look for anything. Let yourself be moved.

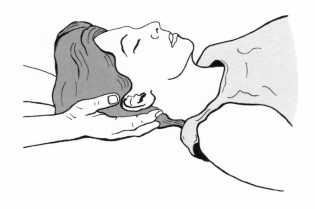

7.6 Occipital cradle hold

Sensing the Fluid Tide

III. Palpation via the Sacral Hold

1. Once you have perceived the fluid tide from the occiput, change position and move to a *sacral hold*. Remember to negotiate your contact. First tell the person what you are intending to do and how your hand will be placed. The pelvis can be a very vulnerable area, and you must be clear in your intentions and in your communication with the patient.

2. In this hold, you will be sitting at the side of the patient. Place your chair towards the foot/cau-

dad end of the table pointing diagonally to the opposite shoulder of the patient. Then ask the patient to lift the pelvis off the table. Place your hand under the sacrum with your fingers pointing cephalad and your hand and wrist more or less lined up with your arm. Your elbow should be under or near the knee. This is a very comfortable and nonconfrontational way of holding the sacrum. Be sure that your hand is comfortably placed under the sacrum and that the person's body is not tilted to one side or the other. Be sure that the heel of your hand is not creating pressure against the sacrum. Spread your fingers apart under the sacrum, but don't create tension in your hand. Reestablish your practitioner fulcrums. Sometimes this can be a very vulnerable area and you may have to give the patient a lot of space by projecting or imagining that your hand is under the table as it

holds the sacrum. You still want to have the feeling that you are floating on the tissues of the sacrum, within fluid, even though there is the weight of the patient on your hand. (See Figure 7.7.)

3. From this vantage point, again see if you can sense the arising and receding of the fluid tide as you float on the structure of the sacrum. You may sense this in inhalation as a filling up or welling up of potency and fluid under your palpating hand, and in exhalation as an emptying or receding. See if you can sense the force within this. In inhalation, you may sense a strong force arising and in exhalation, a sense of emptying as this force recedes. In the inhalation and exhalation phases, this is expressed by cerebrospinal fluid as the rising and sinking of the fluid tide.

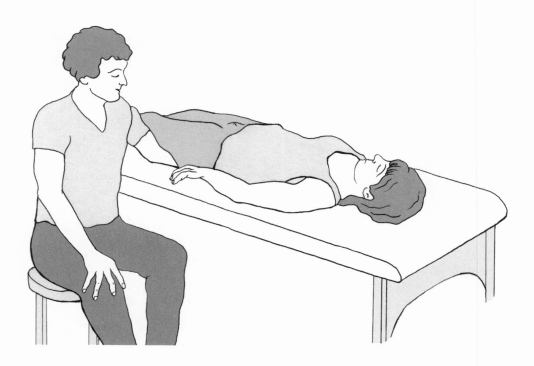

7.7 Sacral hold

Sensing the Fluid Tide

IV. Palpation via Sacrum and Occiput

1. Have the patient move to a side lying position. You may want to place a small cushion under the patient's head and place his or her knees in a comfortable position. Find a comfortable sitting position at the side of the table facing the person's back. First place one hand, with your fingers pointing caudad, over the sacrum. Once you negotiate and establish that contact, place your other hand over the occiput with your fingers pointing cephalad. In this position, you are in relationship to two poles of the classical primary respiratory mechanism. (See Figure 7.8.)

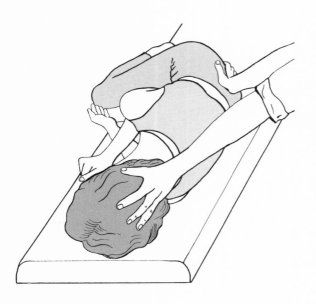

7.8 Sacrum and occiput hold,
side lying

2. Again, let your contact float on the tissues and within fluids. Establish your wide perceptual field to include the whole of the biosphere. See if you can sense a welling up under each hand in inhalation and an emptying or receding in exhalation. See if you can sense the rising and sinking of the fluid tide in each phase and the force within it. Simply listen to the relationships and dynamics of the system from these vantage points. Float within the fluids and let motion and an awareness of force come to you. Again, don't look for anything, just listen and allow. This process of deeply listening to the system at these two poles at once can be very integrative and can be useful at the end of session work.

Clinical Highlight

The quality of a patient's constitutional resources can be sensed by the skilled practitioner. This may be perceived as the driving force within the patient's fluids called *fluid drive*. The quality of fluid drive is related to the ability of the system to express its inherent potency as force or usable energy. It is the potency of the Breath of Life, which drives the fluid tide. The ability of the system to maintain a highly potent fluid system and to express that potency as drive is crucial to discern. If the system cannot express its potency, or does not express it well, then the practitioner knows that the patient may not have the resources to skillfully process inertial patterns. Clinical work may then concern the resources of the system. These must be liberated and their expression encouraged. We will introduce these ideas in more detail in the next chapter.

Clinical Application: Sensing the Fluid Tide in the Body as a Whole

In this final section, you will extend this investigation from the core of the primary respiratory system into the body as a whole. You will extend your listening posts to other relationships. You will see if you can perceive the inhalation and exhalation phases of primary respiration in the body as a whole. In the section below, you will be listening from the shoulders, diaphragm, pelvis, and feet. In the inhalation phase, the fluid tide ascends. You may also perceive that the body generally widens side to side, narrows front to back, and shortens along its long axis. These other motions relate to tissue motility and will be described in detail later. Simply put, as the groundswell of the Breath of Life is expressed, fluids and tissues respond. In the exhalation phase, the fluid tide descends. The body may also be sensed to generally narrow side to side, widen front to back, and lengthen in the exhalation phase. We will describe the specific dynamics of tissue motion and motility in later chapters.

1. You will next monitor the fluid tide from the patient's shoulders, diaphragm, pelvis, and feet. Place your hands comfortably over these areas on either side of the body. Start at the shoulders and work in a caudad direction. Again, establish your neutral at each listening post and hold a wide perceptual field as you allow your hands to float within fluids as they, in turn, float on the tissues. Again synchronize your perceptual field with the mid-tide.

2. Wait at each listening post until you gain a sense of welling up and receding under your hands. Here we are focusing on the sense of drive or force, rather than on tissue motion. When you arrive at the patient's pelvis, place your hands over the iliac crests. You are allowing your hands to float on these areas of the body and are waiting to sense the nature of the body's expression of primary respiration. Again, you are waiting to sense a quality of force that is welling up and receding under your hands.

3. As you sense this in the various body locations, move through the relationships and listen until

you have some sense of this dynamic. For now, it is important that you have a sense of the fluid fluctuation throughout the body and the biodynamic potency that moves it.

Summary

In this chapter, you began your process of learning to palpate the Health within the system. You started with a very general, open listening without too much information. You then worked with different perceptual exercises. These were geared to introduce you to an awareness of transmutation, to the various tidal unfoldments, and to the fluid tide, a particular expression of Health. As we unfold concept and clinical experiences within the context of this book, we will build on this perceptual experience. It is again important to remember that you are learning to be in direct relationship, through your palpation, to the health and vitality of the system. This simple reflection of Health, through the quality of your touch and presence, is one of the foundations of the healing process in the cranial concept. In the next chapter, we will introduce concepts of resources and the stillpoint process.

1. James Jealous, "Around the Edges," quoted with permission of author.

2. Ibid.

3. Original matrix is a term coined by Dr. Jim Jealous, D.O. Originality is a concept also developed by Dr. Erich Blechschmidt, one of the great embryologists of the twentieth century. He convincingly postulated that early development is not a function of the action of genes, but of forces at work. These forces express the Originality, the intentions of life, within the context of embryological development. Genes are responsive and interactive with this imperative. They are not proactive.

4. This approach to developing an awareness of transmutation was first developed and described to me by Dr. Martin Hunt, M.D.,

formerly one of the course tutors at the Karuna Institute.

5. Jim Jealous, "Around the Edges," quoted with permission of author.

6. "Fountain spray of life" is a term coined by Dr. Randolph Stone, D.O., to denote the qual-ity of the midline expression of the Breath of Life within the notochord, or primal midline.

7. W. G. Sutherland, *Teachings in the Science of Osteopathy* (Rudra Press).

8. For a fuller discussion of "beginners mind," see Suzuki Roshi, *Zen Mind, Beginner's Mind*.

8   Resources, Stillness, and Stillpoints

This chapter introduces the concept of resources. Resources include the constitutional, psychological, and emotional assets of a person and his or her system. After a general discussion on resources, we will use a few exercises to help students begin an inquiry into their own resources. After this, we will spend time discussing and working with resources within the cranial context. We have already seen how the potency of the Breath of Life is the most fundamental resource within the human body-mind. We will discover that stillness is the key to accessing and liberating this most basic ground. Within this context, the role of stillness in the development of constitutional resources will be stressed. To introduce this, we will explore a process known as *stillpoint*, a term used when the various rhythms generated by the Breath of Life become still. For the practitioner, the role of stillness is essential to understand. Dr. Sutherland stressed that it is within the *stillness* of the Tide that its power resides.[1] In this context we will also talk a bit more about the Dynamic Stillness, the stillness at the heart of the human condition.

In this chapter we will:

- *Introduce the concept of resources.*
- *Introduce the concept of stillpoints and stillness in the system.*
- *Learn to facilitate stillpoints via intention.*

Resources

When you practice in the cranial field, you will constantly be confronted with the effects and affects of trauma and suffering. Traumatization has physiological roots, which can be powerfully addressed in this work. A somatic understanding of trauma is essential in this context. The work of Dr. Peter Levine is especially useful in the promotion of a clinical awareness of trauma and its affects within the human system.[2] We will look at some of his concepts within a cranial context in a later chapter. In his work, Dr. Levine stresses the importance of *resources,* an extremely important concept to grasp in clinical practice. Resources are the spiritual, psychoemotional, and physical/constitutional aspects of a person's makeup that support and nurture their being in the world. Resources are strengths that a person can draw upon when in threatening or dangerous circumstances, whether these are internal, such as pathogens or toxicity, or external, such as accidents, abuse, or emotional shock. Within the cranial context, the most fundamental resource is the potency of the Breath of Life and its expressions within the human system.

Resources can be appreciated and cultivated in many ways. Resources can be both external and internal. They may be about how people create their home environment, or the friends they have and the associates they share experiences with. They may be about their inner life, how they deal with fear or other feeling tones. They may be about how their thinking processes work. They may revolve around their spiritual life and their inner journey. Almost anything can be a resource. For instance, it may be important to notice how a person protects herself. For example, if a person automatically and habitually reacts to stress by withdrawing or running away, this behavior can be experienced more consciously and used as a skillful option in circumstances that may feel overwhelming. What was a habitual reaction can become a conscious choice and a resource. If a person reacts to stress by dissociating, once she learns what it feels like to be in the body and to connect to its sensations, then even dissociation can be a conscious option and a resource.

The quality of inner sensation that a person is experiencing can also be a resource for him. If a person is only aware of uncomfortable sensations, then he can be more easily overwhelmed by arising shock affects. The concept of space is interrelated to this. If a person is aware only of uncomfortable sensations, then there may not be any space in his system to allow shock affects to process in a nonoverwhelming way. The perception of space generally relates to sensations that are perceived as spacious, warm, open, or calming. Spacious, resourced sensations can allow a person to approach the edges of difficult or frightening sensations without being overwhelmed.

Resources allow a person to meet the experiences of life in ways that are appropriate and skillful. Resources can be anything that gives strength and ground to the ability to move through life in ways that are fulfilling and satisfying. Helping people recognize how they already resource themselves can be very empowering. For instance, noticing simple things, like the favorite clothes they wear or a particular piece of jewelry, can be therapeutic. Likewise, helping a person acknowledge her resources in friends and activities, and a reminder to use them, can be helpful. Bringing a person's attention to these kinds of things, *and to the sensations that are associated with them*, can help her get in touch with inner resources. The usefulness of this kind of inner awareness can be clearly seen within the therapeutic situation. If a patient experiences the arising of a trauma affect during a session, like emotional flooding, a perceptual shift to more resourced sensations can help contain and slow down the process. This can have extremely valuable clinical outcomes. We will discuss this in more detail in a later chapter.

Within the cranial context, the most basic resource of life is the Breath of Life and its expressions within the human system. The potency of the Breath of Life centers the conditions of our lives. It is a universal resource. The same potency within me is within you. The same Original matrix is at work. It is the role of the cranial practitioner to help the patient's system reconnect with and liberate this essential ordering principle. Within the cranial concept, we work with the interrelationship of the experiential or conditional forces of life and the inherent biodynamic forces of the system, which maintain its integrity and balance. The inquiry into resources is thus part of a wider exploration into the nature of life itself. Next we will look at some simple exercises that help to encourage an awareness of resources.

Appreciating Your Resources

In the following sections we will introduce an exercise that may help you appreciate some of your resources. In this process, we will look both at external resources such as environment and friends and at inner resources such as sensations and images. Once appreciated, these can be remembered and elicited within the clinical setting when appropriate. Let's first set up a simple exercise. Holding a pad of paper and a pen, sit in a comfortable position. On one page write the heading "external resources" and on a second page, write "internal resources."

On the first page list all of the external resources you can think of. These may include objects in your home like pictures, images or sculptures, your home itself, or spaces you like to be in. Resources may include places you like to go. These may be places of natural beauty, parks, buildings, even coffee houses—whatever creates a resourced space for you. External resources may also include activities you do, such as listening to music, sports, exercise, meditation, relaxation processes, and so forth. They certainly include the people in your life, family, friends, associates, therapists. It is the "people, places, and things" of your life that resource you.

On the second page, list all of the inner resources that you can think of. These may include meditative processes, awareness processes, qualities and states of mind, qualities of sensation, how you perceive yourself, your self-view, your strengths, what has helped you through difficult periods, and so on. If you are aware of your defensive strategies, note how these have been resources in the past. These might include what arises when you meet stress, how you mobilize yourself to meet stressful situations, how you deal with your angry boss, how you protect yourself from pain, and so on.

Start the inquiry by letting yourself become as still as possible. Take a deep breath: slow down. Begin with "external resources." Simply let your mind flow with the question, "What resources me in my life? What people, places, and things resource me?" Take time with this and you may be surprised what flows out. Then shift your inquiry to inner resources, bringing attention to the sensations and images within your body-mind, float the question, "What tells me I'm okay?" See what arises. Again you may be surprised at the answers. You might also float the question, "How am I protected? How do I protect myself?" Your body-mind may have some interesting things to share with you about this. After you spend some time with this inquiry, meet in small groups to share what you discovered.

As you work with these ideas, you will notice how your external and internal resources are a continuum of process. They are not really separate. The exercise above is simply a beginning, a way to begin to appreciate how we "do ourselves" and the resources we have developed in life. Resources unfold as session work unfolds. They go very deep. These

include our most basic resource, the Breath of Life and its action within the human system. Because of this, we can trust the system and its resources; it is simply a matter of accessing them.

Resourced Sensations

In this section we will explore the quality of our inner sensations more directly. In this process, the intention will be to access *resourced sensations*, sensations and feeling tones that tell us we are okay. Again, this has therapeutic value. It is not uncommon for people to access shock affects during a session. When a patient experiences shock affects within the system, such as emotional flooding, this can be very upsetting and sometimes terrifying. The ability to slow down and access some sensations that are more resourced can help contain and process the arising affects.

Let's look at a simple exercise that usually helps access resourced and spacious sensations. In this process you will work with both imagery and sensation. The first step is to sit in a comfortable position and to practice this internally on your own. The next step will be to practice this on the session table in pairs. Get comfortable and take a deep breath. The first thing to do is to find your way into a relationship to the sensations within your body. To do this, you might first become aware of your breathing. Follow your breath into your body, as we did in a previous exercise, and then notice the sensations you encounter. Use the breath to anchor your awareness within the sensations of the body, and then simply notice the arising sensations. Take a few minutes to simply become aware of your inner sensations.

Once you have a relationship to your inner sensations, imagine within your mind's eye a person, place, activity, or thing that you really like that really resources you. If it is a person, choose a person who truly represents a resource to you. You may find that your relationships hold a lot of ambiguity, and it may be better to use a place, an activity, or an object the first time you try this exercise. Bring the image of this resource into your mind's eye. Then notice the quality of sensation that arises within your body. What is the *felt sense* of this resource? Where in the body do you sense it? Describe it. Are the sensations/feeling tones familiar? Once you sense the resourced sensations and have described them, try to remember them. You can later use the image to access these sensations within the clinical context. This is not as artificial as it sounds. All that is happening is that you are accessing sensations that you already know. The intention is to make them readily available. It is just a matter of becoming skillful in sensing and allowing them. At times of overwhelming sensation, this can be a godsend.

In the rest of this chapter, we will introduce one of the most important concepts within the cranial concept, that of stillness. You will discover that stillness is the most fundamental resource of the system as the Breath of Life may be directly perceived within the stillness of the Tide. Indeed, as you mature in the work, you will discover that all intentions of the Breath of Life arise from what is known as the Dynamic Stillness, the basic ground of our life process. This may sound esoteric, but it can be a direct perceptual experience if one is willing to be still and know.

Dynamic Stillness

As we have discussed in earlier chapters, a Dynamic Stillness is at the heart of the arising of life. In all of the great spiritual traditions, stillness is the ground of emergence of all of life's functions. The spiritual traditions focus on the importance of stillness as a perceptual experience. In the Christian monasteries of the Middle Ages, inner stillness, a darkness of knowing, was an essential step towards unity with God. An appreciation of stillness has always been considered essential in spiritual journeys, even in our own Western traditions. Stillness deepens beyond the conceptual mind and its conditioned state to the roots of our human condition. This understanding has always been a keystone of the Buddhist tradition. In the Zen text, Chinul's

"Straightforward Explanation of the True Mind," Chinul (1158–1210) writes,

> . . . the basic substance (essence) of the true mind transcends causality and pervades time. It is neither profane nor sacred; it has no oppositions. Like space itself, it is omnipresent; its subtle substance is stable and utterly peaceful; beyond all conceptual elaboration. It is unoriginated, imperishable, neither existent nor non-existent. It is unmoving, unstirring profoundly still and eternal. . . . Neither coming nor going, it pervades all time, neither inside nor outside, it permeates all space . . . all activities at all times are manifestations of the subtle function of true mind.[3]

This is the best description of the Dynamic Stillness that I have ever encountered. It speaks to the roots of my condition. In the Zen teaching *true mind* is the heart of awareness itself. It is our basic ground of existence, our Originality. It is the essence of a human being. It is profoundly still, yet all function arises from it. It permeates all space, and all activities and forms are manifestations of its subtle function and action. Within the cranial concept an understanding of this ground of emergence, the Dynamic Stillness, has become part of some practitioners' experience. This brings us to the essence of things, the basic essence of true mind. The Dynamic Stillness can be thought of as the ground from which this essence emerges and acts within the world of form. The Dynamic Stillness is this ground of emergence, an implicate realm of potential from which the creative winds of the Breath of Life arise. The Breath of Life is a subtle manifestation of true mind within the active expression of life and conveys its inherent Intelligence. The Breath of Life unfolds from a profound Stillness and its power is found in this Stillness. Stillness is profoundly healing. It liberates the potency of the Breath of Life in its ordering and healing function. Within the cranial concept, the clinical practice of *accessing a state of balance* reflects this truth. It is about a dynamic equilibrium, a dynamic stillness, in which the forces at work can be expressed in ways beyond the patterns and compensations held. It leads to deeper sources, deeper origins. It is when there is no "coming or going" within the mind of the practitioner that this process can be discerned. This truth is with us from the moment of conception to the moment of death. Indeed, even at the time of death Stillness is profoundly healing. It brings us to what the Tibetans call the "clear light," our essential nature. It helps align our consciousness to the mystery of our existence and to the unfolding of life itself.

Stillpoints

As we have seen, tidal rhythms are expressed in reciprocal phases of motility and motion. There are times when this reciprocal expression of the Breath of Life becomes still. This stillness is commonly called stillpoint. The term *stillpoint* denotes a period of stillness in which tidal phenomena become still. During stillpoint, the potency of the Breath of Life becomes more accessible. It may be liberated beyond the conditions being centered within the system. In this stillness, a deeper connection to the potency of the Breath of Life can be experienced. The fluids of the body have the opportunity to potentize with what Dr. Rollin Becker sometimes called the *Breath of Life factor*. This Breath of Life factor, or potency, is the inherent resource of the system. As we have seen, cerebrospinal fluid is considered to be its initial recipient and it is conveyed by all fluids generally. It is the motive power that moves the fluids and generates the fluid tide. The potency of the Breath of Life lays down the Original matrix as a neutral within the system around which the fluid, cellular, and tissue world organizes.

Potency functions as an inherent ordering principle for all anatomical and physiological processes. Its biodynamic interplay within the human system maintains integrity and balance.[4] Deepening into stillpoint is a major way, at a primary respiratory level, for the system to access this inherent resource. Stillness liberates potency. In stillness there is revitalization. Stillness is about reconnecting to and ex-

pressing our most inherent resources. During stillpoint, the cerebrospinal fluid, and the fluids within the system generally, will potentize with the Breath of Life factor. A sense of greater drive within the fluids may then be perceived. Within the stillpoint, potency that has become inertial due to disturbances in the system may be expressed beyond the conditions being centered, and healing work will be done. During stillpoint, potency can become more available as a biodynamically active force for physiological functioning.

Stillpoint is a natural process and the system will express stillpoints spontaneously. A stillpoint may last anywhere from a second to many minutes. The system will stay in stillpoint as long as it needs to, or as long as it can, given its state of congestion or depletion. In a depleted, congested, or traumatized system, the body may not be able to access its resources or to enter stillness easily. This is especially true in cases of shock traumatization and dissociation. Traumatization, congestion, and resistance in the system can set up a vicious cycle in which the system desperately needs to access stillness to revitalize itself, yet cannot due to the very trauma that it is being centered and compensated for in some way. Within the cranial context, the practitioner can facilitate the expressions of stillness. This can have very deep clinical consequences. As you go along in this book, you will be made aware of the interplay among trauma, resistance, stillness, and healing resources.

The Experience of Stillness

As you become familiar with the stillpoint process, you will notice that stillpoints can have different qualities and different depths. Essentially, you will learn that stillness has depth and, as the system sinks into deeper depths of stillness, different potentialities become accessible. As the system goes into stillpoint, it will tend to enter stillness at the depth that is possible for it at that time and at the depth that is needed for healing purposes. You will thus notice that the system can express different depths of stillness and that these depths have different qualities. Stillness can be thought of as being enfolded within all unfoldments of the Breath of Life. Indeed, Stillness is the ground of all manifestation. The Dynamic Stillness lies at the heart of the groundswell of the Breath of Life itself and is inherent within all phenomena. It is even said that the Dynamic Stillness is the fulcrum for the Breath of Life. When the practitioner's mind becomes profoundly still, deep, and wide, an awareness of a Dynamic Stillness becomes a true possibility.

In the following section we are going to talk about the *relative* experience of stillness. Stillness, at its essence, cannot be talked about in terms of depths or levels. Stillness is nonlinear and Whole. Stillness is Stillness. It is the ground of all unity. We can, however, talk about our relative experience of the system as it deepens into stillness. However, when we are truly within the Dynamic Stillness, words fail. Here we will use words that speak to the relative experience of depth and leave it at that. Within this context, some traditional cranial practitioners talk about "seven depths of stillness." This is an attempt to describe an experience of the unfolding of stillness within the human system. There are clear differences in the *tones* of stillness experienced within the system and the schema of seven depths attempts to describe these unfolding qualities and tones as a perceptual process. Each depth has a certain tone and *range* of quality within it. For instance, there might seem to be a very superficial physical quality to a stillpoint, but this can shift into a deeper quality or depth of stillness within the physical. Thus there is a range of unfoldment in every level of experience. When we are talking about depths of stillness, we are not talking about the Dynamic Stillness. The Dynamic Stillness permeates all form and organization; it is inherent. Here we are talking about our relative experience of the function of Stillness as it unfolds its healing intentions.

These depths may seem esoteric and unscientific, but they do seem to accord with perceptual experience. There is more to human nature than the physical self, and this schema attempts to acknowledge

this via the direct perceptual experience of both practitioner and patient. We must remember that as we encounter the Breath of Life within the human system, we are encountering the intentions of a universal Intelligence within the interplay of consciousness and form. This interplay has depth. At the roots of our being-ness, concepts of energy and matter break down. Movement resolves into stillness, and stillness is found to be at the heart of all form.

> ## The Seven Depths of Stillness
>
> - *the physical level*
> - *the emotional level*
> - *the mental or psychological level*
> - *the heart or urge level, or level of karmic tendencies*
> - *the mind level, or level of archetypal mind*
> - *the spirit or soul level, or the level of being-ness*
> - *the Source, or the level of unity, emptiness, or God*

The Seven Depths of Stillness

The first three depths of stillness directly relate to the general dynamics of the autonomic nervous system, the limbic system, and the cerebral cortex:

1. The *physical level* can be thought of as the first depth of the experience of stillness. There may be a sense of a deep stillness throughout the body. Physical resistance may resolve as inertial fulcrums are processed and you may perceive pulsations of potency, lateral fluctuations of fluid, and reorganization of tissues. The *autonomic nervous system* and brain stem may discharge autonomic traumatization and shock affects. The practitioner may perceive this as subtle tremblings in the tissues and as perturbations within cerebrospinal fluid.

2. The *emotional level* may be perceived as a stillness of emotional tone and of the emotional charge that may be held in the system. A deep sense of emotional well-being may arise here. Conversely, the *limbic system* may discharge traumatic emotional affects during this level of stillness, and patients may sense the release of emotional energies during treatment sessions. The outward expression of emotional process is not the object here. It is ideally a gentle and subtle processing of the energies that arise. The resolution of emotional energies may be experienced as streamings of energy.

    It has become common to encourage patients to experience an *emotional release*. The assumption is that this is inherently healing. It is, however, important to point out that the expression of strong emotional trauma affects may not be healing at all. It may even be re-traumatizing. Within this context, it is important that you understand how to therapeutically relate to shock traumatization in the human system. We will introduce a basic understanding of this in a later chapter.

3. The *mental* or *psychological level* is stillness at the level of psychological patterning, the developmental and psychodynamic layer of the conditioned self. In this layer of stillness, the conditioned mental sets of the *cerebral cortex* may open and shift. Insights into one's historical and reactive self may arise and a deep letting go of the automatic reactions of developmental trauma may be possible.

    The next levels really begin to take us deeper into the unconscious and unknown reaches of the human psyche:

4. At the *urge* or *heart level* the deeper tendencies of our personality system may enter stillness. This is the layer of karmic tendencies, the conditioned urges and instinctual imperatives of our psyche. It is the conditioned push-pull of the system. It is the level of the "it" of Sigmund Freud, usually translated into English as the "id." This is a level of deep, unconscious conditioning, the basic instinctual energies of the human system, and the complex karmic tendencies of the person. At this level of stillness past-life memories may arise, and generational tendencies, sometimes called miasmas, may be stilled and processed. Karmic tendencies may be resolved. Life issues revolving around the unconscious may begin to become more conscious and the potential for insight, clarity, and resolution may come to the fore.

5. At the *mind level* there is a depth of stillness possible that resonates with the archetypal underpinnings of our reality. It is the level of Big Mind. It is a level of transpersonal possibilities and experiences. Archetypal energies and images may emerge. At this level of stillness the potential of greater interconnectiveness and a more holistic experience of life unfolds. The mutuality and inter-being of human life process can be experienced and appreciated. A deep sense of compassion for the human condition will arise. An understanding of the mutuality of suffering and a concurrent arising of great joy may be experienced. Along with this, a deep experience of universal connection, love, and inner warmth may arise.

6. At the *spirit level* such a deep sense of stillness and peace may arise that the sense of a personal self, is lost and issues of separation and duality melt into unity and openness. The inherent openness and spaciousness of the human condition is deeply experienced and appreciated. A basic sense of the openness of life and an abiding in a nondualistic experience of unity and spaciousness may arise here. An experience of what is sometimes called cosmic consciousness may arise where boundaries and divisions are ended and a deep sense of unity is realized.

7. Finally, at the level of *Source* there is depth that is beyond descriptive terms and has to do with the inherent truths that the great spiritual traditions point to. Here is the potential for the appreciation of what has been called Godrealization, satori, nirvana, Dao, and so on. It is the realization of the basic emptiness and openness at the heart of all unfoldments. It is about the Still heart of creativity itself. It is an emptiness that is complete and has all possibility enfolded within it. Time is meaningless as past, present, and future are mutually enfolded.

This may be a lot to take in at this point of our exploration, but it is important to note that the human system has deep spiritual roots and that any depth process of healing always, in its own way, must acknowledge and refer back to these roots.

In all of this, it is the Breath of Life, in its groundswell of expression, that is unfolding from a depth of stillness, and all that is really needed is to deeply appreciate this. In every unfoldment there is the groundswell and in every layer of its depth, there is the Dynamic Stillness that permeates everything.

Consequences of Stillpoints

Let's talk about the nitty-gritty physiological outcomes of the stillpoint process. Stillpoints facilitate physiological healing processes. During stillpoint the system has the opportunity to access its potency and vitality. Within stillness the fluid potency of the system is amplified and its fluid drive is enhanced. The potency, the fluid within the fluid, is expressed with greater clarity. In essence, there is a potentization within the system and more resources become available.

On a physiological level, during stillpoint fluid exchange is encouraged. Enhanced fluid exchange helps the body eliminate anything that it needs to. For instance, toxins may be discharged and eliminated. During stillpoint, there is also a general tendency to take care of unfinished business. As we

shall see in later chapters, potency will become inertial in order to center and compensate for unsolved issues within the system. As inertial potencies are activated within stillpoint, the system will attempt to process patterns and pathologies currently being centered in some way. Pathologies that previously could only be held in compensation may be processed due to the increase in the availability of potency that occurs during stillpoint. Thus, as the potency of the system amplifies generally, potencies within inertial fulcrums may initiate healing processes.[5] Old injuries may complete their healing cycle. Cysts, abscesses, boils, and anything that the system could not previously process may be processed and healed.

Transmutation, Potentization, and Fluid Drive

Within stillpoint, there is a potentization, or potentiation, of the fluid system with the potency of the Breath of Life. This is a function of transmutation. We have discussed transmutation in the previous chapter. Dr. Sutherland stressed that there is a transmutation of potency within the fluids of the body. During stillpoint transmutation is intensified. As a consequence, the healing resources of the system, its inherent healing potency, is also intensified. This can be experienced as an increased vitality throughout the system. During stillpoints the healing resources of the system are augmented and the drive and vitality of the system increases.

One of the first things you might become aware of when palpating a patient's system is the quality and strength of the person's fluid tide. The potency of the Breath of Life is the driving force of this unfoldment. Potency manifests within the cerebrospinal fluid and creates the cerebrospinal fluid tide. The inherent fluctuation of cerebrospinal fluid is thus driven by the groundswell of the Breath of Life expressed as potency within its fluids. The amplitude and power of the longitudinal fluctuation of the fluid tide is an expression of this potency. The term *fluid drive* is generally used to denote the local phenomenon of fluids "driving" within states of balance as healing potencies are expressed. As you may have already experienced, the fluid drive may kick in when the state of balanced tension has been attained. The state of balance is like a mysterious gateway through which something can pass. That something is the potency of the Breath of Life, which is expressed as a driving force within the fluid system. It is the potency that generates fluid fluctuation and conveys the ordering action of potency to all cells and tissues in the body.

The term *fluid drive* is also sometimes used to denote the overall quality of the drive, or strength and clarity of the fluid tide. Fluid drive can thus denote the overall quality or strength of potency that is expressed within the fluid system. This being said, it must be remembered that the fluid drive is an expression of a deeper phenomenon, the groundswell of the Tide, which is, in turn, generated by the intentions of the Breath of Life. If the fluid system can fully express the potency within it, then its fluid drive will seem to be strong and full. If, however, there is much inertia in the system, potency will be bound up in centering it, and the power of fluid drive may seem less intense. At the heart of inertial fulcrums are the biodynamic forces of the Breath of Life centering the inertial forces of trauma and disease processes. If the system is holding many inertial fulcrums and patterns, there can be a large amount of potency bound up in centering the disturbances and maintaining compensations. This can be very debilitating and exhaustion may eventually result. If, however, the potency within the system can be generally enhanced, then these inertial potencies, centering and maintaining the disturbances in the system, may be liberated.

Thus within stillpoint, the potency of the system is augmented and inertial potencies, which are centering various disturbances, can be initiated to express something else beyond the compensation held. The healing forces of the body intensify in their action, inertial forces resolve, and the system can reorient to its natural fulcrums. Tuning into to the strength of the fluid tide can give you, as practitioner, a baseline from which to sense the patient's system and to sense changes before, during, and after session work. It must be remembered that the fluid tide is not the Tide per se.[6] It is a longitudinal fluctuant motion generated by the action of the potency of the Breath of Life as it transmutes within the fluids. It is a useful starting point to sense how the system can express these deeper resources.

Facilitation of Stillpoints

Although stillpoint is a natural process, it is possible as practitioner to encourage its expression and to thus influence the vitality and potency of the patient's system. In facilitating a stillpoint, you will be encouraging something that the patient's system would naturally express on its own, if his potency was not bound up in compensating for resistance and past trauma. In the following sections you will be introduced to the possibility of facilitating stillpoint via potency and fluids. This is a concept that may be new to some readers. Most students are initially taught to facilitate stillpoints via the tissues. I find that if students first learn this process via potency and fluids, a deeper appreciation of its subtlety and potential will occur. When you later learn to facilitate stillpoints via tissues, you will retain this subtlety in your work. We will revisit stillpoints in a later chapter and then learn more traditional approaches called CV4 and EV4.

The concept is very simple. Tune into the patient's system and become aware of the fluid tide. As you do this, you will notice how it expresses the potency within it. You will try to hear the quality of the potency within the fluids. You may sense this as a force or drive within the fluids. You will listen to this for a number of cycles. You will especially become aware of its *exhalation* phase. This will be the phase in which you will initially learn to encourage stillpoint. You will first learn to facilitate stillpoint in the exhalation phase to get used to the responses of the system in this phase. Stillpoints facilitated in either the exhalation or inhalation phases have different biodynamics. I would like you to first focus on the exhalation phase to get used to its dynamics before later exploring stillpoints in the inhalation phase.

Facilitation of Stillness via the Fluid Tide

In stillpoint, the various tidal phenomena will become still. Stillness allows a potentization within the fluids to occur. Other life processes, such as the beating of the heart and breathing, are still occurring. They may indeed be influenced by the stillpoint and may change in their expression as the system expresses stillpoint. In the section below, you will be encouraging stillpoints via the fluid tide as you follow its welling up and receding. Learning to facilitate stillpoint via the fluids will sensitize you to the subtlety of the process. In a later chapter, you will also learn to facilitate stillpoints by following via tissue motion. This is the first time in this book that you are moving to an active intention, and it is important to acknowledge this. Let's begin to explore this important process.

Clinical Applications: Facilitating Stillpoints via the Fluid Tide

In the practical work outlined in this section, you will first sense the fluid tide from the cranium as you did earlier. After sensing the quality of the longitudinal fluctuation of fluid and its drive, notice the receding of the tide footward in its *exhalation* phase. You will then follow the fluid tide to its furthermost exhalation excursion. It is the place where you sense a boundary to the excursion of the fluid tide in that direction. Your intention will then be to encourage the system to wait or idle at this edge. Holding that intention to wait, as a subtle *intention* in your hands,

will be like asking a question: Do you want to enter stillness just now? It is a negotiation, not a demand.

You will be placing a very subtle intention of compression into the fluids at the boundary of its excursion. You will not, however, be making a demand on the system. Rather than making the system enter stillness, you will be starting a conversation with it. "Can you enter into stillness here? Can you access your resources here?" You will not be holding the system at the boundary of its excursion, nor will you be creating any barrier to its expression as commonly taught. You will simply be initiating a conversation with the fluids about the possibility of stillness and potentization.

Within that intention, you may sense certain dynamics, which will be explained below, telling you, as practitioner, that the system is expressing a stillpoint. You may also sense the therapeutic processes that are initiated. This is an important point. In this process, I will ask you to hold the biosphere of the person within your field of awareness. You will be accessing the mid-tide level of perception (the 2.5 cycles a minute tide). As you do this, you must also be actively and keenly listening. Clinical work is based on your perceptual ability to discern the nuances of what is happening.

Stillpoint Facilitation via the Occipital Cradle

1. With the patient in the supine position, place your hands in the vault hold. Allow your perceptual field to synchronize with the mid-tide. Establish your practitioner neutral and negotiate contact. Extend your perceptual field to include the whole of the biosphere, the person's body and the energy field around him or her.

Widen your perceptual field to include the biosphere and hold the intention to listen. As you do this, your mind will tend to become still. The mid-tide of 2.5 cycles a minute will start to make itself known.

2. Listen to the fluids within the mid-tide. The fluid tide will start to clarify. Sense the welling up and receding of the fluid tide under your hands. Try to get a sense of the strength or potency of its expression. This will give you a baseline to come back to at the end of the stillpoint process. You will then be able to compare the quality of the fluid tide and its longitudinal fluctuation before and after the stillpoint process.

3. Next, change your hand position. Gently cup the patient's occiput in your hands. Your hands should be comfortably under the patient's occiput, gently touching at the little fingers, or slightly apart. The patient's head should be resting on the palms of your hands and your fingers should be pointing inferior. Be sure that the heels of your hands are not pressing against the occiput. (See Figure 8.1.) This hold is sometimes

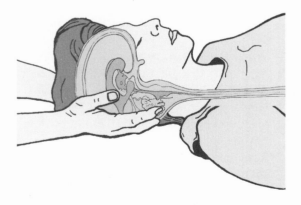

8.1 Occipital cradle holding the occiput
as an entry point into the fluid system

called the *occipital cradle*. In this position, reestablish your neutral and wide perceptual field. Then negotiate your distance in relationship to the patient's system. Give the person's system plenty of space to express its dynamics. Imagine that your hands are sinking under the table as you give the patient's system space.

4. Tune into the fluid tide from this vantage point. Sense the arising and receding of the fluid tide under your hands. In the inhalation phase you may sense an arising of the tide, a welling up under your hands. You may also sense a widening of the cranium transversely and a widening of the occiput. In the exhalation phase, you may sense a sinking and receding of the tide, a transverse narrowing of the cranium, and a narrowing of the occiput. Notice that the drive of the fluid tide occurs in the inhalation phase. The exhalation phase may be sensed to be more of a receding and settling.

5. Focus your attention on the receding of the fluid tide caudad. This is its exhalation phase. Sense both the fluid fluctuation and the potency within it. Notice the boundary of the excursion of the exhalation phase. See if you can sense its furthermost boundary from which the motion shifts from exhalation to its inhalation, welling-up phase.

6. When you become familiar with this boundary, suggest the option of waiting there. At this edge, place a subtle intention of wait within the fluids. This is a subtle back pressure, or compression, against the shift of the fluid tide into the inhalation phase. Do this as a question, an inquiry. You are initiating a conversation, not making a demand. When you ask if the system can enter stillpoint via your subtle intention, you must listen to the answer. The fluids will respond to this suggestion. If the system does not want to enter stillpoint, do not force it. There is

an intelligence even in this response. Be patient. The fluid tide may need to express a number of cycles before it enters stillpoint. Negotiate the intention of stillness.

7. Notice what happens as you hold this suggestion at the boundary to the excursion of the fluid tide. You may sense a number of things occurring at this edge. First of all, you may sense that the fluids go deeper into their exhalation phase. If they do, follow this motion and take up the slack in the system by waiting at the new edge. This may occur a number of times in the process. You may then notice a disorganization of the fluid tide. The coherency of the fluid tide breaks down and its longitudinal fluctuation disorganizes. You may sense this as fluctuations and pulsations of fluid, which can take almost any shape and expression.

8. As you listen to this, you may then notice the system deepening into stillpoint. The disorganization of the longitudinal fluctuation generally heralds the shift of the system into stillpoint. If the system is not particularly inertial and congested, it may deepen into stillpoint in a gentle and fluid way and may not express this disorganization. What you may sense, as the system goes into stillpoint, is a deepening into a felt sense of stillness. You may initially sense this as an absence of the motion of the fluid tide and as a general sense of stillness in the system. You may sense this in your own body as a resonance with stillness and may even access stillpoint yourself. This process of resonating with stillpoints and then going into them is sometimes called entrainment.

9. Remember, in stillpoint the tidal unfoldments become still. Other rhythms such as the cardiac and respiratory rhythms must still be expressed by the system. They may, however, slow down or change in some way, in resonance with the stillpoint. For instance, the person's breath may slow down and deepen. In deep stillness it may even be barely perceptible. Once the system enters into stillpoint, you do not have to hold it there. You can let go of your suggestion to wait and simply listen to what is happening.

10. Sometimes you may sense a quality of stillpoint that seems very superficial; you may not sense the system accessing its potency, and the stillness may seem to have a flatness to it. This is usually because the system is holding inertia and congestion in ways that make it difficult to express a depth of stillpoint. It is possible to encourage a deeper expression of stillness. In this case, encourage a deepening of the stillpoint by deepening the suggestion of stillness in your hands.

11. To do this, again use your hands to create a subtle back pressure against the fluid tide within the superficial stillpoint. You are changing the question in your hands from "Can you access stillness here?" to "Can you deepen here?" As you enter into this conversation with the system, you may then sense the system shifting into a deeper level of stillness, which has more quality of potentization and potential within it. There are depths within depths within stillness.

12. When the system comes out of stillpoint, you will notice that the fluid tide has started again. This may be sensed as a surge against your hands as the system starts to express the inhalation phase of the Tide. Do not prevent this. Let the system express itself as it needs to here. Remember that once the system enters into stillpoint, you do not have to hold it there. You can let go of your suggestion to wait and just listen to what is happening. Likewise, as the system comes out of stillpoint, you are listening and are not opposing the expression of tidal forces.

Stillpoints may last for a few seconds to several minutes. Stay with the sense of the stillpoint as an appreciative fellow traveler. Notice what is happening during the stillpoint. The system will use the increase of potency that occurs during stillpoint to help heal itself. You may sense pulsations of cerebrospinal fluid. These may express patterns of spirals, figure eights and lateral fluctuations of many sorts. This can be an expression of fluid motion around sites of inertia. It is also an attempt by the system to bring increased healing potency into relationship to the inertial fulcrums and trauma impacts held in the body. As this occurs, you may also sense the expression of the inertial potencies within organizing fulcrums. You may sense heat, pulsation, and permeation of fluids and potency around and within the site. You may also sense tissue patterns changing, softening, and expanding. This may all occur during the stillpoint process. You may even sense potency expressed from the primal midline as a kind of radiance. Potency will manifest in an attempt to heal and resolve inertia in the system. It is your role to appreciate all of this and to pay attention to it. As you become more familiar with the primary respiratory system and its dynamics, you will realize that a wealth of information is being communicated to you by the system during stillpoint. Remember the *depths of stillness* described above. Did you have a sense of the depth of stillness that the system was able to access?

When the system comes out of stillpoint, you may sense that the potency within the fluid tide has changed. Its fluid drive may be stronger and fuller. There may be a sense of greater resources in the system. This is important to note and monitor clinically as sessions unfold. You can apply this process to any vantage point in the body. For instance, you might want to work with these intentions at the sacrum. In the sacral hold learned earlier, again follow the inhalation and exhalation expressions of the Tide. You

will sense a welling up and receding of fluids within the sacrum and along the dorsal midline. In the exhalation phase sense its deepest excursion and again suggest/intend wait. You will then be engaged in the same quality of conversation as described above.

In this chapter we introduced the concept of stillpoint and accessed it via your relationship to the fluid tide. We started you off with an appreciation of the subtlety of the process via an awareness of fluids and potency. In a later chapter, you will continue this exploration and learn to relate to tissues in your facilitation of stillness. The important thing to remember, as you later shift to tissues, is to maintain your awareness of this subtlety.

1. W.G. Sutherland, *Teachings in the Science of Osteopathy* (Rudra Press).

2. Peter Levine, *Waking the Tiger—Healing Trauma* (North Atlantic Books, 1997).

3. Thomas Cleary, *Kensho, the Heart of Zen* (Shambala Press, 1997).

4. The term *biodynamic* denotes the understanding that there are inherent forces at work, which both organize and maintain the human system in its functioning.

5. See chapters on the *state of balanced tension* for a discussion of variant and inertial potencies and their functions.

6. See the previous section in which it is stated that the "Tide" refers to the Long Tide and its organizing action. The Tide creates "tidal effects" in potencies and fluids (e.g., the various tidal motions of potency and fluid are created by the action of the underlying power of the Tide).

9

Introduction to Tissue Motility

In previous chapters we introduced the concept of inherent respiratory motions driven by the intentions of the Breath of Life. We introduced the idea of tidal motion and of the fluid tide. In this chapter you will begin an inquiry into the tissue components of these respiratory motions. As we have seen, in a biodynamic approach to the cranial concept, the organization and inherent motions of fluids and tissues are seen to be a function of the Breath of Life. Its potency manifests as an inner or primary respiration, which has been called the primary respiratory impulse. It is the function of primary respiration to organize life. Cellular cycles of inhalation and exhalation are organized around the Breath of Life and its Tide and groundswell. In this chapter we will introduce some concepts relating to the inherent motion of cells and tissues. We will also give an overview to a teaching approach used in courses in order to help students gain an appreciation of tissue motility

and motion. In the next chapter, you will focus on the individual motility and motion of the major cranial bones and the sacrum. In this exploration, we will also introduce the fundamental relationship of the cranial bones to the reciprocal tension membrane.

Tissues, Motility, and Mobility

I want to acknowledge that in this section, I will be describing a view of tissue motility and motion that is not commonly described in most other books. I know that my words will not do justice to my perceptual processes, but I will try my best to convey what I need to here. This view challenges the idea that bones and other tissue structures move as individual forms around separate axes of rotation. Instead, my view is that the human system is whole and that all tissues express their motility as a whole. The human body is organized and moved by the Breath of Life in its creative intentions as a true unit of function.

The potency of the Breath of Life is expressed within fluids as an embodied reality and interfaces with all cells and tissues. This interface begins from the moment of our conception and continues throughout life. As the groundswell of the Tide is expressed within the body, respiratory motions are generated. As the Breath of Life manifests its intentions, a subtle inner motion within tissues called

---

In this chapter we will:

- *Discuss motility and mobility of tissues in general*
- *Discuss the nomenclature used in describing tissue motion*
- *Discuss the cranial bowl*
- *Discuss teaching approaches*

---

motility is generated. Motility is an expression of the potency of the Breath of Life as an inner breath within every cell. Tissues, which are cell aggregates, also express this inner motility. Tissue motility is thus a direct manifestation of the action of potency and the inherent Health of the system. It is the *universal* expressed within each cell and tissue. It is what orients and centers their existence. The action of the potency within the fluids continually orients each cell and tissue to their Original intention and holds the key to their proper functioning.

The Breath of Life generates tidal forces within the human system. At the mid-tide level of action, these forces can be sensed as tidal potencies within the fluids that make everything move. This process is nonlinear; it occurs all at once everywhere in the body. Tissue motility and motion is a direct expression of these tidal forces and manifests as a *unit of function*. In other words, the motility of all tissues is expressed within the body as a whole all at once. In holographic terms, motility is a direct expression of the reference beam, the action of the Tide unfolding within all of the fluids and tissue structures of the body.[1] The practitioner may perceive this inner motility as a sense of a subtle yet powerful welling up and receding within the cells, tissues, and structures being palpated. Along with this sense, particular motions of individual structures can also be perceived.

In the explorations of the next few chapters, you will be listening to the motility and motion of structures within both a CRI context and a mid-tide context. For me, perceiving at the CRI level of action is like looking from the outside in. Bony structures may be perceived to be separate forms moving around separate axes in relationship to other structures. These motions have become known as craniosacral motion. But when one's perceptual field is resonant with the slower tidal rhythms, tissue motility is perceived much differently. Motility is sensed to be an expression of tidal forces at work within the human system. This is actually true for all tissue structures within the body, be they bone, membrane, fascia, or viscera. In our initial inquiries into bony

motion, we will discover that there are both *intraosseous* and *interosseous* motions involved. Intraosseous motion is motion expressed within the bone itself. It is cellular. It is an inner breath expressed within every cell and tissue of the body. *Interosseous motion* is the motion expressed *between* tissue structures. Both intra- and interosseous motions are generated by the action of tidal potencies within the fluids of the body.

Let's expand on this idea. In previous chapters you learned to listen to the fluid tide. You may have sensed its welling up and receding as a function of primary respiration. Here we are simply including the tissues within this field of listening. When you include tissue structures, you may then sense something like this: On palpating the system, you may perceive an inhalation surge arising. This is an expression of potency surging and rising within the fluids and the body as a whole. The tissue structures being palpated seem to well up and widen within your hands. You may have a sense of an intraosseous expansion and widening within the bones and tissues being palpated. As this occurs, more space is also generated within their sutural, joint, or connective tissue relationships, and interosseous motion between structures is also expressed. It is a welling up within every structure all at once in which space and motion is generated. Everything wells up and widens at once. Indeed, the sutures are designed to let this happen. As the inhalation surge occurs within the system, there is an intraosseous welling up within tissues while space is also generated within each suture and joint. This allows individual structures to express this inner motility in relationship to each other. Thus both intraosseous and interosseous motions are a factor of the action of potency within the fluids of the body.

Perhaps a metaphor may be helpful here. Imagine you are holding two balloons, which touch each other and are full of water. More water is pumped into them while you are holding them. You may sense a welling up within the balloons, while at the same time, the balloons move in relationship to each other. These inner and outer motions are not separate; they are a factor of the force generated within the internal fluids. I know that this is hard to describe and hope that as our explorations progress, these ideas will take on some palpable reality. As we shall also see, as the practitioner deepens into an awareness of this whole, the overall information that becomes available is more precise and the nature of the inherent treatment plan begins to clarify. We will expand upon these ideas and place them in a experiential framework later. (See Figure 9.1.)

Thus, when you deepen into the slower tidal rhythms, tissue motility is perceived to be a unified field of action. Individual tissue structures and their motions are clearly discernible, yet these motions are perceived to be part of a much wider tensile field of action. Nothing is really separate here. A perception of structures as separate entities, which move around separate axes of rotation, transforms into an awareness of holistic form and motion. This is most clear within the inhalation phase of the Tide. Listening within the mid-tide, there may be a sense that, as structures are moved in inhalation, an intraosseous motion within all tissues is generated. There is a true intraosseous expansion and widen-

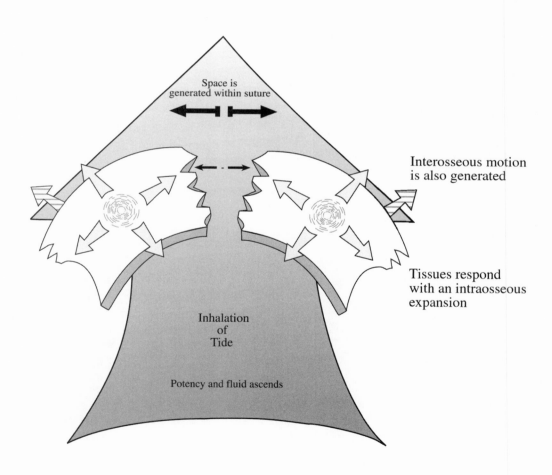

Space is generated within suture

Interosseous motion is also generated

Tissues respond with an intraosseous expansion

Inhalation of Tide

Potency and fluid ascends

9.1 Inhalation of the Tide generates cellular and tissue motility

ing within every tissue structure. As this occurs, interosseous motion—motions between structures—is also generated.

Both intraosseous and interosseous motion have been called *involuntary motions* in the cranial concept. Involuntary motion means that motion is generated by a force from within, not from without. Thus inner motility, and resultant tissue motions, are generated by the action of the potency of the Breath of Life. The relationships of primary respiration, such as the five classical functions of the primary respiratory mechanism, have been called the *involuntary mechanism* by teachers and clinicians. It is, however, important to remember when using this kind of terminology, that the system is far more than a mechanism, it is a living expression of Intelligence at work.

Mobility is another issue. Mobility is about the *ease* of the relationships of the parts. The quality of tissue motion palpated by the practitioner is an expression of both motility and mobility. If the ease of motion between structures is compromised, then mobility is compromised. Joint relationships are obvious examples. Equally at issue are the relationships between connective tissues and organ structures. Mobility is about the ease of relationship and motion between any tissue structure. This includes ease of joint motion, connective tissue motion and visceral motion. All of the structures of the body should ideally express a fluidic state of ease in their relationships. One of my osteopathic teachers used to say that "mobility is ability." Mobility is the *ability* of the individual structures to move in relationship to each other. That simply sums it up. When issues of "ability" arise between structures, you then get mobility issues. When you have mobility issues, you will have motility issues also. In other words, when you get mobility issues, interosseous motion is effected. This in turn will effect the *ability* of cells and tissues to express their intraosseous motions also. As we shall see in later chapters, when there are unresolved forces within the body, such as those generated by pathogens, trauma and accidents, the potency of the Breath of Life will become inertial

in order to contain them in some way. As potencies become inertial, so does the fluid and tissue world. Motility and interosseous motion will become compromised. The related tissues will not be able to express their motion as easily. In all mobility and motility issues, we will discover that it is essential to perceive and understand the forces at work. It is relatively easy to perceive resistance; it is another thing to perceive the forces around which they are organized. It is still another thing to perceive the Health that centers it all. Tissue resistances are expressions of deeper potencies and inertial forces at

---

The Breath of Life Generates Motility and Motion

The groundswell of the Tide
The groundswell of the Tide arises and the tidal rhythms are generated.

▼

The potency
The potency of the Breath of Life is expressed, via transmutation, within the fluids of the body.

▼

The fluids
The fluids are moved by, and convey, this potency.

▼

Intraosseous cellular and tissue motility are simultaneously generated
The potency is expressed within every cell and tissue as an inner *breath* called motility.

▼

Interosseous motion between structures is expressed

As the inhalation surge of the Tide is expressed, space is generated within sutural relationships and interosseous motion is expressed between structures. This is really a factor of the deeper forces at work within the body. It is nonlinear and happens all at once.

work, and we will unfold an understanding of this as we go along.

A Living Anatomy

As we are now entering the realm of form and tissues, it is essential to speak about anatomy. When you meet another person's system, you are meeting that person's living anatomy. Many students find the study of anatomy to be boring or removed from their direct experience. It is important to understand anatomy is a direct expression of life. Like life itself, our living anatomy is in motion and is grounded in the Stillness from which all motion arises. It also is important to realize that anatomy is the language of the body. It is a precise language. The more you are familiar with anatomy, the more it will speak to you. If you have the ears to hear, the body will speak to you, but you must learn its language. The living anatomy will directly communicate the experience and history of the person. It will show you how all of that is being expressed in the present moment and how Health is centering it all.

A visual knowledge is most helpful. A clear visual sense of the parts of the body and their interrelationships is essential. I'm not so concerned with nomenclature, although that is helpful. It is the clear visual *felt sense* of anatomy that is important. Once you have a growing visual knowledge of anatomy, it is important that you don't overlay your images onto a person's system. Simply know the territory and listen in a space of unknowing. Let your knowledge of anatomy be a background, and the living anatomy will exactly describe the shape of things to you. What is communicated will be a particular expression of that person's experience and of the Health that centers it.

The Cranial Bowl, Vault and Base

The cranial bowl is composed of the bones of the cranial vault and base and their articular relation-

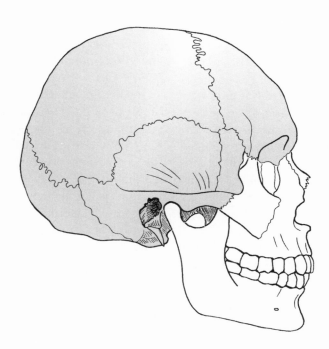

9.2 The cranial bowl

ships. These include the vault bones; the frontal and parietal bones and the bones of the cranial base; the temporal, occipital, sphenoid and ethmoid bones. (See Figure 9.2 above.) The bones of the cranial vault are formed in membrane, while the bones of the cranial base are formed in cartilage. Although this division is generally correct, it is important to remember that the squama of the occiput and temporal bones are formed in membrane, as are the greater wings of the sphenoid bone.

Also remember that bone is a connective tissue and is essentially fluidic in nature. Bone, like any connective tissue, is formed in a fluidic ground substance. Remember that the bone we palpate is living, is fluid, and is breathed by the Breath of Life. It is thus in the nature of bone to express the action of the Tide as a fluidic and tensile structure. This is ideally perceived an inner intraosseous motility within each bony structure palpated. As we shall later see, the respiratory cycles of the Tide generate motions within the tissues of the body called reciprocal tension motions. This means that tissues express a tensile motion, first in one direction and then in another, within the phases of primary respiration. Bone, like any tissue, will express reciprocal tension motion, or tensile dynamics, within its tissue structure.[2]

As we unfold our palpation sense, it is important to remember bone and membrane are a unit of function. In other words, they are whole and move in unity. The periosteum of the bones are continuous with the outer layer of dura within the cranial bowl and their dynamics are inseparable. In terms of the reciprocal tension membrane, the vault bones, the frontal bone, and the parietal bones have most contact with the falx cerebri. The temporal bones have most contact with the tentorium cerebelli, and the occiput has a mutual contact with the falx and tent as their leaves meet on its squama. In terms of the dynamics of the sphenobasilar junction, the tentorium directly stretches from the clinoid processes of the sphenoid bone to the squama of the occiput. (See Figure 9.3.)

The Cranium and Its Sutures

The cranium is basically a sphere, or bowl, composed of bones that are interrelated through joint relationships called sutures. A suture is not like any other joint relationship in the body. A suture is composed of two margins of bone connected by an extremely thin layer of fibrous, vascular connective tissue. This connection allows for subtle movement. A suture consists of a number of layers of relationship. The two outer layers are sometimes called *uniting layers*. They are essentially continuations of the periosteum of the two articulating bones. At a suture, the periosteum of the articulating bones splits into two layers. The outermost layers from both sides of the bones involved continues across the suture and unites the bones; the innermost layers turn around the edges of the articulating bones to form a fibrous capsule that covers their edges. Between the capsules, which are made from this turning in of the periosteum, these is a *central zone* of connective tissue, which has fine fiber bundles running in all directions and has sinusoidal blood vessels within it. Free nerve endings have also been observed within sutures. This zone is vascular and fluidic in nature and allows mobility in sutural relationships.[3] (See Figure 9.4.)

If you remember, it was the possibility of the mobility of cranial articulations that started Dr. Sutherland on his lifelong journey. He sensed, via both palpation and experiment, that the cranial bones do indeed have mobility, and this eventually led him to the profound truths of primary respiration and the fundamental ordering principles of the human body. He discovered that sutures were not naturally fused, but were mobile and that the whole cranial bowl moved in a unified dynamic. Thus a suture contains living connective tissue with blood supply, fluid dynamics, and movement functions. This is important to stress. The cranial bones are not fused together, but are connected by living tissues, which allows motion. The living tissue within the suture is also, in our terms, expressing primary respi-

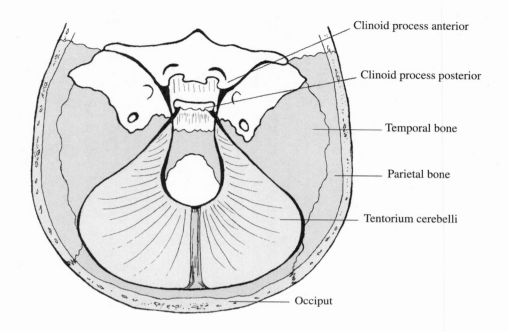

Clinoid process anterior

Clinoid process posterior

Temporal bone

Parietal bone

Tentorium cerebelli

Occiput

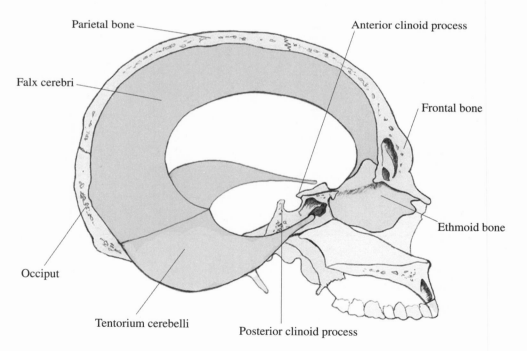

Parietal bone

Anterior clinoid process

Falx cerebri

Frontal bone

Ethmoid bone

Occiput

Tentorium cerebelli

Posterior clinoid process

9.3 The relationships of the falx and tentorium

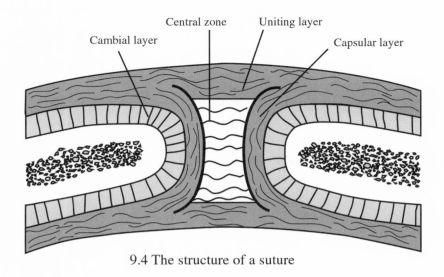

9.4 The structure of a suture

ration as an inner life breath. Within the inhalation phase of the Tide, space is generated within the suture and expansion is allowed. Interosseous motion between bones results.

There are a number of kinds of sutures to be found in the cranium. Sutures are classified depending on the relationship of the bones of the articulation. (See Figure 9.5.)

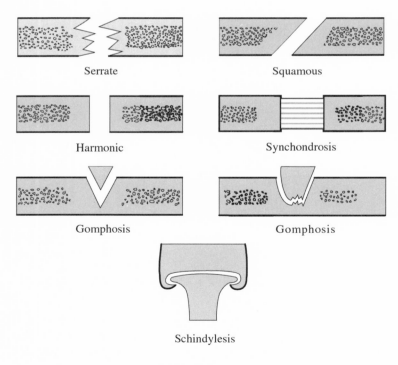

9.5 Types of sutures

- **Serrate sutures**—Sutures that meet in an interdigitizing, "sawtooth" fashion such as the sagittal suture.

- **Squamous sutures**—Sutures that meet in an overlapping fashion such as the squamosal suture between the temporal and parietal bones.

- **Squamoserrate sutures**—Sutures that combine aspects of serrate and squamous relationships such as the coronal or lamboidal sutures.

- **Harmonic sutures**—Sutures that meet end to end such as the lacrimo-ethmoidal suture.

- **Gomphosis sutures**—Sutures, or parts of sutures, that meet in a peg and socket arrangement such as the great wing of the sphenoid with its body, or the temporoparietal pivot point, where a peg from the parietal bone meets the socket of the temporoparietal notch.

- **Irregular sutures**—"Unclassifiable" sutures that meet in irregular arrangements such as the frontosphenoidal and parietomastoid.

- **Schindylesis**—Sutures that meet in a plate and fissure arrangement such as the alar surfaces of the vomer as it meets the rostrum of the sphenoid.

- **Synchondrosis**—Sutures that are formed by a cartilaginous bridge such as the sphenobasilar junction.

Classical Nomenclature

As we have seen, within a craniosacral biodynamic viewpoint, the Breath of Life and its potency is considered to be the basic ordering principle of the human system. It maintains the order and integrity of the mind-body and enlivens all tissues with its potency. The tissues of the body are permeated by this inherent ordering principle and express it as motility, motion, and functional vitality. This ordering principle is first expressed within the embryological development of the human system. All natural fulcrums and axes that organize tissue motility and motion in the adult system are derived from the developmental processes driven by the potency of the Breath of Life. All tissue motion has its roots in this unfoldment. The tissues and structures of the body express their motion in specific rhythmic cycles, or phases of motion: a primary respiratory inhalation and exhalation within the body's cells and tissues. It is thus important to remember that tissue motility and motion is organized and enlivened by the bioelectric matrix and its potency, which is, in turn, generated by the intentions of the Breath of Life. Fluid and tissue motility is an expression of this groundswell. The fluid tide and the motility and motion of tissues are therefore expressions of the Health of the system. They are not just mechanical processes, they are an expression of the unfoldment of life itself. Inherent tissue motion is an expression of these deeper forces at work. These outer motions are derived from the deeper expression of motility within the cells and tissues of the body.

The respiratory phases of tissue motion were given very particular names by Dr. Sutherland. These can be confusing if you don't understand their origins and intentions. The first thing we have to do is to explain the nomenclature he used and to describe the basic dynamic. This nomenclature came from the osteopathic setting in which Dr. Sutherland was working. He took the nomenclature used in his field and modified it to describe the motions he was sensing. In his use of this nomenclature, tissue motions are related to the two phases of primary respiration. These terms are meant to clarify the motion of different structures for practitioner observation. They give a way to talk about these dynamics, but they do not really describe the respiratory motions of tissue structures. Respiratory motion is not mechanical: it is organic and fluidic in nature. In reality, all tissue structures are responding to the potency of the Breath of Life in some way. In inhalation, there is welling up, expansion, and widening: and in exhalation, settling and narrowing.

Let's discuss Dr. Sutherland's use of classical nomenclature. In the inhalation phase of the Tide, the tissue motions generated are called *flexion-external rotation* and in the exhalation phase, they are called *extension-internal rotation*. It is important to understand that these motions were named by Dr. Sutherland according to the relationship between the sphenoid bone and the occiput at the cranial base. Furthermore, the nomenclature is derived from the relationship of their *inferior* aspects at the cranial base. Classically, all tissue motion in the entire body is named in relationship to the dynamics of the inferior aspect of these two bones. What's more, bony motion is always related to *axes of rotation* in some way. For instance the sphenoid bone is said to rotate around a transverse axis. Once again, this is an attempt to help practitioners gain clarity and have a relationship to tissue motion. But I must say that bones don't really rotate around axes: their motion is actually much more fluidic. Bones express inner, intraosseous motions within the phases of the Tide. In inhalation this is perceived to be expressed by expansion and widening, and in exhalation by settling and narrowing. All cells and tissues within the body express this all at once. Motility is a true unit of function. As potency wells up within the system, space is also generated within sutures and interosseous motion is allowed. Again, this occurs all at once. These tissue motions are sometimes called craniosacral motion.

Thus, in this book, I am taking the position that classic axes of rotation are at best just an approximation of reality. They help orient practitioners to tissue motion. But remember that within the deeper tidal rhythms, this motion is seen to be more holistic and fluidic. Tissue motion is really a function of a deep inner breath arising within each and every

cell of the body. Individual tissue structures are perceived to be part of a greater tensile field of action. By this I mean that individual interosseous motion is sensed to be part of a more holistic motion dynamic. All tissue structures are perceived to be part of a unified tissue field, which moves as a whole. Rather than sensing individual structures moving around separate axes of rotation, you may sense more of an inner motion within each structure, which is not separate from the inner motion of other structures. It has more of the sense of flower petals opening. You sense the whole of the flower as it opens yet each flower petal is also distinct. Tissue motion is sensed to happen all at once as a unified field of action. Within this awareness, the individual bones and structures of the body are still discernible in their particular motion dynamic, but this dynamic is sensed to be more fluidic and part of a greater field of action. In reality, when the practitioner listens within the slower, deeper tidal rhythms of the system, concepts of axes of rotation become irrelevant. I am using the classic descriptions of axes of rotation in this book with this very important proviso.

So let's have a look at how tissue motion is classically described. In the inhalation phase of the Tide, the sphenoid and occiput are said to rotate around transverse axes in opposite directions. Their inferior surfaces move closer together and the sphenobasilar junction rises. This is called *craniosacral flexion*. This nomenclature relates to the moving together, or *flexion* of the inferior aspects of these bones. As this occurs, the greater wings of the sphenoid and the lateral aspects of the occipital squama also widen apart and rotate/dive caudad (footward). (See Figure 9.6.)

In the exhalation phase of the Tide, the reverse process occurs. The sphenoid and occiput rotate in opposite directions around transverse axes in the reverse direction. Their inferior surfaces move apart and the sphenobasilar junction sinks. This is called *craniosacral extension*. This nomenclature relates to the moving apart or *extension* of the inferior aspects of these two bones. The greater wings

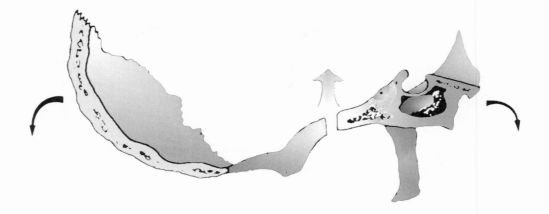

Flexion around the sphenobasilar junction

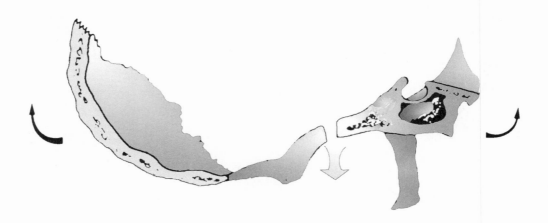

Extension around the sphenobasilar junction

9.6 Flexion extension around the sphenobasilar junction (SBJ) of the sphenoid and the lateral aspects of the occipital squama narrow and rotate cephalad (headward) as this occurs.

In the classic concept, the sphenoid bone is considered to be the keystone of the cranium and of bony motion generally. The occiput and all other single midline bones are said to rotate in the opposite direction to the sphenoid. It is as though the sphenoid is the major gear around which all other midline bones must key off. In this gearing process, they must move in the opposite direction to the major gear, the sphenoid bone. (See Figure 9.7.) All

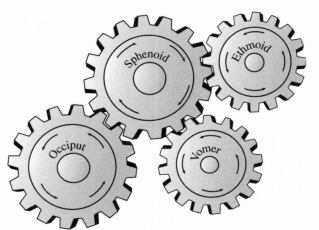

9.7 The "gears" of the cranium

midline bones and structures thus express flexion-extension in relationship to the sphenoid and sphenobasilar junction. Within the primary respiratory mechanism, these include the occiput, ethmoid, vomer, and sacrum. Again, within the classic concept, as the sphenobasilar junction rises and the sphenoid rotates around its transverse axis in flexion, all of the other midline bones rotate in the opposite direction around their own transverse axes. In flexion, the bones also widen transversely and narrow anterior-posterior; in exhalation, they express a narrowing transversely and an anterior-posterior widening. Within a mid-tide level of action, these inner motions are much more prominent.

At the same time, all paired bones express a related motion called external-internal rotation. As the sphenoid expresses inhalation/flexion, the paired bones rotate around their own axes and generally express an outward/lateral rotation or widening/flaring called external rotation. In the exhalation phase the reverse occurs. As an example, the parietal bones express external rotation as they widen and flare apart at their lateral aspects while the sagital suture between them sinks. (See Figure 9.8.)

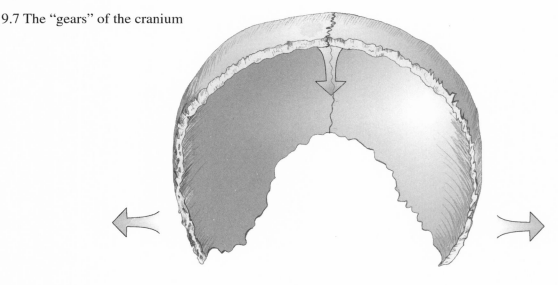

9.8 External rotation of the parietal bones

General Summary of Tissue Motion

Classical Craniosacral Flexion and Extension

Inhalation: flexion-external rotation

- Midline bones express a flexion motion as a rotation around transverse axes. The sphenoid is considered to be the major gear of this motion. As the sphenoid rotates one way, the other midline bones rotate the other way. This occurs around transverse axes.

- Paired bones express an external rotation motion around specific axes. This can be generally perceived as a rotation, flaring out, and widening of the structures.

- The body as a whole expresses a general widening side to side, narrowing front to back, and shortening top to bottom.

Exhalation: extension-internal rotation

- Midline bones express an extension motion in the opposite direction to flexion, as described above.

- Paired bones express their internal rotation motions around specific axes in the opposite direction to external rotation, as described above.

- This yields, in the body, a general narrowing side to side, widening front to back and lengthening top to bottom.

Overview of Teaching Approach

When Dr. Sutherland was a student, he was holding a temporal bone in his hands and was struck by a monumental thought: "Bevelled like the gills of a fish for primary respiration." Dr. Sutherland claimed that this thought sent him off on a lifetime journey. I can imagine him asking himself, "What on earth is *primary respiration* and what does it have to do with the health of the human system?" This is a question that we must also continually ask ourselves as we travel on our own journey of exploration.

In the clarification of the work over many years, the main tool of the clinician has been observation and listening. In our initial approach to the tissue system, we want to empower students to listen and observe for themselves. It is not initially helpful to tell students what they should perceive, but it is helpful to create a context in which students explore their unique perceptual experiences. The following outlines the teaching approach we initially take in observing tissue motion. It is useful to share this here because the following chapters are laid out to support this process.

Within the classroom situation, we initially take a two-step approach in observing tissue motion. First, with minimal information and a review of anatomy, students are shown a way to hold the bones and are asked to simply listen. In this dynamic act of listening, they are asked to observe how primary respiration is expressed within the bones. Students are asked to observe the following: How do the bones express an inner motility? How does intraosseous motion manifest? How is this expressed as an outer interosseous motion? Do you sense motion, pulsation, movements of any kind? The students then meet as a large group and share what was discovered via palpation. From this exploration, tutors build up a picture of the motility and motion of the bone in question.

Tutors present the classical understanding of the motion of that bone in a lecture format. With this information, students then enter a second palpation session and see what has been clarified. In this session, tutors place their hands over the students' hands to amplify and clarify their palpatory experience. Students then meet in a small group with a tutor to clarify what they have experienced. The following information assumes this basic approach.

In the classroom situation, each new relationship will be explored in this manner. The major cranial bones and their relationships, the sacrum and the reciprocal tension membranes, are explored in this format. In later seminars, once students have a clearer grasp of tissue dynamics, this inquiry may be undertaken in one step, information may be directly presented, and palpation sessions then undertaken.[4]

In many courses, you may be first introduced to the dynamics of the SBJ, then to the reciprocal tension membrane and cranial vault, and then the paired bones. In the next chapter, we will begin our journey with the temporal bones. I find that the dynamics of the SBJ are not easily perceived until some felt sense of craniosacral dynamics has already occurred. Thus we will first listen to the temporal bones, then the frontal bone and the parietal bones, before approaching the SBJ and its dynamics. In the following chapters I am introducing the concept of tissue motility and motion. I would like to start our journey into tissue motion from the same vantage point from which Dr. Sutherland gained this most profound initial insight, the temporal bones. In this initial introduction into craniosacral dynamics, you will not be taught to *do* anything. You will simply learn to listen to tissues and their expressions of Health. The inherent motility and mobility of the bones are an expression of the organizing principle of the Breath of Life. These tissue expressions become patterned relative to our experience of life. Before you can appreciate clinical approaches to inertia and congestion within the human system, you must appreciate how its underlying Health is never lost. The work then becomes a matter of hearing the Health and facilitating a reconnection to it. In the next chapter, you will simply be listening to the tissues and noticing, in that simple act of listening, what occurs. In later chapters, we will learn the various skills and approaches that allow a conversation to occur with both the Health and the history of the person. These facilitation skills rest on the ability to listen and to hear how Health manifests.

1. See previous chapters on the holographic principle.

2. We will describe the nature of reciprocal tension motion in detail in later chapters.

3. See H. Magoun, *Osteopathy in the Cranial Field* (The Journal Printing Company, 1997) pp. 12–13 for an interesting discussion of sutures.

4. I want to acknowledge the work of Paul Vick in emphasizing the importance of student exploration and empowerment within the teaching context.

10

Tissue Motility Continued

The previous chapter introduced concepts of motility and mobility within tissue dynamics. We also introduced a particular learning approach. In this approach we first give minimal information about classical understandings of motion dynamics. We ask students to simply listen and see what they discover. We then meet to see what was found and then give more specific information. From this base, another palpation session is undertaken. In this session, tutors offer their hands-on feedback to help amplify what students are palpating. We also honor the particular rhythmic and tidal unfoldments that students naturally perceive. Some will naturally sense the CRI, some the mid-tide with its tidal potencies and fluid tide, and some the Long Tide. The intention is to help a student know what level of unfoldment they naturally hear, to clarify these, and to help them shift their perceptual fields to other levels.

In the following chapters, we will describe the motion dynamics at the beginning of each new relationship. This book is meant to be a reference book for students and practitioners and is not a training course or self-taught course. Please understand this. In this chapter, we will begin to come into relationship to specific tissue dynamics. The chapter begins with an exploration of the dynamics of the temporal bone. It then extends this exploration into the dynamics of the frontal and parietal bones. In this learning process, the challenge will be to simply listen to how Health organizes the motions being palpated. Here we are beginning an exploration into how Health expresses itself via the motility and motion of the tissue system. We are not yet worried about the unresolved issues within the system, nor its patterns of suffering, resistance, and protection. We must first learn to hear the Health that centers all of this.

In this chapter we will:

- *Describe and listen for the motility and motion of the temporal, frontal, and parietal bones.*

Fulcrums, Levers, and Palpation

Before you attempt to palpate tissue motility and motion, I'd like to review some aspects of our previous perceptual work. In earlier chapters, you learned to establish a relational listening field and to establish a presence. This process has a ritual-like quality to it.[1] In this process you first went inward. You checked out your own inner state. You accessed a sense of stillness within. You then moved towards the patient's system and made physical contact. This contact was negotiated as to quality of touch and distance of attention. You then set up a field of listening, a perceptual field. This initiates the creation of a relational field, a field in which both patient and practitioner are mutually engaged. An initial aspect of this process was the concept of the practitioner fulcrum.

The concept of the fulcrum is used over and over again in the cranial field. A simple extension of the use of fulcrums will aid you in feeling and perceiving tissue motion. As you hold the patient's cranium, leave enough room at the head of the table for your elbows and forearms to rest. Let your elbows be fulcrums for sensing tissue motions. Place the weight of your shoulders gently on your elbows and allow your hands to be comfortably relaxed. It is as though your hands are floating off your elbows. In this process, you are creating *elbow fulcrum points* to aid your palpation skills. Palpate or view the patient's system from these elbow fulcrums rather than from your hands. In this case, the idea is to create a longer lever, with your hands as extensions of the lever, as you palpate the patient's system. As you know from basic physics, the longer a lever is, the greater a movement is amplified and the less force is needed to generate it. Hence, as you lengthen your levers and follow the patient's dynamics from your elbows, you are effectively amplifying the movements that you are palpating and perceiving via your hands. Very subtle movements and pulsations in the patient's body will become amplified and can even seem quite large. Another aspect of this is that, as you settle into your elbow fulcrums, your hands can float more freely on the tissues and you don't have to narrow your listening into your hands or fingers. This helps to maintain a wider field of listening and gives the patient's system more space to express itself.

Note that in establishing these elbow fulcrum points, your palpating hands still maintain their gentle contact. Once this is established, just let the tissues come to you. In essence you are floating on and riding the tissues as they move in their unique patterns. Your elbow fulcrum points allow your hands to float within fluids and on the tissues. Notice how the tissues move you. As you gently deepen into your elbow fulcrum points, you deepen your relationship to the tissues being palpated. Allow the tissues to come to you, rather than looking for anything. As you experience this, you will find that the qualities of tissue motion and function begin to speak to you and you can hear their story more clearly.

You can even carry this idea another step. Allow the earth fulcrum you earlier created to be the fulcrum from which you perceive the system. Imagine that your hands are perceiving movement from this fulcrum point in the earth. The patient's primary respiratory motions will then seem greatly amplified. As you deepen into your earth fulcrum, you will also deepen your relationship to the tissues being palpated. As you establish your fulcrums and relationship to the patient's system, imagine/sense that your hands are floating on corks, floating within fluid. Once you have a clear sense of tissue motility and motion and you become more experienced in your palpation skills, you can allow your hands to float within the fluids and to be moved by the potency of the Breath of Life itself.

Shifting Perceptual Fields

Earlier chapters introduced the idea of shifting your perceptual field to the various unfoldments of the Breath of Life. In the following explorations, you will be shifting your perceptual fields to both the CRI level and the mid-tide level of perception. The intention will be to first sense the motion of the specific structure at a CRI level and then to shift to a mid-tide level to see how that effects your perception of motion. Let's remind you of these basic perceptual shifts.

In the first perceptual process, you will shift, or synchronize, your attention to the CRI level of action. To do this, you will allow your hands to float on the tissues like corks on the water. Use whatever image helps you to sense this. The image of corks floating on water helps many people. After negotiating your contact, you will then narrow your perceptual field to the bones and membranes being palpated. Get interested in how these bones and membranes are moving. Let your hands float on the tissues and let them show you their motions. Don't grab onto the tissues. If you do this, even subtly, you will actually restrict their motion and lock up their structure and function. Listen, don't look for anything, and don't expect anything. Let it come to you. See if the faster rhythm, the CRI, comes into your field of awareness. Notice how the particular bone expresses this in its motion. After sensing the motion of the structure at a CRI level, you will then shift, or synchronize, your awareness to the mid-tide level of action.

To do this, you will shift your imagery and widen your perceptual field. In the CRI level of perception, your hands were floating on the tissues. In this shift, let your hands also *float within fluids*. Maintaining the same hold on the structure being palpated, imagine/sense that your hands are now floating in a wider field of fluid as they palpate the tissues. Your hands are immersed within this fluid field. Now also widen your perceptual field to hold the whole of the person and the field around the person. Dr. Rollin Becker, D.O., called this the *biosphere*. The biosphere is the whole of the person, the body, and the field of potency and environmental exchange around the body. It is the wider bioelectric matrix around the person and the physical body within that field. In this process, you widen your field of awareness from the individual tissues and structures palpated above to include the whole of the person and the wider field of potency around the body. Within this field you are sensing the fluids and tissues of the body *as a whole*.

As you do this, you may find that your mind settles and becomes relatively still. Your quality of awareness is wider and softer, yet you also maintain a keen precision within your listening. You are now holding the *whole* of the person within your field of attention. See if the slower rhythm of the mid-tide, 2.5 cycles a minute, begins to unfold its presence. In this process, you are still sensing the particular bone or structure, but within the context of the whole. You may sense a deepening and slowing of the rhythmic unfoldment. You may sense a subtle shift in how the bone expresses its motion. It may be perceived to be more of an inner motion which is part of a wider dynamic, than just a particular motion of a particular bone. Once you have a clear sense of perceptual field and your listening process, you will find that you can hold a very wide field and information will more naturally come to you. You will also learn to modulate your own perceptual field with the patient's energetic field. The perceptual structure described here aids learning and gives practitioners an entree into these perceptual experiences. Let's start this process with the temporal bone.

The Temporal Bones

The temporal bones are extraordinary in their visual beauty and in their intricate relationships within the cranial base and with the rest of the system. (See Figure 10.1.) It was while gazing at a temporal bone that the incredible thought, *Bevelled like the gills of a fish for primary respiration,* struck Dr. Sutherland. He believed that it was a divine insight given to him, which set the tone and direction for the rest of his professional career. It seems an appropriate starting point for our own explorations.

The temporal bones have important functions both in orthodox physiology and in the cranial concept. They contain our hearing mechanisms and the mechanisms that maintain our sense of balance relative to gravity. The temporal bones articulate with the occiput, the parietals, the sphenoid bone, the zygomatic bones and the mandible. They are very much part of the cranial base and will directly reflect cranial base issues in their dynamics. The temporal bones have an important position in the cranial base. They fill the wedge-shaped lateral spaces between the occiput and sphenoid bones. (See Figure 10.2.) As the temporal bones rest in the wedge-shaped spaces between the sphenoid and occiput, any inertial issue held within their dynamics will be directly transferred to the sphenobasilar junction and vice versa. The temporals can become

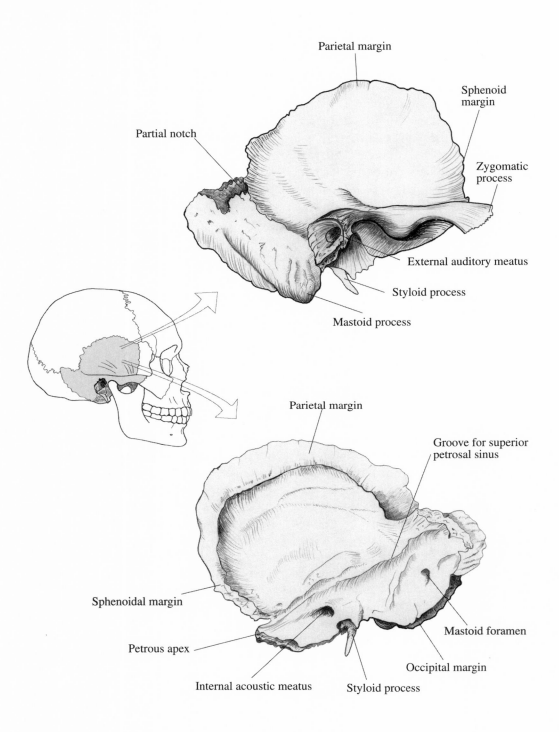

10.1 The temporal bone

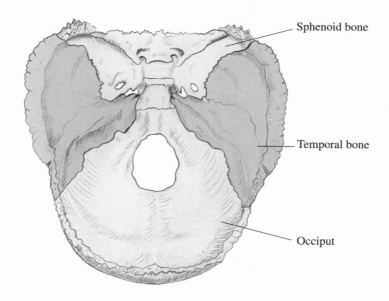

10.2 Temporal bone in cranial base

medially compressed within their wedged-shaped spaces. It is also common for them to hold intraosseous compression within their bony tissue. Some common experiences that may generate compression in the cranial base include birth trauma, shocking experiences, and accidents or falls. The temporomandibular fossas of the temporal bones create the articulatory surfaces for the condyles of the mandible. Due to this anatomical relationship, temporal bone dynamics will directly effect temporomandibular joint function. Compressive issues within their dynamics will be directly transferred to the TMJ and will commonly influence TMJ function in some way.

The temporal bones have an important relationship to the reciprocal tension membranes. The tentorium cerebelli, the horizontal aspect of the reciprocal tension membrane, stretches directly between them. Remember that bone is a connective tissue. All connective tissues are in continuous anatomical relationship. The periosteum of the cranial bones are continuous with the outer layer of dura mater within the skull. The temporal bones are thus directly continuous with the horizontal aspect of the membrane system. (See Figure 10.3.) It is important to understand that bone and membrane are one dynamic. Bone is a specialized connective tissue just as membrane is. They are a continuous unit of function. The dural membranes, in turn, are continuous in their functioning with all other connective tissues in the body. Thus, in a wider context, all connective tissues are a unit of function and represent one unified dynamic. As we will see, at the midtide level of perception, it is possible to perceive the connective tissues of the body as a unified tensile field of action. Furthermore, because the temporal bones have a direct relationship to the horizontal aspect of the membrane system, they will also have a direct relationship to the horizontal structures of the body generally. Their dynamics will thus reflect the overall state of gravity line balance throughout the body. Thus issues held within all horizontal structures, such as major joints, the pelvic diaphragm, the respiratory diaphragm, and the thoracic inlet, will be mirrored within the dynamics of the temporal bones. Their motility and mobility and

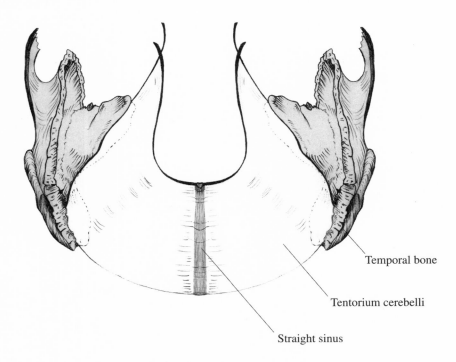

Temporal bone

Tentorium cerebelli

Straight sinus

10.3 Temporal bone and tentorium

related structural issues will be effected by these relationships. (See Figure 10.4.)

Due to their direct continuity to the membranes, their dynamic relationship to all horizontal structures, and their complicated articular surfaces within the wedge-shaped space they occupy, they are sometimes called the "trouble makers" of the craniosacral system. It is not so much that they are troublemakers, more that they express a dynamic equilibrium relative to structural issues within the body as a whole. Issues of traumatization and shock are often reflected in their dynamics, which commonly express compression and torsion. They are key elements within the foundations of the cranial base, which can directly reflect many of our most traumatic experiences. Their positions relative to each other and to the body as a whole are commonly compensations for fulcrums located almost anywhere within the system. As they will compensate for almost any connective tissue and joint dynamic within the body in some way, it is also common for the temporal bones to be out of synchronization in their expression of motion. This is not natural, but is so common that it is sometimes thought to be. Within the phases of the Tide, they naturally widen and narrow in synchronization like flower petals opening and closing.

Motion of the Temporal Bones

Like all tissue structures, the temporal bones express an inherent motility as an inhalation and exhalation within their cellular dynamics. This is expressed as an intraosseous widening in inhalation and a settling and narrowing in exhalation. This inner breath, or motility, is an expression of the potency of the Breath of Life at work and is the most important aspect of cellular and tissue motion. It is important to remember that motility within the body is expressed as a unified dynamic. All tissue structures are moved by the action of potency at the same time, as a whole. It is important to think of the

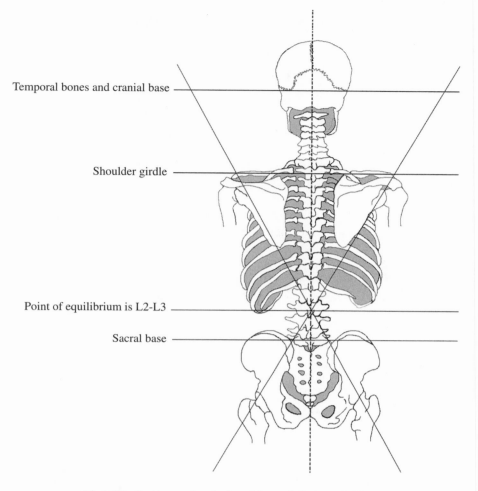

Temporal bones and cranial base

Shoulder girdle

Point of equilibrium is L2-L3

Sacral base

10.4 The horizontal relationships of the cranial base,
temporal bones, shoulder girdle, and sacral base

entire body as a unity expressing a unified motility all at once. The *spirit-mind-body* of a human being is whole. As this inner motility manifests, interosseous motion between individual structures is also generated. As each structure expresses inhalation and exhalation, outer motions between them are generated. This is like an inner force generating external motion. At the CRI level of perception, structures may be perceived to express an 8–14 cycles per minute motion. This motion is a conditioned expression of the life experience of that particular person. It is an expression of unresolved suffering.

At the mid-tide level of action, structures are perceived to express a slower, deeper rhythm of 2.5 cycles a minute. At this perceptual level, the unity of potency, fluid, and tissues is more clearly perceived. The forces at work within fluids and tissues are more easily perceived. Potency is the motivating force. This driving force is expressed as a transmutation within the fluids. As this force moves within the fluids, tissue motility is also generated. Potency is the ordering and driving force, fluid is its medium, and cellular and tissue organization and motion is generated by its action.

As you listen to the motion of the temporal bones, they can be perceived to express *external and internal rotation*. Classically, each temporal bone is said to move around an axis of rotation, which starts within their mastoid portions and follows the petrous ridge to the petrous apex towards the sphenobasilar junction. In the inhalation phase, the temporal bones express an external rotation by rotating around this imaginary oblique axis. The superior aspect of its petrous ridge rotates anterior-laterally and its squama drops outward as its superior aspect also moves anterior-laterally. As you palpate both bones together, you will sense that in external rotation, the temporal bones expand and widen as their squamas drop anterior-laterally and are sensed to widen apart, while their mastoid portions move medially and superior and come closer together. Within the mid-tide, this will be perceived to be expressed as an intraosseous expansion and widening. In-

terosseous motion between the temporal bones and the bones around them are allowed as, within inhalation, space is also generated within all sutures and joints. Dr. Sutherland described this motion as "wobbly wheels." In the exhalation phase the reverse occurs. (See Figure 10.5.)

In your palpation sessions, you must also remember that this motion is in direct relationship to the reciprocal tension membranes, especially the tentorium cerebelli. As the temporal bones express their motion, the tentorium cerebelli is also flattening and widening. Bone and membrane are an inseparable unit of function. As you tune into the motion of the temporal bones below, see if you can sense this unified dynamic. The craniosacral dynamics of the temporal bones, in common with all other cranial bones, are organized around Sutherland's fulcrum, ideally located within the anterior straight sinus.

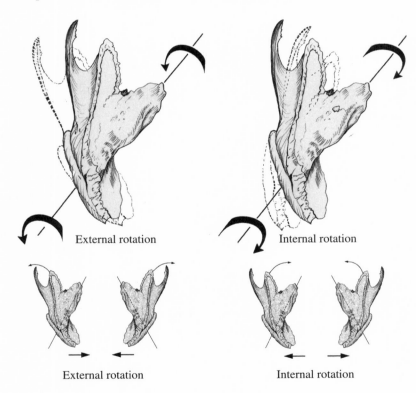

10.5 External and internal rotation of temporal bones

Classic Motion of the Temporal Bones

- *The two bones express an inner expansion expressed as external and internal rotation, classically said to occur around oblique axes.*

- *In external rotation the squama of the temporal bones will be sensed to widen apart and drop anterior-laterally as the mastoid parts are sensed to narrow together, as they move medial and superior. In internal rotation, the reverse may be sensed.*

Mid-Tide Awareness

Within the mid-tide you may have a clearer sense that the temporal bones express their motion as a widening and expansion from within. Basically, in inhalation, there is a cephalad surge of potency and fluid within the system, an expansion and widening occurs within the cells of the temporal bones, and the motions called external rotation are generated. As this happens, more space is also generated within the sutural relationships and interosseous motion between a temporal bone and the structures around it is allowed.

Clinical Application:
Palpating Temporal Bone Dynamics

In this section, you will begin your exploration into tissue motility and mobility. You will start this process by making a relationship to the temporal bones. You will learn a particular way of holding the temporal bones, the *temporal bone hold,* in which the middle finger of each hand is placed in the external auditory meatus (ear canal). You will be asked to tune into the motion of the temporal bones and to sense their inner motility. First you will be asked to enter the CRI perceptual field. After listening to the bones within the CRI level, you will then shift your perceptual field to the mid-tide level of action. We will remind you of the process of shifting perceptual fields below.

1. Move to the temporal bone hold. Place the middle finger of each hand in the ear canal (external meatus). Place your ring fingers posterior to the ear over the mastoid portions of the temporal bones. Place your index finger anterior to the ear over the zygomatic processes of the temporal bone. Your little finger is comfortably placed over the occipital squama. Your thumbs are lightly placed wherever they comfortably

rest. (See Figure 10.6.) In this position, negotiate your relationship with your patient. As you place your hands in the temporal bone hold, be sure to allow space. If there are medial compressive issues within the cranial base, the patient may need a lot of space in the negotiation of contact. You can allow this by imagining your hands farther apart. While maintaining your light contact with the tissues, imagine/intend your hands farther apart. Do not lose actual physical contact while you do this.

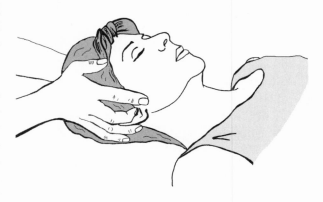

10.6 Temporal bone hold

2. In this position, synchronize your perceptual field with the CRI. Let your palpation contact be as though you are floating on corks, which, in turn, are being moved by the underlying tide. Narrow your perceptual field to the tissues being palpated. Get interested in how the temporal bones are moving. Allow the tissues to move you as you listen. Do not look for anything; just simply listen and allow yourself to be moved. *Any other intention will engage the system's response to you.* You want to see if the tissues will show you their dynamic as though you were not there.

3. In this position simply float and listen. Do not look for anything. Let yourself be moved. You may sense an external-internal rotation dynamic. Let you hands float and be moved by it. Note the dynamics that unfold as you listen. Be open to any expression of motion. It will most likely not be as classically described.

4. Once you have had a sense of the motion of the temporal bones at the CRI level, you then synchronize your perceptual field to the mid-tide level of perception. Do this by allowing your hands to float in fluid as they float on the bones. Then widen your perceptual field to the biosphere as previously learned. The biosphere includes the whole of the person's body and the field around it. Listen within this wider field of awareness. First become aware of the fluid tide, the fluid element within the mid-tide. Then include the tissues. Let the tissues move you as you listen to the whole of the system within this wider perceptual field. Does this change the quality of what you are perceiving? How? Do you sense deeper, more holistic motions? Do you have more of a perception of forces at work?

5. In a class situation, you would do the above observational process twice, first with minimal in-

formation and then with a clearer understanding of the classical context and tutor feedback.

In the next section, you will shift your attention to the cranial vault. You will again initiate a listening process with the tissues as outlined above.

The Cranial Vault

The cranial vault is composed of bones that were largely formed in membrane during their embryological development. The cranial vault is mainly composed of the frontal and parietal bones. It also includes the squama of the occiput and temporal bones, and the greater wings of the sphenoid. In the following sections you will be exploring the motion dynamics of the frontal and parietal bones, which are the major bones of the cranial vault. (See Figure 10.7.)

These bones are in most direct contact with the falx cerebri. The falx is composed of two parts, the *falx cerebri,* which is located above the confluence of sinuses, and the *falx cerebelli*, which is located below the confluence of sinuses. The falx cerebri, as its name implies, is located in relationship to the cerebral hemispheres, and the falx cerebelli is located in relationship to the cerebellum. The falx is the vertical aspect of the intracranial dura, and its dynamics can be thought of as directly continuous with that of the dural tube below. (See Figure 10.8.)

The Frontal Bone

The frontal bone is formed from two bones at birth, which later fuse at their metopic suture, a midline suture. The midline of the frontal bone is most in contact with the falx cerebri, the superior-anterior aspect of the reciprocal tension membrane. Its dynamic will thus directly effect the membrane system at this most anterior superior pole. Likewise, the patterns held within the dynamics of the reciprocal tension membrane will also directly effect the frontal bone and its local dynamics. The frontal

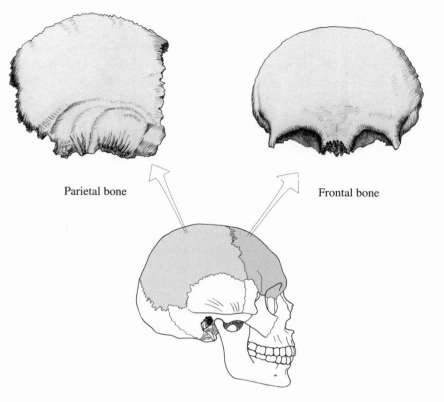

Parietal bone

Frontal bone

10.7 Frontal and parietal bones

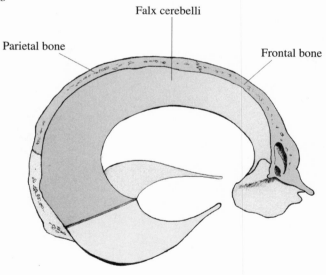

Falx cerebelli

Parietal bone

Frontal bone

10.8 Parietal and frontal bones and continuity to falx

bone has articular relationships with twelve other bones. These include the ethmoid bone, the sphenoid bone, the parietal bones, the lacrimals, the maxillae, the nasal bones, and the zygomatic bones. The frontal bones are thus intimately related to facial dynamics. These dynamics will be explored in chapters on the dynamics of the face and hard palate in Volume Two. (See Figure 10.9.)

Inertial issues relating to the dynamics of the frontal bone commonly arise during the birth process. The frontal bone may experience strong compressive forces during birth, especially in its later stages or in posterior presentations or android pelvic shapes. Overriding of the metopic suture can occur and compression and torsion between the parts of the frontal bone at birth can later be expressed as intraosseous lesions. See the chapters on birth dynamics in Volume Two.

Motion of the Frontal Bone

Embryologically, the frontal bone is largely formed in membrane as two separate bones. They are separated by the vertically oriented metopic suture, which ossifies by five to six years of age. (See Figure 10.10.) Although the frontal bone fuses at the metopic suture, there is still flexibility and motion allowed. Because of this, the frontal bone will still ideally act as though it is two bones. It expresses its motility and motion as a paired bone. In about eight to ten percent of adults the metopic suture is not completely fused.

In the inhalation phase, the two sections of frontal bone express their inhalation motions as though there is still a metopic suture in place. Classically this is called external rotation and is said to occur around vertical axes roughly from the center of each orbital

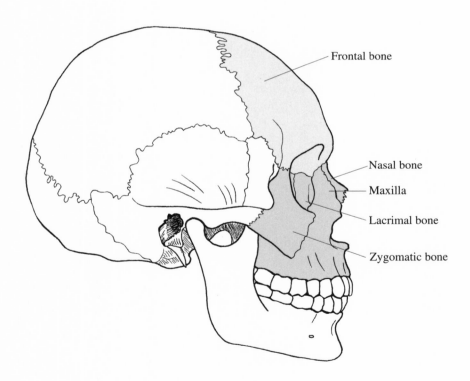

Frontal bone

Nasal bone

Maxilla

Lacrimal bone

Zygomatic bone

10.9 Frontal bone relationships and facial structure

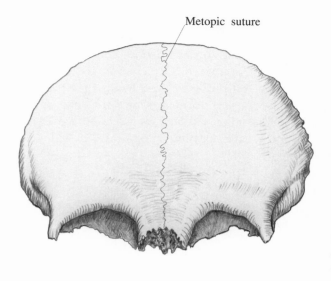

Metopic suture

10.10 Frontal bone and metopic suture

sense a reciprocal tension motion first in one direction and then in another. If you are listening within the mid-tide level of perception, you will sense a deeper inner motility at work. In this unfoldment, the frontal bone will seem to be part of a greater whole and will be perceived to express an inner tidal motility. Its motion will have more of a welling up and receding quality to it and will be perceived to be part of a greater expression of motility throughout the body. This will be sensed to be part of the whole motion of the cranium and even of the body as a whole. In foundation courses in the cranial field, if students naturally listen through the mid-tide, trying to sense the CRI and its faster rate of motion can be frustrating. It is the role of the tutor to help the student know the level they are listening to and to help them shift their perceptual fields to other tidal unfoldments.

In the following palpation session, you will simply listen to the tissues and see what they have to tell you. Do not come to the frontal bone with any preconceptions. Listen for how those tissues are or-

plate through each frontal eminence. The midline of the frontal bone, at the glabella, follows the sickle of the falx posterior as it deepens and moves posterior. The lateral aspects of the frontal bone mirrors the tentorium and the greater wings of the sphenoid in flexion and widens laterally and anterior. All of this generates a flaring out action in external rotation. The upshot of this is that the frontal bone acts as though it is two separate bones, each rotating around a vertical axis at its midline. (See Figure 10.11.) In external and internal rotation, there is said to be a hinge-like action at the metopic suture. Within the mid-tide, the frontal bone may be sensed to express an inner motility or intraosseous motion. In the inhalation phase, you may sense that the bone widens as its lateral aspects flare apart. There is a posterior deepening at the metopic suture as this occurs.

Within the CRI, you may sense the frontal bone to be expressing a relatively fast rate of motion. It may seem to be a separate tissue structure moving in relationship to other separate structures. You may

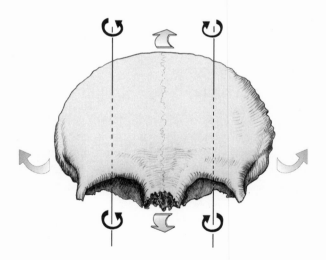

Inhalation external rotation

10.11 Craniosacral motion of the frontal bone

ganized around Health. How do they express the groundswell of the Breath of Life as motility and motion?

Classic Motion of the Frontal Bone

- *The frontal bone expresses its motion as though it is still two bones.*

- *In the inhalation phase, the two sections of frontal bone express a hinge-like external rotation.*

- *This is said to occur around vertical axes roughly from the center of each orbital plate through each frontal eminence.*

- *The midline of the frontal bone, at the glabella, follows the sickle of the falx posterior as it deepens and moves posterior.*

- *The lateral aspects of the frontal bone widen laterally and anterior.*

- *All of this generates a flaring out and widening action in external rotation.*

- *The opposite occurs in internal rotation.*

Clinical Application: Palpating Frontal Bone Dynamics

In the following session, the intention is to make a relationship to the frontal bone and to simply listen to its dynamics. In this listening, you may perceive both its motility and its interosseous motion. You may sense an inner breath and an outer motion. We will start at a CRI level of action and will then shift to the mid-tide in order to sense the different perceptual experience within each unfoldment.

1. First place your hands in the vault hold, establish your practitioner fulcrums, and tune into the system. Next, change your hand position to a *frontal hold*. Your hands are placed over the frontal bone with your thumbs crossed and your

fingers in gentle contact with the frontal bone via its anterior and lateral aspects. Your fingertips are just overlapping the orbital ridge. Your thumbs do not touch the cranium but act as fulcrums, which allows your hands to act as one unit. You are not just using your fingertips to make contact, but have as much of your fingers in contact as possible. (See Figure 10.12.)

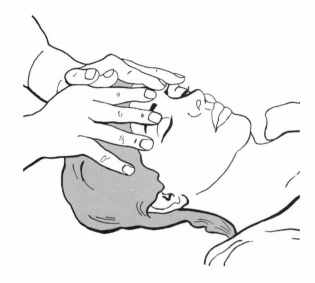

10.12 Frontal hold

2. Remember to establish your practitioner fulcrums and to negotiate your relationship to the patient's system. Start with the CRI level of action. Let your contact be as though you are floating on corks, which are, in turn, floating on water. Narrow your perceptual field to the tissues being palpated. Get interested in how the frontal bone is moving. Allow the tissues to move you as you listen. Simply float lightly on the patient's system. As you are listening to the frontal bone, see if you can sense its external-internal rotation. See if you can sense the unit

of motion of the falx and the frontal bone. As the sickle of the falx curls posteriorly at the crista galli in flexion, can you sense the reciprocal motion at the frontal bone? Remember, these are relatively subtle motions. Be open to any possibility. Do not try to find anything. Do not look for anything. Simply listen, observe, and notice how you are moved.

3. Once you have had an experience of the CRI level of action, shift your perceptual field to the mid-tide level of perception. Do this by allowing your hands to float in fluid as they float on the bones. Then widen your perceptual field to the biosphere, the whole of the person's body and the field around the person. Let your mind settle into listening to the *whole* of the person's system. Listen within this wider field of awareness. As you do this, do not lose awareness of the frontal bone within that larger field. First listen to the action of the fluid tide, and then include the tissues of the frontal bone in this listening. Does your experience of motion change? Do you begin to sense a deeper motility at word? Do tidal forces at work become more obvious?

In a classroom situation, you will do the above observational process twice, first with minimal information and then with a clearer understanding of the classical context with tutor feedback.

Parietal Bones

The parietal bones are paired structures that make up a large part of the superior aspect of the cranial vault. Each parietal bone articulates with five other bones. These include the other parietal bone, the frontal bone, the temporal bone, the sphenoid bones, and the occiput. (See Figure 10.13.) The parietal bones tend to accommodate in their position and motion dynamic any patterns held within the cranial base. They will also clearly reflect pelvic patterns in their dynamic. The sagittal sinus and

parasagittal area is the main location for arachnoid granulations through which the cerebrospinal fluid is drained from the cranium. Any inertial issues held within parietal dynamics will affect this drainage process. The parietal bones may experience different levels of trauma because they commonly take on the forces of head bumps, falls, and even birth forces. They are intimately in contact with the falx cerebri, and any strain pattern held within the system will be transferred to their dynamic in some way.

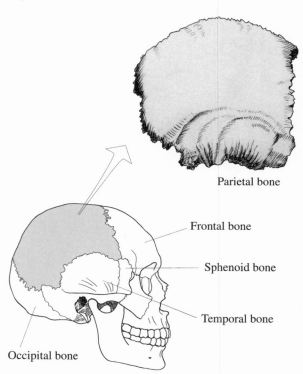

Parietal bone

Frontal bone

Sphenoid bone

Temporal bone

Occipital bone

10.13 Parietal bone relationships

Motion of the Parietal Bones

In this section you will shift your exploration to the parietal bones. In this, you will again simply listen to their motion dynamics. As you listen, the inner motility and motion of the parietal bones may be communicated to you. Remember that the parietal bones have a direct relationship with the falx cerebri. By including an awareness of the falx cerebri in your listening, you can get a sense of the direct continuity of cranial bones with the reciprocal tension membrane.

The parietal bones express their motion as paired bones that have an internal/external rotation motion and relationship. Basically, in the inhalation phase, the lateral aspects of the parietal bones widen apart as the sagittal suture moves inferior and deepens. Classically, each bone is said to have its own axis of rotation. Motion is said to occur around an axis from a point on the coronal suture, just lat-

eral to the bregma, which runs posterior-laterally to the related parietal eminence.

As the two parietal bones express external rotation, they rotate around these axes and their lateral aspects widen apart as their sagittal borders move inferior and also widen apart. This widening apart at the sagittal suture occurs especially at its posterior aspect. This can be clearly seen anatomically, because this greater posterior motion is accommodated by the deeper serrate articulatory surfaces in the posterior aspect of the suture. As this occurs, the falx cerebri is shortening front to back, deepening and sinking, and the tentorium cerebelli is flattening and widening. (See Figure 10.14.) Again, within

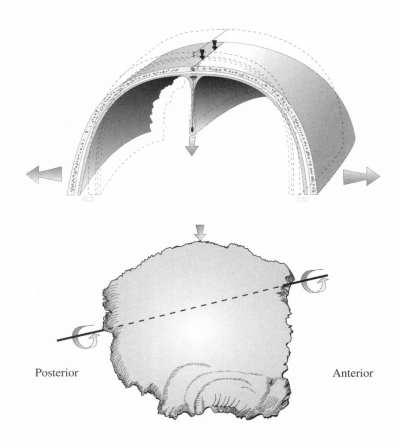

Posterior   Anterior

10.14 Cranionsacral Motion of the parietal bones in inhalation the mid-tide level of action, you may sense a more intraosseous expression of this dynamic. A parietal bone may be sensed to expand and widen from within the inhalation surge of the Tide.

Clinical Application:
Palpating Parietal Bone Dynamics

In this section, you will continue your exploration into the motility and mobility of cranial bones and their continuity with the membrane system. In this process, you will learn a new hold and will explore the dynamics of the parietal bones. The intention is to listen and to allow the dynamics of the parietal bones to speak to you. This process calls for an quality of listening in which you are open to the unknown and do not bring any preconceptions or judgments to this unique encounter.

1. After generally sensing the dynamics of the system from the vault hold, shift to a parietal hold. Cross your thumbs and hold them above the sagittal suture. Your thumbs do not actually touch the bones. They float above them to create fulcrums, which allows your hands to function as one unit. Place the finger pads of each hand on the parietal bones above the squamosal suture. Your fingers are placed close together to ensure that you are just on the parietal bones. (See Figure 10.15.)

2. Settle into your practitioner fulcrums, negotiate your contact with the patient's system, and sense the quality of its potency and resources. Start at the CRI level of perception as in the exercises above. Again, float on the tissues and let them show you their dynamic. As you listen to the parietal bones from this vantage point, do you start to sense their motion at a CRI level? See if the motion of the parietal bones comes into your awareness. Again, do not look for this; simply float on the tissues, listen, and let the tis-

sues move you. Simply appreciate how they express their motion.

3. You might sense a widening apart of the two bones as they express external rotation in their inhalation phase. Allow your hands to just float on the bony structures and notice how they move within the membranes. Can you sense the continuity of motion between the falx and the parietal bones? As the falx deepens in inhalation, can you sense the deepening at the sagittal suture? Does this motion seem balanced? Can you sense the continuity of their motion with the motion of the reciprocal tension membrane?

4. Once you have a sense of the motion dynamics of the parietal bones within the CRI, shift your perceptual field to the mid-tide level of perception as explored in the exercises above. Let your hands float in fluid and widen your perceptual field to the biosphere. Does this change your perception of parietal motion? Do you have a sense of a wider field of action? Do you begin to sense a deeper motility at work? Do tidal forces at work become more obvious?

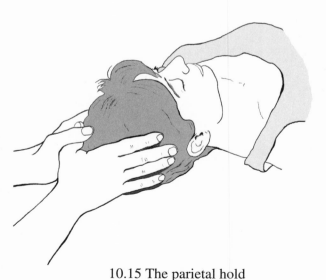

10.15 The parietal hold

Classic Motion of the Parietal Bone

- *In the inhalation phase, the lateral aspects of the parietal bones widen apart as the sagittal suture moves inferior and deepens.*

- *This motion is said to occur around an axis through each bone from a point on the*

coronal suture, just lateral to the bregma, which runs posterior-laterally to the related parietal eminence.

- *As the two parietal bones express external rotation, they rotate around these axes and their lateral aspects widen apart as their sagittal borders move inferior and also widen apart.*

In the next chapter you will begin to explore the basic motion dynamics of the cranial base and sphenobasilar junction. In this process you will explore the motion of the sphenoid and occiput. The next chapter introduces the sacrum and the sacrum's motion dynamics.

1. I'd like to acknowledge the work of Dr. Michael Shea in understanding the shamanistic and ritualistic nature of healing work and of work within the cranial field.

11

Introduction to the Dynamics of the Sphenobasilar Junction

In the previous chapter, you listened to the motility and mobility of the temporal bones, the frontal bone, and the parietal bones. The intention was to simply allow an awareness of their dynamics to come into your perceptual field. In this section you will continue with that intention and turn your attention to the dynamics of the sphenoid and occiput around the SBJ. This is a common starting point in many courses. In a class situation, you will first be given minimal information before an initial palpation session. The anatomy will be introduced, but not a description of motion. You will then exchange short palpation sessions. After the session, you will meet in the large group to see what you have discovered. Then the classical understanding of tissue motion is presented and a further palpation session is undertaken with tutor feedback. In following sections, we will first review the dynamics of the SBJ and then explore some palpation work.

In this chapter we will:

- *Review the classical dynamics of the SBJ, occiput, and sacrum.*

- *Present some palpation sessions in which to explore these. The Sphenobasilar Junction*

The sphenobasilar junction (SBJ) is a joint of particular interest within the cranial concept. It is the junction where the basiocciput and the body of the sphenoid bone meet. The motion around the SBJ is considered to be an important focus within the cranial concept. In the inhalation phase, as potency and fluid rise within the system, the SBJ is also said to rise. It is like the center of an underwater flower, which rises with the rising tide. As this occurs, both the sphenoid and occiput bones express their motility and motion in relationship to the SBJ and to Sutherland's fulcrum. The sphenoid bone, as previously discussed, is said to act like a major gear within bony motion dynamics. It articulates with twelve other bones. These include the occiput, the temporal bones, the parietal bones, the frontal bone, the ethmoid bone, the palatines, the vomer, and the zygomatic bones. The occiput, in turn, articulates with six other bones. These include the sphenoid bone, the temporal bones, the parietal bones, and the atlas. (See Figure 11.1.) In inhalation, as the SBJ rises, all of these bones, like flower petals opening, express expansion and widening.

In the adult, the SBJ is a synchondrosis, which allows the sphenoid and occiput to express motion. The sphenobasilar junction is classically considered to be a central focal point for flexion-extension motion of all bony structures within the cranium and within the body as a whole. The motion dynamics

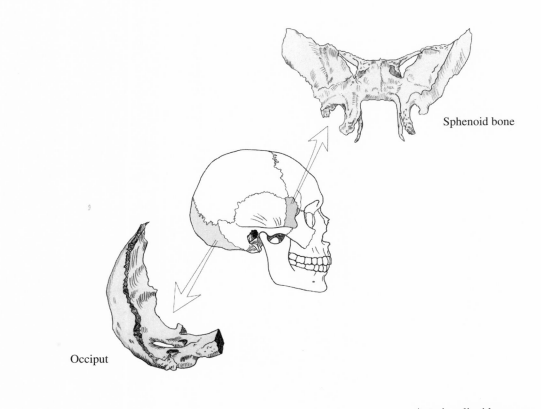

Sphenoid bone

Occiput

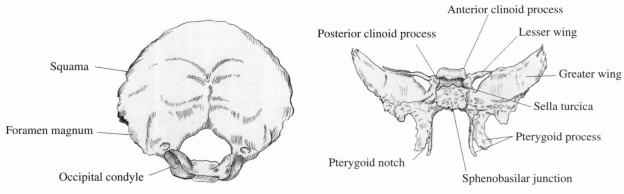

Squama

Foramen magnum

Occipital condyle

Occiput

Anterior clinoid process

Posterior clinoid process

Lesser wing

Greater wing

Sella turcica

Pterygoid process

Pterygoid notch

Sphenobasilar junction

Sphenoid bone

11.1 Sphenoid and occiput

of all bones are thought to key off the SBJ. In other words, all bony motion in the craniosacral system is ideally at a point of balance around the SBJ. All of the dynamics of bony motion within the cranium will be expressed as some kind of organization around the SBJ. Remember that the tissues of the body form a unit of function. They express their motility in relationship to the expression of potency within the fluids as a whole. Tensile tissue motions are generated throughout the body all at once. You might consider the SBJ to be an ideal point of balance within this overall tensile motion. As we shall see, due to this wholeness, any inertial pattern held within the SBJ will be expressed in some form throughout the cranium, and indeed throughout the rest of the body. Inertia held anywhere within the cranium and body will also be expressed at the SBJ in some way. It can be said that the dynamics of the SBJ encapsulate our entire life history as patterns of shape, form, and motion. Having said this, it is again important to stress that bone is a connective tissue and is part of a greater connective tissue field. Bone and membrane are a unit of function, and the natural fulcrum for the entirety of their unified dynamic is Sutherland's fulcrum. All connective tissues exhibit a unified dynamic organized around Sutherland's fulcrum, a point of potency within the anterior aspect of the straight sinus. Sutherland's fulcrum is an expression of the midline organizing intentions of the Breath of Life and is embryologically derived. Awareness of its dynamics can give the insightful observer critical clinical information as to how the system has organized itself and how it is resolving its inertial issues. We will explore the dynamics of Sutherland's fulcrum in later chapters. In this chapter, we will explore the natural motility and motion of the sphenoid bone and occiput around the SBJ. We will describe clinical approaches to their common inertial patterns in the chapter on cranial base dynamics in Volume Two.

Motion Dynamics around the SBJ

In this section we will describe the classic motion dynamics around the SBJ in more detail. As we have seen, tissue motion is related to the two phases of primary respiration. In each phase of primary respiration, there are related tissue motions. These tissue motions are classically called *flexion-external rotation* and *extension-internal rotation*. Flexion is expressed in the inhalation phase of primary respiration, extension is expressed in the exhalation phase. It is important to understand that these motions were named by Dr. Sutherland according to the relationship between the sphenoid bone and the occiput at the cranial base. Furthermore, the nomenclature is derived from the relationship of their inferior aspects at the cranial base. Thus, all craniosacral tissue motion in the entire body is named in relationship to the dynamics of the *inferior* aspect of these two bones. In the inhalation phase of the Tide, the sphenoid and occiput are said to rotate around transverse axes in *opposite directions*. Their inferior surfaces move closer together and the sphenobasilar junction rises. This is called *craniosacral flexion*. This nomenclature relates to the moving together or flexion of the inferior aspects of these bones. As this occurs, the greater wings of the sphenoid and the lateral aspects of the occipital squama also widen apart and rotate/dive caudad (footward). (See Figure 11.2.)

In the exhalation phase of the rhythm, the reverse process occurs. The sphenoid and occiput are said to rotate in opposite directions around transverse axes in the reverse direction. Their inferior surfaces move apart and the sphenobasilar junction sinks. This is called *craniosacral extension*. This nomenclature relates to the moving apart or extension of the inferior aspects of these two bones. The greater wings of the sphenoid and the lateral aspects of the occipital squama narrow and rotate cephalad (headward) as this occurs. (See Figure 11.3.)

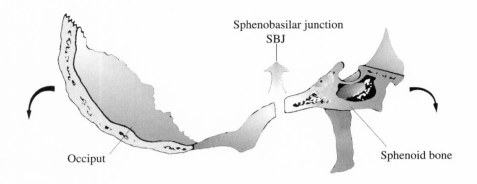

11.2 Motion of the sphenoid and occiput in inhalation / flexion

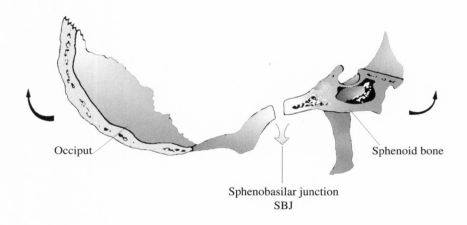

11.3 Motion of sphenoid and occiput in exhalation / extension

Within the mid-tide level of perception, you may sense a more holistic action. The sphenoid and occiput will not be perceived to be separate from the other structures within the cranium, nor will axes of rotation be relevant. A unified tensile field is perceived. In inhalation, a welling up within all tissues may be sensed simultaneously. The SBJ will be sensed to rise with the rising tide. The sphenoid and occiput will be sensed to express both their intraosseous and interosseous dynamic within this context. It has more of the sense of a flower opening. Imagine an underwater flower. The flower is immersed in fluid and supported by that fluid. As the tide surges within the waters, the center of the flower rises as the flower petals open within the fluid field. The individual petals are part of a unified flower-field, which flowers open inexpansion/widening. As this occurs, each flower petal is still discernible in its inner and outer motion. In exhalation, the flower-tissues settle within the fluid field and you may sense the flower petals settling and closing. Cranial bones are like this. The inhalation-exhalation motions of the cranium may be perceived in a similar way to a flower opening and closing within a fluid field. The inner intraosseous motion of each bone will be discernible, as will the interosseous motions between bones. Another analogy might be kelp beds at the bottom of the sea. As the tide surges, the kelp beds within the waters open and float with the tidal force. As the tide recedes, the kelp beds sink and settle.

Palpating Motion: The Vault Hold

In this section, we will use the vault hold to begin to tune into and appreciate the motion around the SBJ. Let's first remember the specific placement of the hands in the vault hold. There are two classic applications of the vault hold. One is sometimes called "Dr. Sutherland's Hold," or the classic vault hold, and the other, "Dr. Becker's Hold," or the modified vault hold. In the classic vault hold, your index fingers should be over the greater wing of the sphenoid which is located in the hollow behind the corner of the eye. Your middle fingers should be in front of the ear over the zygomatic process of the temporal bone, your ring fingers should be behind the ear over the mastoid portions, and your little fingers should be on, or as near as possible to, the occiput. The rest of your hand should be gently cradling the head with as much gentle contact as possible. You can pick up a huge amount of information from the palms of your hands, which are over the parietal and frontal bones. Your thumbs are gently resting on the parietal bones. This hold gives a global sense of the cranium and its dynamics. A variation on this hold is to have the index fingers at the greater wings while all the other fingers are behind the ear over the mastoid processes and occiput. (See Figure 11.4.) In Dr. Becker's vault hold, you gently place your thumbs at the greater wings of the sphenoid bone and your little fingers over the occipital squama. The rest of your hand gently cups the cranium behind the ears. This hold can more

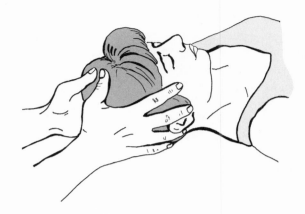

11.4 Dr. Sutherland's hold; classic vault hold

specifically tune you into the dynamic between the sphenoid and occiput at the SBJ, but also will give a global sense of the system within the mid-tide level of perception. (See Figure 11.5.)

Your quality of physical contact should be as though you are floating on corks, which are in turn floating on water. You do not want to place any pressure on the corks, or you will stop them from

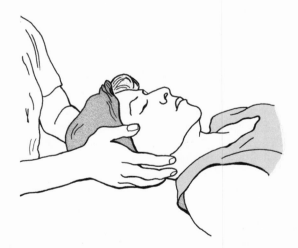

11.5 Dr. Becker's hold; modified vault hold

171

doing what they would naturally do if you were not in contact with them. Allow your hands to be taken by the tissues and fluids on a journey of discovery. You may perceive their motion dynamics to be amplified as you sense from the fulcrum you established in your elbows or from the earth. The longer the lever, the greater will the movement be perceived. Establish a fulcrum to listen from and note the amplification of your proprioceptive sense. In your listening process, you want your physical contact to be neutral. You do not want to introduce forces into the system. You do not want to grab onto the tissues or fluids, and you do not want to lock up the structure and function of the tissues. Finally, you do not want to unconsciously grab onto the tissues with your attention. You must have a clear understanding and experience of negotiating your contact and that includes the contact you make via your attention field. As we have said many times, the first step is to simply *listen*. Just listen in an actively receptive state of being. Stay neutral and receptive and allow yourself to be moved by the patient's system. Don't narrow your attention down into your hands. Remember to listen from a negotiated distance. As you palpate the patient's system, hold a light gentle attention. Don't look for anything, but *listen* and let the tissues come to you. That is really important. Don't look for anything, but be in a receptive state and *listen*. Allow the tissues to come to you. Be patient. You will be surprised at the information that is communicated and the insights that arise. As you palpate the motions at the sphenoid and occiput, you may notice two basic dynamics in your hands. In the inhalation phase the greater wings and occipital squama will take your palpating hands caudad (footward). As you sense this, you may also sense that your hands are transversely widening apart. In the exhalation phase, you may sense the reverse. Your palpating hands will be sensed to float cephalad (superior) and a narrowing between your hands may also be sensed. Remember that in inhalation, as the tissues express flexion, the sphenobasilar junction is rising. As this occurs, the flower petals are opening and

the parts of the bones that you are palpating are widening and moving caudad. Classically it is said that the sphenoid and occiput rotate around transverse axes. As they do this, the greater wings and occipital squama are sensed to rotate caudad under your palpating fingers. The reverse occurs in exhalation. (See Figure 11.6.)

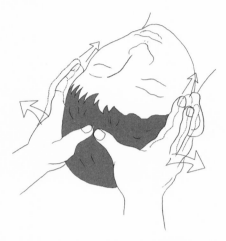

11.6 Motion sensed via palpation
in inhalation / flexion

Classic Motion of the Sphenoid and Occiput

- The sphenoid rotates around a transverse axis within its body just anterior to the floor of the sella turcica; in inhalation the anterior aspect of its body rotates inferior, while its posterior aspect rises; as this occurs the greater wing and pterygoid sections widen.

- The occiput rotates around a transverse axis located just cephalad and anterior to the center of the foramen magnum at the level of the sphenobasilar junction; in inhalation, the basiocciput rotates cephalad with the rising of the sphenobasilar junction and the occipital squama rotates caudad. As this occurs there is also a widening of the occipital squama.

In the inhalation phase:

- The greater wings and occipital squama will take your palpating hands caudad (inferior/footward). As you perceive this, you may also sense that your hands are transversely widening apart.

In the exhalation phase:

- You may sense the reverse. Your palpating hands will be sensed to float cephalad (superior/headward), and you may also perceive a narrowing between your hands.

Clinical Application:
Palpation via the Vault Hold

I. Motion at the SBJ

1. In either vault hold described above, negotiate your contact with the patient's system and tune into the fluid tide and resources of the system. Now shift your perceptual field to the CRI and to the tissues under your palpating hands. Become interested in how the tissues under your palpating hands are moving. Gently become aware of the motion at the greater wings of the sphenoid and at the squama of the occiput. To do this, become more aware of the motion under your index and little fingers (or under your thumbs and little fingers in the modified vault hold). As you do this, don't narrow down your attention. Sense from your fulcrums with the whole of your hands. Remember to maintain a negotiated distance. Allow the tissues to come to you. Don't close things down by narrowing your attention. Imagine/sense that your hands are floating on the tissues, which are floating on water.

2. In the inhalation phase, the two bones normally express craniosacral flexion. You may sense that their greater wings and occipital squama float inferior/caudad. This may seem as if the sphenoid and occiput are diving inferior/caudad towards the feet. In the exhalation phase, you may sense that the two bones are floating superior/cephalad towards you as you sit at the head of the table.

3. Again, try not to place too much attention in your index and little fingers, because this may be sensed as intense pressure by the patient. Rather, try to perceive with your whole hand with an awareness of the greater wings and occipital squama. Listen from your fulcrums and let the tissue motions come to you. Again, as you listen to flexion-extension, be sure that you are not grabbing onto their system with your attention. Let their tissues take you. Float. As you listen to the caudad/cephalad motion at the greater wings and occipital squama, don't forget that the sphenobasilar junction is rising in inhalation-flexion and sinking in exhalation-extension. You may be able to bring this awareness into your hands as you watch the motion at the greater wings and the occipital squama.

4. After you have had some experience of the motion around the SBJ within the CRI level of perception, shift your perceptual field to the mid-tide level of perception. Widen your perceptual field to include the whole of the biosphere. As you float on the tissues, allow your hands to be immersed within a fluid field. Float on the bones and membranes as though they are living kelp, which are in turn floating within fluid and moved by the Tide. If you place too much pressure on the kelp (i.e., the tissues), you will stop them from showing you their inherent motions. First sense the fluid tide, then include the tissues and their movement. As you begin to palpate these motions, see if you can sense the potency that moves them. Again, see if the

experience of motion is perceived differently within this mid-tide or tidal potency level of perception. You may have a more holistic sense of motility and a more integrated experience of cranial dynamics. You have more of a sense of tissue motion like that described above, like a flower opening and closing. As the potency and fluids surge in inhalation, the SBJ may be sensed to rise as the flower petals open and widen apart. Do you sense the bones breathing? Do you sense their inner motility? This inner breath is the expression of how the bones express the potency of the Breath of Life. This is an expression of health at work. Does your experience of motion change here?

Palpation via the Occipital Squama

II. Motion at the Occiput

1. In this application we will return to the *occipital cradle hold* learned earlier. In this hold, place your hands under the patient's head with your little fingers touching, hands and fingers spread and pointing caudad. The fingers of your hands should be comfortably cradling the patient's head. Do not generate any pressure against the patient's occiput with the heels of your hands. (See Figure 11.7.) Again, imagine and sense that your hands are on the tissues being palpated. Synchronize your perceptual field with the CRI level of perception as outlined above.

2. From this vantage point, listen to the tissues that you are palpating. You are now listening to the tissues directly under your palpating hands. Do not narrow down your attention; listen from a negotiated distance. Again, allow your hands to float on these tissues which are in turn floating on fluid. Get interested in how the occiput is moving. You may then begin to sense the motion of the occiput. Just let your hands listen and be taken by the patient's tissues into their motions. You may sense the squama widening in

the inhalation phase as it is perceived to settle inferior. Classically, it is said that the occiput rotates around a transverse axis. This axis is located just cephalad and anterior to the center of the foramen magnum at the level of the sphenobasilar junction. It is not located within the bone itself.

3. Let your hands gently float on the tissues and be taken by them as they express their motion. Let the motion come into your hands. Let your hands be moved by it. Don't try to look for motion; just listen and let your hands float on the tissues. Although I have described an ideal motion of the occiput, be open to anything. There may indeed be very little motion expressed due to inertial issues and compressive patterns.

4. Again, once you have had some experience of the motion of the occiput within the CRI, shift your perceptual field to the mid-tide level of action. Let your hands float within fluid and widen your perceptual field to the biosphere. How does this change your experience of motion as you listen to the *whole* via the occiput? You may have a sense of an inner breath expressed as an intraosseous expansion and widening within the bone itself. A more holistic sense of motion may

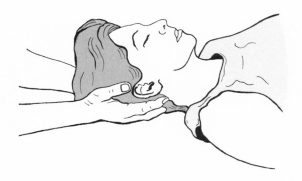

11.7 Occipital cradle hold

predominate. How does the occiput express primary respiration? As you synchronize your attention with the mid-tide field of action, how does this change your perception of motion?

The Sacrum

The sacrum is a large wedge-shaped bone at the base of the spine. It is something like a curved upside-down pyramid. It articulates with the last lumbar vertebra at the lumbosacral junction, with the ilia at the sacroiliac joints, and with the coccyx

below. (See Figure 11.8.) At birth the sacrum is in five parts, which are five modified vertebra. The sacrum ossifies fully in adulthood. Its two most superior components ossify between the seventh and eighth year of life. Intraosseous lesions of the sacrum are often seen and commonly arise during birth or in early childhood. These are due to the presence of unresolved compressive forces within the tissues of the sacrum. The sacrum and coccyx rest at the inferior pole of the midline and inertial issues held within their dynamics can strongly affect the quality of potency and drive within the

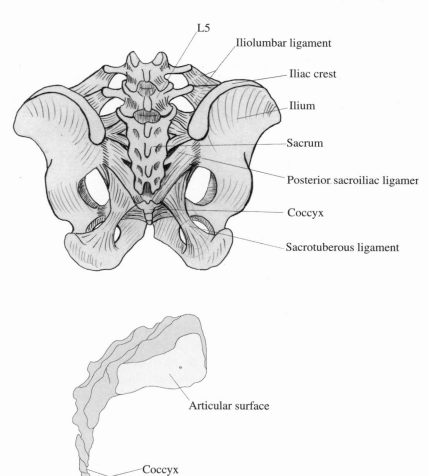

L5

Iliolumbar ligament

Iliac crest

Ilium

Sacrum

Posterior sacroiliac ligamer

Coccyx

Sacrotuberous ligament

Articular surface

Coccyx

11.8 The sacrum

system. If the sacrum is compressed within its articulations, the central nervous system can become tethered in its expression of motility, because the spinal cord is anchored to the coccyx via the filament terminale, an extension of pia mater and dura. We will discuss the dynamics of the sacrum and the central nervous system in more detail in Volume Two.

Motion of the Sacrum

We are including an introduction to the motion dynamics of the sacrum here because its expression is directly related to the SBJ above. The dynamics of the SBJ and sacrum are a clear unit of function, because they are located at the superior and inferior poles of the midline. The notochord midline has its most inferior pole within the coccyx and its most superior pole within the body of the sphenoid. The craniosacral dynamics of each will be directly mirrored within the forms of motion expressed at each pole. The sacrum expresses its motion as a midline bone. Like all midline bones, it is said to rotate around a transverse axis in the opposite direction to the sphenoid bone. Its motion is ideally in synchrony with the occiput above. Like all bony structures, sacral motion is ideally organized in relationship to the midline and to Sutherland's fulcrum above. It will also express its motion dynamic in relationship to the SBJ and its dynamics. In inhalation, as potency surges and the SBJ rises, you may perceive a subtle cephalad lifting of the sacrum, then a rotation of its superior aspect posterior and superior. You may also sense an intraosseous widening and uncurling of the sacral, segments which is an expression of inner motility. This is classically called *craniosacral flexion*. As the sacrum expresses its inhalation motion, you may perceive a filling in your hand. In exhalation, you may perceive a subtle caudad settling of the sacrum, then a rotation of the superior aspect of the sacrum anterior and inferior. You may also sense an intraosseous narrowing and curling up of the sacral segments. This is called *craniosacral extension*. As the sacrum expresses its exhalation motion, you

may perceive an emptying or receding in your hand. (See Figure 11.9.)

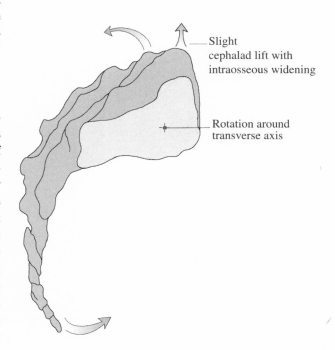

Slight cephalad lift with intraosseous widening

Rotation around transverse axis

11.9 The motion of the sacrum in inhalation

The motion of the sacrum is totally integrated with the other dynamics of the primary respiratory system. Remember that bone is a connective tissue. Think of bone as being continuous with all of the connective tissues of the body. All connective tissues form a unified tensile field of action. Thus the sacrum and dura are part of the same field of motion. The sacrum should literally be perceived to float within the sacroiliac joints. In inhalation, as the potency surges, the sacrum may be sensed to subtly float cephalad. Along with this, the dural tube also rises in inhalation. As the dural tube expresses its rising action, there is a subtle superior lift at its inferior pole of attachment at S2. As this occurs there is also a superior and posterior rotation of the sacrum at its base. (See Figure 11.10.)

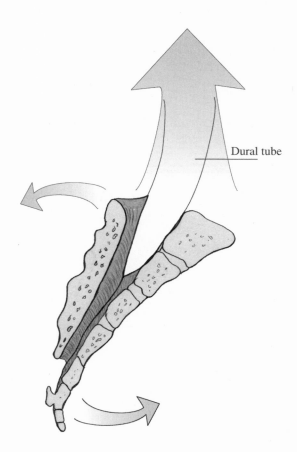

11.10 Dural tube rises
in inhalation

The central nervous system is also directly related to the dynamics of the sacrum. The central nervous system is anchored at its most inferior pole within the vertebral canal at the coccyx. The pia mater which surrounds the spinal cord pierces the dura within the sacral canal, becomes the filament terminalis, and attaches to the coccyx. This filament is also invested with a thin coating of dura. If the sacrum is compressed in any of its joint relation-ships or is holding inertial issues of any kind, the motility of the CNS will be directly effected. There will be a tethering of the spinal cord in its motility and mobility, and an inertial force will be introduced within CNS dynamics. CNS motility will be effected. (See Figure 11.11.) We will explore the dynamics of the sacrum and pelvis in much more detail in Volume Two. Within the mid-tide level of perception, all of this motion, that is, of bone, membrane, and neural tissue, can be perceived to be a unified field of action, a whole. Indeed, within the mid-tide the motion of potency, fluid, and of *all* tissues can be sensed to be a unified dynamic.

Motion at the Sacrum: Palpation via the Sacral Hold

After you have gained a clear sense of the craniosacral dynamics at the vault and occipital cradle holds, shift your vantage point to the sacrum. Here you will listen for the motion of the sacrum and for its expression of motility.

1. Begin the session at the sacrum. You will use the sacral hold as described earlier. Move your chair to the footward end of the table. Sit so that you are facing the patient's opposite shoulder. Place your hand under the sacrum with your fingers spread. Do not place any pressure on the sacrum with the heel of your hand. Your elbow should be more or less under the patient's knee with your wrist relatively straight. (See Figure 11.12.) Settle into your relationship with the patient, establish your practitioner fulcrums and negotiate your distance to the patient's system. Allow your palpating hand to float on the tissues of the sacrum, even though the weight of the body is on your hand. Soften and relax your palpating hand and imagine that it is floating under the table. This gives your patient a sense of space in the contact and allows you to have a sense of floating on the tissues of the sacrum.

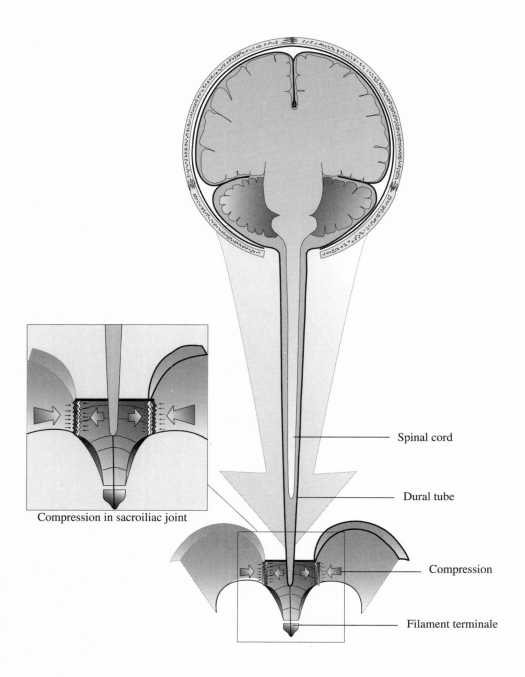

Compression in sacroiliac joint

Spinal cord

Dural tube

Compression

Filament terminale

11.11 Central nervous system and tethering

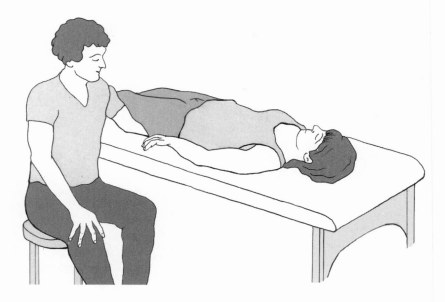

11.12 Sacral hold

2. Once again, you will first synchronize your perceptual field to the CRI level of unfoldment. From this vantage point, allow yourself to simply listen and be moved by the tissues of the sacrum. Remember the dynamics of the motility and mobility of the sacrum as earlier described. Notice the quality of the motion of the sacrum within the CRI level of action. Notice its ease of motion, or mobility. Mobility is its ability to express motion within the sacroiliac joints between the ilia, and motility is a deeper sense of primary breath as an inner respiratory motion. In the inhalation phase, you may perceive a subtle floating of the sacrum superior and a rotation of the base of the sacrum superior and posterior into your palpating hand. It may have a sense of filling your hand. In the exhalation/extension phase you may sense the sacral base receding from your palpating hand.

3. Once you have a sense of the CRI level of motion, again shift your perceptual field to the mid-tide level of perception as practiced above.

Allow your hands to float within fluid and widen your perceptual field to the biosphere. See if a sense of inner breath is communicated to you within this unfoldment. This inner motility is a direct expression of the Health of the system at work. It is important to remember that in this work we are always looking for how the system is expressing its Health and its healing resources. See if you can be aware of the inner motility of the sacrum as it widens and uncurls in its inhalation phase and narrows and curls up in its exhalation phase. In inhalation, you may sense a subtle rising of the sacrum and a widening and uncurling within your hand. You may sense that your hand is being filled. How does the perceptual shift change your sense of the motion of the sacrum?

Palpation via Sacrum and Occiput

In the last palpation session of this chapter, you will listen for motion and motility via both the sacrum and occiput. You will hold the two poles of the midline at the same time. The intention will be to see if you can sense the nature and quality of the integrated motion at both poles. All motility is a unit of function. Inhalation and exhalation happen all at once everywhere at once. See how the system can express this "one-thing-ness." In inhalation you may sense that the sacral base and occipital squama widen into your palpating hands. Your hands may have a sense of being filled. You may also begin to sense the continuity of the dural membranes under your hands. You may sense a rising of the membranes in inhalation and a sinking in exhalation. Imagine/sense that bone and membrane are one thing. How does this one thing express motion? Within the CRI level of action you may perceive the tissues to act as separate structures, which express a rate of motion anywhere from 8 to 14 cycles a minute. At a mid-tide level, the motion of the tissues will be sensed to be more of a unified field of action. You can sense the individual motions, but they seem to be part of a greater tensile field of action. You may also sense a surge filling and welling up within the tissues in inhalation, and a settling in exhalation at the slower rhythmic expression of 2.5 cycles a minute. You may also perceive the rising of the fluid tide within inhalation and its sinking within exhalation.

1. Have the patient move to a side lying position. You may want to place a small cushion under the patient's head and to place the knees in a comfortable position. Find a comfortable sitting position at the side of the table facing the patient's back. First place one hand, with your fingers pointing caudad, over the sacrum. Once you negotiate and establish that contact, place your other hand over the occiput with your fingers pointing cephalad. In this position, you are in relationship to two poles of the classic primary respiratory mechanism. (See Figure 11.13.) Again, let your contact float on the tissues and get interested in the motions of individual bones and membranes. Synchronize your perceptual field with the CRI. Listen and see if

you can discern the motions at each pole. Do you have a sense of the continuity of membrane between your hands? Is the motion balanced around the midline?

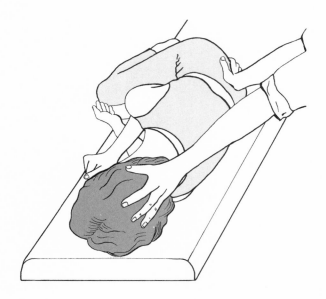

11.13 Sacrum and occiput hold; side lying

2. Now synchronize your attention with the mid-tide level of perception. Establish a wider perceptual field to include the whole of the biosphere. Does this change your perception of motion? See if you can sense a welling up under each hand in inhalation and an emptying or receding in exhalation. See if you can sense the rising and sinking of the fluid tide in each phase and the *force* within it. How do the tissues express this as a tensile field of action? How do you perceive the tissues expressing reciprocal tension motion within this slower 2.5 cycles a minute rhythm? Is this motion balanced around Sutherland's fulcrum and the midline? Simply listen to the relationships and dynamics of the system from these vantage points. Float within

the fluids and let motion and an awareness of force come to you. Again, don't look for anything, just listen and allow. This process of deeply listening to the system at these two poles at once can be very integrative and can be useful at the end of session work. In the next chapters, we will expand on these experiences of motility and motion and will begin to unfold some of the semi-

nal clinical skills of the cranial concept. These include the *point of balanced membranous tension* and the *state of balanced tension*.

12
Reciprocal Tensions

In this chapter, we will discuss the concept of reciprocal tension and reciprocal tension motion in some detail. We will introduce the idea of tensile fields, automatically shifting fulcrums, and reciprocal tension motion. In this chapter we will focus on the nature of the reciprocal tension membrane, although it must be borne in mind that all tissues are part of a unified tensile system, and all of the tissues within the body express reciprocal tension motion. It is also important to remember that potency and fluids, as tensile fields of action, also express reciprocal tension motion. We will discuss the motion dynamics of the reciprocal tension membrane in more detail than previously. The intention of this chapter is to deepen your perception and understanding of reciprocal tension motion dynamics. To this end you will engage in a number of palpation sessions and see what you discover.

In this chapter we will:

- *Discuss tensile fields, automatically shifting fulcrums, and reciprocal tension motion.*

- *Describe and listen for the reciprocal tension motion of the reciprocal tension membrane.*

- *Listen to the dynamics of the falx and tentorium.*

In a structured course these sessions would be approached in two stages. In the first you would be asked to palpate reciprocal tension motions with only a short review of the anatomy of the reciprocal tension membrane. After that session you would meet in the large group and see what you discovered. There would then be a discussion of the classical understanding of these dynamics and a second palpation session would be undertaken with tutor feedback. Let's unfold some of the concepts.

Tensile Fields
and Reciprocal Tension Motion

All of the tissue systems within the body act as tensile fields. A tensile field is a field of action that always holds a natural tension. In other words, there is a natural tension expressed throughout its form. What's more, all tensile fields express an inherent motility or motion, as a whole field of action. As an example, all of the tissues within the body are not separate; they are truly whole, a unified field. This unified field is moved by the respiratory action of the Tide, through its bioelectric potency. This is expressed as cycles of *reciprocal* motion, first in one direction and then in another. In other words, a reciprocal motion of the whole tissue field is expressed within the inhalation and exhalation cycles of the Tide. This manifests as a unified *tension* dynamic, which manifests *all at once* throughout the whole field. This kind of tensile motion is called *reciprocal tension motion*. We shall see that all of the tissues within the body function as a unified tensile field, and this field expresses a tensile motion orchestrated by the creative intentions of the Breath of Life and the action of its Tide. As the Tide manifests its respiratory cycles, the whole tissue field is moved. At the mid-tide level of action, this is perceived as a 2.5 cycles a minute tidal motion. In this chapter we will focus particularly on the dural membrane as a unified field of action. The internal aspects of the dura within the skull were called the reciprocal tension membrane by Dr. Sutherland. Their motion and function is critical to understand and is the first step in sensing and appreciating the concept of reciprocal tension motion. Although we are focusing on the reciprocal tension membrane, please remember that all of the tissues within the body are a unified whole and also express this kind of dynamic. That means that the dural membranes are not separate in their action from the rest of the tissues within the body. It must be also understood that fluids and potency, as unified fields of action, also express reciprocal tension motion. This is obvious when you remember that all tissue organization and motion is orchestrated by the organization and motion of the *potency* within the fluids. As we shall see, potency, fluids, and tissues are unified fields of action, and their dynamics can be perceived and have vast clinical importance. All three function as unified fields that express reciprocal tension motion. This is most obvious at the mid-tide level of action.

Suspended Automatically Shifting Fulcrums

All motion is organized by fulcrums, concentrated points of potency that govern the organization and motion of form. Each field of action has a natural fulcrum around which it is organized and by which it is moved. If fulcrums were not present, all would be chaos. They define the natural tensions and boundaries of every field of action. They are gener-

ated by the action of the Breath of Life as the Original matrix of a human being is laid down. A fulcrum gives the whole field of action, be it tissues, fluids, or potency, a focus that maintains order and coherent relationship. These points are concentrations of potency, which are still places within a whole field of action. The fulcrum both organizes the field and is the point around which it moves. Natural fulcrums are expressed embryologically and maintain order throughout life. All reciprocal tension motion is organized and generated by the action of these fulcrums.

Naturally occurring fulcrums were called *suspended automatically shifting fulcrums* by Dr. Sutherland. A suspended automatically shifting fulcrum is a point of potency, a stillness within a wider field of action, which is suspended within its wider field, and which automatically shifts within the inhalation and exhalation cycles of the Tide. Automatically shifting fulcrums are natural points of reference laid down by the intentions of the Breath of Life. They arise within the Original matrix as concentrations of potency that organize form and motion. Their action even governs the overall motion and balance of the embryological development of cells and tissues.

The Long Tide lays down the ordering matrix for human form. As we have seen, this is a stable field of bioenergy, or potency. Points of potency within this field are expressed as organizing fulcrums for different fields of action. These are essentially points of stillness. The idea is that all form and motion is organized by stillness. These points of stillness are fulcrum points, natural points of balance, within the overall action of the field in which they manifest. They are fulcrum points that organize these fields and around which the field moves. These points of stillness are not static; they move, or shift, within the cycles of the Tide. The Long Tide expresses a respiratory cycle of 50-second inhalations and 50-second exhalations. This respiratory action generates the bioelectric matrix and its primal midline. From the midline, suspended automatically shifting fulcrums are naturally generated. These move within the respiratory cycles originated by the action of the Tide. From these phenomena, other tidal rhythms and related reciprocal tension motions are also generated. The potencies, fluids, and tissues, as unified tensile fields of action, are all organized and maintained in balance by the action of these naturally occurring fulcrums. As the fulcrum moves, so does the whole field of action.

As we have seen, automatically shifting fulcrums are suspended within the field they organize. As they move, the whole field moves. All of the motion of the field, be it the reciprocal tension membrane, the tissue field as a whole, or the fluid field, has a natural point of balance around automatically shifting fulcrums. The fulcrum, the moving point of stillness, centers the field of action. Its presence controls the action of the field and also generates its natural boundaries. If the fulcrum were not present, energy would dissipate and form could not coalesce. Order would descend into chaos. Its presence also generates the natural tensions within the field. The centering action of the fulcrum generates a natural tension throughout the whole field. Thus, as described above, the whole field of action is also called a *tensile field*. As we shall see, all three functions of potency, fluids, and tissues are tensile fields of action that are organized around suspended automatically shifting fulcrums. As the fulcrum naturally shifts with the intentions of the Tide, the whole field that it is part of moves, and reciprocal tension motions are generated. All of the tensions held within the field are also naturally balanced around these fulcrums.

Summary of Concepts

Let's review some concepts here. All automatically shifting fulcrums are suspended within the field they organize. Imagine a field of potency, a living bioenergy field the shape of the human body. Then imagine a point of concentrated potency within the midst of this larger field. This concentrated point of potency is not separate from the field. It is a concentration *within* the field. It is a concentration of

potency suspended within its own field of action. Its function is to organize, control, and give boundary to the field it is part of. These points of concentrated stillness also generate the natural tensions within the field. The fulcrum generates and organizes a tensile field of action and defines the boundaries of that field. Again, imagine a bioenergy field the shape of a human body. As bioenergy, or potency, concentrates within its wider field to form a fulcrum, a drawing in towards this concentration occurs throughout the whole field. A field of tensile potency, so to speak, results. As fluids and tissues are organized by the action of potency, a tensile fluid-tissue field is also generated.

The unity of bioelectric phenomena and the fluid-tissue field has been explored in orthodox research. Remember our discussion in Chapter Five about the liquid crystalline nature of the human body. The fluids and tissues of the body literally form a unified fluid-tissue matrix due to hydrogen bonding both between the water molecules themselves and between water molecules and the peptide side chains of connective tissues. There is literally a unified fluid-tissue matrix, a one-thingness, which expresses the unity of the human system. Also remember our discussion about the quantum level of organization of this fluid-tissue matrix. Quantum fields of action have been noted within this unified fluid-tissue matrix. The fluid-tissue field has been seen to be ordered by subtle quantum fields of action, which include the movements of light photons within the fluids.[1] This is just another language for the perception of the unity of potency, fluid, and tissues within the human system.

Let's imagine that a piece of cloth represents the unified fluid-tissue field. Imagine that this piece of cloth is taut. As you gather or pinch the center of the cloth together, a tension is generated within the whole field, that is, the whole piece of cloth. This pinching represents the action of the potency within this unified field which acts to generate its tensile organization and which also acts to generate its motion. All natural fulcrums move with the inhalation and exhalation cycles of the Tide. Another way to say this is that they move with the *intentions* of the Tide. They are not static. They automatically shift in their location as the Tide manifests its inhalation and exhalation motions. These fulcrums are still places that naturally shift within the inhalation and exhalation cycles of primary respiration. As they shift, the whole tensile field organized around them also shifts. Again imagine a taut piece of cloth. You pinch the material at the center of the cloth. As you move the pinched center, the whole field, that is, the whole piece of cloth, moves with it. Reciprocal tension motion of *the whole field* is generated by and organized around the moving fulcrum.

Clinical Highlight

An awareness of suspended automatically shifting fulcrums gives the practitioner a wealth of information. If the practitioner is aware of the dynamics of these natural fulcrums, then the overall organization of the system can be tracked. As you will see, all inertial issues within the system are centered and balanced by the Breath of Life as a whole. All of our unresolved life experiences are centered as a unified dynamic within the system. When an inertial issue is resolved and the traumatic or pathological forces that organize its presence are dissipated, then the fluid and tissue world is free to realign to its natural suspended automatically shifting fulcrums. The practitioner can track this reorganization and be sure of the clinical results of the session work. Another important clinical indicator, as we shall see, is the quality of potency that the system can express and manifest. These ideas will be developed in later chapters.

The Power Is in the Fulcrum

Automatically shifting fulcrums organize the natural reciprocal tension motions of both fluids and tis-

sues. These natural points of balance are expressed and perceived at every level of the system. Within the CRI they are perceived as points or locations within the tissues. Within the mid-tide they are perceived as points of potency, which have the power to organize and move the field in which they are suspended. This is closer to their true nature. Suspended automatically shifting fulcrums are, in essence, points of concentrated potency suspended within a larger field of action. These still concentrations of potency have the power to organize and move whole fields of action. Thus the fluid and tissue world and its organization and motion, is organized around these suspended and still concentrations of potency. As these suspended fulcrums move with the intentions of the Tide, so do the fluid and tissue fields. Reciprocal tension motion is then generated. All fields of action are thus naturally organized and balanced around these suspended automatically shifting fulcrums.

The power to organize and generate motion is concentrated within the fulcrum. It is important to understand that it is the *power* found within the fulcrum that organizes and generates all reciprocal tension motion within the body. Within the heart of every fulcrum point there is a kernel of potency that has the power to organize. This is expressed as a *stillness* that organizes motion. As discussed above, an automatically shifting fulcrum is a point of potency that has condensed and become still within a wider field of action. It is suspended within that field. Imagine that potency is a unified bioelectric field within which cells and tissues are organized. Thus potency, fluids, and tissues are a unified field of action. Within this field, potency condenses and becomes still. This *concentration of potency* is the key to understand. Potency naturally condenses within its own field of action in order to generate organizing fulcrums. These points of condensation and stillness within the wider bioelectric field become organizing points for cellular and tissue fulcrums, motion, and function. These points of condensed potency are a concentration of power and are still part of a wider field of action. Power is concentrated so that organization can evolve and life can take shape.

To summarize, the point of concentrated potency, a stillness within the wider bioelectric field, shifts automatically with the organizing imperative of the Breath of Life. These organizing fulcrums, points of potency and stillness, shift with the cycles of inhalation and exhalation generated by the Tide. The whole tensile field of potency shifts with the respiratory intentions of the Tide, and all automatically shifting fulcrums are part of this dynamic. These organizing fulcrums are the *stillness* at the heart of all natural tensile motion and motility. All natural reciprocal tension motions are generated, organized, and moved by the power concentrated within these fulcrums. This concept is also found within Chinese medicine and Daoist philosophy. Within the heart of all motion is a stillness that organizes. Stillness is at the heart of all polarities and polarity motions, such as the classic *yin* and *yang* polarities. Reciprocal tension motion is also a polarity motion. This motion is organized around the stillness of the potency found within automatically shifting fulcrums. Let's now focus our attention on the membrane system. The reciprocal tension membrane is a classic example of a tensile field of action organized around a suspended automatically shifting fulcrum.

The Reciprocal Tension Membrane

Let's begin to explore the dural membrane system. The dural membranes are the outermost layer of the meninges. Its outer surface is continuous with the periosteum of cranial bone. It is essential to understand that bone and membrane are a true *unit of function*. The reciprocal tension membrane is continuous in its structural and physiological functioning with the bones of the cranium. It is impossible to discuss bony motion without understanding that this motion is expressed in direct relationship to membranous motility and motion. Cranial bones move within and in relationship to the reciprocal

tension membrane. Remember that bone is a connective tissue and all connective tissues within the body are in continuous relationship. Classically, it is thought that the role of the reciprocal tension membrane is to guide and control the motion of the cranial bones and of their articulations. The bones were thought to ride within the membrane system. All motions of bone and membrane are thus *membranous articular* motions.

Embryologically, the cranial bones develop within the same mesenchyme from which membrane arises.[2] First the mesenchymal fields are generated, then the membranous fields within which the bone condenses. Cranial bone develops in relationship to the developing membrane within its stretches and condensation fields. Thus cranial bone and membrane develop from the same mesenchyme and this embryological oneness is maintained throughout life. So not only does cranial bone "ride" within the membrane, but bone and membrane can truly be considered to be a unified dynamic.

In the cranium, the reciprocal tension membrane system is composed of the falx cerebri and cerebelli and the tentorium cerebelli. The sickles of the falx and tentorium can be thought of as *arising* from their meeting place at the straight sinus. (See Figure 12.1.) The falx cerebri has its anterior pole at the crista galli of the ethmoid bone and its posterior pole at the occipital squama at the internal occipital protuberance (See Figure 12.2.), while the tentorium has its lateral poles of attachment at the temporal bones and its anterior-posterior poles at the occipital squama and the clinoid processes of the sphenoid bone. (See Figure 12.3.) The dural tube can be thought of as being continuous with the falx and tentorium and having a completely integrated dynamic. All of these membranes are continuous in their structure and function and are part of a unified *reciprocal tension membrane* (RTM) system. The various parts of this reciprocal tension structure function and move as one thing. The membrane structure is under natural and continual tension. The RTM expresses its primary respiratory

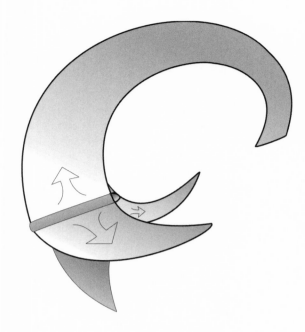

12.1 The falx and tentorium arise from the straight sinus

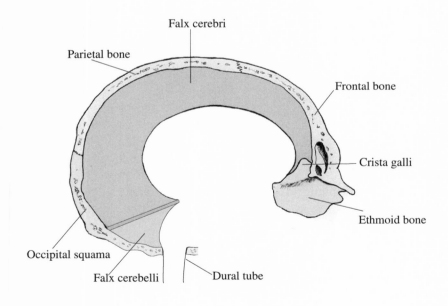

12.2 Poles of attachment of falx

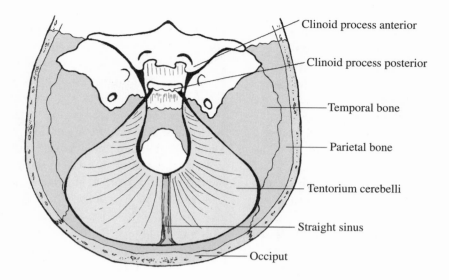

Clinoid process anterior

Clinoid process posterior

Temporal bone

Parietal bone

Tentorium cerebelli

Straight sinus

Occiput

12.3 Poles of attachment of tentorium

motion in reciprocal cycles of tensile motion, first in one direction, then in another.

Reciprocal Tension Motion and the Membrane System

As you palpate the tissue system, the reciprocal tension membrane is perceived to express the two phases of inhalation/exhalation as a reciprocal tension structure. The membrane system is always under tension as it expresses primary respiration, first in one direction and then in the other. Remember that all fluid and tissue motion is organized by the action of the potency of the Breath of Life. As discussed above, organizing fulcrums called automatically shifting fulcrums are laid down during early embryological development. Around these fulcrums the natural motility and tension dynamics of the system are organized. These fulcrums are a factor of the Original bioelectric field laid down by the action of the Long Tide. Potency becomes concentrated within this field and tissue fulcrums are generated. The organizing fulcrum for the osseous-membrane system is ideally located within the anterior aspect of the straight sinus. Due to its

importance, it was called *Sutherland's fulcrum* by Dr. Harold Magoun. The movement of bones and dural membrane have an ideal point of balance, or fulcrum point, in Sutherland's fulcrum (ideally located within the anterior straight sinus just where it meets the greater vein of Galen). As Sutherland's fulcrum shifts in its dynamics, membranes and bones move with coherence and integration around it. The power to organize and move rests in the action of the potency within these fulcrums.

Remember that Sutherland's fulcrum is an automatically shifting fulcrum. It is a fulcrum that automatically shifts in location as it follows the organizational imperative of the Breath of Life. At any moment, it is the natural point of balance for the reciprocal tensions held within the membrane system. A practitioner will ideally perceive reciprocal tension motion as a shift within tensile dynamics around Sutherland's fulcrum. In inhalation and exhalation, you may sense a reciprocal tension motion, first in one direction and then in the other. Ideally this will be sensed to be balanced and easy in both directions around the automatically shifting motion of Sutherland's fulcrum. We will describe the action of Sutherland's fulcrum in more detail below.

The most anterior pole of the falx cerebri is the

189

crista galli of the ethmoid bone, and its posterior pole is located at the inion and the occipital squama. In its inhalation-flexion motion, as Sutherland's fulcrum shifts, the anterior aspect of the falx cerebri shifts towards the crista galli of the ethmoid bone. As it does this, it follows the arc of its sickle and the aspect of it that is curled under and attached to the crista galli moves posteriorly. Its posterior pole at the occipital squama moves anteriorly. As this occurs, the falx generally shortens front to back, deepens and lowers. This is classically called the flexion motion of the reciprocal tension membrane. Its dynamics are completely integrated with the dynamics of the frontal and parietal bones, which have a direct relationship to the falx. As the anterior aspect of the falx curls posteriorly, the metopic suture also moves posterior. At its superior aspect at the sagi-

tal suture, as the falx deepens in its inhalation phase, the sagital suture also deepens.

The tentorium has its anterior poles of attachment at the clinoid processes of the sphenoid bone, its lateral poles at the petrous ridges of the temporal bones, and its posterior pole at the inion and the occipital squama. In its inhalation phase, the tentorium cerebelli generally moves anteriorly and flattens. Its most anterior poles at the clinoid processes of the sphenoid move superiorly and posteriorly. The motion at its anterior pole is integrated with the motion of the posterior aspect of the sphenoid. At its lateral poles, the petrous temporal bones, the tentorium shifts superiorly and anterolaterally, and it generally flattens and widens as the temporal bones express their inhalation/flexion motions. (See Figure 12.4.)

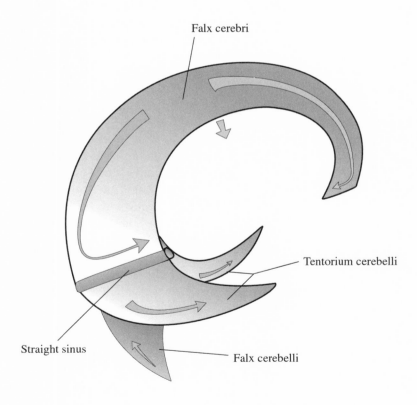

12.4 Motion of reciprocal tension menbrane in inhalation flexion

To summarize, as the tentorium expresses its inhalation-flexion motion, its most anterior aspect moves posteriorly and superior as it generally flattens and widens side to side and narrows front to back. This relates to the general shortening of the cranium front to back and widening side to side in the inhalation-flexion phase of primary respiration. All of these dynamics occur as the membranes express the shift in Sutherland's fulcrum as a reciprocal tension motion.

Summary of the Craniosacral Dynamics of the Reciprocal Tension Membrane in the Inhalation/Flexion

- In the inhalation phase, the anterior aspect of the falx cerebri shifts towards the crista galli of the ethmoid bone. Its anterior aspect shifts anterior, inferior, and posterior as it follows the arc of its sickle at the crista galli. Its posterior aspect moves anteriorly in an integrated dynamic with the occiput, the sphenobasilar junction, and the shift in the dynamics of its natural fulcrum within the straight sinus. The falx shortens anterior to posterior and deepens caudally.

- The tentorium flattens and widens as its lateral poles express an integrated dynamic with the petrous ridges of the temporal bones, and its most anterior poles, at the clinoid processes of the sphenoid, move superior-posterior.

- This motion occurs around the natural fulcrum of the straight sinus, which has been called Sutherland's fulcrum. As the membrane system expresses its inhalation-flexion motions, there is an automatically shifting fulcrum located within the straight sinus. The reciprocal tension membrane follows the shift in Sutherland's fulcrum in cycles of balanced tension as do the cranial bones generally (see below).

Mid-Tide Dynamics

The practitioner, when listening via the cranial rhythmic impulse (8–14 cycles a minute), may perceive the various tissue motions as separate relationships moving in a hopefully integrated dynamic. When listening through the action of the mid-tide (2.5 cycles a minute), you may perceive a wider dynamic. You may perceive reciprocal tension motion throughout the body as *one thing*, as a whole. Within this context, the reciprocal tension membrane will be perceived to be a unified structure. It will be sensed to express a unified tensile motion that is not separate from any other tissue within the body. Within this wider listening, bones, membranes, and fluids may be perceived to be expressing one unified tensile dynamic. The cranium may be sensed to be more fluid and its motility will be perceived more as a whole. You will also be in more direct relationship to the forces that make everything move. The drive of the potency of the Breath of Life within the fluids will be more of a living experience.

As you listen through the mid-tide, you may sense a reciprocal rising of the membranes in inhalation and a settling in exhalation. It is as though they rise within the fluid tide in an inhalation surge and settle in exhalation once the surge ceases. It is like kelp being moved by tidal forces within the depths of the ocean. You will be more aware of the continuity of tissue, fluid, and potency at this level of unfoldment. Bony and membranous motion may be more directly perceived as unified dynamic with fluid and potency. You may perceive the surge of potency within the inhalation phase to be the driving force of tissue motility. The practitioner will be more aware of these forces at work when listening through the mid-tide level of unfoldment. You will experience the reciprocal tension dynamics described above as a true unit of function expressed at every level. You will still sense the reciprocal tension dynamics of the RTM as described above, but they will be perceived to be part of a whole, a unified tensile tissue dynamic sensed throughout the body. You will perceive that tissue, fluid, and potency express their reciprocal tension dynamics as one thing. You will also have a more precise access to the history of your patient and a clearer awareness of the resultant inertial forces and fulcrums around which the system has had to organize.

Remember that there are three functions discernible within the mid-tide. They are potency, fluids, and tissues. Each function can be perceived to express a reciprocal tension dynamic. Within the fluids, this motion dynamic is called the fluid tide. Awareness of the fluid tide gives you a more direct access to the nature of the resources within the person's system. A strong fluid tide may indicate a vital system, which can access its potency, while a weaker fluid tide may indicate that there is much potency bound up in centering the unresolved history and current disturbances within the person's system. A practitioner may have to work to assist in the liberation of inertial potency and help the system build up its resources. Stillpoints are a classic example of an approach to this area.

Sutherland's Fulcrum

The reciprocal tension membrane is a unified tensile field of action. Its inherent reciprocal tension motion is moved and organized by the action of a suspended automatically shifting fulcrum. As we have mentioned, this fulcrum is called Sutherland's fulcrum. Sutherland's fulcrum is ideally located within the anterior aspect of the straight sinus. This point is suspended within the whole osseous-membranous field and the whole field is likewise suspended from it. It is a point of potency suspended within all of the tension factors within the tissue field. Think of the membranes as a tensile field of action. They always hold tension, and this tension has its balance point around the fulcrum suspended within its midst. All of the natural tension within the membranes is balanced and reconciled around this suspended fulcrum. Sutherland's fulcrum is the natural, suspended automatically shifting fulcrum of the membranous *and* connective tissue systems. Sutherland's fulcrum is a dynamic point of stillness around which the motion of the RTM is naturally

organized. Sutherland's fulcrum, like all natural fulcrums, moves, or automatically shifts, within the phases of primary respiration. As it moves, the whole membrane system moves, and reciprocal tension motion is generated. Remember that an automatically shifting fulcrum is a point of potency, a stillness, which has the power to organize and move the field within which it is suspended. Think of Sutherland's fulcrum as a point of potency that is ideally located within the anterior aspect of the straight sinus and reciprocally shifts in the inhalation and exhalation cycles of the Tide. As this occurs, the whole membrane system also shifts and reciprocal tension motion is generated. This may initially be a hard concept to grasp. Let's expand this idea.

At any moment, Sutherland's fulcrum is the natural point of organization for the RTM and is the ideal point of tension balance within its reciprocal tension motion. This is important to understand. Sutherland's fulcrum is not just a membranous fulcrum, but is the major fulcrum for the whole of the membranous-articular mechanism of the cranium. As Sutherland's fulcrum moves, the whole membranous-articular system moves and is organized around its automatically shifting action. As the RTM expresses reciprocal tension motion, the membranes move as though they are suspended from the straight sinus, which has an automatically shifting suspension fulcrum within it. As we have seen, this fulcrum organizes their tensile motion. At any moment, this fulcrum is the ideal balance point for the reciprocal tensions held within the membrane system.

Thus the reciprocal tension membrane is so arranged that the sickles of the leaves of its membranes are suspended from a shifting fulcrum point of balance within the straight sinus. The integrated motion of the reciprocal tension membrane is naturally organized around the shifting action of Sutherland's fulcrum. (See Figure 12.5.) One way of understanding these dynamics is to visualize the leaves of the falx and tentorium as arising and being suspended from the straight sinus. As bone and

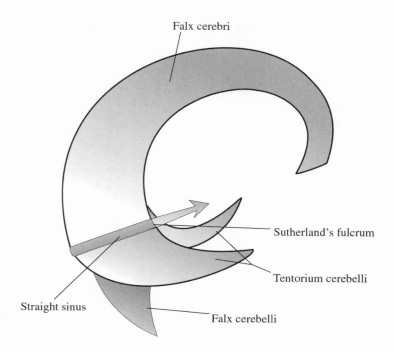

Falx cerebri

Sutherland's fulcrum

Tentorium cerebelli

Straight sinus

Falx cerebelli

12.5 Sutherland's fulcrum in inhalation

membrane are a unit of function, the whole of the bony-membranous system of the cranium can be thought to be suspended from the straight sinus. No matter what position the head is in, the fulcrum in the straight sinus acts as a *tension balance point* both in the motion dynamics of the membranes and in their structural relationships. This is an important concept. The falx and tentorium are arranged so that they are suspended from the straight sinus. As the cranial bones are in direct, continuous structural relationship to dural membrane, the cranial bones also move in direct relationship to Sutherland's fulcrum and are also, in essence, suspended from it.

As we noted above, since the periosteum of cranial bone is continuous with dural membrane, bone and membrane are a *membranous-articular unit*. Bone and membrane are a true unit of function. Sutherland's fulcrum, within the straight sinus, is therefore a fulcrum point of balance for the entire membranous-articular system. Sutherland's ful-

crum, as a point of potency and stillness in any given moment, will also shift to compensate for any strain or inertial force that is unresolved in the system. As it does this, the tensions generated by inertial forces and strain patterns are balanced and compensated for in the system as a whole. Thus, as Sutherland's fulcrum organizes the motion of bone and membrane, the whole membranous articular system will also move in compensation for unresolved issues. The classic *membranous articular strain* pattern results.[3] More on this in the next chapter.

Hence, if there is a shift in the action of this fulcrum due to traumatic or pathological circumstances, then the whole system will be effected. Any shift in Sutherland's fulcrum will effect the whole of the cranial membranous-articular system and, indeed, the whole tensile-tissue field of the body. Indeed, since all connective tissues within the body function as an integrated unit of function, Sutherland's fulcrum can be considered to be the organizing fulcrum for *all* connective tissues in the body! Any pattern of motion or restriction within connective tissue–membranous-articular relationships will be expressed in some way at Sutherland's fulcrum, and any shift in the fulcrum will affect the dynamics of the whole body. It is common for this crucial fulcrum point to shift away from its natural position within the straight sinus. This occurs as the system accommodates and compensates for the inertial issues being centered by the action of the Breath of Life. The point of potency must shift to accommodate and compensate for the tensions generated by unresolved experience.

Visualizing the Dynamics

Let's try a visualization here. Review your anatomy of the dural membranes and cranium. Visualize the reciprocal tension membrane (the falx cerebri and cerebelli and the tentorium cerebelli) within a skull. Imagine them as being suspended from the straight sinus. Include their continuity with the bones of the cranium in this image. Remember that these membranes are part of the total dural membrane system within the cranium and are continuous with the periosteum of the cranial bones. See the bones as floating within the membranes. Furthermore, remember that the membranes are always in tension and that their action is one of reciprocal tension motion. Now visualize what happens as the automatically shifting fulcrum within the straight sinus shifts back and forth. Notice, in this visualization, the reciprocal motion of bone and membrane as they float within fluid and express a unified reciprocal tension motion, flexion-external rotation, and extension-internal rotation. Notice this action as the automatically shifting fulcrum within the straight sinus moves anterior and posterior.

Now, imagine that you are standing within a huge cranium just anterior to the straight sinus. The brain has been removed; the membranes and the cranial bones surround you. Imagine that you are standing on the sphenobasilar junction and face posterior towards the straight sinus. In this position, hold the point where the falx and tentorium meet, just where they meet the great vein of Galen. Imagine that you are pulling this juncture anterior/superior with your hands. What happens to the reciprocal tension membrane as you do this? Notice how the membranes are moved in their reciprocal tension motion around the point you are pulling and how the bones are, in turn, moved and express motion. You now may have a sense that as the fulcrum moves, so moves membrane and cranial bone. Move this fulcrum point anterior and posterior in your mind's eye for a number of cycles.

The reciprocal tension motion of both bone and membrane is, as we saw above, a unit of function that has an automatic shifting fulcrum within the straight sinus. Sutherland's fulcrum is an important point of balance for the functioning of both. Furthermore, the power or potency to move everything is concentrated in the fulcrum. This is a classic concept. It is the fulcrum that organizes and moves everything. Perhaps our great journey in this life is to discover this. What is the fulcrum that organizes and moves our lives? What is the fulcrum that organizes and moves everything?

Tuning In to the RTM

Let's now spend some time with the simple intention of just listening to the motion dynamics of the reciprocal tension membrane (RTM). To do this, you must have a clear anatomical image of these membranes in your mind. If you are clear about your anatomy, the system will be able to clearly communicate its motions and patterns to you in its own language. In the following process, the intention will be to float within fluid on the cranial bones and the reciprocal tension membrane. The idea is to sense the whole of that movement as a unit of function in your hands. In this you may begin to sense the integrated motion around Sutherland's fulcrum.

Cranial bones and dural membranes move as a unit in related respiratory cycles. Thus, when you palpated the motion at the sphenoid and occiput earlier, you were also in direct relationship to the reciprocal tension membrane and its fulcrum point of balance within the straight sinus. In the application below, you will be asked to include the reciprocal tension membrane and its motion dynamic in your perceptual field. In this, you may also discover a more global sense of the reciprocal and unified motion of both bone and membrane in the cranium. Classically, the motion dynamic of the reciprocal tension membrane is said to guide and control the reciprocal motion of the cranial bones. The bones are limited in their excursion by the reciprocal tensions within the membrane system whose motion is in turn organized around Sutherland's fulcrum. On a deeper level, it can be perceived that it is the potency of the Breath of Life that is moving and guiding everything.

Clinical Application:
Tuning In to the Reciprocal
Tension Membrane

In the following exploration, you will start at a CRI level of action, then shift to the mid-tide. The intention will be to build up a perceptual awareness of reciprocal tension motion at both levels of perception.

1. Place your hands in the vault hold as outlined earlier. Establish your practitioner fulcrums and settle into your relationship with your patient. Synchronize your perceptual field with the CRI. Let your hands float on the tissues and narrow your field of awareness to the motions of bone and membrane. Now become aware of the motion at the sphenoid and occiput. Settle into this motion as above and let yourself be taken by the tissues. Settle into the respiratory expressions of flexion and extension at the SBJ.

2. Now include the reciprocal tension membrane (falx and tentorium) within your perceptual field. Don't try to visualize this, but let the tissues and their dynamics come into your hands. Shift from just palpating bones and include the membranes within your perceptual field. See if you can sense the reciprocal tension motions of the membranes along with the general motions of the bones. See if you can sense their motion as one thing. Allow the falx and tentorium to carry you along in their motion. As you allow this, you may discover a wider awareness of the overall motion of the reciprocal tension membrane. See if you can let the reciprocal motion come into your palpating hands. Don't look, just listen. Allow the tissues to come to you. Allow yourself to be moved. As you do this, you are perceiving the continuity of relationship between cranial bone and membrane. They are a unit of function and cannot be separated. Imagine that the bones are just denser places in the membranes and follow their unified dynamic.

3. Note the quality of this motion. How does the reciprocal tension membrane express the respiratory cycles generated by the Breath of Life? Is there balance in the reciprocal tension motions? Can you sense any of the dynamics described above? Does there seem to be any eccentricities to their excursion as you palpate their motions? Just allow yourself the luxury of listening and not having to do anything. Let the system do the doing. Finally and most importantly, can you sense the motion around the automatically shifting fulcrum within the straight sinus, Sutherland's fulcrum?

4. Once you have had an experience of the reciprocal tension motion at a CRI level, synchronize your perceptual field with the mid-tide level of action. Let your hands be buoyant as they float on the tissues. Sense that your hands are immersed within fluid. Widen your perceptual field to the biosphere. Listen to the system as a whole. Listen to the tensile action of the tissues as a whole. Notice how your perception

of reciprocal tension motion may change. Are you more aware of potency and fluid here? Do you sense the drive of the potency within the fluids as the tissues express reciprocal tension motion? Do you sense the tissue motion as a unified dynamic? Do you sense the inhalation surge and exhalation settling of a unified tensile tissue field?

Do not be discouraged if these relationships are not immediately clear to you. This will take many palpation sessions. The more you bring attention to the system in this way, the clearer it will become. It is a gradual process of increasing your sensitivity to the system and its dynamics. If you are more aware of bony motion, use the cranial bones as handles into the reciprocal motions of the membranes. Remember that they are a unit of function and in palpating one aspect, you are also in direct relationship to the other. Whatever you do, do not crowd the system in your listening. Remember your practitioner fulcrums and hold a wide perceptual field. If you crowd the system, it will not speak to you. Let it all come to you. Also remember that, in essence, tissue, fluid, and potency are a unified dynamic, a unit of function. See if this begins to becomes a living reality for you.

Summary of Key Concepts

The cranial bones, their sutures, and the reciprocal tension membrane are a unit of function. They express an integrated craniosacral dynamic. Their expression of motility and mobility are intimately integrated and interdependent. The reciprocal tension membrane is composed of the falx cerebelli, the falx cerebri, and the tentorium cerebelli. It is important to remember that the periosteum of the bones of the cranium are continuous with the dural membranes and that the bones and the membranes are one functional unit. As the dural membranes express a reciprocal respiratory motion, the bones express their motion. The dural membranes act as relatively inelastic bands, always under reciprocal tension, which classically serve to guide and control the bones in their expression of motion. When you are in relationship to bony motion, you are therefore also in relationship to the reciprocal motion of the reciprocal tension membrane. One way to relate to this is to sense that cranial bones are denser places within the membranes. They always express their motion dynamic as a unity. Remember that this dynamic is generated and organized by the potency found within automatically shifting fulcrums, in this case, Sutherland's fulcrum.

Breaking Down the Unit of Function

Sometimes it is useful to break down the unit of function into smaller parts for observation. As we do this, it is important to remember that we are always perceiving the whole of a human being. We can break this whole down into smaller units for the purpose of observation and learning, but it is essential to remember that this is artificial and that we are always, in essence, palpating this whole. In the following sections, you will learn a new hold, the fronto-occipital hold, to listen more particularly to the motion of the falx and its continuity with cranial bone. The motion of the frontal and parietal bones and the falx is an integrated dynamic. As the falx expresses its flexion and extension motions, the frontal and parietal bones express their external and internal rotation motions. You will also palpate the unit of function of temporal bones and tentorium. Here we are breaking down the unit of function in order to more particularly perceive the local unit of temporal bones and tentorium.

Clinical Application:
The Fronto-occipital Hold

Let's first review the basic craniosacral dynamics described above. In inhalation, the falx cerebri shifts towards its anterior pole at the crista galli of the ethmoid bone. As this occurs, it follows the arc of its sickle, and the aspect of it that is curled under and attached to the crista galli moves posteriorly. As this occurs, the glabella area of the frontal bone is carried posteriorly as their lateral aspects flare and widen in external rotation. (See Figure 12.6.) Its posterior pole at the occipital squama moves anteriorly as it follows the shift in Sutherland's fulcrum. As this occurs, the falx generally shortens front to back, deepens and lowers. This is a part of a general shortening of the cranium from front to back and from its vertex to its base in the inhalation phase. The deepening and lowering of the falx carries the sagital suture and the parietal bones inferior at the midline, while their lateral aspects widen laterally as the tentorium lowers and widens. The rear of the sagittal suture has more motion as the parietals express external and internal rotation. (See Figure 12.7.)

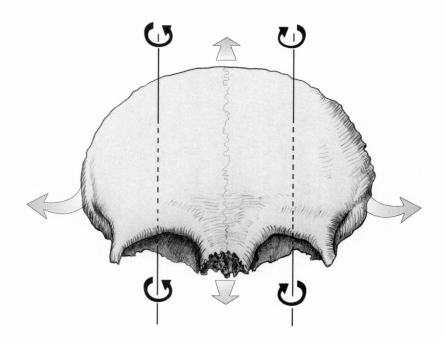

Inhalation external rotation

12.6 Craniosacral motion of the frontal bone

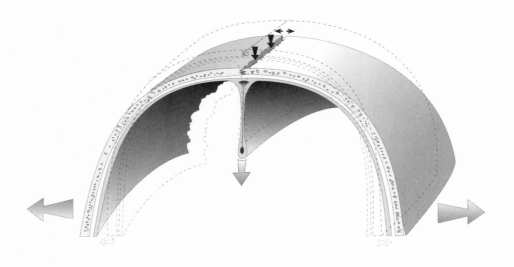

12.7 Cranionsacral motion of the parietal bones in inhalation

1. Place your hands in a fronto-occipital hold. In this hold you will have the falx and the unit of occiput-falx-frontal bone between your hands. The intention will be to sense the reciprocal and integrated motion between these relationships. Place one hand in an occipital cradle with your fingers spread and pointing inferior. The occiput rests on your fingers and on the palm of your hand. Balance the occiput on your hand. Do not place pressure on the occiput with the heel of your hand. Place your other hand over the frontal bone with your fingers spread and pointing inferior. Your fingertips are placed just over the orbital ridges of the eyes. Have as much contact with the flesh of your fingers on the frontal bone as possible. Maintain a gentle, light, floating contact. (See Figure 12.8.)

2. Shift your perceptual field to the CRI level of motion. Get interested in what these structures are doing. From this vantage point, hold bones and membranes as a unit within your perceptual field. Sense the unit of function among the frontal bone, the falx, and the occiput. See if you can sense their integrated craniosacral dynamic.

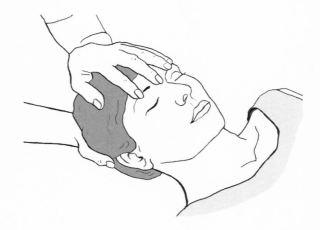

12.8 Fronto-occipital hold

3. Can you sense the reciprocal motion of the falx and the frontal and occiput bones? Can you sense the falx curling posterior at the crista galli in flexion? Can you sense the reciprocal motion of the frontal bone as it deepens at the glabella? Can you sense the unit of motion of frontal bone–falx-occiput? Does it seem to be one thing? Does there seem to be a balanced motion between the bones and through the membrane system? Does there seem to be a balanced motion in relationship to Sutherland's fulcrum?

4. Once you have a clear sense of the motion dynamic viewed through the CRI, repeat this exercise and synchronize your perceptual field with the mid-tide level of perception to sense how that changes your perceptual experience.

Temporal Bones and the Tentorium as a Unit of Function

We can apply the same process of *breaking down the unit of function* to the dynamics of the tentorium. You will be in relationship to the unit of temporal bones and tentorium. In the following process you will use the temporal bone hold already learned. Remember that as the temporal bones express their external and internal rotation motions, the tentorium expresses flexion. This occurs as a unified dynamic. In inhalation, the temporal bones express external rotation as they rotate around an oblique axis through their petrous portions. Their squama widens apart as their mastoid portions narrow together. While this occurs, the tentorium flattens and widens between the temporals as described earlier. (See Figure 12.9.)

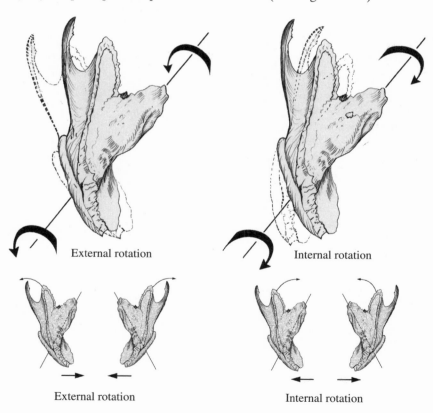

External rotation

Internal rotation

External rotation

Internal rotation

12.9 Craniosacral motion of the temporal bones

1. Place your hands in the temporal bone hold learned earlier. Your middle fingers are gently in the ear canal, your index fingers are over the zygomatic arches, and your ring fingers are over the mastoid portions. (See Figure 12.10.)

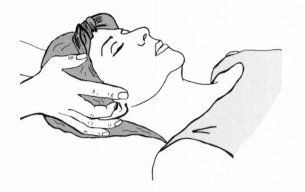

12.10 Temporal bone hold

2. Again synchronize your perceptual field with the CRI. First bring your attention to the temporal bones. See if you can sense their motion. Once you sense this, include the tentorium within your perceptual field.

3. Allow the unified dynamic between the temporal bones and the tentorium to come into your awareness. What do you sense? How do the tissues under your hands express their craniosacral dynamics? How is this organized around Sutherland's fulcrum?

4. Once you have a clear sense of the motion dynamic viewed through the CRI, repeat this exercise and synchronize your perceptual field with the mid-tide level of perception to sense how that changes your perceptual experience.

In these perceptual exercises, the intention was to deepen your awareness of the dynamics of the reciprocal tension membrane and of the unit of function of cranial bone and membrane. Please continue with this process in your practice sessions and simply be open to the truths that the human system unfolds to you.

1. Mae-Wan Ho, *The Rainbow and the Worm, the Physics of Organisms* (World Scientific).

2. See E. Blechschmidt and R. F. Gasser, *Biokinetics and Biodynamics of Human Differentiation* (Charles C. Thomas).

3. For a classic description of this see Magoun, Harold, *Osteopathy in the Cranial Field,* The Journal Printing Company, (1966) (1976)

SECTION THREE
Essential Clinical Skills

13

Forces and Fulcrums

In the next few chapters, we will discuss some of the most important healing principles found within the cranial concept. These are the concepts of the *fulcrum* and of *states of balanced tension*. In this process, you will begin to explore how the human system organizes itself. Organization is always twofold. There is the universal within us, the Breath of Life and its potency. The cellular and tissue world naturally organizes to this universal as does the mind when it is still. Then there are the forces of our experience. The cellular and tissue world must also organize relative to its experience and potencies will respond. On the level of mind, mental forms and self-constructs are generated; on the emotional level, emotional affects are held; and on the tissue level, inertia is generated. In the following sections, you will explore how potency becomes inertial in relationship to trauma and pathology, and how these

are centered and compensated for within the bio-dynamics of the system. You will also learn to relate to the inherent forces that both maintain and center the unprocessed disturbances held within the system. In this chapter we will outline some basic principles before introducing the concept of the state of balanced tension.

Introduction

In the next few chapters, you will learn some fundamental clinical concepts that will allow you, as practitioner, to relate to patterns of experience within the human system. These skills encompass:

- the ability to sense a pattern of inertia in the body,

- the ability to follow the motion dynamics of that pattern,

- the ability to sense the inertial fulcrum that organizes that pattern,

- the ability to access and relate to the inherent forces or potencies within the heart of that fulcrum, and

- the ability to access what is known as the state of balanced tension, a state of dynamic

---

In this chapter we will:

- *Introduce the concept of the fulcrum.*

- *Introduce the concept of biodynamic and biokinetic forces.*

- *Introduce the concept of inertial fulcrums.*

- *Introduce the palpation of tissue motion and fulcrums.*

---

equilibrium, within which the inherent forces can be expressed beyond the containment and compensation present.

The intention of this work is to help the system reestablish its relationship to the Breath of Life and its inherent ordering principle. The main focus of this is an appreciation of what is known as the state of balanced tension, a state of dynamic equilibrium of the forces and tension patterns involved. Basically, the state of balanced tension is a state of dynamic stillness in which the inertial forces and potencies that maintain and center the disturbance within the system can be resolved. You will learn that in the state of balanced tension the healing potency of the system naturally expresses itself.

In ongoing courses, these skills are taught in a graduated way. The next few chapters mirror that teaching intention. In this chapter, I will discuss the concepts of biodynamics and inertial fulcrums. In later chapters we will learn the classical approach to what is known as the *point* of balanced membranous tension. Finally, we will deepen into these concepts and begin to relate to the *state* of balanced tension in more open ways. The intention will be to relate to the intrinsic forces at work within patterns of distress in the human system, not just to the resultant tissue or fluid resistances and congestion. To this end we will introduce concepts from the work of Dr. Rollin Becker, D.O., and lead you through a number of perceptual exercises, which will build and deepen your clinical awareness of these concepts.

Biodynamics

In most basic cranial courses the teaching emphasis is on the CRI level of action and perception. The focus tends to be on craniosacral motion at this rate of expression, on the dynamics of structures involved, and on the release of tissue resistance. There is an orientation to patterns of resistance and inertia within the tissue system. The clinical intention is to diagnose, analyze, and treat these patterns of resistance. Healing processes become lesion and resistance oriented. Some practitioners also become focused on emotional release as an end in itself. In this endeavor, they don't necessarily have a grounding in trauma theory or skills. Patients are encouraged to "unwind" patterns and to express strong emotions without necessary discernment as to whether these processes are healing or retraumatizing.

In a *biodynamic* approach to work in the cranial field, the initial focus is on the inherent Health of the system. A perceptual experience of the unfoldments of the Breath of Life becomes the foundation of the work. Practitioners learn to listen to the dynamics of the Breath of Life as the fluid, cellular, and tissue world organizes around it. The potency of the Breath of Life is perceived to be the biodynamic ordering principle within the human system. This principle is *epigenetic* because its functions underlie or precede genetics. This force arises at the moment of conception and is with us as an intrinsic ordering force throughout life. The cellular and tissue world is constantly organizing around its imperative. This is the intrinsic Health of the system. It is the force that drives embryological development and organizes cellular growth and differentiation from conception until death. Practitioners can learn to perceive this ordering principle at work. It continually arises in the present moment. Its intentions unfold in the eternal present and every moment of our life is a moment of creation. This Health is a universal. The same Health at work within me is at work within you. Within this wider context, practitioners also learn to relate to the *history* of the patient. These are the conditional processes within the human system. Practitioners can become very skilled in the perception of the shape and form of personal history, pathology, and resistance in the body. Thus the interplay of the universal and the conditional is the ground of inquiry in the work.

In this framework, practitioners learn to relate to the *forces* at work within the human system. These forces maintain and center the organization, patterns, and resistances within the body-mind. The focus is not just on the results of these forces, such as tissue resistances, congestion, fixation, and pathology, but on the actual forces that organize them. Practitioners learn that at the heart of every inertial issue are present both the biodynamic potencies of the Breath of Life and the experiential forces of trauma and disease states. In order to clinically relate to these, students learn to access a *neutral* within the system. This neutral is expressed as a *state of balanced tension* within which the healing forces of the system come into play. A deep appreciation of stillness arises and the truths of the healing processes of the system become more obvious. In the following sections I would like to introduce some of these relevant concepts.

Natural Fulcrums

The *fulcrum* is an important concept in classical osteopathic practice and in the cranial concept. Motility, and all inherent tissue motions within the body, are seen to be organized by natural fulcrums. All motion in the human body, indeed, all of life's processes, are organized around fulcrums. A fulcrum is a still place around which motion occurs. It is the focal point around which motion is organized. Simply put, *fulcrums organize motion*. Without fulcrums all would be chaos. Power is concentrated within the fulcrum. Fulcrums have the power, or potency, to organize. Within the body, they act as the loci for organized and cohesive structure and motion.

As we saw in the last chapter, fulcrums are manifestations of potency. The human system is organized via intricate bioelectric or bioenergy fields of action, and potency concentrates within these fields to form organizing loci, or fulcrums.[1] These fulcrums have the power to organize and move the cellular and tissue world. Patterns of motion, whether they are the natural reciprocal tension motion of tissues and fluid or inertial patterns relating to trauma, are organized in their form and motion by fulcrums, places of concentration of forces and potencies. We will discuss this idea in some detail below. For now it is important to understand that at the heart of the

concept of a fulcrum is an awareness of bioenergy or potency. Potency is concentrated within a fulcrum and around this concentration of power the cellular and tissue world organizes. In other words, fulcrums have the potency to organize motion and function.[2]

The cellular and tissue world will naturally organize around condensations, or loci of potency. Potency is a factor of the Breath of Life and natural concentrations of potency occur around which cells and tissues organize. Again, think of the potency of the Breath of Life as a bioelectric field phenomenon. This is an Intelligent field. It is not mechanical or sterile. Think of an Intelligent bioenergy field as the organizing foundation of the human system. Think of natural fulcrums as condensations, or concentrations of potency within this wider field of action. These focal points of potency become organizing factors for the cellular and tissue world. Tissues fulcrums are then generated around which motility and motion are naturally organized.

Thus:

- there is a living, Intelligent bioelectric field of potency or bioenergy,

- there are condensations or concentrations of potency within this field,

- there are natural tissue fulcrums generated by these condensations of potency,

- and tissue motility and motion are organized around these places of condensation.

In essence, all tissue fulcrums are organized by coalescences of potency or bioenergy, and potency is a biodynamically active ordering force within the human system. Potency, as it concentrates within its own field of action, becomes a still place within its wider bioelectric field of action. This is a *dynamically acting stillness*, as all natural fulcrums automatically shift with the respiratory cycles of the Tide. A fulcrum is a locus of stillness around which fluid and tissue activity and motion are organized.

It is a concentration of power, which expresses the organizing intentions of the Breath of Life. The power to organize is thus a factor of precise concentrations of potency within the bioelectric field. These places of dynamic stillness are the heart of the organization and natural motion of the fluids, cells, and tissues of the human system. Natural fulcrums are precisely expressed within the tissue system. For instance, as we saw in the last chapter, one very important natural fulcrum within the body is called *Sutherland's fulcrum*, ideally located within the anterior aspect of the straight sinus. Sutherland's fulcrum is the organizing fulcrum for membrane, bone, and connective tissue both within the cranium and within the body as a whole. (See Figure 13.1.) Likewise, the motion of the central nervous system is naturally organized around the anterior wall of the third ventricle, the lamina terminalis of the embryological neural tube. The central nervous system, in its embryological formation, develops in relationship to the lamina terminalis and it remains the organizing fulcrum of its motility throughout life. (See Figure 13.2.) As we saw in the last chapter, natural fulcrums are *suspended automatically shifting fulcrums*. A natural fulcrum is a point of potency, a stillness within a wider field of action, which is suspended within this wider field, and which automatically shifts with the inhalation and exhalation cycles of the Tide. In the next section we will introduce a type of fulcrum that does not automatically shift with the Tide, the inertia fulcrum.

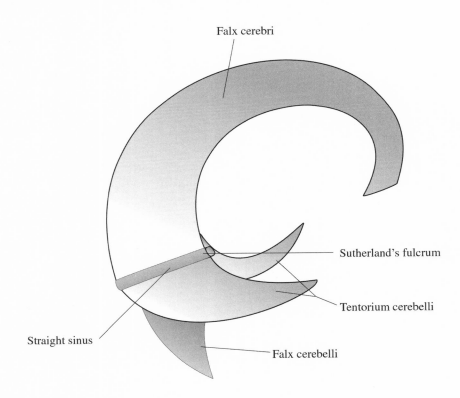

Falx cerebri

Sutherland's fulcrum

Tentorium cerebelli

Straight sinus

Falx cerebelli

13.1 Sutherland's fulcrum

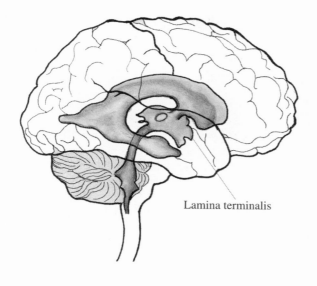

Lamina terminalis

13.2 Lamina terminalis

Inertial Fulcrums

Above I introduced the idea of the fulcrum as an organizing principle. Here I will introduce the concept of the *inertial fulcrum. Inertia* simply means something that naturally expresses motion has become still, and will tend to remain still, unless the forces that maintain the inertia are resolved. Within a cranial context, when inertia arises within the system, potencies, fluids, and tissues, which ideally express a natural motility and motion, become still. They manifest resistance to movement, or inertia. Resistance to movement within the human system is organized by what are known as inertial fulcrums. Like the natural fulcrums of the system, inertial fulcrums are loci of potency and force. But unlike natural fulcrums, which express reciprocal tension motion generated by the Breath of Life, these do not. They are organized not just by the potency of the Breath of Life, but also by the forces of our experience. Natural fulcrums are concentrations of potency and express a dynamic stillness, but they are not inertial, they automatically shift within the in-

tentions of the Tide. Natural fulcrums are automatically shifting fulcrums. Inertial fulcrums are not. Inertial fulcrums do not automatically shift with the intentions of the Tide. They are an expression of inertia. Remember that all motion is organized around fulcrums. Thus inertial fulcrums will also organize fluid and tissue motion. Eccentric and conditioned motility and motion will result.

At the heart of the inertial fulcrum are potencies or forces that have become inertial. Every experience we have has its potency, its energy. If these experiential forces cannot be resolved by the system, they will have to be contained and compensated for by the Breath of Life in some way. If potencies become inertial within the system, tissue and fluid inertia will follow. Boundary, fixity, and strain arise as the potencies, fluids, and tissue elements become inertial. An inertial fulcrum forms when a force or stress of some nature overwhelms the system and cannot be resolved. Dr. Rollin Becker, D.O., called these forces *biokinetic forces*. Dr. Becker used this term in a specific way. The inherent biodynamic potencies of the Breath of Life organize motion. The biodynamics of the system naturally organize cellular and tissue motion and motility. These natural motions can be called biokinetic motions. The motility and motions generated by the intentions and actions of the Breath of Life are thus natural *biokinetic motions*.[3] Biokinetic forces are forces taken on by the system, which effect its natural biokinetic motions in some way. Thus the term *biokinetic forces* means that forces which are not natural to the system have been introduced into its dynamics, and these forces then effect or condition the natural biokinetic motions of cells and tissues in some way.

For instance, let's imagine that a person has a traumatic motorcycle accident and sustains head injuries. A blow enters his cranium as a physical force. This may entail a powerful impact, let's say 100 pounds per square inch. This is an overwhelming force for the system to deal with. Due to the overwhelming nature of the experience, the forces involved may become entrapped. This is classically called an *entrapped force vector*. If these forces cannot be resolved within the immediacy of the experience, the energy of this vector will become lodged within the system. It will become inertial. The potency of the Breath of Life will, in turn, also become inertial in order to contain and compensate for the action of the unresolved force vector. A site of inertial potencies and forces results. At this site, an *inertial fulcrum* will be generated. This orb of inertia includes the inertial potencies and forces involved and the resultant fluid and tissue organization. As the tissue and fluid world naturally organizes around the potency of the Breath of Life, if potency becomes inertial, tissues and fluids will also become inertial. The cellular and tissue world, which naturally organizes around the fulcrums laid down by the Breath of Life, will now also have to organize around these inertial forces. The natural biokinetic motions of the cells and tissues will be effected. The force vector, which has become lodged within the system, could thus be called a *biokinetic force*. In other words, if it remains unresolved within the system, it has the power to effect the natural biokinetics of the fluid, cellular, and tissue world.

In this example we described a traumatic accident, but experiential forces are multifaceted. They can include those of genetics, pathogens, environmental issues, toxins, and any other force overlaid upon the natural organization of the system. These are all biokinetic forces. If unresolved, they all have the power to effect the natural biokinetics of the system. The important point to remember here is that inertial forces organize inertial tissues and fluids. Thus at the heart of an inertial fulcrum forces are at work. These are the potencies of the Breath of Life *and* the forces of the unresolved experience.

Osteopathic Lesions

When tissues and fluids become inertial, the classical osteopathic lesion will result. The term *lesion* is used differently in osteopathy than in orthodox medicine. An *osteopathic lesion* is classically a site of pathological tissue and fluid change. The term

describes an orb of tissue and fluid stasis and change. More recently the term *somatic dysfunction* has been used in some quarters in place of the term osteopathic lesion.

Osteopathic lesions are composed of:

- compression and fixation in tissue relationships,

- changes in the nature of the tissues involved, such as dryness, densification, or thickening of the tissues,

- fluid congestion,

- edema and poor fluid circulation around and within the site, and a buildup of toxicity locally,

- possible nervous system facilitation.

These changes will compromise the functioning of the involved tissues, organs, and tissue relationships effected. Commonly, osteopathic lesions relate to fixations in joint or sutural relationships, but they are also expressions of any disruption and disorientation in tissue structure and function. A vertebral fixation is a classic example of an osteopathic lesion. You will find structural fixation, tissue compression and adhesion, qualitative tissue changes, fluid stasis, and nerve involvement. The important point here is that these tissue and fluid changes are the result of deeper forces at work. In a biodynamic approach the clinical intention is to relate to the organizing forces involved, not just to the resultant tissue and fluid changes. In essence, we are talking about the interplay of the universal forces of the Breath of Life and the experiential forces we met in life. Let's look at these concepts more slowly and introduce some of the language originally developed by Dr. Rollin Becker, D.O.

Biodynamic and Biokinetic Forces at Work

In this book, I am using a particular framework to describe the interface between universal and conditional forces. This framework was originally described by Dr. Rollin Becker, D.O. Dr. Becker wrote a series of remarkable articles in the Yearbooks of the Academy of Applied Osteopathy in the 1960s. He expressed so much that is relevant to the work that I can only encourage practitioners to read and reread them.[4] Each time I do, I discover something more and find myself in continual wonder at his clarity and eloquence. I will share my particular understanding of some of the concepts that Dr. Becker unfolds in his writings. I find that his approach and language helps to clarify the concept of an inertial fulcrum and its bioenergy dynamics.

In these articles, he called the universal forces of the Breath of Life *biodynamic potencies* and the forces of trauma and experience *biokinetic forces*. As mentioned above, I believe that Dr. Becker used these terms in particular ways and I have found it to be an extremely useful nomenclature. It helps students and practitioners become aware of the interplay of the forces at work within any pattern of inertia. Dr. Becker states that within any pattern of disturbance in the body, there are two basic forces at work: the biodynamic potencies generated by the Breath of Life and the biokinetic forces introduced into the system via trauma and life experience.

Biodynamic potencies are the intrinsic forces within the human body. They are the biodynamic forces that maintain order, integrity, and homeostatic balance. They arise at the moment of conception, organize cellular differentiation, and are with us until the day we die. Biodynamic potency is an intrinsic, physiologically functioning ordering force. Biodynamic potency is Dr. Becker's term for the potency generated by the Breath of Life. Thus the potency of the Breath of Life, as the intrinsic biodynamic force of the body, is its inherent ordering principle. As we have seen, potency is literally a bio-electric or biomagnetic *field phenomenon*. There is thus a unified field of Health around which fluids, cells, and tissues organize. As we have also seen, potency is expressed as a unified field of action within the fluid systems of the body. It directs and orders embryological development and continues to manifest order throughout life. It is an expression of the *Original matrix* around which our mind and body naturally orients.

Biokinetic forces are forces that are added to the system from experience and from the environment in some way. They are environmental forces, toxins, traumatic forces, and the forces of pathogens and disease states. We can also add the forces of genetics to this list. Again, in this particular usage of the word biokinetic, Dr. Becker is pointing to *forces* that effect the natural biokinetics of the system. These forces effect and alter the natural biokinetic motions of fluids, cells, and tissues in some way. Dr. Becker stressed that when conditions of trauma and pathology are found within the human system, there have been forces introduced into it which effect its physiology in some way. These forces continue to maintain the diseased or disturbed state. *This is critical to understand.* Patterns of resistance, strain, and pathology are not just about past history. They are about how the system is still organizing around these forces in the present. Whenever resistance, pain, and pathology are present, there are forces at work that act to maintain these patterns and disturbances.

Biodynamic Potencies, Biokinetic Forces, and Inertial Fulcrums

As we have seen, there are biodynamic intrinsic potencies within the body, and there are added forces called biokinetic forces, which are expressions of traumatic experiences, environmental forces, and past history. Natural biokinetic motion, or motility, is normally ordered by the biodynamic potency of the Breath of Life. Biokinetic forces are added forces that effect the natural biokinetic motions of cells and tissues. These forces generate and maintain patterns of resistance and disease states. In essence, the action of these added biokinetic forces generates the formation of inertial fulcrums within the body.

If you remember our discussion of inertial fulcrums above, when biokinetic forces are introduced into the system, the potency of the Breath of Life will attempt to resolve them. If the forces are not resolvable, then the biodynamic or intrinsic potencies of the system will act to contain them in some way. As we have discussed, this occurs as potency becomes inertial in order to contain and compensate for the unresolvable force. Again, potency is expressed as a bioelectric field of action. It is this bioelectric field, or Original matrix, which organizes cellular and tissue form and motion. When forces are added to the dynamics of the system, potency will become inertial within this wider field in order to resolve or contain the biokinetic force introduced. Again, these forces may be generated by an overwhelming accident, by the birthing process, or by the action of toxins and pathogens, to name but a few examples.

The body physiology, organized by biodynamic potency, is continually trying to dissipate, contain, and compensate for these added forces. It is the role of the practitioner to help the system resolve them. It is only when the forces that organize the disturbances within the system are processed that there can be a return to normal function and motion. Dr. Becker claimed that when these forces are dissipated and resolved, he could only perceive the action of the normal biodynamic potencies at work. In other words, when biokinetic forces are resolved by the system, there is a return to the normal action and motion generated by the potency of the Breath of Life. When the biokinetic forces that maintain the disturbance or pathology have been processed and dissipated, only the intrinsic biodynamic forces remain. This is one of the great keys for understanding how the body heals itself as you work in the cranial field.

Dr. Becker also shared that when he treated patients, his attention was placed within the potency of that patient. Dr. Becker wrote,

> My attention, as a physician using diagnostic touch, is on the potency within this patient because I know that within the potency is power and many other attributes around which the disease state or the traumatic condition within the patient is manifesting itself. I know that if a change takes place within this potency a whole new pattern will manifest itself, usually towards health for the patient.[5]

This is so important to appreciate. Dr. Becker is sharing a clinical perspective that is firmly rooted within an awareness of the action of potency within the human system. It is one in which structure and function is the essential starting point, but acknowledges the fundamental role of the potency of the Breath of Life within the human system. He states that within potency lies power. It holds the power to organize and heal the conditions of our lives. Remember that it is the nature of potency to organize. Potency has the power to organize. The disease or disturbance within the system is also organized by the action of potency, both by the intrinsic biodynamic potency of the system and by the added biokinetic forces that it has to resolve or contain in some way. The natural potencies of the system will attempt to organize the added biokinetic forces in ways that are least detrimental to the system. He also states that it is his awareness of a change in the potency that is the key indicator of clinical effect and healing process. Placing attention within the dynamics of potency allows the practitioner a more direct access to the forces maintaining the disease state. It is only when the practitioner perceives a return to a more natural expression of potency and the natural motility and motion generated by it that a return to wellness is considered to have occurred.

Thus it is possible for practitioners to place their attention within the potencies involved in any disturbance or inertial pattern, not just on the results of the action of these forces such as tissue resistance or lesion patterns. It is the potencies involved that have the power to manifest the disease state and also the power to heal it. To summarize, there is within the system the inherent biodynamic potency of the Breath of Life and there are biokinetic forces that the system must resolve or compensate for. Again, when these biokinetic forces are dissipated and resolved, there is a return to the natural condition of health and only the action of natural potencies are perceived. The most important thing to note here is that the practitioner's attention can be with these forces and their interplay. His or her attention is with the organizing factors of both health and disease, not just the results of their presence. The placing of one's attention in relation to these intrinsic forces is a perceptual skill that must be developed by all practitioners. We will outline approaches to these skills in the chapters that follow.

Summary of Concepts from Dr. Rollin Becker

Biodynamic Potency

The potency
   of the Breath of Life

The ordering principle

The Original matrix

Biokinetic Forces

Environmental
   forces, stress

Traumatic forces

Pathogens

Genetics

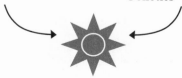

Biodynamic potencies become inertial in order to center the biokinetic forces maintaining the disturbance.

At the heart of every inertial fulcrum are forces at work, the biodynamic potencies centering the disturbance and the biokinetic forces that maintain them. Tissue resistances, tissue changes, and fluid congestion are effects, or results of deeper forces at work.

Fulcrums and Potencies

I would like to summarize some important concepts here. Biodynamic potency acts to center or contain the unresolved experiences still held within the system. These unresolved traumas and traumatic forces, such as accidents, birth processes, stress patterns, and environmental toxins, all have their own potency or power. If unresolved, the system will have to organize around them in some way too. If these forces are maintained within the body, the inherent potency of the system will become inertial within the site of the location of the traumatic force, toxin, or environmental assault. If these forces revolve around more general states of shock and neuroendocrine imbalance, then wider inertial issues will be found within the body. The inherent potency within the system always attempts to contain and compensate for all of these unresolved forces.

Dr. Becker discussed potency in very specific ways. He maintained that potency is a point of stillness within the bioenergy fields of the body. This echoes concepts discussed above and in past chapters. These places of stillness manifest as fulcrums that organize the activities of the body. Potency is a field phenomenon. As we have discussed, within the body physiology there is a unified field of potency, or bioenergy. Within this field are condensations of potency that become organizing fulcrums. They are coalescences of potency within a wider field of action. They organize the motion and function of that field. The intrinsic potencies within the body concentrate to form fulcrums around which the patterns of activity within the body move and function. This is true for the body's natural fulcrums as well as its inertial fulcrums.

The site of a disturbance within the system becomes a site of inertial forces around which cells and tissues must organize. Within this is the stillness or inertia of the biokinetic forces that are manifesting the disturbance in some way. That is, these forces have become concentrated and relatively still within the greater bioenergy or bioelectric field of the system. Within this fulcrum point are also found the potencies of the Breath of Life itself, the intrinsic biodynamic potencies of the body. These inherent potencies initially attempt to resolve the biokinetic forces in some way. If this is not possible, they will also become inertial in order to center and contain them. They will be held in the best possible compensation within the whole of the body physiology. This site of inertial potency will become an inertial fulcrum within the body physiology. These fulcrums maintain and manifest tissue and fluid disturbances. In essence, the biodynamic potency of the Breath of Life will vary from its natural expression in order to contain and compensate for any unresolvable inertial force within the system.

This is an extremely important concept to grasp. The body expresses its health through its inherent potency and this potency, the potency of the Breath of Life, has the capacity to *vary* from its natural expression in order to center and contain the disturbance in some way. The potency of the Breath of Life will become inertial at the heart of any disturbance in order to compensate for and center the biokinetic forces involved. Thus, within every inertial fulcrum there is inertial potency. At the heart of every disturbance there is both the potency of the Breath of Life manifesting the health of the body and the potency of the biokinetic forces that manifest the disease state or strain within the system. The intrinsic biodynamic potencies of the Breath of Life are *centering* the biokinetic forces at the heart of the disturbance, maintaining the best possible compensation for its action.

Thus potency becomes inertial in order to center disturbances and the fluid, cellular and tissue world follows. Inertial fulcrums result. Inertial fulcrums become still places that organize the structure and function of the body and its motility and motion. At the heart of the inertial fulcrum is a stillness, the stillness of the inertial potencies that both maintain and center the unresolvable disturbance. Dr. Becker encourages the practitioner to become aware of these areas of stillness or inertia within the disturbed tissues. These are the organizing fulcrums of the disturbance. Perceiving the stillness at the heart

of a disturbance is to begin to perceive the inertial potencies that are both maintaining and centering it. Perceiving and understanding these fulcrums, potencies, and forces at work is the key to efficient and noninvasive clinical practice.

Forces at Work

- Intrinsic biodynamic potencies within the human system. These are the potencies of the Breath of Life, an expression of the Original matrix.

- Biokinetic forces that overlay the Original matrix and affect the natural biokinetics of the system. These are the genetic, environmental, pathogenic, and traumatic forces of experience and their potencies,

- Biodynamic potencies and biokinetic forces become inertial and generate fields of action and motion organized around inertial fulcrums. The cellular and tissue world will become inertial and organize motility and mobility around inertial fulcrums.

Repercussions of Inertia

The repercussions of all of this are huge. As potency becomes more and more bound up in inertia, reduced vitality will be experienced. Tissue and fluid changes will occur, classical osteopathic lesions will be generated, reduced functioning will result, metabolic fields will become inertial, and pathological processes will have the opportunity to gain a foothold. If the system is holding many inertial fulcrums and patterns, there can be a huge amount of potency bound up in centering the disturbances and maintaining compensations. This will have a depleting effect on the whole system. The more potency that becomes inertial in order to center disturbances, the less will be available for the biodynamics of the system as a whole. As potency becomes inertial, the tissue and fluid world, which is organized around its dynamics, will also become inertial. Metabolic fields will become inertial and body physiology will be affected. Tissue changes, fixation, and pathology will result.

Life Is a Unit of Function

The cellular world can be thought of as a world of metabolic motion. Cells are not separate entities and are obviously not separate from their environment. In essence, a cell is not a thing, but a living process which is always in motion. Furthermore, cellular activities are not isolated processes. As the potency of the Breath of Life is expressed as a unified field phenomenon, the cells of the body can also be thought of as a unified physiological field. Drs. Blechschmidt and Gasser write in their extraordinary book, *Biokinetics and Biodynamics of Human Differentiation:*

> There is good reason for the assumption that every cell represents a field that is called a metabolic field. The concept of a metabolic field is very important. It shows that no cell should be thought of as rigid unity but rather as a momentary aspect of spacially ordered metabolic movement. The same is valid for cell aggregations (tissues), for tissue aggregations (organs) and also for the whole organizm at any stage of development.[6]

This statement has powerful repercussions for healing work of any kind. It stresses that cells, tissues, and organ systems are interdependent metabolic fields, which are expressions of "spacially ordered metabolic movements." In other words, they are not things, they are processes. Furthermore, they are "a momentary aspect" of these fields, which means that cells and tissues live totally in *present time* with the immediacy and impermanence of their interactions being the only reality. This also means that they can only be clinically approached in present time and that our work in the cranial field is totally geared to this present time-ness.

Every cell is an expression of the dynamics of a unified living *metabolic field*. The whole body is one great metabolic field and, indeed, expresses metabolic movements and interchange as a whole. An important aspect of this is that metabolic fields are essentially fluid fields, and that fluids are the ground of all metabolic processes. Metabolic movements are fluid movements, and fluids convey the potency of the Breath of Life. Thus, within our context, metabolic fields are an expression of the unified field of potency that organizes it. Potency, fluid, and tissues are a unit of function, and the unity of the metabolic fields within the body is a manifestation of this. There is the unified field of potency, the unified field of fluids, and the unified metabolic field, which organizes around it. In essence, cells, tissues, fluids, and potency are all an expression of a unified life process, which is impossible to separate into pieces or parts. All parts are an expression of the dynamics of the whole: all life is a unit of function.

Potency, Metabolic Fields, and Inertia

Within the framework of this book, the motility and motion of fluids and tissues is an expression of a living and palpable biodynamic process. This process is orchestrated and generated by the action of the Breath of Life. Motility is a key metabolic motion, which is an expression of this creative intention. At a physiological level, the potency of the Breath of Life acts through the fluid systems of the body. This is what maintains order within all "spacially ordered metabolic movements." When an inertial fulcrum arises within the body physiology, metabolic fields are directly effected. As inertial potencies are generated, fluids will also become inertial. Because metabolic fields are essentially fluid fields, the metabolic processes that occur within them are effected. Stasis arises within these metabolic fields of action as potency and fluid become inertial. In other words, inertia arises within the body physiology. The important point here is that the body functions as a unified metabolic field. Disturbances within that field are a direct manifestation of inertial forces at work. Inertial potencies will generate inertial fluids, and inertial fluids will be expressed as inertia within the metabolic fields of the body. An inertial fulcrum will affect the *whole* in some way, not just the parts within that whole.

As discussed in earlier chapters, recent research has discovered that there are bioelectric quantum-level fields of organization in living organisms. These fields form a unified coherent and dynamic bioelectric matrix, which seems to represent the most subtle level of organization within living systems. This quantum level field phenomenon is a coherent and unified field of action; it is whole. The fluids of the body seem to be intimately associated with its expression. As also mentioned in previous chapters, the interstitial fluids of the body form a unified field or matrix via discrete and coherent hydrogen bonding. This unified field is, in turn, bonded to the peptide side chains of connective tissues, forming a unified fluid-tissue matrix throughout the body. It has been further discovered that disruptions to this field have both local and whole body effects. Local bioelectric disruptions, perhaps due to trauma and disease states, have been noted within the unified quantum-level bioelectric field. These loci of disorder are seen to generate distortion effects within the entire quantum field or matrix. In other words, local inertial fulcrums organize distortions within the whole field! This has been observed through palpation and observation in the cranial field. This information is most available within the mid-tide and Long Tide fields of action. This new research seems to echo the very things we have been describing.

As described in earlier chapters, it has also been found that discrete and coherent quantum wave forms move through this fluid-tissue matrix. The exchange of information at this level is near the speed of light! Furthermore, this local quantum level field is not separate from other fields. Indeed, it can be considered to be a local quantum phenomenon within a much larger field of action. This field of action may be the whole of the universe! This begins to sound like descriptions of how the Long Tide generates the human bioelectric field as a local phenomenon within a vast field of action. The presence of light photons has even been noted within the fluids of the body, especially cerebrospinal fluid. Dr. Sutherland's description of *"liquid light"* is much more than just a metaphor, it is a living reality. Here we see scientific research that echoes the insights gained within the cranial field via observation and palpation.[7]

Mechanisms of Protection

As we have seen, there is an Intelligence at work within the metabolic fields of the human body. Embryological development and cellular differentiation are expressions of this deeper Intelligence. The potency of the Breath of Life lays down the bioelectric matrix and the cellular and tissue world responds. This intelligence underlies all metabolic field relationships. As seen above, metabolic fields are, in essence, fluid fields. Fluid fields hold and convey the potency of the Breath of Life. This potency is at the heart of the metabolic processes of the body. Cellular and tissue structures organize in relationship to these dynamics. Metabolic fields are in essence fields of fluid and potency. Potency, fluids, and tissues form one unified field of action. When the body is placed under stress, disturbances occur within the dynamics of the entire field. Potencies, fluids, and tissues will respond to that stress as a unit of function. Biodynamic forces within the field will attempt to protect the system.

As we have seen, when the system is placed under stress, there will be condensation and coalescence of potency within this unified field. Potency will condense and concentrate, and the fluid and tissue world will respond. The cells and tissues that are expressions of these fields will react to the circumstances imposed upon them. They will respond to the stresses imposed upon the field because they are a unified part of that field. They will respond by contraction and compression. Tissues will contract and compress, and fluids will express stasis and congestion. The natural flow and motility of things is then lost. To paraphrase Dr. Peter Levine, where there is normally flow, there is fixity.

As potency responds to inertial forces, a coiling effect occurs. Locally, as part of the process of condensation, potency spirals or coils in tight centripetal motions. It seems that centripetal or inwardly spiralling motions are the heart of organization within the bioelectric field. Remember from the discussion in Chapter Five that human bioelectric field is generated within a much larger field of action via spiraling, centripetal forces. See Chapter Five for a discussion of this in terms of the works of Victor Schauberger. Even Dr. Sutherland talked about an awareness of spiraling forces active within the fluid dynamics of the system. Inertial fulcrums are generated in the same way. Potencies become inertial by coiling inward via centripetal action in order to contain and center any biokinetic forces that enter the system.

As biodynamic potencies coil and compress in order to contain biokinetic forces and protect the system, tissues will respond via contraction. The most basic way that cell and tissue systems respond to stress is to *contract* to protect their integrity. This can even happen on a microlevel within the cell structure. Microtubules, hollow connective tissues within the cell, have contractile abilities. If the resources of the system are overwhelmed by stress or trauma, then potencies, fluids, and tissues will be effected and this will be expressed within the form of the field (i.e., its cells and tissue systems). Tissues will contract, fluid dynamics will be affected, and "spacially ordered metabolic movements" will become disrupted. Thus in order to counter the unresolved forces of experience, potencies will coil and condense, fluids will become congested, and tissues will contract and undergo qualitative changes. The bottom line is that the relationship to the Breath of Life and the expression of its potency within cells and tissues will become compromised. The cellular and tissue world, rather than orienting to the Original matrix alone, now also has to orient to the stress being centered.

Thus, it is the natural tendency of all cellular and tissue systems, when placed under stress, to defend by contraction. All biological systems will contract to defend themselves when placed under stress. All cells are part of interrelated metabolic fields and will contract when stress is experienced in these fields. The essence of this is that tissue contraction is an expression of the action of potencies. Once again, when biodynamic potencies condense and become inertial in order to meet the biokinetic forces imposed upon the system, potencies will condense, fluids densify, and tissues contract.

A classic example of this is what may happen during birthing processes. During birth the system is placed under extreme compressive forces. If these forces overwhelm the integrity of the baby, then some of the forces involved may not be able to be processed during the birth experience. Potencies will condense to meet these forces, fluids will densify, and tissues will contract to protect the integrity of the organism. In the adult, you may sense fluid congestion and density within the dynamics of the cerebrospinal fluid, membranous and tissue contraction, and compression of structural parts. The fluids may seem dense, the membranes contracted, and the vertebral axis and cranial base compressed. Thus, cerebrospinal fluid will hold the memory of birth compression as density and congestion, and the tissues will express this dynamic as chronic patterns of contraction and structural compression. Again, potencies condense to center the inertial forces involved, fluids densify, and tissues contract to defend the organism.

Contraction also occurs at a macrolevel in the body. The connective tissues of the body will contract as a unit of function when the organism is placed under stress. Potency will become inertial within its field of action in order to center the experience, and the related tissue contractions will be maintained by the interplay of the biodynamic and biokinetic forces involved. If the system's resources are overwhelmed by the experience, these inertial potencies will remain and the protective contractions will be maintained. If the system is traumatized as it responds to its experience, and if there are strong emotional affects, such as fear and anger, at the time of the experience, then it is even more likely that these protective patterns will become frozen and locked into the system's dynamics.

Frozen in Time

These protective responses are essential at the initial time of the experience but, if not resolved, can become locked into the system as deeply ingrained protective patterning. This occurs on all levels. Tissues, fluids, and potency act as a unified field of action. Inertial fulcrums will be generated around which the system has to organize. After a traumatic incident, future stress of any kind may be met by similar inertial responses. The system will tend to protect itself relative to the protective compressions and contractions it is already holding. Along with this protective response, interrelated shock affects are also commonly held within the system. These may include the cycling of stress responses and related emotions, the cycling of autonomic energies, and neuroendocrine imbalances.

This will have repercussions in everyday life. For instance, a bad or stressful day at work might reactivate an existing protective pattern, related stress responses, and familiar symptomatology. These may range from quite mild symptoms to more intense ones such as cervical pain, muscular tension, migraine headaches, and so on. These will also be expressed via emotional and psychological processes. Stress states, such as feelings of anxiety or fear, may arise. These processes are commonly related to past traumatization and its retention within the system. The person becomes "frozen in time" as the experience, its related shock affects, and the need to protect against them is locked into the system. These forms will also be expressed as central nervous system facilitation and shock affects, as fluid congestion, and as chronic tissue tension, contraction, and

organization. We will describe neuroendocrine stress responses and their effects on the system in Volume Two.

All of this is a result of unresolved inertial potencies at work. Biodynamic potencies will become inertial in order to meet and center the biokinetic forces involved. The tissue and fluid world will, in turn, organize around these potencies. Remember, at the heart of every inertial fulcrum forces are at work. These forces will be expressed at every level within the mind-body. Psychological constructs may arise, emotional affects may be held, and tissues will hold protective contractions and fixation. Phew! you might say. How in the world can I, as a practitioner, deal with all of this? I can only answer by encouraging you to trust in the resources of the very system that is experiencing pain and suffering. Trust in the inherent healing forces, which are always present. At the deepest level, Health is never lost and, when given the opportunity, the system will move to higher levels of organization, homeostatic balance and energy. Indeed, within every pattern of resistance and suffering, the inherent potency of the Breath of Life is ever present and is waiting to be accessed.

The Inertial Fulcrum: Concepts Summarized

Let's take a breath! There are a lot of concepts and information outlined above, so a summary here may not go amiss. As we have discussed, the term *inertial fulcrum* is very important. It refers to sites of congestion and inertia within the body. All patterns of fixity and resistance within the system are organized around inertial fulcrums. The term denotes both the *forces and potencies* at work and the *response* of tissues and fluids to them. Within the heart of every inertial fulcrum there are forces at work. These include both the biodynamic potencies of the Breath of Life and the conditional forces of experience. Conditional forces may include the forces of accidents, trauma, pathogens, or the forces of any experience the system has not been able to resolve. The potency of the Breath of Life acts to center these forces in some way. Biodynamic potency is *centering* these traumatic or experiential forces within the system as a whole. Dr. Becker used the term *centering* in a specific way. He said that the biodynamic potencies of the Breath of Life act to *center* the disturbances within the system in some way. *Centering* simply means that the forces maintaining the pattern of resistance or pathology are contained and compensated for in some way by the potency of the Breath of Life.

When experiential forces such as accidents, trauma, or pathology cannot be processed by the system, they become organizing factors and must be contained and compensated for in some way. The potency of the Breath of Life does this by becoming inertial in relationship to the experiential forces involved. Thus, at the heart of any inertial process there are both experiential forces present, which maintain the resistance or pathology, and intrinsic potencies, which attempt to process, contain, and compensate for then. As described earlier, Dr. Rollin Becker, D.O., called the traumatic forces that maintain the inertia in the system *biokinetic forces*. He called the potency of the Breath of Life, which is centering and compensating for these, *biodynamic potencies*. Both come into play in the creation of an inertial fulcrum. Thus within the site of any resistance or pathology found in the system, there are inertial forces at work. These are both the biodynamic potencies of the Breath of Life and the inertial forces that they are centering.

Potency is a unified field within the human system. Potency is whole and within its unified field of expression, sites of inertia arise in relationship to the biokinetic forces taken on by the system. Potency, within its unified field, condenses and becomes inertial in order to center these forces. The forces are centered within the greater dynamics of the system. Potency, in essence, becomes inertial within its own field of action in order to process or center the disturbances present. Thus inertial potency is a condensation within a wider unified field. It is a discrete expression of the Intelligence and Health inherent within the system. In its natural expression of tensile motility, the potency itself will then express eccentric motions around areas of its own inertia. Fluids and tissues will follow. Much potency can become bound up in centering the unresolved forces of experience. Eccentric motion, reduced motility, physiological dysfunction, and lowered vitality result.

An area that has become inertial has lost its natural ability to fully express natural motility and mobility. An inertial fulcrum may be very focal and expressed as a specific site of inertia, like a vertebral fixation or a particular visceral adhesion. It may also have wider manifestations. For instance, the birth process commonly places strong axial forces into the system. These forces may be introduced into the vertebral axis as a whole and large areas of axial compression may result. These are expressions of inertial forces, which have wide action within the body and are centered as a whole. Thus inertial forces may be held within a large area within the body as one unified dynamic. In all cases, whenever inertial fulcrums are generated, the whole tensile field of action is effected. You may perceive the whole tensile tissue field distorting around inertial areas. This is easiest to perceive at the mid-tide or Long Tide level of action. For instance, as you palpate the cranium, you may sense the whole membranous articular field distort around an inertial fulcrum located within a suture. Holding a wider view, you may even sense the whole body, as a unified tensile field, distorting around that particular fulcrum.

Inertial Fulcrums and Automatically Shifting Fulcrums

As we have seen, the natural organizing fulcrums of the system are automatically shifting fulcrums, that is, they shift with the intentions of the Breath of Life. Inertial fulcrums are sites within the system that have lost the ability to automatically shift within the inhalation and exhalation phases of primary respiration. As we have seen, the term *inertial fulcrum* denotes not only a locus of tissue and fluid change, but also includes the forces that both maintain and center the disturbance. These sites include both the tissue changes present and the forces that maintain them. Where there should ideally be fluidity, sites of fixity and density arise. When these are held within the system, the reciprocal tension motion of fluids and tissues will become patterned in some way. Their natural motion will become shaped and their natural orientation to the midline and to embryologically derived fulcrums will be affected.

This is an important point to reemphasize. Ideally tissues and fluids express a natural reciprocal tension motion oriented around embryologically derived, automatically shifting fulcrums. These natural axes and fulcrums are embryologically laid down and are an expression of the blueprint carried by the Breath of Life. These natural fulcrums are called *suspended automatically shifting fulcrums* because they are suspended within their field of action and naturally shift in response to the phases of primary respiration. Inertial fulcrums, however, are not automatically shifting fulcrums. They are locations of inertia and fixity. When inertial fulcrums arise within the body, tissues and fluids will have to reorient and express motion in relationship to these loci too. The biodynamics of the system will have to take these experiential fulcrums into account, and there is a shift away from the ideal expression of motility and motion within the body. A new organization occurs. We will discuss automatically shifting fulcrums in later chapters in much more depth.

Conditioned Shape: Form, Motion, and Quality

I sometimes use the term *shape* to denote inertial or conditioned organization. Conditioned organization is an expression of unresolved experience. *Form, movement, and quality* are aspects of the organization of fluids and tissues within and around an inertial fulcrum. All of these aspects together create the pattern of expression, or shape, that the system has taken. When you sense the shapes of experience within a person's system, it is important not to forget that you are palpating a whole person. Remember that, as you palpate the person's history, you are in relationship to the *whole* of that history and the Health that centers it within the human condition.

The term *shape* is a shorthand to denote the whole of an inertial pattern *and* its inertial fulcrum. Thus a shape is the whole dynamic of an inertial pattern and the fulcrum that organizes its movement and form. As you develop perceptual experience, you will see that *shape* has three basic aspects: *form, motion,* and *quality* organized around an inertial fulcrum. In this work, you will learn to relate to inertial patterns as shapes within the system that have become organized around inertial fulcrums.

First, every conditioned shape or pattern in the body has its *form*. When the body holds an inertial fulcrum, its fluids, cells, and tissues will become organized in relationship to it. The fluids of the body and its tissues, be they membranes, bony structures, or organ systems, will compensate for and habituate to the fulcrum involved. A form expressing that experience will arise. This form will be expressed physically as shapes of tension, density, resistance, and fixation, which are all part of overall cellular and tissue shape. An overall form will be assumed in relationship to the inertial fulcrum that organizes it. This form is unique to that person. It is expressed as a deviation from the ideal or universal design of the system. Even with these dynamics at play, the integrity of this design is still maintained. Even in the most intransigent pathologies, the Breath of Life always functions to maintain the integrity of the whole. The system is still a unity. I remind you of this so that, in the inquiry into the experiential shapes of a conditioned system, you do not get lost in its fragments. No matter how seemingly fragmented and resistant a system is, we must remember that this wholeness is never lost.

Shape also has its *motion* dynamic. All the tissues in the body express primary respiration in cycles of reciprocal tension motion. This inherent motion is ideally organized in relationship to the primal midline and by the natural fulcrums derived from it. However, when inertial fulcrums arise, they will also become organizing factors within the system. Motion will then also become shaped or patterned in direct relationship to the inertia the system is holding. Thus, as we respond to our environment and to the conditions of our life, inertial fulcrums will create unique movement patterns and the tissue world will express its motility and motion in unique and patterned ways. In essence, the whole history of the person will be expressed in the forms and motions (or, indeed, lack of motion) within the system.

Finally, each shape will have its *quality* or qualities. It is important to understand that the qualities of a particular shape are in direct relationship to the qualities of the fulcrum that organizes it. Its quality may have a physical sense to it; dense, light, full, strong, weak, and so on. The tissues may have a sense of heaviness, thickness, thinness, dryness, or congestion. The shape may also have feeling tones and emotional qualities coupled with it, and there may also be processes of memory, image, or thought forms coupled with the organizing fulcrum. There may be shock affects held in the system in relationship to the fulcrum and shape organized around it.

Thus, there may be shock affects, emotions, feeling tones, sensations, mental states, images, and even behaviors that relate to the fulcrum and shape you are sensing. This is critical to understand. You are not just palpating a physical body. You are in a privileged position of trust in which you are literally palpating the whole of a person's life experience and history. Furthermore, you are also in the humbling position of being in direct relationship to the expression of Health, the potency of the Breath of Life, which literally permeates the whole of the human system, including the historical shapes held.

Clinical Application:
Awareness of Inertial Fulcrums

In this first investigation, you will simply begin to sense shapes of experience. These shapes are organized around the inertial fulcrums that the system has had to create in order to center our experience of life. When a trauma or disease condition cannot be fully processed by the system, the Breath of Life will *center* it in some way. At the heart of any tissue or fluid resistance are forces at work, both the forces that maintain the resistance and the forces of the Breath of Life that are centering them. Here the intention is simply to listen to the system with active attention and a wide perceptual field. In this process, you will simply listen to the patterns that arise within your perceptual field and ask the question, "What organizes this?"

In your previous work, you learned to listen to the motility and mobility of tissues. As you did this, I am sure that eccentric motion patterns became obvious. These are patterns that deviate from the ideal motion around natural fulcrums and their midline organization. In this perceptual exercise, you will simply become aware of these and ask the question, "What organizes this?" Let the system answer. As you do this, do not *look* for anything. Listen and let it speak to you. Your intention will be to perceive the still place or fulcrum that organizes this motion. Let your hands make a gentle, floating contact and imagine/sense that your hands are literally floating in fluid. As you ask the question, simply listen for the answer. Notice how you receive the information that returns to you from your perceptual field. In this exercise you will synchronize your perceptual field with the mid-tide level of perception. Here you will receive an overall sense of the system and very precise information can be communicated to you.

1. With the patient in the supine position, place your hands in the vault hold described earlier. Establish your practitioner fulcrums and negotiate your contact and viewing distance. After

negotiating your relationship to the patient's system, be sure that your physical contact is light and stable. As you establish this contact, create a further practitioner fulcrum to clarify your relationship to the system. Place gentle pressure on your elbows. To do this, allow the weight of your shoulders to settle into your elbows. As discussed in previous chapters, this will create *elbow fulcrum points*. This will enhance your perception of the tissue motions being palpated. As you do this, allow your hands to float freely from your elbow fulcrum points. Do not lose the gentle contact you have negotiated with the patient's system.

2. Synchronize your perceptual field with the midtide. Let your hands float on the tissues and be immersed in fluids. Widen your perceptual field to include the whole of the biosphere, the person's body, and the field of environmental exchange around it. Image/sense that your hands are floating within fluids as they float on the tissues. Sense that the tissues are like kelp beds floating within the tidal forces of the ocean. Let your hands float within fluid and be moved by the potency, fluid, and tissues as a unified field of action. Any physical pressure on the tissues will stop them from doing what they would do if you were not there. Let them, in turn, move you. As you hold an awareness of the biosphere, do not lose a perception of tissues and tissue motion.

3. Allow the tissues to come to you, rather than trying to find anything. Be aware of the tissues as a unified tensile field of action. Listen to the whole of the tissues at once. *Listen*, don't look. Sense whatever tissue motion begins to clarify. See what speaks to you. Float within fluids and let yourself be moved. As you tune into this, notice the pattern of this motion. You may notice an eccentric or patterned motion. The system may prefer either inhalation or exhalation, and

this may be expressed in specific ways. You may sense distortions within the tensile tissue field. There may be a sense of torsioning or circling as you follow the tissue motions under your hands. There may also be a sense of pulls or strains as you listen.

4. As you perceive this, see if you can sense how the motion is organized. Ask the question, "What organizes this?" For instance, you might sense a pattern of motion that seems to circle around a particular suture, or you might sense the tissues being pulled into a particular place. It might be in the cranium, or it might even be moving in relationship to some other place in the body. Just be open to motion and motility and allow these to show you the organizing fulcrum. Give yourself the luxury of *not knowing* and not having to do anything. Just listen and see if you can appreciate what organizes the tissue dynamics you are palpating. You are essentially perceiving places of stillness around which motion is organized. You may also receive information from the fluids. Are there fluid fluctuations that communicate anything about tissue organization and related inertial fulcrums?

5. Once you have a sense of this at the vault hold, move your hands to the occipital cradle and sacral holds and repeat the exploration at those vantage points. At each place, first tune in to the general expression of motion and motility and then to its unique patterning. Start a conversation with the tissues; allow them to show you their story. Be open to the possibility that you can sense this. Let yourself guess; allow yourself to be wrong. In time you will trust what you are sensing more and more. The most important thing is not to look for anything. Allow the tissues and their history to come to you. Let yourself listen to them, but don't seek or grasp them. Simply see if you can sense the fulcrums that

organize their motion. Finish the exploration with a sacrooccipital hold to help the system integrate whatever it needs to.

The intention of the above exploration was to help you tune in to tissue motion and motility and to begin to sense what that motion is organized around. Remember that the power to organize is concentrated within the fulcrum, not at the poles of its expression (e.g., not in the shape that is organized around it). Dr. Rollin Becker wrote of the fulcrum as a place of potency and power. Fulcrums have the power to organize and are expressions of potencies at work. Natural fulcrums are expressions of the natural organizing potencies of the Breath of Life. Inertial fulcrums are expressions of the unresolved forces of our experience and how they are centered within the system as a whole.

A Wider View of the Forces at Work

As we simply become still and listen, a wider view of life and of the forces that organize it naturally unfolds. It is a very humbling experience. It is important to remember that a human being is not just physical. We are not just an expression of form and inertia. I believe that we are an expression of the interrelationship among physical form, emotional and psychological process, and the interplay between soul and spirit. An inertial fulcrum can be held anywhere within the dynamics of form, emotional process, and psychological conditioning. People also talk about the wounding of the soul, or "soul wounding." In these terms a deeply traumatic process can be held within the deepest recesses of who we are, our soul organization. Buddhists might call this the karmic organization of our stream of consciousness, or *citta*.

Spirit is the universal at work within the play of consciousness and form. Spirit, in the universal or archetypal sense, is the Intelligent space in which this all unfolds. It is the "Holy Spirit," the divine Intelligence at work within us all. A friend of mine once had a conversation with a Russian Orthodox priest. My friend came from a Catholic background, but had left the faith. He asked the priest about the holy trinity, the Father, Son, and Holy Spirit, which he never really connected with. The priest gave a wonderful explanation. He said that the Father is the divine potential for all manifestation, that the Holy Spirit orchestrates the intentions of the divine, and that the Son is that potential made manifest. The Father is the potential for all of manifestation, the Son is that potential made manifest, and the Holy Spirit orchestrates and connects. Thus the Holy Spirit expresses the intentions of the divine; it connects all to that intention and maintains the wholeness of life. This seems so similar to the idea of the Breath of Life as an expression of a divine Intelligence and intention. This Intelligence is always working to maintain the integrity of our form, and the potency of the Breath of Life is an expression of its function.

Within the Buddhist tradition, Ven. Chogyam Trungpa Rinpoche used the term "brilliant sanity" to express its action.[8] In our terms, the Breath of Life is the brilliant sanity within the play of our conditions. Brilliant sanity has three aspects: spaciousness, clarity, and compassion. When one is attuned to its expression within our human form, these naturally unfold and are our birthright. They are expressions of the interconnectedness and mutuality of all phenomena. When one's mind is truly still and one's perceptual field is very wide, this truth begins to unfold. We are, at essence, beings of clear light. In Tibetan Buddhism, practitioners learn ways to prepare for the dying process when this truth can be seen within the dissolution of form. The clear light, our essential nature, shines through. This is also called *mahamudra,* or Buddha nature; the already enlightened state within each of us. This state is not different in you or me, it is a universal at work and underpins our existence. These are wider issues that we all must inquire into in our own way as part of our unique journey through life. I have no answers here, only the intention to pay attention to life as it unfolds within me and others. Perhaps the great inquiry is, "What is the fulcrum that is at the heart of it all?"

In the following chapters we deepen our exploration of these concepts and explore some of the basic skills of the cranial concept. The most important principle we will explore in the next few chapters is that of the *state of balanced tension* and the *neutral*. In these sections you will begin to extend your understanding of the fulcrum, the potency manifest within it, and the power of accessing the neutral in relationship to it.

1. See the discussion in Chapter Five on quantum-field levels of organization in the body. Coherent, quantum-level bioelectric field phenomena have been discovered within living organisms. Concepts of "life force" or bioenergy are seen in all traditional forms of medicine.

2. For an elegant description of these concepts see R. E. Becker, "Diagnostic Touch: Its Principles and Application, I, II, III, IV" *Academy of Applied Osteopathy Yearbooks* 1963, 1964, 1965; an edited version of these papers is also found in R. E. Becker, *Life in Motion* (Rudra Press).

3. Dr. Erich Blechschmidt wrote about the natural biokinetic movements of cells during embryological differentiation and development. See Blechschmidt and Gasser, *Biokinetics and Biodynamics of Human Differentiation* (Charles C. Thomas 1978).

4. see Becker, R.E. Diagnostic touch: its principles and application I, II, III, IV. *Academy of Applied Osteopathy Yearbooks* 1963,1964,1965.

5. Becker, R.E. Diagnostic touch: its principles and application IV. *Academy of Applied Osteopathy Yearbooks* 1965. Reprinted with the permission of the American Academy of Osteopathy.

6. Blechschmidt and Gasser, Biokinetics and Biodynamics of Human Differentiation, Charles C. Thomas Publisher (1978).

7. Mae-Wan Ho, *The Rainbow and the Worm, the Physics of Organisms* (World Scientific).

8. The term *brilliant sanity* was coined by the Ven. Chogyam Trungpa Rinpoche.

14

The Point of Balanced Tension

In previous chapters we began to explore both the motility and mobility of cranial bones and the motion of the reciprocal tension membranes. We talked about the classical understanding of the reciprocal tension motion and introduced the dynamics of Sutherland's fulcrum. The last chapter introduced the concepts of the inertial fulcrum and shapes of experience. This chapter continues this exploration. I will introduce a classical approach to the resolution of inertial issues, the *point of balanced tension*, one of the most important concepts in cranial work. This introduction will focus initially on the CRI level of action. Within the CRI, we will focus on tissue patterns and the inertial fulcrums that organize them. In the following chapter, I will open up this concept to an understanding that acknowledges the importance of stillness and the unity of potency, fluids, and tissues. You will then explore what is known

as the *state of balanced tension*. In all of this, you will begin to appreciate the importance of accessing a neutral within the inertial dynamics perceived.

The Shape of History

As you enter this inquiry, you will see that each person's system is a unique expression of his or her history, experience and tendencies. As we experience life, our system becomes conditioned and personalized. The conditional is overlaid upon the universal. The Original matrix is ever present, but unresolved experiential fulcrums generate patterns and forms, which shift structure and function away from the ideal. As this occurs, motility and mobility also become conditioned and personalized. The cells and tissues of the body become shaped in ways specific to a person's history. These shapes are expressions of a person's suffering and personal life journey. As we discussed earlier, all of this is always centered by the potency of the Breath of Life in some way, and its potency is always present even within the most seemingly chaotic and chronic situations.

Introduction to Clinical Applications

In the following sections, I am going to introduce some concepts that are at the heart of work in the cranial field. In this exploration, you will begin to learn to relate to inertial fulcrums and the patterns

In this chapter we will:

- *Begin our exploration into shapes of experience.*

- *Introduce the classical concept of the point of balanced tension.*

- *Introduce clinical skills related to the point of balanced tension.*

they organize. You will discover, as a perceptual experience, that within the heart of any inertial process there is Health. As we have discussed, inertial fulcrums are maintained by biokinetic forces, which the system has to process or center in some way. These may be traumatic forces such as accidents, or the forces that pathogens introduce into the system, or even the forces of genetics. If these forces cannot be processed by the system, then the Breath of Life, via its potency, will become inertial in order to center and compensate for the disturbances or distortions in the system. This is the Health manifesting even in the most confused situations. You can visualize this by imagining a field of fluid and potency within the body. As traumatic forces are introduced into this field, the potency within the fluids condenses to meet these forces and becomes inertial in order to resolve, contain, or center them. Thus at the heart of every resistance or pathological process held, there is Health attempting to process, balance, and compensate for these forces.

The intention of this work is to liberate this Health and to allow a reconnection and realignment to the inherent ordering principles it conveys. In this process, potency is freed to express itself beyond the compensations being held and the experiential forces being balanced. You will learn to access what is known as the *point of balanced tension* and the *state of balanced tension*. I am making a distinction between these two concepts. In this chapter you will learn the classical healing process by which the practitioner facilitates a point of balanced tension within the reciprocal tension motions of membranes and connective tissues. In this approach, you will be in relationship to the tissues within the CRI level of action. In this process practitioners facilitate a *point of balanced membranous tension* within the dynamics of inertial tissue patterns. The focus tends to be on the release and resolution of resistance and lesions.[1] In the next chapter, we will introduce a more holistic approach, which broadens and deepens the original concept. In that approach, you will widen your perceptual field and deepen into the tidal potencies and the 2.5 cycles a minute mid-tide. You will

sense the wholeness of the system and the unit of function of tissues, fluids, and potency. As you learn to do this, you will begin to appreciate that the state of balance has depth and breadth and can be the "eye of the needle" to the most formative forces within the human system. The intrinsic biodynamic forces are perceived to be doing the healing. Dr. Sutherland's admonition to allow the intrinsic forces from within to do the healing can be clearly understood. *From that point on, all clinical applications in this book will be described from the perspective of these deeper rhythms and tidal forces.*

As you learn to appreciate these processes, you will see that at the heart of every lesion, or somatic dysfunction, there are forces at work. Within the fulcrum that organizes the conditioned pattern, the organizing principle of the Breath of Life is never lost and the Original matrix, the inherent blueprint of the human system, is always available. Indeed, even in the most chronic and seemingly hopeless clinical conditions, the blueprint for health is never lost and the healing resources of the system are always available. As we shall see, it is within the state of balanced tension that these resources are naturally expressed. We shall see that at the heart of every disturbance or disease state within the body, there are both conditional forces that are maintaining the state, and biodynamic potencies that act to contain and center these forces.[2]

Reciprocal Tensions and Sutherland's Fulcrum

Before we introduce the clinical concept of the point of balanced membranous tension, it is important to discuss the relationship between membranous tension and Sutherland's fulcrum. As we know, cranial bones and membranes are a unit of function. That is, they function as *one thing* and their dynamics cannot be separated. Furthermore, the dural membranes are seen to move in relationship to an automatically shifting fulcrum called Sutherland's fulcrum. We have discussed this dynamic in previous chapters. This automatically shifting fulcrum is located within the straight sinus, just anterior to where the falx and tentorium meet. (See Figure 14.1.) The membranes are always under tension between this fulcrum and their poles of attachment within the cranium.

You may remember that Sutherland's fulcrum is actually a point of concentrated potency, which has the power to organize and move. The action of Sutherland's fulcrum helps generate the reciprocal tension motion within the osseous-membranous system. Membranes manifest their primary respiratory motion as a *reciprocal tension membrane* moving first one way and then the other around Sutherland's fulcrum. (See Figure 14.2.) Sutherland's fulcrum is one of the natural automatically shifting fulcrums within the system. If a person and his or her system had no inertial fulcrums to deal with, then all membranous, bony, and connective tissue motion within

the body would be organized around Sutherland's fulcrum in a balanced and easy way. Since the cranial bones and the membranes are a unit of function, the motions of the cranial bones are also ideally organized around the dynamic of the automatically shifting fulcrum within the straight sinus.

As we have seen, any added force that has not been resolved by the system will generate inertial fulcrums. These also have the power to organize. Unlike natural fulcrums like Sutherland's fulcrum, these inertial fulcrums do not automatically shift within the phases of the Tide. Eccentric tension patterns, classically called strain patterns, and fluid and tissue affects will result. The reciprocal tension membranes will then not express ideal motion and the organization around Sutherland's fulcrum will change. In fact, this point of potency, ideally located within the most anterior aspect of the straight sinus, may actually shift away from its ideal location in

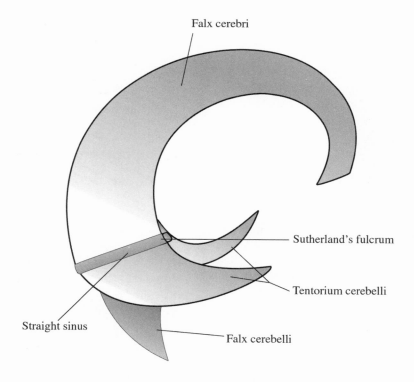

Falx cerebri

Sutherland's fulcrum

Tentorium cerebelli

Straight sinus

Falx cerebelli

14.1 Sutherland's fulcrum

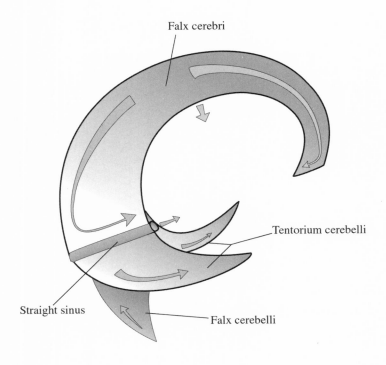

Falx cerebri

Tentorium cerebelli

Straight sinus

Falx cerebelli

14.2 Motion of reciprocal tension menbrane in inhalation

order to center and compensate for the tensions generated by inertial fulcrums.

If you think of Sutherland's fulcrum as a point of potency that acts to balance and resolve the tensions within the membranes, then you will see how it may shift away from its ideal position in order to act as a balance point for all of the tensions present, including those generated by inertial fulcrums. Remember that the power to organize and move rests within the fulcrum. Sutherland's fulcrum, as a point of concentrated potency and power, is still acting to organize and move the connective tissue system and must compensate for all of the tensions held within that system. It will shift from its ideal position in order to do this. If the practitioner has a perceptual awareness of the dynamics around Sutherland's fulcrum, much clinical information becomes available. If an inertial fulcrum and the inertial forces and potencies that organize it are truly resolved, there will be a shift of this fulcrum towards a more ideal location within the straight sinus.

Introduction to the Point of Balanced Tension

The principle of the *point of balanced tension* is one of the key clinical concepts to understand in classical cranial work. The concept was originally used in relationship to cranial lesions and the reciprocal tension membrane system. In this context it is commonly called the *point of balanced membranous tension*, or BMT (balanced membranous tension). It is focused on the CRI level of action and perception. As we shall see, this concept can be widened to encompass all tissues in the body, to the fluctuations of fluid, and even to the potency of the Breath of Life itself. The classical approach is aptly described in *Osteopathy in the Cranial Field*, by Dr. Harold Magoun, D.O.[3] It is the approach that I originally learned many years ago in osteopathic college and in osteopathic apprenticeship.

Since bone and membrane function as one thing, any resistance or lesion found within bony dynamics will be expressed as tension or strain within the membrane system. Likewise, any distortions in membranous dynamics will, in turn, be transferred to cranial bones. Classically, if an inertial fulcrum is located within bony relationships, then the strain pattern is called an *articular membranous strain*. If it is located within the membranes, it is called a *membranous articular strain*. For simplicity, I will generally use the term *membranous articular strain* when discussing these concepts. As a practitioner becomes aware of a membranous articular strain pattern, the intention becomes one of accessing a point of balance, or a neutral, within its tension dynamics. It is thought that this neutral state is the optimum position for the resolution of the strain.

The intention of accessing a point of balanced tension, within this classical context, is to access a neutral within the reciprocal tension dynamics of the tissues. This neutral is the point or state where all the tensions held within the membrane system are at a balance point around their organizing fulcrum. It is a state of *dynamic equilibrium*. It is a point of balance in which there is no push or pull around the inertial fulcrum that organizes the strain pattern within the system. The classic approach is to access a precisely neutral position within the osseous-membranous system in relationship to the inertial fulcrum and the strain pattern it generates. The point of balanced membranous tension is also called a *precise neutral*. The practitioner accesses this neutral via an active inquiry into the tension dynamics of that particular lesion pattern. This precise neutral is considered to be a position in which all of the tension generated by the forces within the inertial fulcrum have found a point of tension balance around the organizing fulcrum. It is considered to be a point of optimum potential for healing processes to be engaged. Once a point of balanced

tension is accessed, then the practitioner holds the tissues at this precise neutral until a release occurs. It is assumed that it is within this neutral state that the inherent healing potencies of the system will come into play and processing of the inertial forces will occur. The intention is to obtain a point of balance, a neutral, in which all the forces maintaining the lesion are balanced and the potential for the self-regulating and self-healing forces of the system come back into play.

This approach was initially applied to membranous articular strains and lesions within the cranium, but can be used anywhere in the body. A cranial lesion is a combination of bony resistance, such as a sutural compression, and the membranous strain that relates to it. The tension created by the lesion is overlaid upon the natural reciprocal tension dynamics of the membranes, and a strain or tension pattern results. Traditionally, the point of balanced membranous tension is a state in which all of the membranous tensions within a lesion pattern are at a balanced point around the fulcrum that originally organized it. In other words, the forces and tensions held within a strain pattern are at a dynamic equilibrium within and around the fulcrum that organizes them. There are relatively no pushes or pulls around the fulcrum, but a point of balance is obtained. It was perceived that at this point the self-correcting tendencies of the system come into play. This concept can be extended to all bony-connective relationships in the body. Outside of the primary respiratory mechanism, the point of balance was called the *point of balanced ligamentous tension*.

The Point of Balanced Membranous Tension: A Dynamic View

As we have seen, within the cranium, the point of balanced tension is classically called the *point of balanced membranous tension*. The term denotes a point within a membranous articular strain pattern where all of the tensions held within the membranes, relative to a specific fulcrum, are at a point of dynamic equilibrium or balance. Classically the point of balanced membranous tension is said to be that point where, within the range of motion of an articulation, such as a suture, the membranes are poised between their natural tensions around Sutherland's fulcrum and the tensions generated by the inertial fulcrum, a fixation within its normal tension dynamics. In this state, all of the tensions generated by the fulcrum or fixation involved are at their absolute minimum, and the possibility for resolution is at its highest potential. The involuntary mechanism is then said to be under the least possible strain and the inherent healing potencies of the system have the most optimum potential to resolve the forces that organize the strain pattern.

Thus, on the level of membranous-articular dynamics, the point of balanced tension is that point where the system is poised between its normal tension dynamic and the tension held due to fixation and trauma. It is a neutral position where all of the tensions held within the pattern are balanced around the fulcrum organizing that pattern. The balance point accessed is in direct relationship to the particular strain pattern being palpated. This is an important concept to grasp. When the point of balanced tension is accessed in relationship to a particular inertial fulcrum, that fulcrum and the pattern it organizes is uncoupled from all other patterns within the system. In essence the whole system is poised around that particular inertial issue. The inherent potencies, both within the inertial fulcrum being palpated and within the whole tensile field of potency of which it is a part, can precisely come into play relative to a particular issue.

In trauma terms this is excellent work. As we have seen, potency is an expression of a unified field of action. This unified field of potency acts *as a whole* to center the inertial issues within the system. The potency of the Breath of Life acts to center the disturbances in the system as a whole. All inertial fulcrums within the body-mind are being centered, contained, and compensated for, all at once. The reciprocal tension motion of the whole system, as a unit of function, reflects this. All inertial fulcrums that affect membranous-articular motion affect it all at once. The tissues will express all of this as a *unified tensile tissue field,* which expresses reciprocal tension motion as a whole. This, all inertial fulcrums, and the tensions they organize, are being compensated for as a *whole* within the system. In this process, when you access the point of balanced tension, you are uncoupling one of these inertial issues from all others. You are not asking the system to resolve everything at once, but are uncoupling one particular issue to attend to. This has great significance.

In the following sections, you will learn to directly relate to inertial fulcrums within the articular membranous system. You do this by learning to access the point of balanced membranous tension within a particular strain pattern. In the next chapter, you will expand this concept by learning to relate to reciprocal states of balanced tension in tissues, fluids, and potency as a unit of function. *Accessing the neutral* is one of the great skills found within the cranial concept. It helps the system express its intrinsic health within inertial fulcrums. As we shall later see, the state of balanced tension is crucial to understand in terms of the biodynamic processes of the body. It is within the state of balance that the inertial potency centering the disturbance is expressed beyond the compensation held within the pattern.

Reciprocal Tensions, Automatically Shifting Fulcrums, and the Point of Balanced Tension

In order to appreciate the importance of the point of balanced tension, you must be able to appreciate the dynamic between Sutherland's fulcrum and the reciprocal tension motion it organizes. As we have seen, all primary respiratory motion within the human system is based on *reciprocal tension motion.* As the Breath of Life generates inhalation and exhalation phases, potency, fluids, and tissues respond by expressing motion in reciprocal cycles. This is especially easy to sense within the dural membrane system. As we have seen, the sickles of the falx and tentorium as a unit of function are called the *reciprocal tension membrane*. They are always in tension and are taut in relationship to their poles of attachment and to the fulcrum that organizes their motion. As seen above, this fulcrum is located within the straight sinus at its junction with the great vein of Galen.

As we have seen, Dr. Sutherland called it an automatically shifting fulcrum. This denotes its dynamic expression of the inhalation and exhalation phases of the Breath of Life. As this fulcrum automatically shifts with the intentions of the Tide, the membrane system moves in relationship to it as a reciprocal tension structure, first one way, then the other.[4] At any time, the tensions held within the membranes are ideally at a point of dynamic balance around Sutherland's fulcrum. Dr. Jim Jealous, D.O., writes,

> As physicians skilled in the recognition of the normal tensile potency and its natural range of motion, we have secondarily become familiar with unhealthy states reflected as inertial phenomena, within the body. We have also become familiar with treatment techniques that will resolve the inertial phenomena if we can properly establish a new state of balance that replicates the suspended automatically shifting fulcrum of a healthy system. This new fulcrum has the quality of a neutral state of balance which when established in the inertial tissue allows the forces from within, that is the self-correcting forces, to shift the inertial tensile forces through a neutral fulcrum back into a moving reciprocal tension.[5]

In this elegant statement, Dr. Jealous is presenting one of the most important concepts in this work. Let's break down this statement and investigate some of its salient concepts. First of all, the ground of our work is to be aware of the health within the system. This is the fundamental truth. Health is

never lost and is with us from the moment of conception until the day we die. The normal "tensile potency" is an expression of this health when it is unimpeded within the human system. The Breath of Life generates potencies, forces with the power to organize, within the fluids and this potency, driven by the inhalation and exhalation phases of the Tide, has tensile qualities. It too expresses motility in cycles of reciprocal tension motion and its "normal tensile" expression is part of the unit of function of potency, fluids, and tissues. All express reciprocal tension motion as a whole, and this dynamic is an expression of the Health of the system.

An awareness of the Health is the ground of the work in this field. In our work we also become aware of how the system has become patterned and conditioned due to the vicissitudes of life. These are expressed and perceived as "inertial phenomena." These sites and patterns of inertia within the body are expressions of the history of the system. They are expressions of the particular, the individualization of the system. In the cranial concept, treatment approaches have been developed to help the system resolve these issues. The most fundamental of these approaches is founded upon the understanding and perception of suspended automatically shifting fulcrums and of states of balance. We have discussed Sutherland's fulcrum and the concept of the suspended automatically shifting fulcrum. These are the natural fulcrums within the system, which are laid down embryologically by the action of the Breath of Life. If no inertial issues are present within the system, all tissues and fluids would naturally orient to these fulcrums. If the practitioner can access a *neutral* within the dynamics of the inertial pattern, the inherent "forces from within" will come into play. This neutral has the "quality of a neutral state of balance," which realigns the tissues, fluids, and potencies involved to their Original intention and to the natural automatically shifting fulcrums of the system. They shift from a state of inertia to once again express reciprocal tension motion around automatically shifting fulcrums. Once the forces within an inertial fulcrum are resolved, the tissues, fluids, and potencies involved are freed to express their natural reciprocal tension motions around automatically shifting fulcrums. Dr. Jealous goes on to say,

> This newly established motion may or may not reach the perfect original Sutherland fulcrum. The motion within this new fulcrum reflects a resolution of inertia but at the same time represents the acknowledgement of the limits of the needs of the entire matrix of the body's tension as a whole and so an ideal may or may not ever be reached. However, even in this somewhat compromised state, all physiological functions that were held static within the inertial pattern are now free to move and restore health to all the tissues of the body. Our work, then, is often to find these inertial conditions and to find a neutral point or fulcrum around which motion can be organised to re-establish health.[6]

The "newly established motion" may still exhibit a compromised motion dynamic. The ideal may never be reached. This is due to the presence of other inertial and tensile issues that the system is still holding and centering. The system is whole and its inertial fulcrums will be expressed within the tensile dynamics of the whole, that is, within "the entire matrix of the body's tension." Nonetheless, the specific inertial issue that was addressed has been resolved, and the potential to express health is once again possible. Dr. Jealous ends this particular paragraph with the important statement, "Our work, then, is often to find these inertial conditions and to find a neutral point or fulcrum around which motion can be organised to re-establish health." This is the focus of these next two chapters, and is the most fundamental clinical skill found within the cranial concept.

Some Other Clinical Concepts and Things to Consider

In accessing the point of balanced tension, a number of perceptual skills are required. All of the previous skills explored in this book come into play. For a depth of clinical work to be possible, the ability to establish a still center within yourself and the ability to synchronize your perceptual fields with different tidal phenomena are of critical importance. Within this context, you must be able to perceive the dynamics of primary respiration within the fluids and tissues of the body. In previous chapters, we have focused on building these basic perceptual skills. You will have, by now, experienced the fluid tide and the motility and motion of some important structures within the body. As you have been listening to the unfoldment of these fluctuations and motions, you also will have noticed how they have become shaped in particular and unique ways. For instance, while palpating the temporal bones, you may have noticed particular motion patterns and may have also sensed the membranous dynamic related to it. So another skill is the ability to perceive motion via palpation and to have a felt sense for the shape and organizing fulcrum of that dynamic.

It is of utmost importance to appreciate that these dynamics are expressed in cycles of reciprocal tension motion. As we have seen, these motions are ideally expressed around Sutherland's fulcrum, the most anterior aspect of the straight sinus. The ability to read the nuances of the membranes as they express reciprocal tension motion is an important clinical skill in this context. As you listen to a dynamic you may notice a number of interesting things. First of all, you may notice that the motion dynamic you are palpating is not purely organized around Sutherland's fulcrum. You may notice eccentric tissue motions, pushes and pulls in membranes and connective tissues, and places of fixity or congestion. You may also notice various kinds of eccentric fluid fluctuations and motions. All of this indicates compensatory motion around inertial fulcrums of some kind. Another critical clinical skill is the ability to sense the inertial fulcrum organizing the pattern you are palpating. This is a skill that develops over time and can become quite subtle.

In this chapter we will focus on the CRI level of action. In the next chapter we will shift to the deeper tidal forces found within the mid-tide, the 2.5 cycles a minute rhythm. There are certain things to consider when working with the point of balanced tension within the CRI level of perception. The CRI level expresses the results and affects of past experience and trauma. Here, practitioners are most aware of the repercussions of unresolved experience and trauma. Issues tend to be perceived in terms of tissue and fluid resistance. The classic osteopathic lesion may become the focus of attention. Shock affects, such as emotional flooding and freezing states, may be more easily activated in an overwhelming way here. It is a level of perceptual work at which the underlying forces at work, and the inherent Health within, are not as obvious. What tends to be more obvious here are results and affects of suffering, such as tissue changes and compressions, fluid congestion, and central nervous system facilitation and shock affect. At this level of work the activation of shock affect is more likely. Shock affects include such things as emotional flooding, dissociation, freezing states, and trembling and shaking without a sense of something clearing in a resourced manner. We will cover clinical approaches to these processes in later chapters. For now it is important to acknowledge them and, if any arise, to simply slow the process down and maintain your fulcrums and presence. Finally, you never know if an inertial pattern is truly resolved unless you can sense the resolution of the inertial forces that organize it. The shape organized around an inertial fulcrum can change without the fulcrum itself being resolved. I have seen many practitioners chasing shapes when ideally they should have been able to appreciate and perceive the forces that both maintain and center their organization. We will focus on these issues more fully in the next chapter when we expand the concept of the point of balanced tension into the state of balance.

Accessing the Point of Balanced Membranous Tension

In this first application, you will be relating to the cranium in the vault hold. You will synchronize your perceptual field with the CRI level of perception. I am starting you here so that you have an experience of this level of work. In the next chapter, you will apply these principles from within the deeper tidal rhythms with a much more holistic outlook. We have used this hold many times now. You have palpated motility and motion from this vantage point with a number of intentions. Here we will simply listen to the unfolding story in a certain way and help access the *point of balanced membranous tension* within the patterns perceived. In classical approaches, the practitioner can be very active in the intention to access a neutral within the pattern being palpated. In one approach, the practitioner senses the motion dynamic of bone and membrane as they palpate from a particular vantage point. He or she then subtly and gently seeks the neutral, or the point of balanced membranous tension, by taking the structures through their range of motion and existing tension dynamics until the point of least membranous tension is obtained. At this point a settling and stilling of the tissue elements will be perceived.

This intention is almost like holding a multidimensional seesaw or teeter totter and attempting to balance it around its fulcrum point. Imagine a children's seesaw as a circular structure that moves around a central pivot point. Now imagine that this seesaw has a number of children sitting on it. Your job is to find the exact neutral point where all the weight is evenly distributed around the fulcrum point and the seesaw accesses a point of balance in which it is still and balanced upon its fulcrum. (See Figure 14.3.)

Similarly, here the practitioner subtly explores the tension dynamics of the bones and membranes being palpated. In this process you will subtly seek the point where the membranous tensions palpated are evenly distributed in relationship to the fulcrum that organizes them. When this is obtained, the practitioner will sense a settling within the tissues and a stillness in the tension dynamic. There will be no push or pull in any direction. You will have accessed the stillness at the heart of the organizing fulcrum, a point of potency that organizes the pattern being palpated. This is the point for optimum potential

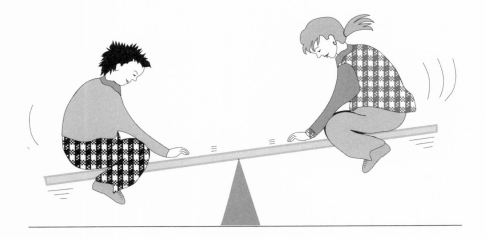

14.3 Point of balanced tension

adjustment in the classical concept. This balance point is actually inherent within the dynamics of the situation. It just has to be accessed. This is important. The practitioner does not create the point of balance; he or she facilitates its access. Classically, this approach is further refined by the practitioner initiating certain motion intentions within the tissue pattern. This will be described later.

A point of balance and stillness has then been reached in which:

1. the inherent healing forces can be expressed,

2. the inertial forces can be resolved, and

3. the tissues involved can realign their reciprocal tension dynamics to natural automatically shifting fulcrums.

Clinical Application: Sensing the Point of Balanced Tension

Before working with this process, let's imagine something else. Imagine that you are looking at a cranium and that the bones are transparent. For this visualization let's remove the brain so that all we visualize are transparent bones, the reciprocal tension membranes, and the cerebrospinal fluid within which they float. Remember that the transparent bones are not hard and solid, but are resilient living tissue. Now imagine that the fluids, bones, and membranes are breathing in reciprocal cycles of inhalation and exhalation. Notice that bone, membrane, and fluid are continuous. They express an integrated unit of function. Now imagine that you are holding this cranium. As you hold the cranium, notice that the membranes are like taut elastic bands holding tension, and, because bone and membrane are continuous, you can sense this tension through the bones and fluids. Let their reciprocal tension motion come into your awareness.

As you let the tissues and fluids move you, you may sense particular patterns of motion. Sense the fluids supporting this motion. Notice that the transparent bones and membranes move as a whole as they express the tensions of the pattern. Notice that their motion is organized around the automatically shifting fulcrum within the straight sinus. As you follow the reciprocal tension motions of bones and membrane, you may sense patterns that are eccentric, that is, not clearly organized around Sutherland's fulcrum. Like the teeter-totter image on the previous page, see if you can imagine subtly guiding and adjusting the tension structures until a point of balance is obtained within the pattern of strain, and you perceive a settling and a stilling within articular membranous dynamics. Let's try this as a clinical application.

1. With the patient in the supine position, palpate the system via the vault hold. Establish your practitioner fulcrums and remember to negotiate your contact with the patient's system. First listen for the fluid tide, listen for the resources of the system, listen for the Health. Then synchronize your perceptual field to the CRI as previously learned. To do this, allow your hands to float on the tissues and narrow your perceptual field to the motion of the bones and membranes being palpated. Do not grab the tissues as you do this. Let the tissues and their motion come to you as previous learned. As you narrow your field of perception and get interested in particular tissue structures, the CRI level of perception will start to come to you. This is the faster rhythmic expression of 8–14 cycles a minute. Let your hands float on the tissue elements and let them show you their motion. Do not look for anything, simply listen. Remember the visualization of the bones as transparent and continuous with the membranes and that they are all floating within fluid. Let yourself come into relationship to all of this. Allow the bones to show you the membranes.

2. Make contact as though you are floating on the tissues. Sense that your hands are literally floating on tissues like corks floating on the tide. Allow yourself to be moved by the tissues that you are palpating. Be aware of the continuity of bone and membrane. Remember that bone and membrane express their motion dynamic as one thing. Sense the membranes as though they are taut elastic bands.[7] Notice their *reciprocal tension motion* as a unit of function. Notice how bone and membrane express reciprocal tension motion as a whole.

3. Follow the motion dynamic under your hands as though you are holding the three-dimensional teeter-totter mentioned above. Let the tissues and fluids show you their motion dynamics and simply notice and follow them. Listen to the story. Do not grab onto the tissues as you listen. Follow the most prominent motion dynamic. You may become aware of the inertial fulcrum that organizes this motion. This may be located within a suture or within another relationship. Remember the earlier exercise around the perception of inertial fulcrums. Simply ask the question, "What organizes this?" This ability to sense the organizing fulcrum will become more and more refined as your learning process and experience builds. Do not worry about it for now, but simply let it be a perceptual possibility. See if you can hold both the shape of the pattern and its inertial fulcrum within your awareness at the same time.

4. As you listen, you may sense that the membranes naturally settle into a point of balanced membranous tension. Their reciprocal tension motion slows down and settles into a stillness. They may not do this, however, without some facilitation on your part. The system is likely to be centering many inertial issues, and it may be difficult for the tissues to access their point of balance in relationship to a particular fulcrum.

In this case, as you listen to the reciprocal tension motion dynamic, notice the shape of its motion. Notice the boundaries of the motion. Follow it in what seems to be its preferred motion and direction. Then subtly slow the motion down. Do not grab onto the tissues as you intend this. As you slow the motion down, you may notice that the tissues involved naturally access a point of balanced tension. You will sense a stilling of the motion dynamic and a settling of the tissues.

5. You may, however, sense that the tissues cannot easily access the point of balance even with the intention of slowing down. You may sense a see-sawing or rocking motion, as though they are seeking a neutral point, yet cannot attain it.[8] If this is the case, then you may have to become a bit more active in your facilitation. Subtly, via your floating contact with the bones, *more actively* seek a point where there is a settling and stilling within the push-pull of the motion dynamic. Slow the motion dynamic down and subtly *seek the neutral* by subtly moving the tissues around their organizing fulcrum. In the analogy above, this is like subtly adjusting the teeter - totter in a children's playground until a balance point is attained. Here you are adjusting the teeter-totter of reciprocal tension motion until a point of balance is obtained. Once this occurs, the tissues will settle into stillness around the organizing fulcrum. Sense that you are subtly balancing the taut elastic bands until the tensions within them are balanced, and a settling into a neutral state is perceived. Do not grab onto the tissues to do this. Let this be a floating within the fluids. Let the fluids carry the bones and membranes as you subtly and gently move and adjust their position in order to seek the neutral. This is as much an intention as a doing. When this point is accessed, you will sense a settling of the tissues into a point of balance and stillness.

6. Listen to what happens within this point of balance. For now, simply listen for expressions of health. You may sense fluid fluctuations and expressions of potency within the stillness of the point of balance. You may perceive softening and expansion within the relationships being palpated. In the next chapter, you will be listening for expressions of health in a much wider and deeper context. Again, within a classical context, at this point of balance the membranous articular complex is held at a *precise neutral* and the opportunity for self-correction is most potent, because the forces that organize the "lesion pattern" are at a point of balance.

7. When the forces organizing the fulcrum have been wholly or partially resolved, you will sense softening and expansion within both the tissues involved and the system as a whole. Remember the discussion in the last chapter about how the system centers and contains inertial forces. Potencies condense and coil, fluids densify, and tissues contract. This leads to a sense of compression within the relationship. When these inertial forces are resolved each function of potency, fluid, and tissue is free to expand and realign as best as possible to the action of Sutherland's fulcrum. When a resolution of forces occurs, motion will also return. When motion returns, notice the new reciprocal tension motion dynamic. Do the tissues express a clearer reciprocal tension motion around Sutherland's fulcrum, the automatically shifting fulcrum of the membranous articular system? Is there a clearer relationship to the midline? Is there greater ease and balance in their motion?

Over a number of practice sessions, repeat this exercise at the various relationships that you have already worked with. Repeat this exercise at the temporal bones using the temporal bone hold previously learned. Palpating the temporal bones can give you a real sense of the continuity between them and the tentorium. See the description of the poles of attachments from the previous chapter. Repeat the exercise at the frontal and parietal bones using the holds previously learned. Palpating the frontal and parietal bones can again give you a real sense of their continuity with the falx cerebri. Also repeat this exercise at the sacrum using the sacral hold previously learned.

Once you are familiar with the process, start in the vault hold and hold an open awareness to the system. Let the tissues and fluids lead you intuitively to a particular relationship. You may sense a particular shape organized around an inertial fulcrum, or you may sense a membranous pull into a particular relationship. Change your hand hold as necessary. As we go on in the book, you will discover that, as you hold a wider perceptual field with a still mind, the system will show you its priorities and the *inherent treatment plan* will unfold.

These explorations should take place over a number of practice sessions. Do not work for more than a half-hour at a time. Work with one relationship in each palpation session.

Taking the Work a Step Further

In the classical model a further refinement to this clinical approach is taken. In this, the practitioner initiates certain intentions that help to access the point of balance in particular ways. Again, Dr. Magoun clearly outlines these classical approaches in *Osteopathy in the Cranial Field*. In this book you will learn the three most common approaches: *exaggeration*, *direct action*, and *disengagement*. We will explore these in later chapters on conversation skills. The first approach is called *exaggeration*. This is the preferred approach used in the majority of the work. It is contraindicated in children under six years of age and in acute illness. We will outline it here and develop it more later. In this approach to accessing the point of balanced tension, a number of concepts are important to review. Let's list these and then look at each in turn:

> • Inertial fulcrums organize motion and affect function.
>
> • Inertial patterns of shape organize around inertial fulcrums. These shapes have form, motion, and qualities.
>
> • Inertial fulcrums give rise to boundary.

The first has to do with the nature of how inertial fulcrums organize motion. As we have seen, when inertial fulcrums form within the system, they effect its organization. Inertial fulcrums do not automatically shift with the intentions of the Tide as do natural fulcrums. When inertial fulcrums form, new tensions are introduced into the system. As new tensions are introduced into the system, automatically shifting fulcrums like Sutherland's fulcrum will also shift in their action in order to center the new tensions within the system and to maintain balance within reciprocal tension motion dynamics. These dynamics now include the new tensions that have been added to the system by the site of fixity. The overall tensile balance within the system must be maintained. The overall reciprocal tension motion dynamic of tissues will also shift away from a pure orientation to automatically shifting fulcrums, to include any inertial fulcrums found within the system. Eccentric and conditioned motion patterns result.

The second and third points have to do with how inertial fulcrums limit motion. When an inertial fulcrum arises in the system, fixity and boundary result. Where natural easy motion once existed, conditioned and limited motion is found. When an inertial fulcrum arises, the natural motion of the tissues becomes bound and limited. The tissue structures are forced to take particular pathways of motion, which have to do with the nature of the inertial forces held in the system. These conditioned pathways become patterns of preferred motion. So inertial fulcrums create boundary and preferred and conditioned motion dynamics result. This tendency to move in a particular direction is an important aspect of the clinical approach outlined below. It was classically called the *direction of ease*. It could likewise be called the *direction of preference*.

The direction of ease is a preferred direction of tissue motion, which arises due to an inertial fulcrum. It is a conditioned and limited tissue dynamic. It is the direction in which the tissues become fixated within their reciprocal tension dynamics. On a macrolevel in the system, it may be the preferred motion dynamic of a vertebra or joint. On a microlevel, motility and motion will become organized around inertial fulcrums and will be expressed in patterned and conditioned ways. The direction of ease is expressed in relationship to the fixations present within tissue relationships. If tissues are limited in their range of motion by an inertial fulcrum, they will be become fixated in the direction that the fulcrum dictates. For instance, if a vertebra is fixed in rotation into a particular direction, it will rotate more easily in that direction, the direction that the fixation dictates. Thus a vertebra fixed in right rotation will more easily rotate into the direction of the fixation, that is, to the right. The direction of ease is the easiest direction for tissue motion to take, given the forces and tissue affects held. It is a tissue and motion dynamic organized around an inertial fulcrum. The reciprocal tension motion of the tissues becomes patterned and fixated in relationship to this fulcrum. The direction of ease is thus really the direction of fixation. The pattern becomes locked or frozen in the system and then becomes its familiar, conditioned way of expression.

As you learn to perceive the direction of ease, you will also notice another important thing. The direction of ease has a *boundary* to its motion. Inertial fulcrums generate boundary. Remember that motion is organized around fulcrums and the nature of the fulcrum will delineate both the pattern of the motion and its boundaries. Natural fulcrums are automatically shifting fulcrums. Inertial fulcrums are not. Again, inertial fulcrums do not automatically shift with the intentions of the Tide. Boundary, fixity, and strain arise as the potencies, fluids, and tissue elements become inertial in order to center the conditions present.

So you will notice that the motion you are palpating and following has a boundary to its excursion. This boundary is classically called its *edge of resistance*. It is the point where the inherent physiological motion of the tissues encounters the resistance generated by the inertial forces involved. It is the point where the membranes are poised between their normal reciprocal tensions and the increased tension and strain present due to the presence of an inertial fulcrum. It is thus the boundary of motion allowed by the tension held within the tissues, due to the presence of the fixation that organizes them. More simply, on a practical level, as you perceive an inertial pattern moving in its direction of ease, you will sense a boundary or edge to that movement. The awareness of these dynamics is essential to understand within the context of the clinical approach called *exaggeration*. Let's next look at this approach

Clinical Application: Exaggeration

In this approach, the practitioner "exaggerates" the inertial pattern by subtly carrying the tissues involved deeper into their direction of ease or preference. In clinical practice, many practitioners simply follow the preferred motion of an inertial pattern, rather than initiating any exaggeration. The main difference between what is described below and what you explored above is a refinement in terms of the particulars of the shape you are following. Classical concepts of *directions of ease* and *boundary* are introduced.

In this process, as the practitioner follows the inertial pattern, he or she notices the edge of resistance, or boundary to the motion. This may be perceived as a sense of boundary to any further motion in that direction. This edge, or boundary, is the point where the membranes are poised between their normal reciprocal tensions and the increased tension and strain present due to the presence of an inertial fulcrum. It is the boundary generated by the tension held within the tissues, due to the presence of the fixation that organizes them.

As you meet this boundary, you are near the point where the membranes can access a point of balance around the inertial fulcrum that is creating the strain. Let's take this into a real situation. Let's say you are palpating the temporal bones and notice a particular inertial pattern unfolding in your awareness.

1. Start with the vault hold and shift your perceptual field to the CRI level of perception. Narrow your attention to the general sense of motion in the cranium. Let your hands float on the tissues as you do this. Do not grab onto tissues or the patterns being expressed. See if the CRI level of perception comes into your field of awareness. Shift your hand position to the temporal bone hold learned earlier. (See Figure 14.4.) Have a good sense of the anatomical continuity between the temporal bones and the dural

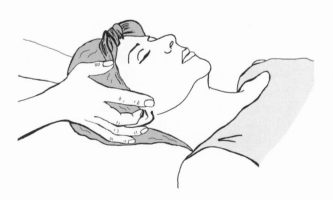

14.4 Temporal bone hold

membranes via the tentorium cerebelli. (See Figure 14.5.)

2. Listen to the reciprocal tension motion dynamic as you palpate the relationships. See if you can sense the motion of the temporal bones, external and internal rotation. Follow this motion dynamic. Does the motion seem balanced in its expression of inhalation and exhalation? Does it express external and internal rotation in a balanced way? Is there a sense of the inner breath or motility? Can you sense the continuity with the membranes? Can you sense the *unit of function* of bone and membrane as you monitor motion? Do you notice any eccentric tendencies? Any fixations? Any eccentric motions?

3. As you follow a particular reciprocal tension motion dynamic, can you sense the fulcrum around which it is organized? Simply ask the question, "What organizes this?" Do not look for the answer; let the tissue motion show you. Let the answer come to you. Remember to maintain a negotiated distance form the patient's system. What organizes this pattern? Is it a suture? Is it within the cranium? Is it somewhere else? If you can't sense the organizing fulcrum, don't worry; this perceptual skill will grow. Allow yourself to guess, trust your intuition, let images come, especially anatomical images.

4. Follow the shape that you are now aware of. It might be a perception of torsion, or an "out of phase" kind of dynamic between the two bones, or a sense of membranous pull. Notice its direction of ease, its preferred, conditioned direction of motion. Follow this. In one approach the practitioner subtly directs the tissues deeper into this direction. This is called *exaggeration*. In this exercise, simply notice the direction in which the tissues prefer to move. Give the system space and follow the tissue motion into its preferred direction. Float on the tissues; do not

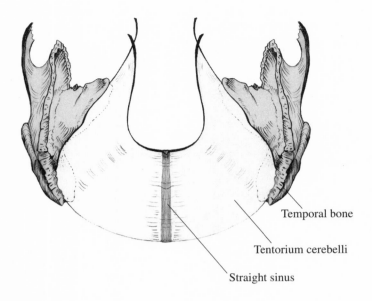

Temporal bone

Tentorium cerebelli

Straight sinus

14.5 Temporal bone and tentorium

grab on. This is in itself a reflective process and helps to uncouple this particular pattern from others in the body.

5. Sense the edge to this motion, the boundary that it does not move past. You may sense a subtle tissue rebound here. You may also sense fluids echoing off the boundary. At or near this boundary, use the bones as handles into the whole of what you are palpating. Remember the visualization above, where we visualized bone and membrane as one thing and sensed the membranes connecting the bones like elastic bands in tension. Sense the membranous tensions within this unity. At or near the boundary perceived, very subtly seek the neutral as described above.

6. Have a sense of floating on the tissues. Let them move you. Near the boundary, subtly, without grabbing onto the tissues, adjust the relation-ship of bone and membrane until you perceive a sense of balance in the membranous relation-ships. This is like subtly moving corks floating on water. Do not place any force on these tissues. Simply imply direction. This can be likened to seeking the point of balance in a children's teeter-totter as described above. When the point of balanced membranous tension is accessed, you will sense a settling of the tissue elements you are palpating. This is the point of balanced membranous tension. Do not hold onto the tissues. Remember that you are still floating on the tissues. If you grab the tissues, the system will begin to react to your presence, and you will stop the self-healing mechanisms from coming into play. You will basically lock up the structure and function of the tissues.

7. Listen to what happens within the point of balanced tension. Listen for expressions of health. These might include the expressions of potency

and fluid fluctuation. See if you can sense a softening and expansion within the tissues you are palpating. After this occurs, do the tissues express a more balanced reciprocal tension motion? Is this organized closer to the ideal automatically shifting fulcrum within the straight sinus, Sutherland's fulcrum?

Repeat this exercise at the sphenobasilar junction (SBJ). Use the vault hold to do this. Float on the tissues and follow a particular motion pattern as it comes into your awareness. Follow the procedure outlined above. It is important to become more and more at ease in palpating the dynamics at the SBJ. We will go into cranial base dynamics in detail in later chapters and more specifically in Volume Two of this book. After you have a clear experience of this process at the temporal bones and SBJ, practice this intention at the other relationships that you have explored so far. This includes the frontal bone, the parietals, the occiput, and the sacrum. Use the hand holds already learned. Take one practice session for each particular bone or relationship.

Once you are familiar with this intention, then try a more open approach to the system. Listen to the dynamics at the vault hold and go to a particular bone or relationship that attracts you. You may sense a motion focused around a particular suture or bone, or you may sense a membranous pull into a particular relationship. Let your intuition come into play and work with the relationship to which you are drawn. This will develop into an important clinical skill in which you will be able to perceive the various inertial fulcrums the system is holding.

In the next chapter, you will expand upon this clinical approach and deepen your appreciation of the state of balanced tension. We will begin to relate to tissues, fluids, and potency as a unit of function and will deepen our perception of the Health as it is expressed within the *state of balance*.

1. See the last chapter for a discussion of the osteopathic lesion.

2. See R. E. Becker, "Diagnostic Touch: Its Principles and Application, I, II, III, IV," *Academy of Applied Osteopathy Yearbooks* (1963, 1964, 1965); and R. E. Becker, *Life in Motion* (Rudra Press), for elegant and poetic descriptions of these concepts.

3. Harold Magoun, *Osteopathy in the Cranial Field* (The Journal Printing Company, 1966, 1976).

4. See previous chapters for descriptions of the motion of the reciprocal tension membranes and Sutherland's fulcrum.

5. From the paper *Reciprocal Tensions,* by Dr. Jim Jealous, D.O., passed on to me by Dr. Jealous via Dr. Joseph Hartmann, D.O.

6. Ibid.

7. Although the dural membranes are tough and relative inelastic when compared to other connective tissues, there is elasticity in their dynamics, and this image has proven useful for teaching purposes.

8. This may be because the tissue pattern is organized around a number of coupled inertial fulcrums, or that the inertia involved is so dense that a neutral is more difficult to attain.

15

The State of Balanced Tension

In this chapter, we will deepen our understanding and appreciation of the point of balanced tension and reframe it as the *state of balanced tension,* or *the state of balance.* You will begin to relate to the processes that unfold as one's perceptual field synchronizes with the mid-tide, the 2.5 cycles a minute tidal rhythm. From this point on, most clinical applications described in this book will start within this perceptual field. With an awareness of the mid-tide field of action, you will discover that tissues, fluids, and potency are perceived as *one thing,* a unified dynamic. All three functions of potency, tissues, and fluids can be perceived to express reciprocal tension motion organized around automatically shifting fulcrums and midline phenomena. Here the concept of a point of balanced membranous tension (BMT) will deepen into an appreciation of an inherent state

> **In this chapter we will:**
>
> - *Review the concept of variant potencies.*
>
> - *Discuss the Health that is never lost.*
>
> - *Reframe the concept of the point of balanced tension*
>
> - *Work with perceptual and clinical exercises in relationship to the state of balanced tension.*

of balance found within every function of the system. When this state of balance is accessed, the potency of the Breath of Life is expressed beyond the compensations held and the inertial forces being centered. To understand this work in context, we will first review some basic concepts: (1) the Health that is never lost, (2) inertial potencies, and (3) altered reciprocal tension dynamics.

Health Is Never Lost

In previous chapters we discussed the idea of Health. I would like to review and expand upon this here. Within this work there is a different understanding of Health than is common in our culture. In this paradigm, Health is seen to be a constant. It is an expression of universal forces at work within each of us. Health is never lost or diseased. Over the years I have seen how easy it is for practitioners to focus on lesions, fixations, resistance, and trauma. These states are relatively easy to perceive and diagnose. Within a craniosacral biodynamic context, it is essential for practitioners to begin to shift their perceptual processes to the Health that centers these disturbances. Our relationship to Health is at the heart of our work in this field. It is of vital importance to understand that Health is never lost, only our relationship to it. It is this deep truth that allows the system to heal itself and the cranial practitioner to facilitate that healing process. The human system is always whole and always in balance. No matter how seemingly entrenched the resistance or pathology, no matter how seemingly fragmented the system seems, this balance within the whole is always present. As we have seen, the potency of the Breath of Life is a unified field of action. Inertia may arise within this field, but the field is always whole and never fragmented. Moreover, it is always maintaining the best possible balance given the inertial issues being centered. One of our life dictums is to maintain balance, no matter how compensated this balance may seem to be. Let's again look at a quote from Dr. Jim Jealous in which he clearly writes about this inherent Health and its ever present availability:

> Health can be defined as the emergence of Originality. The Originality expresses a complete balance of both structure and function as intentionalized in the creation of a human being. . . . This Innate Wisdom which gives the body form and maintains its existence is not a function of any system of the body. Our health is only secondarily controlled through the central nervous system and the cell nucleus. Our existence is totally dependent upon this Original matrix expressing its intention. . . . The Original matrix is a form that is carried through the potency of the breath of life around which the molecular and cellular world will organize itself into the Original pattern set forth by the Master Mechanic.[1]

This powerful statement acknowledges the depth of our potential to heal. The emergence of Originality is the most basic ground of our human existence. It orders and maintains whatever it meets. This is a continual emergence, a continual creation in each moment of our lives. Originality, as an emergent reality, is the Innate Wisdom within the body-mind. It manifests as a precise bioelectric field, an Original matrix, which expresses the epigenetic or universal blueprint of the human system. This matrix is a primal expression of Originality as a field of potency that maintains the creative principle in form. This most primal matrix is the ordering principle of form and function and is never lost; it is a constant. As we have seen, there is a transmutation of this ordering force within the fluids of the body. Within the fluids, the intentions carried by the Original matrix become a truly embodied ordering force. It is through and around these forces that the cellular and tissue world organizes. It is deeply humbling to acknowledge that this interplay is an expression of an Intelligence much greater than our own. This Health, and the Original matrix that is an expression of its precision, is never lost. It is only our relationship to it that becomes estranged and inertial. The Original matrix is an expression of the Innate Wisdom, which organizes the cellular and tissue world and maintains its existence.

The Original matrix is expressed as epigenetic ordering forces within the fluids. It is arises at the moment of conception, is with us throughout life, and is always expressed within present time, that is, within the eternal present. From conception to death, the fluid, cellular, and tissue world organizes around its intentions. Health is maintained in the body by the relationship of the potency of the Breath of Life to all of its tissue systems, not just to the integrity of the central nervous system or to genetic function. In essence, Health is expressed as an inherent blueprint that is carried within the fluids of the body and informs all of its activities. This is echoed by all of the great spiritual traditions in the world and by all forms of traditional medicine. Dr. Jealous continues,

> The health that we talk about in osteopathy is at the core of our being and cannot be increased or decreased to a greater or lesser degree. In other words the health in our body cannot become diseased. The health in the body actually transcends death. The health in our body is one hundred percent available 24 hours a day from conception until death, then it transpires. It does not expire. . . . This health, this Original matrix within the human body, interfaces with every physiological, structural and psychological stress that one con-

tacts. This interface begins as early as our encounter with our genetics and ends at death with
a shift in our perceptual fields.[2]

This health is at the "core of our being" and is never
lost. Health is a constant; it does not increase or decrease. It is a most fundamental ordering principle
and is with us at all times. Health cannot become
diseased but, as we will see, will attempt to contain
and center the unresolved conditions within the
human system. This Original matrix, this inherent
Health, "interfaces with every physiological, structural and psychological stress that one contacts."
Thus, within the heart of all the unresolved stressors
within the body there is Health centering the conditions present. Understanding this is the key to
clinical efficiency. At the heart of every inertial fulcrum within the human body, there is Health manifesting its ordering function. There is potency at
work, which interfaces with and centers any disturbance active within the system. The potency of the
breath of Life always functions to center the disturbance, and is ever present even in the most seemingly desperate situations. Our challenge as
practitioners in this field is to truly acknowledge this
and to form a relationship to Health no matter what
conditions are presented.

It is important to understand that the Health in
the body does not expire at death, but "transpires."
Dr. Jealous states that, "This interface begins as
early as our encounter with our genetics and ends
at death with a shift in our perceptual fields." What
a wonderful description of this life transition. Death
is seen here as a shift in our perceptual fields! This
is so important to perceive, both on a personal level
and as a health practitioner. Death is not a defeat,
but a natural transition, a "shift in our perceptual
fields." This understanding has always been part of
traditional health and spiritual systems. It is a
shame, I believe, that most modern physicians do
not seem to have a connection with this deep inherent truth. We as health practitioners must take
some responsibility in the preparation of patients
and their families for this great life transition.

Perhaps the first step in this process is for health
practitioners themselves to deeply be with these issues and to clearly and perceptually prepare *ourselves* for that inevitable transition.

Inertial Potencies Reviewed

I feel that it is important to review some concepts
here before we launch into the rest of the material
in this chapter.[3] In previous chapters we discussed
the nature of the biodynamic potency that organizes
and supports the human system. The expression of
potency within the human system is always whole.
Potency is expressed as a unified bioelectric field
phenomenon. This unified field is a bioenergy field,
which supports the wellness of mind and body. Dr.
Becker called the potency expressed within this
field biodynamic potency. In the chapter on inertial
fulcrums, we introduced Dr. Becker's concepts of
biodynamic and biokinetic forces. Biodynamic potencies are the intrinsic organizing forces generated
by the actions of the Breath of Life. Biodynamic potencies generate the natural biokinetic motility and
motion of cells and tissues. Biokinetic forces are inertial forces that are overlaid upon the system and
that affect the normal biokinetic motions of fluids,
cells, and tissues in some way. These include the
forces of trauma, pathogens, toxins, and even genetics. Biodynamic potency will become inertial within
its wider field of action in order to center these biokinetic forces. As we have seen, at the heart or core
of every disturbance within the human system, there
are biodynamic potencies at work. These potencies
have the ability to resolve or contain the inertial or
traumatic forces maintaining the disturbance. In
other words, they *center* the disturbance. This centering occurs within the context of the whole system. Inertial issues are held, or centered, within the
context of the whole field of potency, fluids, and tissues as a unified dynamic. Life is forever whole.

Dr. Becker called inertial potency *variant potency*. In this process, the potency of the Breath of
Life has had to *vary* from its natural expression in
order to meet and center the unresolved experiences

and traumas of life. In order to do this, potency concentrates and becomes inertial to meet the forces that are generating or maintaining the disturbance in the system. Potency thus has the ability to vary from its natural expression in order to center the disturbances found within the system. It does this by concentrating, or condensing within its wider field of action. In other words, it concentrates and varies from its natural expression in order to contain and center the traumatic or pathological forces at work within the body. These variant or inertial potencies will also maintain compensatory processes as they respond to the unresolved traumas or disease states held within the body.

Thus, within very inertial fulcrums, there are inertial or variant potencies and forces at work. When the system meets the forces of our experience, the potency of the Breath of Life will attempt to process the experience or to center it in some way. The experiential forces introduced into the system must be met and compensated for in some way, in other words, they must be *centered*. They are centered in relationship to the whole. This idea of centering is important. Inertia fulcrums are not separate from the system in which they manifest. They are centered by the Breath of Life as part of the wider dynamics of the system. The human system is thus always whole and never truly fragmented. Visualize a unified field of potency, fluid, and tissue. As traumatic or stressful forces are encountered by the system, potencies within this unified field will condense, concentrate, and become inertial in order to meet the forces involved. These inertial potencies and forces are then centered within the dynamics of the system as a whole, and the best compensations for their action are maintained.

Potency concentrates and becomes still within its wider field of action in order to contain the traumatic or pathological forces at work within the system. Potency within the heart of a disturbance expresses stillness. Remember that fulcrums are still places that organize motion. Stillness holds the power to organize. Within inertial patterns, stillness centers the disturbance. One of the roles of the practitioner is to access this stillness. It is the gateway into deeper forces and healing processes. This expression of Health within the most seemingly chaotic and disoriented fluids and tissues is always present and can always be palpated, accessed, and experienced. As we shall see, it is within the state of balanced tension that this stillness is accessed. Within the stillness, something happens. Forces are engaged and inertial potencies are activated beyond the containment and compensations held, and the wider field of potency can come into play. A permeation of potency into the inertial site can then occur.

When the precise neutral of the state of balance is obtained, potency is naturally expressed within the fulcrum that is organizing the resistance or disorder. In this state, all of the forces maintaining and centering the pattern of resistance are at a dynamic equilibrium where options are again available and healing resources can be expressed. Thus the state of balance is like "an eye of a needle through which something can pass!"[4] That something is the ordering principle and potency of the Breath of Life. As we shall later see, potency has tensile qualities and will be concentrated precisely within the inertial fulcrum when the state of balanced tension is accessed. It is our job not just to recognize tissue resistance, but to perceive the forces that both maintains and centers it.

Altered Reciprocal Tension Motion

Tissues, fluids, and potency are three functions, which are an inseparable unity. The three express a totally unified dynamic. This is easily sensed within the action of the mid-tide. Potency is the organizing factor, fluid is the medium, and the cellular and tissue world is the physical ground. As we have also seen, all motility and motion within the human system is naturally organized around suspended automatically shifting fulcrums. All three functions of potency, fluids, and tissues will express reciprocal tension motion around automatically shifting fulcrums. Ideally, tissues, fluids, and potency naturally express their reciprocal tension motions in an easy and balanced way. Within the mid-tide level of perception, you may sense this as tensile cycles of *surge* in the inhalation phase and *settling* in the exhalation phase. This motion is ideally oriented to the groundswell of the Tide, its midline function, and the natural automatically shifting fulcrums within the system.

However, as we have seen, as we meet the forces of experience, new fulcrums may be generated, which alter or condition the natural reciprocal tension motions of the system. These altered shapes are organized around the forces that generate them. These forces give rise to inertial fulcrums, sites of inertia, congestion, and resistance to the natural dynamics of the system. As we have seen, inertial fulcrums are sites of fixity, which do not automatically shift with the intentions of the Tide. They are not automatically shifting fulcrums. Due to these sites of fixity, altered and strained tension dynamics are fed into the system. Altered reciprocal tension motion results. These new fulcrums and the tensions they generate have to be taken into account and centered in some way within the body physiology. In your work with patients, you will learn to perceive and read these dynamics as patterns of altered reciprocal tension motion and to respond to them clinically. Simply remember that altered reciprocal tension motion is organized by inertial fulcrums. Simply ask the questions, "What organizes this? What are the origins of this?"

You have already begun to appreciate the normal reciprocal tension motion dynamics of the fluids and tissues of the body. You have listened to the reciprocal fluctuation of CSF and to the motility and mobility of tissues. As you came into relationship to these dynamics, you may have also noticed how they have become conditioned. Perhaps you noticed a tendency to prefer one phase of primary respiration to the other? Or perhaps you noticed particular fluid fluctuations within the overall expression of motion? These fluctuations may have been perceived like the eddying of the ocean waters around obstructions, such as breakers, built into the natural contours of the beach. Or perhaps you noticed eccentric tissue motion, or membranous pulls and tensions? All of these phenomena are expressions of the shapes of our conditioned experience. They are organized around inertial forces, unresolved patterns of experience, from genetics to the various environmental issues and life experiences we meet.

These forces must be resolved or centered in some way. The system will compensate for its inertia and these compensations become part of its overall dynamic. There is a price to pay for this in lost vitality and limited options. Potency becomes inertial within its field of action and lowered vitality results. Once we become locked into conditioned patterns of expression, then the potential of the system becomes limited. We become bound by the limits of our own conditions. In the processes outlined below, you will be in relationship to altered patterns of reciprocal tension motion. Please remember that *altered reciprocal tension motion* is always organized by inertial fulcrums. Inertial fulcrums are not automatically shifting fulcrums. Because of this, they generate altered reciprocal tension motion. Coupled with this will be changes in motility and in the quality of fluids and tissues. You will learn to follow these patterns within a wider context than previously presented.

In the last chapter, you learned to explore the *point of balanced membranous tension*. This is an important entry point into a clinical awareness of natural healing processes. In this chapter, you will extend this inquiry. You will, within the context of the mid-tide, explore the *state of balanced tension* in which all three functions of potency, fluids, and tissues access a *state of balanced stillness* around the organizing forces generating the altered reciprocal tension motions within the system. This is a state of *dynamic equilibrium* between the forces present and the altered reciprocal tensions they generate.

The State of Balanced Tension and Transmutation

In the classical concept of the *point of balanced membranous tension*, the focus is strongly on tissues, especially membranes and connective tissues. The focus is on accessing the point of balance in membranous or connective tissue relationships, and the perceptual field is commonly within the CRI. As we saw in the last chapter, the intention is to access a neutral within the tensile dynamics of the membranes, ligaments and connective tissues being palpated. This is a powerful concept within itself. However, here we are going to expand this understanding to include a more holistic perceptual awareness. In accessing the point of balanced membranous tension, the practitioner's awareness is on the tensions within the membranes or connective tissue fields. These tensions are the results of the organizational forces involved. Inertial fulcrums will generate tensions within the tissue field, and this is what the practitioner's attention is focused on. In other words, the practitioner is focused on results and effects, not on the forces that generate them. In the last chapter you were advised to follow these tension patterns in their preferred direction to the boundary of their motion. You were then asked to facilitate the point of balance at or near that edge. This was seen to be a delicate negotiation with the altered reciprocal tensions within the tissue field. In this chapter we will shift away from a narrow focus on tissue tensions, to a wider listening process. We will synchronize our perceptual field with the mid-tide and open to an awareness of the forces which generate these tensions. As we do this, the quality of clinical work will also shift. The intention will be to have a more conscious awareness of the energy dynamics involved and to perceive the unit of function of potency, fluid, and tissues. The idea is to have a more direct sense of the potencies and forces within the inertial fulcrums and the expressions of Health that arise relative to them.

As discussed earlier, as the Breath of Life unfolds within the human system, a transmutation process takes place.[5] There is a transmutation of potency within the fluids of the body. Potency is expressed, via transmutation, as an embodied ordering force within the dynamics of the human system. It is also possible to talk about transmutation, or changes in state, within a wider context. The process of holographic, nonlinear unfoldment from a Dynamic Stillness to embodied form can be spoken of in terms of enfolded transmutations. The Breath of Life orchestrates this holomovement.[6]

In the first transmutation from Stillness, an intention arises. This creative spark generates motion within a huge field of action. The Long Tide, the Original motion, manifests the creative intention of the Breath of Life as motion. The Long Tide carries the blueprint energy, or the Original matrix, into the world of form. From this Original motion the bioelectric field is organized and force or potency, is generated. This is not a dull electric force, but a creative Intelligence that permeates everything. There is then a transmutation of this factor within the fluids of the body. The Original matrix is laid down within the fluid field and there is then a transmutation of force within the fluids around which every cell and tissue of the body is organized.

When potencies become inertial in order to center disturbances within the system, stasis results. Within the dynamics of an inertial fulcrum, the transmutation intention can become compromised. Although there is always a kernel of Health centering the conditions, a site of stasis is generated. Within the state of balance, there is a stillness. It is within this stillness that the potency of the Breath of Life is liberated beyond the conditions present, and the transmutation process is facilitated. As we learn to access a state of balance within the potencies, fluids, and tissues of the system, we are bringing the natural intrinsic motions of these functions into a balance point, a state of *dynamic equilibrium.* This balanced state relates directly to the pattern and inertial fulcrum being palpated. A dynamic equilibrium is attained relative to the forces present. As this occurs, the entire field of bioelectric potency is balanced around and focused upon this particular issue. It is literally a state of balanced stillness. The ordering intentions of the Tide come to balance directly in relationship to a particular fulcrum and pattern. Potencies will then come into play within the dynamics of the specific inertial pattern being palpated. A transmutation takes place within the disordered area and a change in the potencies involved occurs. This process of transmutation liberates the inertial potencies involved to do something else beyond the containment and compensations held.[7]

Thus as the state of balanced tension is reached, a dynamic equilibrium is attained in which all three functions of potency, fluids, and tissues have settled into a dynamic stillness directly related to the forces within the inertial fulcrums being palpated. Remember that the potencies, fluids, and tissues within the body are a truly unified tensile field of action. In a state of balance, all three functions (potency, fluids, and tissues) enter a state where a dynamic equilibrium is attained around a particular inertial fulcrum and its organizing forces. Remember that within an inertial fulcrum are inertial forces and potencies at work. These inertial potencies and forces are not separate from the unified bioelectric-fluid-tissue field. Within a state of balance, this field as a whole is dynamically balanced around an inertial fulcrum. When this unified field of action reaches a dynamic equilibrium relative to the inertial potencies and forces involved, then the whole field of potency can come into play in direct relationship to that particular site of inertia. In essence, the whole field is dynamically balanced around its own inertia and healing mechanisms come into play directly in relationship to a specific issue. This is a powerful process to understand and perceive. It is precise. As we shall see, this dynamic is most easily appreciated within the mid-tide level of perception.

The State of Balance and Automatically Shifting Fulcrums

Another way to describe this is in terms of suspended automatically shifting fulcrums. Natural fulcrums are suspended automatically shifting fulcrums. They are suspended within their field of action, and naturally shift with the inhalation and exhalation cycles of the Tide. They are not static. They *automatically shift* in their location as the Tide manifests its inhalation and exhalation motions.

Another way to say this is that they move with the intentions of the Tide. As they shift, the whole tensile field organized around them also shifts. Inertial fulcrums, as we have seen, do not automatically shift with the intentions of the Tide. They are static and inertial. They are sites of condensed potency and inertial forces. There is a loss of motion due to their presence. They become organizing fulcrums, which are not natural to the system. Inertial fulcrums generate altered reciprocal tension motion and strain patterns. As you will see, when the state of balance is attained, there is a realignment of the forces within the inertial fulcrum to natural, automatically shifting fulcrums and the Original matrix, or the bioelectric ordering field. As this occurs, there is a transmutation of potency within the inertial fulcrums being attended to. The forces of the whole literally take over. This is critical to understand. There is a transmutation process that naturally arises within the human system and this process is the key to its organization and functioning. It is within the state of balance that the potency, a stillness at the heart of the disturbance, can be accessed and healing potencies engaged.[8] Within the stillness of the state of balance, the potency and power of the Tide acts *through* the fulcrum and a transmutation takes place. There is a change in the potency. This initiates the inertial forces involved and inherent healing potencies come into play. Dr. Sutherland used to stress that the power of the Tide is found within its stillness. There is a stillness within the Tide and there is potency within this stillness. This potency has the power to organize and heal. Indeed, it is the accessing of stillness that is the key to the healing processes within the body-mind. Stillness resonates with stillness. Within stillness, potency is liberated. Within stillness, there can be a permeation of potency into the seemingly chaotic conditions present.

This stillness is not a dead or void quality. It is an alive and dynamic stillness. It has potency and power within it. It is the ground for the generation and organization of the human system. It can be perceived and experienced. As we shall discover, the state of balance, a stillness, can be like a mysterious gateway into deeper and deeper experiences of stillness, even into the Dynamic Stillness itself. Once accessed, the healing intentions of the Breath of Life take over. In our work, we must begin to understand and appreciate the functions of stillness within the human system. It is humbling. It is much easier and less challenging to follow motion and perceive problems, but can we access the Stillness, the ground of Originality itself? This is our great challenge and the key to understanding the principles and forces at work as we enter into relationship with the human system. There is an intrinsic and Dynamic Stillness from which the matrix of our existence arises, and it is within stillness that its ordering principles are apprehended. All spiritual traditions that I am familiar with acknowledge this truth.

The State of Balance, Fluid Drive, and Permeation

Within the state of balance there is optimum potential for healing processes to come into play. When they are accessed, the potential for reconnection and healing is initiated. Within the state of balance, you will notice a *stillness*. Within the stillness, the potencies that organize form can be accessed and their potential expressed. Something happens within the stillness and there is a change in the potencies involved.[9] You may then sense expressions of Health. These expressions may include various manifestations of potency, various kinds of fluid fluctuations, increased fluid circulation, and various kinds of tissue responses. For instance, within the stillness, you may sense a drive of potency through the fulcrum being attended to. As potencies are initiated within the state of balance, the *fluid drive* of the system may kick in, as a surge of potency literally moves through the fulcrum being palpated. This drive of potency may have a sharp and directive quality to it. Again, you may literally sense a drive of potency through the fulcrum being palpated as the healing intentions of the Breath of Life are expressed. You may also sense the fluids following this drive as a directive healing force. Hence the term *fluid drive*. It is a unitary experience. You may also sense a softer permeation of potency through the area and the fulcrum being attended to. This has a different quality to it. It is more of a field phenomenon. You may sense the whole field of potency come into play. A building and welling up of potency may be perceived. It is as if a shift within the whole field of potency is occurring. As the system is poised within a state of balance around a particular fulcrum, the whole field of potency organizes around this particular inertial issue. A movement of potency throughout its field towards the inertial fulcrum may be sensed. As this occurs, a soft permeation of potency may be perceived within the area and fulcrum being palpated. It is like water soaking a dense knob of sand and melting it away. As you will later see, when you synchronize your perceptual field to the mid-tide of 2.5 cycles a minute, these forces and potencies at work become more obvious. Dr. James Jealous, D.O., writes,

> It is the permeation of the Breath of life into disoriented tissue that re-establishes the Original matrix. The Original matrix is a form that is carried through the potency of the breath of life around which the molecular and cellular world will organize itself into the Original pattern set forth by the Master Mechanic. The perception of this "Original idea" permeating the tissue (e.g. the Breath of Life) should be a direct sensory experience.[10]

This is an eloquent and precise description of the inherent healing processes within the human system and of a fundamental intention of this work. Within this context, we appreciate the unfoldment of the Breath of Life in the human system as it permeates disoriented tissues and reestablishes the Original matrix. The Original matrix holds the "Original idea" or intention of a human being. It organizes the molecular and cellular world and is conveyed within the fluids of the embryo. It precedes genetics and holds the intention of our human embodiment. The

Original matrix of the Breath of Life maintains this original intention throughout our lives. It is the *life force principle,* which orders the unfolding of our embryology and is with us until the day we die. In the quote above, Dr. Jealous is pointing to the possibility that the Original intention of cellular and tissue organization can be reestablished via a permeation of this deepest life principle. Within this state, the practitioner can have a direct perceptual experience of this ordering principle at work. Dr. Jealous continues,

> One can bring the "idea" into the process of a neutral, through the fulcrum; it can pass like light through the eye of a needle. Think about the point of balance as the eye of a needle through which something can pass! [11]

This statement is, in my experience, not just an elegant and poetic metaphor. It is a description of a direct perceptual experience of what actually occurs as the system accesses its inherent Health. Within the state of balance a deep stillness is accessed. This fulcrum point of balance, the stillness, is like the eye of the needle through which something can pass. Through it, potency is naturally expressed via transmutation and permeation. Within the process of a neutral the "Original idea" can permeate the relationship. It can pass right through the fulcrum established by the state of balance, like light through the eye of a needle. Within this neutral, the Breath of Life will permeate the disoriented tissues and restore the "Original idea" or intention to them. The Original matrix is an expression of the Original intention of a human being in form. Dr. Stone, D.O., called it the "blueprint energy." Indeed, this Original matrix is always present and is an expression of the inherent Health of the human system. This Health, as we have discussed, is never lost, but can and does become obscured in our daily life experience. The Health in our system can be sensed as a felt experience. This is a powerful concept, one of the themes that runs throughout this book and which we will expand upon later. Thus the state of balance is like the eye of a needle through which the "Original idea" is expressed and the Original matrix reestablished.

In the following sections, we will focus on the state of balanced tension as the state in which the healing processes of the system can be directly accessed. It is within the stillness of the state of balance that the inertial potencies are accessed. It is within the stillness at the heart of the inertia that the transmutation process is found. As inertial potencies are initiated, and become active, the transmutation process is initiated. In the following sections we will attempt to enter this exploration and to plumb the depths of our abilities to be still, to know, and to appropriately respond to the human condition. Concepts outlined above will become clearer as we develop them below.

Introduction to the Three-Step Healing Awareness

In the next few sections, you will undertake some clinical and perceptual exercises. These will reframe the concept of the *point of balanced membranous tension* into the *state of balance,* and give rise to a more dynamic and holistic perception. In this section, we will look at the work of Dr. Rollin Becker and his *three-step healing awareness.* This framework comes from a series of papers Dr. Becker wrote in the early 1960s. The descriptions are based upon my personal clinical and teaching experiences. I encourage you to read and reread these papers, put the ideas into practice, and come to your own understanding and clinical evaluation. In this exploration, you will begin to have a more open relationship to the state of balanced tension and begin to appreciate the unity of potency, fluids, and tissues. Healing will be perceived to proceed from the "without to the within and the within to the without." [12] In this process, you will more openly relate to the potency, fluid, and tissue elements and begin to appreciate the deeper forces at work.

As you learn to be in relationship to the system

in this way, the healing processes that are initiated will become known to you. Initially, it is important to establish your practitioner neutral and to synchronize your perceptual field with the mid-tide level of unfoldment of 2.5 cycles a minute. Within this deeper unfoldment, the unit of function of tissue, fluid, and potency will become more obvious. You may sense the wholeness of their function and the unified tensile field they share. Within this unfoldment you will experience tissue motility as a unity. Tissue patterns and their altered reciprocal tension motions will be sensed as distortions within whole tensile fields.

The following description is based on the writings of Dr. Rollin Becker mentioned in previous chapters and above. Dr. Becker wrote about particular perceptual experiences. These were gained after years of listening to patients' systems and healing processes within a clinical context. I find his insights to be particularly helpful in clarifying the stages of healing process that relate to states of balance. I also find his insights especially relevant for processes perceived within the mid-tide (2.5 cycles a minute) field of action. I find that his writings clarify the experience of many practitioners in the field. Similar concepts were described by Dr. Randolph Stone, D.O., and others. Dr. Stone use to say that "all healing occurs at the fulcrum, not at the poles." He encouraged practitioners to access the neutral within any relationship. It is within this neutral that healing occurs. In these writings Dr. Becker emphasizes the role of the neutral and an awareness of potency as a field phenomenon. He uses the term *bioenergy field* to denote the manifestation of potency as a unified field of action. Various other researchers into human energy fields, such as Dr. Wilhelm Reich, Dr. Alexander Lowen, and Dr. Randolph Stone have also used this or similar terms to denote this level of action and organization. Dr. Becker writes,

> Through the years, I have learned that there are bioenergy fields of activity within body physiological functioning and that is possible to learn to feel these bioenergy fields, to analyse them, to in-

terpret them, and to re-evaluate them in anatomical-physiological terminology for diagnosis and treatment.[13]

Work in this field, as we get to the depths of clinical practice, is essentially energetic in nature. Here Dr. Becker is pointing out that it is possible to sense the bioenergy fields in action within the human system and to evaluate and treat from this perspective. It is these bioenergy fields of potency that order and maintain the human system. This perspective does not mean that an understanding of structure and function is not necessary. Far from that. A clinical awareness of tissue relationships and their organization is essential for effective and efficient clinical work. An awareness of the bioenergy underpinnings of structure and function, however, deepens the nature of this work and clarifies the healing processes set in motion by the deeper intentions of the Breath of Life.

The Three-Step Healing Awareness

For many years I struggled with a way to give a simple framework for teaching about the state of balanced tension in foundation courses. It is one of the most important principles in clinical practice. In rereading Dr. Becker's work, I realized that he described a wonderfully straightforward way to lead students into a clear relationship to this principle. In his writings, Dr. Becker tells a story about his early work. He says that after training in the field and practicing for a number of years, he realized that he did not really know what was happening. It wasn't that he was not getting results; he was. But they were variable, and he did not have a sense of what the healing process truly was. He then did what I consider to be a courageous thing. He stopped doing anything to his patients and began to simply listen. He shared that after seeing 40,000 patients, the healing process began to clarify. I find this a wonderful example of someone with consummate integrity. As this healing process unfolded, its straightforwardness became apparent. The three-step process as I describe it below is derived from the insights Dr. Becker obtained with his still and present listening. I find it an excellent way to frame the teaching of the state of balanced tension in a foundation course. It gives clarity to the discussion of the process and a framework for students and practitioners to relate to.

I am going to describe this listening process in terms of the *biosphere*. Dr. Becker used this phrase to denote a wider field of action, which includes the *whole* of the person and his or her human condition. In this process, the practitioner establishes a particular field of listening. This field includes an awareness of the whole of the person's body and the field of environmental exchange, or the bioenergy field around it. As a practitioner palpates a patient's system, within a wider field of listening, certain phenomena can be perceived. It can be seen that the potencies, fluids, and tissues go through three basic phases of the healing process as the healing intentions of the Breath of Life manifest.[14]

Stage One

(i) As the practitioner palpates a specific inertial pattern within the body, he or she will sense the bioenergy field, and the fluid and tissue elements within it, seeking a neutral. It will seem like the potencies, fluids, and tissues involved are working their way towards a state of balance, a neutral particular to the specific pattern being sensed.[15]

Here you are in a clinical relationship to the bioenergy fields of the body. This is the unified field of potency, which establishes and expresses the Original matrix within the human system. As you silently listen, a precise process is engaged. The inherent treatment plan begins to emerge. Dr. Becker used to say that the *treatment plan is inherent within the disturbance.* As you listen with a negotiated contact, something will begin to emerge after a time. This may take ten minutes, or occur over a number of sessions. Within a gentle field of listening, and with

appropriate contact by the practitioner, the treatment plan will begin to emerge. It will seem as if something engages from within. The whole field of potency begins to organize around a particular fulcrum, a particular issue. There is a precision to this. All inertial forces within the system are centered by the Breath of Life in a precise way. The order of treatment is also precise. As you listen with a wide awareness, something, among all the issues carried by that person, will clarify. Listen; resist the urge to do anything or to follow any movements. Don't get in the way. Gradually a particular will clarify. You may sense that the whole tensile field of action distorts around a particular inertial fulcrum. Tissues, as a unified tensile field of action, are experienced in a more fluid way. For instance, you may sense the whole cranium, as a unified tissue field, distorting spontaneously around a particular site. As you perceive this, listen for the organizing fulcrum as described in an earlier chapter.

In this first stage the system may show you a particular pattern of distress. Something engages from within and the whole system begins to organize around a particular inertial issue. All or any of the three functions may show you this. Potency, fluid, and the tensile tissue field will begin to organize around a particular fulcrum. You may sense a distortion within the whole tissue field around a particular inertial fulcrum, you may sense eccentric fluctuations of fluid around it, or even a more energetic shift of bioenergy/potency towards and around the inertial site. A pattern is expressed around an inertial fulcrum and you notice a movement within the tissues towards a state of balance for that pattern. You may sense that potencies, fluids, and tissues express motions that indicate a *seeking of the neutral*. The three elements, potency, fluids, and tissues, will seem to be working their way towards a state of stillness or balance within that particular pattern. These may be expressed as fluid fluctuations and tissue motions such as rocking or idling, like a teeter-totter rocking around its fulcrum seeking a balanced state. As you shall see, as a practitioner, you can gently facilitate this state of balance. In this process, you will learn to subtly help the system access a neutral. As we have seen, it is the neutral that allows something else to occur beyond the forces being centered and the tissue affects that result.

Stage Two

(ii) As the practitioner listens to the bioenergy, fluid and tissue elements, he or she will note that a neutral is attained, that is, the state of balance is accessed as the fluid and tissue elements settle into a stillness. The state of balanced tension is perceived to be a stillness, a dynamic equilibrium accessed within the conditions present. When the inertial fulcrum being attended to goes through the stillness, a change occurs within the potencies involved. Accessing this stillness within the heart of the inertial pattern is the main object of the work. Within the stillness, healing processes engage. Changes take place within the inertial potencies involved, and within the whole living bioenergy field. Healing forces are engaged beyond the conditions and compensations held.

In the second stage, the state of balance is attained and potencies, fluids, and tissues express a stillness particular to the pattern being attended to. Within the mid-tide level of perception, you may have a perceptual experience that the entire field of potency, fluid, and tissue comes to balance around the organizing fulcrum, and a stillness is accessed directly related to that fulcrum. A state of balance is accessed. The state of balance is a state in which a dynamic equilibrium is attained between the inherent potencies centering the disturbance and the inertial forces maintaining it. *Dynamic equilibrium* is a state in which all forces involved in the generation of an inertial fulcrum are in balance. It is not a static equilibrium, but an alive and dynamic state of balance and interchange. As a dynamic equilibrium is attained between the forces within an inertial fulcrum, the potency of the Breath of Life is freed to express itself beyond the containment of the biokinetic forces, which are maintaining the disturbance

within the system. The whole field of potency comes directly into play in relationship to that particular issue. That is the power of this process. It is precise. This occurs within the stillness of the state of balance. It is this stillness, a dynamic and alive equilibrium, that can lead one to the deepest healing intentions of the Breath of Life.

Remember the chapter on inertial fulcrums. We discussed Dr. Becker's concepts of biodynamic potencies and biokinetic forces. At the heart of every inertial fulcrum within the body-mind, there are biokinetic forces of experience, forces added to the body physiology in some way, which maintain the disturbance within the system. Coupled with these and containing their action in some way are the biodynamic potencies of the Breath of Life. Remember that potency becomes inertial within its own field of action in order to center the unresolved forces present within the system. Inertial fulcrums result. Fluid and tissue changes also result, as does the classic osteopathic lesion. It is within the state of dynamic equilibrium, a state of balanced tension, that the biodynamic potencies can be expressed in ways that can lead to the resolution of the biokinetic forces present.

The state of balance is a *stillness* at the heart of the fulcrum being attended to. Within this stillness forces are engaged. You will be in a direct perceptual relationship to the forces that organize that pattern. A stillness is attained. In the stillness, potency is accessed and healing processes come into play. A neutral is generated within the overall dynamic. The neutral is, in essence, a new fulcrum around which the whole system is poised. The state of balance establishes a new fulcrum for the potencies and forces involved to relate to. As this occurs, there is the potential to process the inertial forces maintaining the disturbance within the system. Within the stillness, there is a change in the potency. Inertial potencies are activated, the whole bioenergy field comes into play, and expressions of healing may be perceived. A change in the potency occurs, and the inertial forces *go through* this newly established fulcrum as healing potencies come into play. Self-correcting phenomena arise. There is an expression, in some way, of biodynamic potencies and biokinetic forces within the fulcrum. Within the state of balance, they are freed to do something else beyond the conditions and compensations held. Within the stillness you may perceive many expressions of Health. This is the heart of the healing process. You may sense a sharp, directive drive of potency and fluid through the area. This is called the fluid drive of the system. Or you may perceive the whole field of potency come into play as the inertial forces are activated. This quality of potency has more of a sense of permeation. It is both soft and gentle, and clear and powerful. It has the sense of welling up and permeation, rather than of directive force. As you learn to access the state of balance, listen for these expressions of healing potency. They are the key to clinical efficiency at this level of work.

Within the state of balance, the whole field of action is now focused upon this one issue. It is thus uncoupled from all other inertial issues and can be more safely dealt with. The intentions of the Tide are now focused on this particular issue. The potency is now freed to resolve the inertial forces beyond the containment and compensations held. Remember that potency is a unified field phenomenon and as the condensation of potency within this field begins to express itself, the whole field comes in play. As described earlier, potency, within the whole bioenergy field, will condense, concentrate, and become inertial in order to contain and center any unresolved biokinetic force within the system. As potency, within a state of balance, is once again free to express itself, its whole field of action comes into play. A perception of field phenomena is common here. The practitioner may perceive a literal permeation of the potency of the Breath of Life directly into the disordered area. This is an expression of transmutation. Potency shifts in state within the fluids and healing resources become an embodied reality. This occurs as the inertial potency within the fulcrum is freed to express itself beyond the containment of the traumatic or inertial forces, which are maintaining the disturbance.

To summarize, within the state of balance a precise neutral is accessed in which a particular inertial fulcrum is uncoupled from others within the system. A specific fulcrum can be focused upon without necessarily activating the inertial forces found in other fulcrums. This leads to more precision in clinical work and less activation of symptoms and emotional affects. The stillness within the state of balance allows potency to express itself beyond the forces being centered and the compensations being maintained. Within the stillness of the state of balanced tension, potency will permeate disordered cells and tissues. It is a transmutation process. There is a transmutation of the Breath of Life, accessed within the state of balance, which initiates the healing process. It is like a mysterious gateway through which the light of the Breath of Life passes. The state of balance, accessed within a wider perceptual field than the point of balanced membranous tension, has a feeling of depth and breadth to it. Within its stillness there is a sense of deepening, and there may even be a perception of very formative ordering forces and power being engaged. Remember that the power of the Tide is in its Stillness, and the stillness within the state of balance can be like going through a gateway to deeper forces and mysteries.

Dr. Sutherland called the potency within the fluids *liquid light*. This is not just a metaphor, it is a perceptual experience. Within the state of balance, the cellular and tissue world can reestablish its relationship to the "Original Idea," the universal blueprint of a human being. As we have seen, the biodynamic forces that Dr. Becker wrote about are the physiologically active potencies of the Breath of Life. These bring the Original matrix, the embryological pattern energy of a human being, into direct relationship to every cell and tissue throughout life. When Dr. Jealous writes, "Think about the point of balance as the eye of a needle through which something can pass," this something is the Breath of Life and its intrinsic ordering intention.

Dr. Rollin Becker taught that within the stillness of the state of balance, *something happens*. Something happens, and expressions of Health manifest.

Something happens as the inherent potency of the Breath of Life expresses itself within the state of balance. Within the stillness, there is an activation or initiation of potency within the inertial fulcrum and its pattern of disturbance. As the state of balanced tension is attained, inertial potencies are initiated and there is a welling up, or permeation, of the life principle within the heart of the disturbance. As this occurs, biokinetic forces are dissipated back into the environment and, ideally, the biodynamic potencies of the Breath of Life are all that remain. In this process, you may perceive force vectors literally leaving the body, or sense pulsation, heat, expansion, and energy being released as the biokinetic forces are processed. Within this whole process, Dr. Becker encouraged practitioners to have their attention on the *potency* within the system. It is this potency that has the power to maintain balance and to contain unresolved traumatic forces. It is also this potency that has the power to resolve these issues. Dr. Becker wrote,

> My attention, as a physician using diagnostic touch, is on the potency within this patient because I know that within the potency is power and many other attributes around which the disease state or the traumatic condition within the patient is manifesting itself. I know that if a change takes place within this potency a whole new pattern will manifest itself, usually towards health for the patient.[16]

Dr. Becker knows that, "if a change takes place within this potency a whole new pattern will manifest itself, usually towards health for the patient." An awareness of these kinds of bioenergy changes gives the practitioner a wealth of information and is humbling. It is not we who do the healing, it is the unerring forces from within. If you are able to sense the changes within the bioenergy field, you will also sense how the system has been able to reorganize its fluid and tissue relationships after the resolution of the inertial potencies. This is an extremely important clinical awareness to cultivate. This takes us to stage three, outlined below.

Stage Three

(iii) When biokinetic forces are resolved, and the relationship to the ordering matrix is re-established, then the bioenergy, fluid and tissue elements begin to express their inherent motions again. In other words, the potencies, fluids, and tissues come out of the state of balance and stillness, and again express primary respiratory cycles as motility and motion. As this occurs, a new pattern of motion unfolds which is closer to the ideal. Motion may be perceived to be more balanced around natural fulcra, such as Sutherland's fulcrum, and the midline.

The third stage is one of realignment, reorientation and reorganisation. It is about a reconnection to the Original intention of the ordering matrix and the Breath of Life that generates it. The inertial forces and their tissue affects are ideally resolved, artificial boundaries soften, and potencies, fluids, and tissues reorient to the midline function and natural, suspended automatically shifting fulcrums. This is critical to understand. When the forces of inertia are truly processed, potencies, fluids, and tissues will naturally reorient to suspended automatically shifting fulcrums. It is important to allow this stage of reorganisation to occur. Give it time, be patient, and trust the Intelligence expressed within the system. The tissue field and its individual parts will ideally reorient and reorganize so that their motility and motion are expressed with greater harmony in relationship to the fulcrums and the midline function within the body. You may, for instance, sense the motion and motility of bone and membrane to be in a more harmonious relationship to Sutherland's fulcrum and to be more balanced in relationship to the structural and primal midline.

The three-step healing process is, in essence, one in which the centering and ordering intentions of the Breath of Life are expressed within states of dynamic equilibrium. Bioenergy, fluid, and tissue elements, within a particular inertial pattern, seek a neutral. A stillness is attained, a state of dynamic equilibrium specific to that particular pattern. As the state of balanced tension is attained, the variant, or inertial potency within the inertial fulcrum, has the opportunity to be expressed. Potencies are initiated, and the whole field of potency comes into play. Within the stillness, the potency has an opportunity to express its healing and ordering function

---

Summary Dr. Becker's Three-Stage Healing Awareness

- A particular fulcrum and pattern of organization clarifies as the inherent treatment plan is engaged. Within this pattern, tissues, fluids and potencies naturally seek a neutral, a state of balance, around the fulcrum being attended to. There is a sense that the potencies, fluids, and tissues are working their way towards a state of balance, a neutral. There is a movement towards a state of *dynamic equilibrium* within the forces.

- The state of balance is accessed, a stillness is attained. *Something happens* within the state of balance. There is a change within the potencies involved. Biodynamic potencies and biokinetic forces are initiated. Expressions of Health are perceived. The state of balance may be perceived to be the eye of a needle, or the mysterious gateway, through which something can pass. There is a permeation of potency and inertial forces are resolved.

- Tissues, fluids and potencies reorganize/realign to the primal midline and suspended automatically shifting fulcrums. A more balanced and natural pattern of motion may be perceived.

---

beyond the original compensation that centers the disturbance. Literally, something else can happen. The potency of the Breath of Life expresses itself beyond the conditions and compensations present and the biokinetic forces of the trauma or disease state are resolved and dissipated back to the environment. The permeation of the potency of the Breath of Life reestablishes the relationship to the Original matrix, or blueprint, of a human being. As we have seen, this original organizing principle was present at the time of conception and continues to maintain the ordering principle throughout life. It was expressed within the fluids of the embryo as an embodied force and continues to be expressed within the fluids of the body until the day we die.

Within the mid-tide level of perception and action, healing is perceived as a function of transmutation. Within the state of balanced tension, the transmutation and activation of inertial potencies is perceived to herald the beginning of a healing process. Healing is perceived as a resolution of the inertial forces that are maintaining the disturbances within the system. This occurs via the action of an inherent biodynamic potency within a larger field of action. Potency is perceived to be expressed as a whole tensile field of action within the fluids. A transmutation, or shift in state, of potency within this field can be experienced within the inertial fulcrum as the inertial forces are processed. A change happens within the potencies involved, and healing processes are initiated. When this occurs there is a reorganisation of tissues, fluids, and potencies to the primal midline and natural fulcrums. The Original intention is reestablished.

Working through the Mid-Tide: Trauma, Emotional and Psychological Processes

When working through the CRI, the results and affects of past traumatization may become activated in an overwhelming way. Examples may include emotional flooding, dissociative processes and numbness, or freezing states. These kinds of processes may seem to be healing, but can actually deepen the inertial forces involved. The system may experience the process as a new traumatic episode and more potency will become inertial in order to contain it. Intensification of symptoms is also more likely here. When you are working within the mid-tide, you are more in relationship to the patient's Health and resources. The action of potency within patterns of distress and traumatisation becomes more obvious. Unlike the CRI level, where activation of shock affect may be overwhelming, at the mid-tide, releases tend to be milder and containable. The interplay of biodynamic and biokinetic forces are more obvious.

In clinical practice, as you listen through the mid-tide level of perception, you may also notice other important and related phenomena. Work within the mid-tide tends to bring the inherent resources of the system, the biodynamic potency of the Breath of Life, into play. With the engagement of these potencies, the unresolved traumatic forces are more likely to be safely processed. This occurs in a way that encourages a resolution of traumatic affects, rather than a potentially retraumatizing recycling of past experience and shock affect. Emotional charge will resolve in a more resourced and gentle manner. If there is an emotional charge coupled with the fulcrums, the patient may feel emotional tones and energies being processed within the stillness. This may take the form of subtler emotional tones arising and clearing. The patient may experience a streaming of energies and feeling tones, commonly from the core to the periphery.

On a basic level, resolution occurs in a gentler way here because the process is more grounded within the resources of the system. Strong emotional releases tend to be associated with the CRI level of processing, where the affects of experience come more easily into play and the underlying forces tend to cycle rather than resolve. Within the mid-tide, the patient may also experience the reso-

lution of shock affects as streaming of energies and gentle or strong trembling within the tissues. The practitioner may also perceive the processing of traumatic energies as perturbations within the cerebrospinal fluid. These are experienced by patients as a perception of resource and empowerment, and as a completion of unfinished business. On a psychological level, memories may arise and insights be gained. Some of the deepest shifts seem to occur quietly and almost imperceptibly. I have heard over and over again from patients something like, "It's like I look over my shoulder and that's not there anymore." People notice things like personality patterns changing without having to do anything about them and the felt sense of "myself" shifting without having to go through great cathartic releases.

This is important. It is worth repeating. There is a great difference between a true emotional completion and an emotional process which is spinning and cycling traumatic energies. In one, the history is completing within a resourced and grounded context. In the other, dissociative states arise, traumatic energies cycle, and retraumatization may occur as the history and its related energies spin. The biokinetic forces of the trauma are not resolved and the system may even experience the process as a new traumatic episode. More potencies then become inertial in order to center the new experience, and the traumatic holding deepens. Here the traumatic energies may even intensify and become more entrenched. The tricky thing here is that dissociation and associated emotional releases can "feel good" as dopamine and endorphins flood the system. The patient may even experience what seems to be a transpersonal experience which may only be an expression of dissociative processes. True spiritual experiences are grounded in present time, and the patient will not lose the ability to be in contact. They will not feel dissociated to you. They are a blessing and humbling to witness. The key to sensing the difference as a practitioner is to be aware of signs of overwhelm and dissociation. We will discuss dissociative processes and emotional releases in a later chapter.

Shifting Perceptual Fields

It is important that you review a perceptual process that was described in Chapter Seven on palpating the tides. Please go back to it and do some practice with it before the following exercise. This perceptual process is a foundation for all your clinical explorations. We return to it over and over again. It is critical to review and continually explore this process as you palpate different systems. It gives you clinical access to different levels of information and healing processes within the system. As you learned, in this process you use different modes of intention and a widening perceptual field to help gain access to the different tidal unfoldments. You can work within the three basic unfoldments of the CRI, the mid-tide, and the Long Tide. The CRI tends to express itself anywhere from 8 to 10 cycles a minute. The mid-tide expresses itself at a more stable 2.5 cycles a minute, and the Long Tide at 100-second cycles (50-second inhalation and 50-second exhalation). Refer back to Chapter Five for a detailed discussion of this process. Later, we will explore entrées to the Dynamic Stillness itself. A summary chart is repeated below:

Clinical Application:
The Three-Step Healing Process

In the following application of the above concepts, you will simply listen for the three-stage healing process that Dr. Becker describes. The perceptual exercise reviewed above is an essential starting point for this exercise. In this process, you will synchronize your perceptual field to the mid-tide level of perception. This is the 2.5-cycles a minute tidal rhythm where the unit of function of potency, fluids, and tissues is more obvious. Within this particular rhythm the healing dynamics described by Dr. Becker become clear. Here you are in relationship to tidal potencies as they manifest in the fluids of the body. Listening within this particular rhythm, you may also notice that there is a natural tendency for tissues to access the state of balance. As the inherent treatment plan engages, you may simply perceive the potency, fluid, and tissue elements accessing a state of balance in relationship to the inertial pattern and forces present. Although this is a natural tendency when listening within this particular tidal unfoldment, you can also help the three functions of potency, fluids, and tissues to access the state of balance by simply slowing things down.

Summary of Access to Perceptual Levels

CRI

8-14 cycles a minute
- **Hands** float on tissues like corks on water.
- **Perceptual field** narrows to tissue, bone, membrane.
- **Mind** is interested in individual structures and relationships of structures/parts.

Mid-Tide

2.5 cycles a minute
- **Hands** are immersed/float within fluid.

- **Perceptual field** widens to hold the whole of the person and the biosphere. (The body and the field of potency and environmental exchange around it)

- **Mind** is relatively quiet, holds a wider field, and is in relationship to whole of person.

Long Tide

100-second cycles
- **Hands** are immersed/float within potency (the fluid within the fluid).

- **Perceptual field** widens to the horizon.

- **Mind** is expansive and still, breathes with the Breath of Life.

This is a different process than when working with the point of balanced membranous tension. In that process you followed the tension patterns within the membranes or connective tissues in the direction of motion preferred, and accessed the point of balanced tension near the boundary of that motion. That placed you in a direct relationship to the *tension patterns* within the membranes. The intention was to access a dynamic tension balance within all of the tension factors present. In the following approach, you will be listening within the mid-tide. Here you may discover that the state of balance is inherent within the forces involved. The intention will simply be to listen to the pattern of motion as it arises and to hold a wider listening field. You will discover that, at most, you will need to simply slow things down. The intention is to relate to the potencies and forces at work, rather than to the tension patterns generated by those forces. This is a subtle process of negotiation and settling. If you worked as in the point of balanced tension and followed a pattern to a boundary or edge of resistance, you may find that you lock the whole process up. Instead of accessing a state of balance that has depth, you end up waiting in a stillness which is a factor of the inertia present. This can be both frustrating and confusing. Within the mid-tide you will have access to all three functions, potency, fluids, and tissues, and will notice that within a state of balance all three settle into a state of dynamic equilibrium.

Let's first review how to synchronize your perceptual field with the mid-tide level of perception and then listen for the three-step process to unfold.

Accessing the Mid-Tide Level of Perception

1. Start in the vault hold. Negotiate your contact with the patient's system. Let your hands float on the tissues like corks on water. Synchronize your perceptual field to the mid-tide. This is a perceptual shift, which allows an initial access to the deeper forces at work. Let your hands be immersed in fluid and widen your perceptual field to the biosphere. Let your awareness widen and hold the whole of the person within your perceptual field. The biosphere includes the whole of the patient's body and the energy-environmental field around it. When you have established this wider field, bring your awareness to tissues, fluids, and potency. Imagine that your hands are floating within fluids and that the tissues are like kelp beds being moved by the Tide. Do not look for tissues; let them come to you within this wide field of perception. Let your mind settle into this relationship and become relatively still. You can't make your mind become still. Simply extend a wide perceptual field, settle into yourself and listen. In the listening, your mind will begin to settle.

2. As you widen your perceptual field to hold the whole of the person, and as you become aware of the fluids within that field, a deeper tidal phenomenon will start to unfold. You may now sense the deeper, slower tidal impulse of 2.5 cycles a minute, the mid-tide. Here you are in a more direct relationship to the dynamics of the potency within the fluids. Potency, fluids, and tissues may be perceived to be a unit of function. As you establish your wider perceptual field, do not lose awareness of the tissues and tissue motion within it. Tissue motility will be perceived to be a unified dynamic. You will perceive reciprocal tension motion as a tensile shift of the whole tissue field. This may be sensed as a surge and settling as tissues express their dynamic as a whole. At this level of perception, inertial fulcrums are perceived via the inertial potencies that organize them. The information thus perceived will be more precise than at the CRI level. You will perceive inertial fulcrums via distortions within whole tensile fields, not just as resistance between parts. Within this tidal unfoldment, you will be in direct perceptual relationship to organizing forces and potencies. You can have a clearer relationship to the forces that

maintain and center the disturbances within the system, the biodynamic and biokinetic potencies Dr. Becker describes.

The Three-Step Awareness

(i) The bioenergy field and the fluid and tissue elements seem to be seeking a neutral, a state of balance within a particular pattern around its organizing fulcrum.

1. Maintain this wider perceptual field and relatively still mind. You may perceive tissue motion as a whole. All tissue structure and motion will be perceived to be a unified dynamic. You may also perceive the particular motions of structures like the sphenoid bone, but their motility and craniosacral motion will be sensed to be part of a greater whole and, within this field of perception, will express the slower 2.5 cycles a minute rhythm. Simply let your hands float within fluid and listen. Sense the tissues as though they are tensile kelp beds being moved by the Tide. Do not lose awareness of tissue motion within this wider perceptual field, and do not grab onto the tissues or crowd the system with your awareness. If you do this, the system will react to your presence and you may find yourself chasing shadows.

2. Do the kelp beds and the tidal forces move you? How is this organized around the midline and around Sutherland's fulcrum? Is there a sense of balance? Have patience. It may take some time for the treatment plan to engage. Do not go to patterns; do not follow them. Simply notice and let go. It will seem as though something engages from within. A particular pattern, around a particular fulcrum, clarifies. Remember the previous exercise when we explored an awareness of inertial patterns. Within the midtide these patterns may be perceived to be distortions of the whole field around particular sites. For instance, you may sense the whole tensile tissue field of the cranium distorting around a particular suture. An inertial pattern will have its potency, fluid, and tissue elements. Track these motions within the larger field. Again, do not grab onto the tissues, simply float within the fluids and maintain your wide perceptual field. Do not try to analyze anything. If your lose your wide perceptual field and relatively still mind, if you start to look for things, you will begin to shift back to the CRI level.

3. As you follow a particular motion dynamic via the tissue field, you may notice the fulcrum that organizes it. Simply bring the question to your hands: "What organizes this?" See if you can sense the inertial fulcrum that organizes the movement. Remember that inertial fulcrums are not automatically shifting fulcrums. They do not shift with the respiratory cycles of the Tide. They are still or inertial places within a greater field of action.

4. Notice the motion dynamic organized around the inertial fulcrum. As you do this, you may notice the bioenergy field and the fluid and tissue elements moving towards a state of balance. You may notice subtle tissue and fluid motions like rocking, idling, and swirling. These elements are *seeking a neutral* in relationship to the forces that organize their dynamics. You may also sense eccentric fluid fluctuations as the neutral is sought. The neutral is inherent within the organizing fulcrum, and the fluid and tissue motions are an attempt to attain it.

(ii) The potencies, fluids, and tissue elements settle into a state of balance around the organizing fulcrum. A neutral is accessed within the overall dynamic. This establishes a new fulcrum for the forces to relate to. A stillness is accessed. This is the heart of the potency centering the inertial forces present. A change in the potency occurs, and the inertial forces go through this newly established fulcrum as healing potencies come into play. Within the stillness, inertial potencies are activated, the whole bioenergy field comes into play, and expressions of healing may be perceived.

5. As you maintain your wide perceptual field, you may then perceive potencies, fluids, and tissues naturally settling into a state of balance. This a stillness within which all motion apparently ceases. (although there is always a *kernel* of potency expressing motion within the heart of even the most dense inertia). At deeper levels, the *neutral* resonates with Stillness and the Original matrix, which is never lost. The state of balance is a gateway through which a reconnection to the inherent ordering principles of the system can occur.

6. If the potency, fluids, and tissues do not settle into the state of balance, you can assist this process. With your hands floating within fluid, simply slow things down. Follow the potency, fluid, and tissue motions in the direction they take you and subtly slow things down. Let the action of the potency show you the fulcrum. Go with the action of the potency. Slow things down until a settling into stillness is sensed. Again, this is a very subtle intention. You do not grab onto the tissues, or the fluids, or the potency to do this. It is an inquiry into the possibility of stillness. Simply slow things down with the question, "Can you access stillness here?" It is a subtle intention of inquiry in your hands, with no physical force. You do not narrow down your field of perception as you do this. This will simply lock up the potencies, fluids, and tissues being sensed.

7. Once the pattern settles into stillness, listen for expressions of Health. In the stillness of the state of balance, you will perceive the forces that center and maintain the inertia. The biodynamic potencies and biokinetic forces will be initiated or called into action. A change will take place within the potency. You sense a

buildup of potency within the fulcrum. You may sense pulsation and fluctuation as this occurs. As potencies are initiated within the state of balance, the *fluid drive* of the system may kick in, as a surge of potency literally moves through the fulcrum being palpated. This drive of potency may be sharp and directed. You may also sense a softer permeation of potency through the area and the fulcrum being attended to. This has a different quality. It is more of a field phenomenon. You may sense the whole field of potency come into play. A building and welling up of potency may be perceived. As the system is poised within a state of balance around a particular fulcrum, the whole field of potency organizes around this particular inertial issue. A movement of potency throughout its field towards the inertial fulcrum may be sensed. As this occurs, a soft permeation of potency may be perceived within the area and fulcrum being palpated. It is like water soaking a dense knob of sand and melting it away. You may literally sense a welling up of potency within the whole tensile field, which moves right through the inertial fulcrum you are palpating. Remember that the inertial potencies are still part of that wider field. You may sense a welling up and permeation of potency into the inertial area.

(iii) When inertial forces are resolved, there is a return to motion within the potencies, fluids, and tissues of the system. This is a period of reorganisation and realignment to natural fulcrums and the midline.

8. Once the inertial issues are resolved, you will sense potency, fluid, and tissue moving again. You may initially sense expansion. Once the biokinetic forces are dissipated back to the environment, inherent potency, which condensed to center the inertial forces, now is freed to expand. When potency expands, tissues will also expand. You may sense an expansion within the tissue elements involved in the inertial issue.

You may then sense reorganization processes. This may take some time. Again, have patience. This is not a new inertial pattern being expressed. Do not engage it. Give the system space to complete its reorganization process. When biokinetic forces are resolved, potencies, fluids, and tissues are free to organize around their natural fulcrums and the primal midline (the primal or notochord midline is the primary ordering axis of the human system). Do tissues now express motion dynamics more aligned to the action of Sutherland's fulcrum? How do the tissues express their motion around the primal midline? Is there more balanced motion around this midline? Basically, when inertial forces resolve, there is a natural tendency to reorient to the intentions of the Breath of Life and its imperative. Potencies, fluids, and tissues will reorganize to natural automatically shifting fulcrums and to the midline function of the Breath of Life.

You can practice this intention using the various bony and membranous relationships already learned for experience and feedback over a number of sessions. This is a key understanding and perceptual process to cultivate. Have patience with the process and with yourself. This one of the key healing principles to understand, and you will come back to it again and again. Be still and listen. It will become more and more obvious to you. All of the other skills are simply ways to initiate and engage this healing principle. Remember that the intention here is to become aware of the inherent potencies and forces at work within the human system. The potency of the Breath of Life has the power to organize life and has the power to heal its most desperate conditions. Dr. Becker wrote,

> The bioenergy of wellness is the most powerful force in the world. It is a force field that begins with the moment of conception and continues to the last moment of death.[17]

Quick Clinical Reference Guide: Dr. Becker's Three-Step Healing Awareness

(i) Listen for the inherent treatment plan to begin to unfold. A particular pattern and its inertial fulcrum will clarify. A particular organization will be perceived. The bioenergy field, and the fluid and tissue elements, will seem to be seeking a neutral, a state of balance for a particular pattern around its organizing fulcrum. Notice this; at most slow things down. Do not grab on. Do not get in the way of this process.

(ii) The potencies, fluids, and tissue elements settle into a state of balanced tension around the organizing fulcrum. A neutral is accessed within the overall dynamic. This establishes a new fulcrum for the forces to relate to. A stillness, a dynamic equilibrium, is accessed. This is the heart of the potency centering the inertial forces present. A change in the potency occurs, and the inertial forces go through this newly established fulcrum as healing potencies come into play. Within the stillness, inertial potencies are activated, the whole bioenergy field comes into play, and expressions of healing may be perceived. You may perceive fluctuations of potency and fluid, a permeation of potency into the inertial site, and an expansion of potency and tissue elements.

(iii) When inertial forces are resolved, there is a return to motion within the potencies, fluids, and tissues of the system. This is a period of reorganization and realignment to suspended automatically shifting fulcrum and the midline. Listen for this and give this reorganization process space. This is not a new inertial issue being expressed. It is a reorganization. Do not engage it. Let it be, give it time to complete. Notice the new organization that results. Is it more balanced in relationship to suspended automatically shifting fulcrums?

It is easy to forget this fact in the midst of clinical diagnosis and the mental and physical discomfort of our patients. Let's remember these words when our minds get too busy, or when we think we know what is best. It is the magnificent human system that knows best, and it is the potencies that organize its structure and function that have the power to heal. It is our role to help generate the circumstances for something else to happen beyond the conditions being centered, but we must engage in this process with a deep reverence for life and an ability to listen and to wait. The Breath of Life will show us the way, if we have the patience to listen. Dr. Becker wrote about the *inherent treatment plan* and it is up to us to be able to hear its unfolding.

Advanced Processes

In the next sections, we will take alternative approaches to exploring the state of balanced tension. These build upon what we have already discussed. In the first approach, I will outline an exploration that asks the practitioner to become aware of reciprocal states of balance within potency, fluids, and tissues. In the second approach, I will present an important exploration, which will become a theme in this book, the state of balance as the "eye of the needle," or the "mysterious gateway," into the deeper organizing forces and intentions within the human system. As we will discover, when one is holding a very wide perceptual field, the state of balance can lead both patient and practitioner to the most formative organizing forces and principles in life itself.

Reciprocal Tension Motion Revisited

In the first approach, we will look at the reciprocity between potency, fluids, and tissues. One way to appreciate the state of balance is to break down the unit of function of potency, fluids, and tissues and look at each in turn. As you do this, you will discover that each expresses reciprocal tension motion and each, within the state of balance, expresses the neutral. All three express reciprocal tension motion

as tensile fields of action, and all three also express a synchronous state of reciprocal tension balance. As we have seen, the term *reciprocal tension motion* classically relates to the motion of the reciprocal tension membranes. You may have already experienced their reciprocal tension motion around a suspended automatically shifting fulcrum, Sutherland's fulcrum. It must be understood, however, that the potency, the fluids, and the tissues all express reciprocal tension motion as a unified field of action. One of the beautiful things about the Breath of Life is that it is an expression of a universal within the system. Its laws hold at every level of manifestation and within all functions. It makes things very simple. Its action is the same no matter where you look. The Breath of Life generates reciprocal cycles of primary respiration in all functions and relationships. Dr. Randolph Stone, D.O., used to stress in his teachings that polarities, or reciprocal tension motions, are how everything in the universe manifests form and function.

Every level of the system expresses reciprocal tension motion as a whole. In this process, the potency of the Breath of Life is taken up by the fluids, and tissue motility, motion, and organization are generated. Tissues, fluids, and potency are a unit of function. These three functions cannot be separated. Potency is the organizing factor, fluids are the medium, and the cellular and tissue world is the physical ground. The organization of tissues is based on the continuity of this relationship. Tissues, fluids, and potency are thus one dynamic. All are moved by the intentions of the Breath of Life and all express reciprocal tension motion. These are all expressed as self-limiting tensile fields of action. The tensile fields generated by the Breath of Life all have boundaries and are thus limited in their field of action. Life naturally limits its expression. If this were not so, energies would endlessly expand and form could not coalesce around the expressions of potency.

All fluid and tissue motility is driven by the cyclical expression of the Breath of Life via the action of its Tide. This is the root of primary respiration.

Tissues, fluids, and potency express the reciprocal cycles of primary respiration, inhalation and exhalation, as a whole. They exhibit a unified motion dynamic. They are moved as a unit of function in cycles of reciprocal tension motion. Reciprocal tension motion is set up within the fluids, cells, and tissues of the body by the action of the Breath of Life. All of this motion is organized around automatically shifting fulcrums suspended within tensile fields. The tissues, in their natural motion, express reciprocal tension motion as a tensile field. This is expressed in cycles of reciprocal tension motion, which is limited in its excursions. Likewise, the fluids act as a whole to express longitudinal and transverse fluctuations as a tensile field, first in one direction, then another. Although tissue boundaries help to generate this tensile fluid field, it is really created by the action of the potency within the fluids.

Finally, potency itself is expressed as a unified tensile field which expresses reciprocal tension motion. This is really the heart of the matter. Potency is expressed as a tensile field within and around the body. This field has limits. It is limited by the relationship of the potency to the midline. The midline organizes the expression of potency, and the whole field of potency must always refer back to it. The relationship of the potency to the primal midline is one of a reciprocal tension field to its ordering axis. Thus potency is expressed as a tensile field and is self-limiting. It is because of this fact that potencies can concentrate within their own field of action. As you have already perceived, within the state of balance, potencies naturally coalesce and concentrate. This can occur because potency is expressed as a self-limiting tensile field. If the expression of potency were not self-limiting, it would manifest in endless expansion and dissipate. It would not then be able to concentrate or coalesce within its own field of action to form organizing fulcrums, whether natural or inertial.

Reciprocal tension motion is thus a universal expression of organization seen at every level of manifestation. These motions are naturally organized and balanced around the primal midline and the automatically shifting fulcrums organized along its axis. Within the perceptual field of the mid-tide, automatically shifting fulcrums are perceived to be suspended points, or coalescences, of potency within a greater field of action. The Long Tide generates the bioelectric matrix and the primal midline is generated within this wider field. This arises, as discussed in earlier chapters, via centripetal action and the spiraling of potencies to form a stable tensile field. The primal midline is the organizing axis for all tissue motion and motility. From this midline the tensile fields of the human system are set up and reciprocal tension motion around automatically shifting fulcrums are generated.

Automatically shifting fulcrums not only occur within tissues, but also within the fluids and potency. A unit of function is whole and universal principles apply in all parts. Tissues, fluids, and potency all express reciprocal tension motion organized around automatically shifting fulcrums. This can be perceived no matter where reciprocal tension motion is found. Dr. Randolph Stone used to teach that life force moves from a source and must return to that source in tensile cycles of polarity motion. Potencies are expressed in outward centrifugal motions from the source and return back to the source in inward centripetal spirals. Life spirals out to express form and spirals in to both generate form and to return to its source. Within this greater field of action there are centripetal motions, the Original motion of Victor Schauberger, which generate specific bioelectric matrices for form to coalesce within. This process generates form and boundary. Life is a self-limiting and self-generating system. Thus we see:

- The Breath of Life expresses its intentions by generating potency, an organizing and ordering force,

- the potency manifests as a unified tensile field of action which expresses reciprocal tension motion,

- fluids and tissues organize around the imperative carried by the potency,

- fluids and tissues respond to the reciprocal tension motions of potency and, in turn, express their own reciprocal tension motions, and

- all of this is organized around suspended automatically shifting fulcrums, which are, in essence, points of concentrated potency within a wider field of action.

In the clinical sections below, we will try to unfold these ideas within a perceptual framework. You will gain an experiential felt sense of these concepts.

Reciprocal Tension Balance

In the next clinical explorations, you will inquire into the nature of reciprocal tension as a field of action. You will open to the dynamic within potency, fluids, and tissues and listen for states of reciprocal tension balance within each function. As you do this, you are breaking down a unit of function into its component parts for observation and clarity. Visualize a unified field of potency, fluid and tissue. Imagine a unified field of potency within which fluids and tissues organize. Each aspect is a function of increasing density. First there is a bioelectric field, then a fluid field, and then a more physical field of cells and tissues. Each is a tensile field in its own right and all interact and manifest a unified tensile dynamic. You will simply listen, in turn, first to the reciprocal tension motion of tissues, then to the fluids and their field of fluctuant action, and finally to the bioelectric function of potency within its own tensile field. We will apply Dr. Becker's observations to each layer in turn. Dr. Jim Jealous describes this clinical concept beautifully:

Suppose instead of saying reciprocal tension membrane, I said to you reciprocal tension fluid and let this idea of reciprocal tension fluid sit in your mind and at the same time envision your experience with the reciprocal tension membrane. Reciprocal tension fluid. Would we not have a suspended automatically shifting fulcrum at the point of balance in the fluid? Would we not have a fulcrum around which the potency of the fluid drive was able to manifest its hydraulic forces? [18]

Again, suspended automatically shifting fulcrums are at work at every level of organization. Thus the fluid field is a tensile field of action just as the tissue field is. It too expresses a reciprocal tension action around an automatically shifting fulcrum. In the following clinical exploration, you will first tune into the reciprocal tension dynamics of the membranes. You will listen to their reciprocal tension patterns in the light of Dr. Becker's work as we explored above. As they settle into a state of balanced tension, notice the state of reciprocal tension balance within the tissue field. You will then include an awareness of the fluids and also notice what is happening within its tensile field of action. Notice reciprocal balanced fluid tension. Notice how fluids also settle around the fulcrum and express reciprocal tension balance. The heart of all of this is the potency and its expression of balance within its own tensile field. Dr. Jealous goes on to say,

If you ask the same question about potency and if I say to you reciprocal tension potency, or if I said to you tensile potency, or reciprocal tensile potency, or reciprocating tensile potency and you think about the fluid and the membrane and their reciprocal tensions and you hold all of that in your mind, what do you come to? Could we not say that the concept we used for the reciprocal tension membrane and the reciprocal tension fluids could also apply to the tensile forces of the potency? The potency has a tensile quality. Potency is reciprocally balanced around a fulcrum and it is limited in its range of motion to the needs of the function of the entire system and the geometric pattern of that system which we call anatomy.[19]

Again,˙ potency, the organizing bioelectric form within the system, manifests an automatically shifting fulcrum within its wider field of action. All reciprocal tension motion is organized around these automatically shifting fulcrums, even the action of potency as a tensile field. As you notice reciprocal tension balance in tissues and fluids, you will then include the potency within your field of inquiry. Potency is also expressed within a tensile field. Reciprocal balanced potency tension brings you to the heart of the forces at work within the pattern being investigated. Do you sense reciprocal tension balance within the potency? Can you sense the potency as a tensile field in a state of balance? Let's see! In the following sections you will again explore the clinical concept of states of balanced tension and hopefully widen your perceptual understanding. You may also note that the neutral accessed within the fluids and potency is qualitatively different to that accessed within the membranous level. A depth arises as the stillness deepens within the unit of function, and the forces at work are initiated.

Clinical Application:
Reciprocal States of Balanced Tension

In the following clinical application, you will inquire into these ideas. Remember the work you have already done with reciprocal tension membranes and with Dr. Rollin Becker's concepts. All come into play here. In the following, you will artificially separate the three functions of tissue, fluid, and potency and will more consciously include all three in your inquiry. When these three functions (tissues, fluids, and potency) come into a synchronous state of balance, when their neutrals align, so to speak, you will find yourself within the heart of the inertial fulcrum and its potencies. Within each of the three functions, as you listen to the settling into stillness, remember the perceptual work you have already explored.

Synchronize your perceptual field with the mid-tide level of unfoldment. Obviously, Dr. Becker's three-stage healing process will be expressed within all three functions.

1. In the vault hold, establish a wide perceptual field and let your hands float within fluids. Hold the whole of the biosphere within your awareness. Settle into the mid-tide level of perception. As above, listen to the reciprocal tension motions of the tissues. Allow an inertial pattern to make itself known to you. Allow the healing intentions of the Breath of Life to clarify. Be patient here. You may sense this as a *distortion* within the whole tissue field being palpated. Hold a wide perceptual field and allow a tensile pattern to clarify within it. Be patient: give it time to do so. As you track tensile tissue motions, see if you can sense an organizing fulcrum.

2. Explore reciprocal tension membranous balance. Within a wide perceptual field notice the tissues, as a tensile field, settling into a state of reciprocal tension balance around their organizing fulcrum. Bring a wide awareness to the tissue elements as they seek a neutral within their reciprocal tension motions. Maintain your awareness of the biosphere as you do this. You can facilitate the state of balance by simply slowing the motions down. Again, do not grab the tissues to do this.

3. Now include the fluids within your field of awareness. Notice how the fluids express a reciprocal tension motion around the organizing fulcrum. See if you can sense the fluids accessing a state of balance. Note *reciprocal tension fluid balance*. This may be perceived as a deepening into the state of balance, a further settling into stillness. You can likewise facilitate this settling by slowing down any fluctuant phenomena. Do not grab the fluids to do this. Clear intention and space is necessary.

4. Now include the potency within your field of awareness. Notice how the potency is expressed as a tensile field. You may sense this between your hands as an bioelectric field phenomenon, a field of bioenergy. Notice how this tensile field of potency also moves to a state of balanced tension in relationship to the organizing fulcrum. Remember that this fulcrum is an expression of inertial potencies. The potency is simply accessing a neutral within its own field of action. Simply explore reciprocal tension potency balance, or reciprocal tension balance within the unified field of potency. Again, if necessary, slow the fluctuant potency down bioelectrically within your hands. Do not grab the potency to do this.

If you grab onto any of the three functions (tissue, fluids, and potency) they will have to respond to your presence and the state of balance will not be accessed. You will be chasing shadows, the system's response to your intervention, not the inertial fulcrum and pattern the Breath of Life is centering.

5. As the three layers deepen into the state of balance, a *synchronous neutral* with depth may be noted. Simply give space and listen. You are now at the heart of the inertial forces, which both maintain and center the fulcrum being explored. The potency, and the inertial forces involved, will move through the new fulcrum generated within the deepening stillness. A change in the potency will be perceived. You are at the heart of the potential to reconnect to the Health that is never lost.

6. Listen for expressions of Health, for resolution of inertia forces, and for the reorientation of the three functions to the midline and to the natural fulcrums of the system.

Explore this concept from different vantage points within the system. Use the holds and relationships learned previously to deepen your understanding.

In your practice sessions, start with the classical intention of balanced membranous tension as described earlier. Then, in further sessions, explore the state of balance and Dr. Becker's concepts as outlined above. Finally, in sessions after that, explore reciprocal states of balance within tissues, fluids, and potency in order to separate the three functions for greater clarity and a deeper clinical awareness of the healing process. As you do this, the possibility of perceiving a synchronous state of balanced within all three functions will clarify.

Epigenetic Potencies

As we have seen in earlier chapters, potency, in its most fundamental expression within the human system, manifests as an epigenetic ordering matrix. This bioelectric matrix is laid down by the action of the Long Tide as it moves to generate the template for the human system. This ordering template maintains the integrity of form and function throughout life. These forces or potencies are with us at the moment of conception and generate the matrix around which cellular differentiation and development occur. They are epigenetic forces and underpin the later involvement of genetics. Epigenetic forces are organizing forces, which are not tied into genetics; they precede and underlie genetic expression. These are the biodynamic potencies of the Breath of Life in their most primal and fundamental expression. Their interplay precedes genetics and is the bioelectric template within which genetics function.

Genetics is about the particular and the individual. It is about the detail of the species. Genetics helps maintain constancy *and* variation within the species. Epigenetic forces are about the whole. They hold the larger picture. They orchestrate overall patterns and development and generate the template for the particular species without dictating a rigid form. For instance, epigenetic forces hold the template for a particular organ or shape and its function, like a liver or a nose. It holds that template within the context of the whole. Genetics gives that form a particular shape, like the shape of nose particular to that family or cultural line. Epigenetic forces lay down the template for that liver; genetics may modify its function, like making it less efficient, more resilient to certain toxins, more prone to particular disease states, and so on.

As we shall see, the state of balance may become a gateway into a relationship with these most primary potencies. The state of balance is a state of *dynamic equilibrium*. It is a stillness within the dynamics of the forces that organize an inertial pattern. When this state of dynamic equilibrium is attained, a stillness is accessed. The state of dynamic equilibrium is an inherent stillness found within all of the conditions present. It is a dynamic state of reciprocal tension balance which takes you to the heart of the fulcrum being palpated. It is attained within all three functions of potency, fluids, and tissues in relationship to the inertial forces present. This state of dynamic equilibrium resonates with all states of inherent balance within the organization of a human being.

This stillness can be like a mysterious gateway into the deeper epigenetic potencies at work within the human system. Like the eye of a needle, it can take you to the Original matrix itself. The Original matrix is a stable living bioelectric field, a template for organization. The stable field represents a dynamic state of equilibrium within the centripetal and centrifugal action of the Long Tide. This dynamic equilibrium manifests as an alive stillness within the field. The state of balance, like a mysterious gateway, can take you to this stillness and to the inherent organizing matrix of a human being. It is here that the epigenetic organizing potencies are encountered. The Long Tide, like a great wind moving through space, generates this template. Within a state of balance, as you listen within a very wide perceptual field, you may sense these forces at work like a great wind moving right through the fulcrum being palpated.

As your relationship to the state of balance deepens, a reconnection to this inherent ordering principle may occur, and cells and tissues may realign to their Original intention. It is like dropping through

a mysterious gateway to a deeper level of organization and order. The Original intention has to do with universal creative intentions at work. Our organization as a human being is thus not solely determined by genetics.[20] It is within this deeper level of work that the fluids, cells, and tissues of the human system may remember what they are and realign to the ordering matrix and the creative winds of the Long Tide. Accessing the dynamic equilibrium of the organizing matrix, a stillness within the field, can become another gateway to the Dynamic Stillness itself.

Epigenetic Forces and the Mysterious Gateway

In this section we will explore the eye of the needle, or the mysterious gateway, into these deeper potencies at work within the human system. It is a shift from a relationship to form and results to a more primal level of organization. It is hard to give an analogy for what occurs. It is literally a shift in your perceptual field, like moving through a mysterious gateway to a whole other perception of what is occurring within healing and ordering processes. This section may help you open to a wider and deeper perception and appreciation of the forces at work within the human system. The state of balance can, like the eye of a needle, be the gateway to these deeper forces at work. It can lead you to a more direct perception of the potency of the Breath of Life as it unfolds within the system. Within the state of balance, a stillness, a dynamic equilibrium, is accessed. This stillness is the gateway to the mysteries of the human system.

Within the state of balance, as your relationship to stillness deepens, you may experience a perceptual shift. One aspect of this is the perception of the Original matrix, and the organizing winds which generate it, as a primal field phenomenon. By primal, I mean a principle of order, which is with us from the moment of conception until the day we die. It is a manifestation of the ever present-ness of the creative process. You may also sense the stillness, which is the ground of this matrix. Stillness is the heart of its stability. Within this wider field of awareness you may, in turn, sense the potency of the Breath of Life rising through the midline, through the tensile fields of the body, right through the fulcrum being palpated. The potency that permeates the fulcrum may be experienced to arise from "outside in" and "inside out"—from very deep sources indeed. The state of balance can thus be the eye of the needle, or a mysterious gateway into deeper and deeper healing and ordering intentions.

As the practitioner deepens into stillness, a darkness may arise. This is a descent into a space of unknowing. Within the Dynamic Stillness everything is enshrouded in a darkness. It is a state of perception without a perceiver. Here healing processes are about resonance and reconnection. There is Originality in its most primal form. This is a level of total potential, a ground of emergence. It is a subtle essence from which motion arises and to which it returns. As you move through the eye of the needle, perceptual shifts and deeper experiences of wholeness arise. It is a moment of total compassion within the darkness of the known mind. A quote from Rumi, the great Sufi sage, speaks to this,

> *This moment this love comes to rest in me*
> *many beings in one being.*
> *In one wheat-grain a thousand sheaf stacks.*
> *Inside the needle's eye, a turning night of*
> *stars.*[21]

What was isolated and particular is now wholly part of a "turning night of stars." As we widen our perceptual field and deepen into stillness, a resonance occurs with the deeper ordering intentions of the Breath of Life. A mystery unfolds its magic to us. It is the magic of life itself, and it is a humbling experience. In essence it allows us to touch, even so briefly, the compassion of life and the love that is the universal, which generates its movement. The overriding sense of this for me is a compassionate warmth, which is not about need or desire. It simply is.

The state of balance can be the eye of the needle in many ways. As we open to its stillness, it becomes the eye of the needle through which our perception can pass. As we deepen our relationship to stillness, we naturally begin to appreciate the human condition as a whole. The stillness within the state of balance is one gateway to deeper and deeper levels of reality. We can directly see how potency, fluids, and tissues are a true unit of function and how the inherent forces of the system heal from within. It helps shift the practitioner from a tissue- and lesion-based perception to a more open relationship to the inherent forces at work. This "eye" will also allow us to appreciate even deeper forces at work. We can move through the eye to the ordering matrix and the winds of the Long Tide as form is organized and generated. A dawning appreciation of the transmutation process begins to clarify. With a deepening relationship to stillness this eye can even lead to the Dynamic Stillness itself. Another mysterious gateway, perhaps the "true" gateway, opens here. Thus as we deepen and broaden our perceptual field, the Dynamic Stillness itself may unfold the answers to its own questions, within a cloud of unknowing and a depth of vibrant stillness.

In the context of the work described below, the first perceptual shift within the state of balance relates to epigenetic organization. These are principles of order beyond the realm of genetics. Here we are widening the concept of the state of balance to include the *epigenetic* intentions of the potency of the Breath of Life. By this I mean opening to the possibility of having a deeper and more direct relationship to its potency. First you may discover that potency can be perceived as a deeper phenomenon within the system. This is the level of the bioelectric matrix, a stable form generated by the organizing winds of the Long Tide. This organizing matrix is more perceptible within the Long Tide field of action. It is a level of action in which the Original matrix is laid down and the stable bioenergy field is generated. This is the function of the "winds of the vital forces" as described in Tibetan medicine.

At this level of perception, you may become aware of the *epigenetic* action of biodynamic potency. By this I mean that genetic processes are secondary   to its action. You are now beneath the mid-tide level of forces at work and have a more direct perception of the ordering matrix itself. You may sense the radiance of the potency of the Breath of Life more directly. You may form a relationship to the matrix of potency that orders form and generates function. It may also open you to clinical processes and forces grounded in the perception of the Original matrix and its potency as the Breath of Life establishes the priorities within the human system. Here the inherent treatment plan is more directly sensed.[22] Here there is nothing to do except to remain keenly aware of the healing priorities of the system as they unfold. The alive stillness within this matrix can, of itself, be another eye into the Dynamic Stillness itself. Again stillness resonates with stillness. Here it is a question of depth of space and stillness, not of motion or form. From within this Dynamic Stillness, the mystery of life begins to speak to us. Within this Stillness there is perception without a perceiver, and healing is a matter of resonance and direct reconnection. It truly has nothing to with "me."

Clinical Application:
The Mysterious Gateway, Epigenetic Forces, and the State of Balance

In this last exploration you will again access the state of balanced tension and work to explore the state of balance as the eye of the needle or the mysterious gateway to these deeper forces at work. You will do this by shifting your perceptual fields within the stillness accessed via the state of balance. You will shift your perceptual fields while settling deeper into the state of balance, a dynamic equilibrium not just within the patient's system, but also within your state of consciousness. In this exercise, you will again start within the mid-tide level of perception. This process calls for a quality of listening in which you are open to the unknown and do not bring any preconceptions or judgments to a unique therapeutic encounter. You will first facilitate the state of balance within the mid-tide level of perception and then widen your perceptual field towards the horizon. This may open your perceptual field to the Long Tide level of action and to the Original matrix, which underlies the organization of form. As you widen your perceptual field, you will listen for any phenomena that arise within the state of balance.

The first step is to establish a safe and trustworthy space. Review concepts presented in Chapter Six. Gently negotiate your relationship and be open to listening within a context of unknowing. It is important to establish your practitioner fulcrums. This gives the patient's system a relational ground from which healing processes can be established. It is also important to establish a still clinical space. Let your mind still within its wide perceptual field. This contains, initiates, and holds the patient's process. It is a call to the deeper forces and Intentions at work within the human system. It is a call towards a relationship to the mystery of the Breath of Life itself. So remember your practitioner fulcrums, come into breath and sensation, let your mind still and hold a wide and natural field of listening. This establishes a safe therapeutic space and is a call to the deeper healing resources within and beyond the conditional forces being centered. Much more important, it is a humbling entrée into a healing process, which is a mutual journey for both therapist and patient.

1. Start at the vault hold and negotiate your contact with the patient's system. In this position, synchronize your perceptual field with the mid-tide (2.5 cycles a minute), phenomenon. Do this by allowing your hands to float in fluid as they float on the tissues. Then widen your perceptual field to the biosphere as previously learned.

2. Within the biosphere, notice reciprocal tension motion as a unified motion dynamic within tissues, fluids, and potency. Listen to this as the cycles of primary respiration are expressed. Notice the tissue field as it expresses its tensile motion. Let the treatment plan engage. Give the system time to clarify its intentions. Notice any distortions or inertial patterns within that field. Notice what organizes that motion. Notice Dr. Becker's three-step process. Listen to the tissues as they seek a neutral. Subtly slow their motions down until a state of balanced tension is obtained as learned earlier. Do not grab onto any function (tissues, fluids, or potency) as you explore reciprocal tension balance within tissues, fluids, and potency. Maintain an awareness of the inertial fulcrums and state of balanced tension within the biosphere. Do not narrow your perceptual field as you listen. Listen within this wider field of awareness. Include the tissues, fluids, and potency as a unified tensile field. Notice the three functions accessing the state of balance. Listen for forces and potencies at work. Listen for expressions of Health.

3. Now, within the state of balance, gently shift your perceptual field towards the horizon. Let your hands float in potency and widen your perceptual field towards the horizon. Widen your field to wherever it is sensed to be safe and tolerable. Do not lose awareness of the state of balance and fulcrums being palpated as you do this. It is like holding a dual awareness, a wide perceptual field and an awareness of the particulars within it. Let this awareness settle and deepen.

4. As you do this, you may sense the deeper, slower tidal phenomenon of the Long Tide. It may seem to be all around you. It may seem as if you are in the Tide. The midline imperative of the potency of the Breath of Life may also become more obvious here. Listen within the stillness of the state of balance to the inherent

biodynamic forces as they begin to express their healing intentions. You may actually have an experience of an uprising potency moving into the midline, arising through the tensile fields of the body, right through the inertial fulcrums being attended to. You may literally have the experience of the potency of the Breath of Life moving through the inertial fulcrum like light through the eye of a needle. Like a mysterious gateway, the shift in your perceptual fields can bring you to the most formative organizing forces at work. The state of balance can bring you, like the eye of a needle, to the Original matrix itself. Biodynamic, epigenetic forces are perceived more directly here. The phenomenon of permeation of the potency right through the inertial fulcrums may be clearly experienced here. Experiences of radiance, luminescence and field phenomena are common here. The practitioner may have a sense of being in the ocean in the midst of huge tidal forces at work. This is directly perceived to part of a greater whole, a universal process of Original motion coming into play.

5. As your mind synchronizes with a depth of stillness and accesses a state of balance in which it is neither coming nor going, another gateway may open for you. You may enter a depth of Stillness from which all things arise. In Daoism it is called the Subtle Essence. It is entered in unknowing, a darkness. The mind is totally at balance and peace. It is wide and deep. Here the Dynamic Stillness, the ground of emergence of the human system, may be appreciated. It is truly a humbling experience. It is a stillness that permeates everything, that is alive with potential. It underpins the unfoldment of life. It is the ground of vibrancy from which particular forms arise. Here healing processes are directly a function of a greater plan and organization beyond the local inertial forces being centered. Perhaps it is like a subtle ground matrix in which all potential is unfolded. Within David Bohm's new

physics context, it is the implicate order from which all form arises. Within this state, what is appropriate to unfold will unfold. As you shift from this state you may again find yourself within the Long Tide and its Original motion. Notice the form of things here. Let healing processes complete. Listen for the midline function to clarify within your perceptual field.

6. As the tissues, fluids, and potencies again express motion, slowly shift your perceptual field back to the biosphere. Allow the reorganization process to unfold. Do not rush this. Wait for a sense of tissue reorganization relative to Sutherland's fulcrum and the primal midline. Listen for a clear expression of the fluid tide to come through. Notice its quality.

With practice, you can hold a very wide perceptual field from the beginning and listen to the unfoldments and healing processes at any level within it. In the next chapters, we will explore further clinical skills as "conversations" held with the tissues, fluids, and potencies of the system. We will discover that

disengagement, decompression, tissue releases, and so on, all come from within; they are not factors of your intervention.

1. James Jealous, "Around the Edges." Quotes used with kind permission of author.

2. Ibid.

3. For a wonderful discussion of these ideas see R. E. Becker, "Diagnostic Touch: Its Principles and Application, I, II, III, IV," *Academy of Applied Osteopathy Yearbooks* (1963, 1964, 1965); an edited version of these papers is also found in R. E. Becker, *Life in Motion* (Rudra Press).

4. James Jealous, "Around the Edges."

5. See sections from Chapter Six, which introduces this process and takes you through a perceptual exercise in relationship to transmutation.

6. *Holomovement* is a term coined by the physicist David Bohm. It indicates the wholeness of all motion, the unfoldment of the universe as a holographic unity.

The Mysterious Gateway: Summary of the Process

- Synchronize your perceptual field with the mid-tide (the 2.5 cycles a minute tide). Widen your perceptual field to the biosphere and listen to the unit of function of tissues, fluids, and potency as a whole unified tensile field of action. Listen for a particular inertial issue to clarify. Facilitate the state of balanced tension. Listen for expression of forces at work.

- Within the state of balance, again widen your perceptual field, this time towards the horizon. See if the Long Tide and the midline function of the Breath of Life become more obvious. Settle into the stillness and allow your mind to

still. Listen for healing to occur truly from the inside out as the Original intention of the Breath of Life clarifies within the system. You may literally have the experience of the potency of the Breath of Life moving through the inertial fulcrum like light through the eye of a needle. Biodynamic, epigenetic forces are perceived more directly here.

- In this process a stillness may be entered in which your mind is neither coming nor going. Mind itself totally settles and enters a state of balance in which the Dynamic Stillness is appreciated. Another mysterious gateway may open here, a timeless state from which the most formative healing processes may arise.

7. See R. E. Becker, "Be Still and Know," Sutherland Memorial lecture, *Newsletter of the Cranial Academy* (Dec. 1965), for a discussion of these concepts. Also in R. E. Becker, *Life in Motion* (Rudra Press).

8. *The Master Mechanic* was Dr. Still's term for God, or the organizing principle of all manifest reality.

9. See R. E. Becker, "Diagnostic Touch: Its Principles and Application, I, II, III, IV," *Academy of Applied Osteopathy Yearbooks* (1963, 1964, 1965).

10. James Jealous, "Around the Edges."

11. Ibid.

12. A favorite saying of Dr. Randolph Stone, D.O.

13. R. E. Becker, "Diagnostic Touch: Its Principles and Application, IV," *Academy of Applied Osteopathy Yearbooks* (1965). Reprinted with the permission of the American Academy of Osteopathy.

14. For Dr. Becker's description of this process see R. E. Becker, "Diagnostic Touch: Its Principles and Application, I, II, III, IV," *Academy of Applied Osteopathy Yearbooks* (1963, 1964, 1965); an edited version of these papers is also found in R. E. Becker, *Life in Motion* (Rudra Press).

15. To read this description in Dr. Becker's own words, please see the articles mentioned in note 14, especially: "Diagnostic Touch: Its Principles and Application, IV," *Academy of Applied Osteopathy Yearbook* (1965).

16. R. E. Becker, "Diagnostic Touch: Its Principles and Application, IV," *Academy of Applied Osteopathy Yearbooks* 1965. Reprinted with the permission of the American Academy of Osteopathy.

17. R. E. Becker, "Diagnostic Touch: Its Principles and Application, IV," *Academy of Applied Osteopathy Yearbooks* (1965). Reprinted with the permission of the American Academy of Osteopathy.

18. From Jim Jealous, D.O., *Reciprocal Tensions*. Used with permission of the author.

19. From Jim Jealous, D.O., *Reciprocal Tensions*. Used with permission of the author.

20. For scientific discussions about these concepts see: Mae-Wan Ho, *The Rainbow and the Worm, The Physics of Organisms* (World Scientific), and also the work of the great embryologist Erich Blechschmidt, *Biokinetics and Biodynamics of Human Differentiation* (Charles C. Thomas).

21. From *Unseen Rain, the quatrains of Rumi,* trans. John Moyne and Coleman Barks (Threshold Books).

22. See Chapter Twenty-four.

16

Stillpoints Revisited

In this chapter, I would like to again explore the stillpoint process and the nature of stillness. In Chapter Eight you used your awareness of the fluid tide to encourage a stillness within its fluid fluctuation. We started you off within the fluid element in order to help you understand the subtleties of this process. In that work, you followed the fluid tide into its exhalation or settling phase and suggested, via your contact, *wait* at the boundary of its excursion. It was a suggestion of a subtle back pressure within the fluids at the furthest excursion of the fluid tide. It was offered as an inquiry into the possibility of stillness. Now that you are more familiar with tissue motility and motion, we would like to add the motility of the tissues to this equation. Please review Chapter Eight, especially the section on depths of stillness.

In this chapter we will:

- *Learn to relate to the tissue layer in the stillpoint process.*
- *Learn the CV4 process.*
- *Learn the EV4 process.*
- *Discuss stillpoints as the **eye of the needle** to deeper stillness and to the dynamic stillness itself.*

The Importance of Stillness

As we discussed in Chapter Eight, the stillpoint process helps the system express its resources. During stillpoint, a settling into a stillness occurs. As seen in Chapter Eight, this process has depth to it. It is not a mechanistic stillness. During stillpoint the system has a chance to access and express its potency. Potency may build within the fluids. This potency then becomes available for healing purposes. The stillness accessed may also bring you into relationship to the Dynamic Stillness itself. A settling into a deeper stillness within yourself occurs, until the inherent ground of Stillness itself is sensed. Then the healing process moves into a whole other dynamic. In this perceptual experience, Stillness is sensed to be whole. It permeates everything and is the ground of emergence for the ordering forces of life. A literal interchange between the Dynamic Stillness, potency, and form may be sensed both by the practitioner and the aware patient. This was discussed in the last chapter. However, once one truly enters the Dynamic Stillness, a darkness arises. This is a darkness of knowing, a literal state of unknowing. Here healing processes are mysterious and are certainly not a function of anything the practitioner can do. This may sound esoteric and far out, but it is the best I can do to describe my sense of it all. It has vast clinical significance. It is just something that is very hard to describe. Once you name it, it is not it. I can only describe my subjective experiences of it, not the Dynamic Stillness itself. It is too vast and too dynamically still for that. Some perceptual experiences of its actionless-action were discussed in the last two chapters.

When the resources of the patient are very low, the stillpoint process is extremely useful, over a period of time, to help liberate those resources. As we have seen, potency will become inertial in order to center the unresolved forces of experience. These forces include trauma, pathogens, shock, even the genetics we take on as we incarnate. The fluids will also become inertial as this occurs. In some cases, a person's system can be holding considerable inertial potency. In other words, there may be a lot of potency bound up in centering the biokinetic forces held within the system. The system may seem to be locked up. Little drive may be perceived either within the fluid tide or within states of balance. The fluid tide may seem flat or locked up in some way. It is the state of balanced tension, a dynamic equilibrium, which allows these inertial potencies to be expressed and encourages something to happen beyond the containment and compensations present. Sometimes the inertial forces are so dense, and the potencies centering them so coiled, that the state of balance has a flatness. It has no depth. It goes nowhere. It does no good to stay there. If nothing is happening, then other conversations must be brought into play. We introduce these other conversations in these next chapters.

One conversation that can be of general help is the stillpoint process. During stillpoint, enough potency may build within the fluids so that when the state of balance is accessed, a sense of depth will occur. There may be a sense of a deepening stillness and of potencies being initiated into action. Potencies will be liberated beyond the conditions present and healing processes will come into play. Again, a depth of stillness may arise, which acts like a gateway into the deeper forces at work within the system. The organizing winds of the Long Tide may come into awareness, and there may be a sense of a Presence so deep that tears come to your eyes. In this chapter we will revisit the stillpoint process and include the tissues and see where that takes our perceptual understanding.

Stillpoints and CV4

In the following process, you will be introduced to the classical concept of the CV4 process. Classically, the term CV4 denotes *compression of the fourth ventricle*. CV4 is a process that was thought to introduce a compression into the fourth ventricle (hence CV4) and to stimulate the brainstem nuclei grouped around it. This was thought to be a factor of the transmutation of potency within the fluids of the fourth ventricle as the fluid system idles in stillness. In the original hold much compression was fed into the system and into the fourth ventricle. Over the years this process has become more and more gentle. In more recent years practitioners have found that the process can be very subtle indeed. A negotiated and gentle approach to CV4 and tissue dynamics has been found to produce even better results than a forced technique. This is clarified and made even more efficient by starting within the mid-tide level of action, rather than within the CRI.

In the following sections you will learn to facilitate stillpoints by relating both to the fluids and to the motion and motility of the tissues. In this process, you will synchronize your perceptual field to the biosphere and mid-tide and to its fluid and tissue elements. As you do this, you will first settle into an awareness of the fluid tide and its expression within the system. You will then include an awareness of tissue motility and motion, and sense the related inhalation-flexion, exhalation-extension dynamics. You will then follow the exhalation direction of fluid *and* tissue motion to the boundary of its excursion and suggest *wait*. You will make this suggestion via a subtle intention in your hands at the boundary of excursion. This is just a suggestion; you will not fight against the tissues or force the system to do anything that it is not ready to do. You will be facilitating a stillness, not forcing it. It is a negotiated process. It is an inquiry into the possibility of stillness. The intention is to offer options, not to force your intentions on the system. If the system cannot access stillpoint, then there is good reason for that. Whatever the issue is, it must be heard and followed up by the practitioner.

CV4: Stillpoints in Exhalation

With this background, let's look at the dynamics of exhalation in relationship to CV4. In the CV4 process, stillpoints are encouraged in the exhalation phase, where fluids and tissues are at the boundary of their excursion. In the CV4 process, you will intend a subtle back pressure at the occiput and cisterna magna in the exhalation phase of the Tide. In exhalation, the cerebrospinal fluid tide is in its descending or settling phase, the ventricles of the brain are narrowing transversely, and tissues express exhalation-extension as the inhalation surge of potency recedes. Thus the system, in CV4, assesses stillpoint in *exhalation,* where the ventricles are narrowed, the fluids are descending, and the tissues are in craniosacral extension. Potency within the exhalation phase is not surging and is held in a still, exhalation intention. Within this stillness, there is the opportunity for potency to build, for the fluids to potentize, and for the vitality of the system to be amplified. Potency builds within the core of the system. Within a CV4 process, there is also the tendency to access deeper and deeper levels of stillness as the system settles into itself.

In stillpoint accessed via the exhalation phase, there is a general potentization and increase of the system's resources. The increased potency tends to be directed to where it is most needed. Fluid exchange and tissue reorganization will result. Thus CV4, and stillpoints in the exhalation phase generally, encourages a general increase in the potency and energetic resources of the system. We will look at stillpoints via the inhalation phase later in the chapter.

Classic Contraindications to CV4

There are a number of classic contraindications for the CV4 process. These contraindications were noted over time in clinical practice. They are especially relevant to the classic CV4 approach at the CRI level of perception, where intracranial pressures are increased due to the pressure of the practitioner's hands. After cranial trauma such as severe blows or cerebral accident (stroke), it is considered inadvisable to facilitate stillpoints via the CV4 process because intracranial pressures may be increased. This is especially so if you are struggling or forcing the system to enter stillpoint via the CV4 hold, or if you generate increased intracranial pressure via your contact. In the stillpoint approach outlined below, you endeavor not to do that. There are also classic contraindications for CV4 in pregnancy. It is believed by some practitioners that CV4 during the first trimester of pregnancy may cause a miscarriage. Others believe that this might happen anytime during pregnancy. This contraindication is

---

As practitioner, during a CV4 stillpoint, you may sense:

- A settling into stillness, which seems to have depth and which is resourcing to the system,

- A building and general increase in potency,

- Fluctuations of potency and fluid,

- A general increase in fluid exchange,

- The resolution of inertial potencies and fulcrums,

- Tissue reorganization.

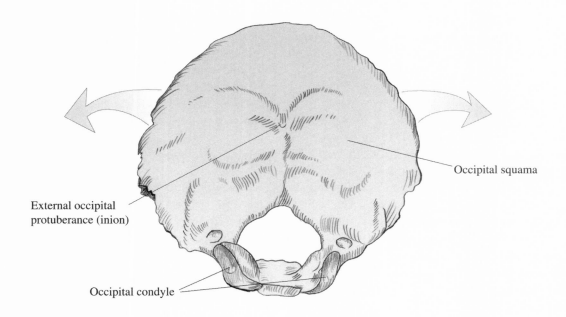

External occipital
protuberance (inion)

Occipital squama

Occipital condyle

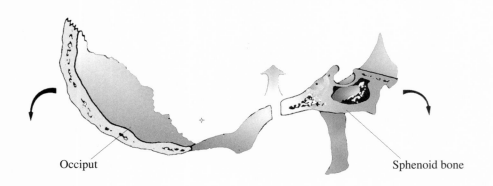

Occiput

Sphenoid bone

16.1 Motion of the occiput in inhalation flexion

one that is debated among practitioners. Some maintain that in CV4 the body will only miscarry if the fetus is damaged or if the mother's life is in danger and a miscarriage will happen anyway. I use a conservative approach and recommend that practitioners facilitate stillpoints via the sacrum during pregnancy. CV4 is, however, very useful during labor because it can speed and ease the birth process for both mother and baby.

Clinical Application: CV4 within the Mid-Tide

Commonly, the CV4 process is taught within the CRI level of action. Students are taught, via their hand hold, to create a barrier at the extreme excursion of the extension motion and to resist the shift into flexion. In our description here, the intention will be subtler and negotiated with the needs of the system. Here you will initiate this process within the mid-tide level of action. As you will see, within this field of action, the work becomes much more subtle. The work has a quality of a clinical conversation and the stillness accessed can go to great depth. It becomes a conversation with form, space, and stillness. It is about the relationship between the organization of form and motion, and the Stillness and potency that support it.

In our first approach to stillpoint in Chapter Eight, you initiated stillpoint via the fluid tide within the mid-tide level of perception. Here, with a new hand hold and relationship, you will simply be adding an awareness of the tissues as you do this. Within the mid-tide (the 2.5 cycles a minute tide) you can sense the tissues to be a unified tensile field. Within this field you can still be aware of specific tissue structures and their motility and motion. The perception of this will, however, be different from that within the CRI. You may sense something like this. The particular structure, in this case the occiput, will express motion as a reciprocal surge and settling within the phases of the Tide. You may sense a welling up and widening within the occiput in inhalation and a receding and settling within exhalation. (See Figure 16.1.) As this occurs, the occiput will express its motion as an expansion at the slower rate of the mid-tide. You will still sense the occiput widening and narrowing within the phases of the Tide, but it will seem to be part of a wider dynamic. The tissues, as we have seen, are a unified tensile field and, at this level of perception, will be experienced as such. The occiput will hopefully express its dynamic in relationship to the midline and to Sutherland's fulcrum. Sutherland's fulcrum itself may be experienced as a moving point of potency, rather than simply as a place within the straight sinus. Let's explore the intention of stillpoint within the mid-tide.

1. The patient is in the supine position. Cup your hands into a cradle so that the fingers of one hand overlap the fingers of the other hand and your thumbs point towards each other with about an inch of space between them. As you place your hands under the patient's head, your thumbs should lie at about the level of C2 or C3. Your thenar eminences are placed under the occipital squama, avoiding the mastoid processes. It should feel comfortable to both you and your patient. In the original hold, the thenar eminences were placed close together and a lot of pressure was introduced into the occipital squama. You do not have to do this. Your hand must be placed more caudad than usually assumed. Your fingers rest under the cervical area. This hold generates a fulcrum, which initiates a particular kind of relationship to the patient's system. The initial inquiry will be into the possibility of stillness within the potencies, fluids, and tissues of the patient's system. (See Figure 16.2.)

2. Settle into your relationship; give the patient space. Widen your perceptual field to the biosphere. Allow the mid-tide to come to you. You

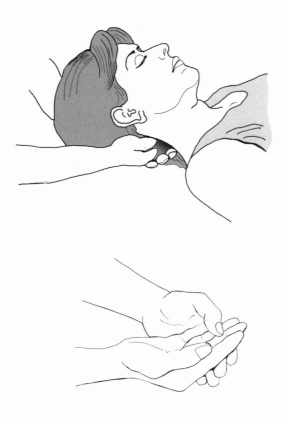

16.2 CV4 hold

settling throughout its tissues? Follow these dynamics. Especially notice the exhalation phase of motion.

3. Notice the boundary of excursion of the exhalation motion. Include both an awareness of the fluids and of the tissues. At this boundary, notice the unified dynamic between tissues and fluids and suggest a back pressure within the occiput and the fluids at the same time. Suggest "wait" through the occiput and the tissue-fluid field as a whole. This is a subtle suggestion, an inquiry into stillness. Be aware of the entry into stillness. Don't force the stillpoint; simply suggest wait via a subtle intention in your hands. It is an offering of an option. *It must be negotiated.* You offer a suggestion as an inquiry, and you must hear the answer from the system. The system may not want to enter a stillpoint at that time. You must respect that. You can again suggest stillness, but it is an inquiry into the possibility of stillness, not a demand. As the system negotiates its entry into stillness, you may sense that the longitudinal fluctuation of the CSF begins to disorganize. You may notice various fluctuant phenomena arise within the fluids. Simply listen to this. On a tissue level, the occiput may go deeper into exhalation/narrowing. If it does, follow it in to the new boundary and again subtly suggest wait. As the system moves towards a stillpoint, you may sense a kind of deepening inward. This is the initial expression of the *stillpoint.* It is important not to fight the system or to try to force a stillpoint on the system.

may first be aware of the fluid tide within its dynamic. The fluid tide is an expression of the action of the potency within the fluids. As you become aware of this phenomenon, include the tissues within your field of awareness. In inhalation the occiput may be perceived to widen laterally and move slightly caudad as you sense a subtle pushing against your hands. In exhalation, the occiput may be sensed to narrow and move cephalad. This will be perceived at the slower rate of the mid-tide (2.5 cycles/minute). How does the occiput express its motility within the fluid tide? Can you sense its widening and narrowing? Can you sense a surge and

4. Be patient. While the tidal rhythm stills, the cardiac and breathing rhythms are still expressed, but might slow down and soften during the stillpoint. Patients may sense a deep sense of relaxation and peace. They may take a deep breath; they might settle into themselves and feel peaceful. You, as practitioner, might resonate with their stillness by sensing relaxation

and peace in yourself. You might even settle into your own stillpoint as the patients express theirs. This process of resonance is sometimes known as "entrainment." As you widen your perceptual field, the system may access even deeper expressions of stillness. You may experience the radiant nature of potency. We will discuss this deepening process later in this chapter.

5. In stillpoint you may notice various self-healing processes arise. These may include the initiation of potencies, the resolution of biokinetic forces, the release of heat, fluid exchange and fluid fluctuations, and changes in tissue organization and fulcrums. Within the stillness you may sense potency building and moving, fluid and tissue motions, and the resolution of inertial forces. The system will take advantage of the stillness and work where it is appropriate according to the inherent treatment plan as it unfolds. Again, if inertial forces are resolved during the stillpoint, tissues will reorganize and realign to the midline. Listen for this dynamic.

6. Wait for the system to express tidal motion again. Do not resist this. As this occurs, you may sense a general increase in resources and a stronger and fuller fluid tide. You may also sense a change in the reciprocal tension dynamics of the tissues being palpated. How has this changed? Is there a more balanced motion relative to the midline and Sutherland's fulcrum?

CV4 Process within the CRI

In the application above, you began the CV4 process within the mid-tide. There are times when it is important to know how to initiate the process within the CRI. Sometimes a person's system is so inertial that all you can sense is a CRI level of action. It may be very hard to make a perceptual shift to the mid-tide. There may be so much potency

bound in centering various inertial conditions that only the CRI is obvious. If you begin to work within the CRI with an attitude of releasing something or changing something, it is very likely that an activation of some kind will occur. This may take the form of increased symptoms, emotional flooding, freezing states, numbness, dissociation, reliving of trauma in an unresourced manner, stress states, and so on. What I recommend to practitioners is to find some way to help the system access its own resources. It is a matter of liberating potency beyond the inertial conditions present within the system. When this occurs, the mid-tide will again become more available to your perceptual field.

One way of approaching this is to work with the CV4 stillpoint process within the CRI and, within the stillpoint to make a conscious shift to the mid-tide level of action. Do this by simply widening your perceptual field to the biosphere and settle into your own mid-tide as you hold the patient within your awareness. It is like going through the eye of the needle to the deeper resources of the system, even if these resources are largely bound up. It is a question of appreciating the qualities of deepening stillness as potency is initiated and accessed. It is within the stillness that the deeper forces and intentions of the Breath of Life can be accessed.

The intention is to offer the suggestion of waiting, or idling, at the boundary of the exhalation-extension excursion of the tissues. You will be bringing this intention to the system via the occiput in the CV4 hold learned above. Perceived at a faster CRI rate of expression, in the inhalation phase, the occipital squama will rotate caudad and widen. In the exhalation phase, the occipital squama will rotate cephalad and narrow. This will appear to occur in the 8–14 cycles a minute range of motion. Simply suggest wait at the boundary of its excursion in extension until a stillpoint is accessed. Even here do not force this on the system; deepen into a stillness, within yourself and a resonance within the field of listening will eventually happen. Do not generate a barrier to tissue motion; negotiate the stillpoint here too. As the CRI settles into stillness, settle deeper into a stillness within yourself and listen for the expression of potency within the system. See if you can make that perceptual shift to the mid-tide and form a relationship to the potency within this field of action.

EV4: Stillpoints in Inhalation

Now let's shift our attention and look at the dynamics of stillpoints facilitated during the *inhalation* phase of primary respiration. This process is commonly called EV4. EV4 implies *expansion* of the fourth ventricle, rather than compression as in CV4. The dynamics of EV4 are different in some respects from those discussed above. In the inhalation phase, the fluid tide is surging and ascending, and an imperative to motion arises within the potencies, fluids, and tissues of the body. As this occurs, particular motion dynamics result. Potencies and fluids are rising, or *longitudinally* ascending in a tide-like fashion. The ventricles of the brain are widening like a bird spreading its wings as it is about to take flight, and the tissues are expressing inhalation as a tensile surge in their motility. This groundswell, generated by the Tide and its impulse, can be sensed to arise from the inferior pole at the sacro-coccygeal complex and lumbosacral cistern.

As you encourage a stillpoint in the inhalation phase, the potency of the Breath of Life is expressing its ascending surge throughout the system, the ventricles of the brain are at their fullest inhalation excursion, and the fluid system is in its ascending fluctuation. Because of this, in stillpoint facilitated via the inhalation phase, the ascending surge of potency within the system is amplified and there is a general movement of potency from the midline into the periphery of the system. In essence, the system, during stillpoint in the inhalation phase, is helped to access and manifest its resources as the inhalation intention of the groundswell is amplified.

In stillpoint facilitated in the inhalation phase, the practitioner may perceive a welling up of potency from the sacro-coccygeal area towards the waterbeds of the cranium. The practitioner may then sense a stronger drive within the fluids and clearer longitudinal fluctuation. During this process, the practitioner may get a sense of the potency as an invisible force within the fluids. EV4 thus helps a person manifest his or her resources. EV4 can also be used in dissociative processes where there has been overwhelm and traumatization. If you meet a person whose system seems empty or vacant, as though his or her consciousness is elsewhere, then EV4, over time, may help in the reassociative process. It is also an integrative process and can be useful at the end of sessions to help the system to integrate clinical work.

The Different Dynamics of CV4 and EV4

Thus there are differences between the dynamics of CV4 and EV4. Stillpoints accessed within the exhalation phase via CV4 encourage a general potentization of the system along with a deepening into depths of stillness. Potency builds within the core. Stillpoints accessed within inhalation via EV4 encourage the system to manifest its potency from the midline into the periphery. CV4 is about potentization and deepening, and EV4 is largely about the manifestation of resources. Basically, in CV4, while the system is held in exhalation, there is an idling without the surging intention of the inhalation phase. Potency is concentrated within the core of the system. In this idling, there is the potential for deepening into stillness and for a general potentization of the system. (See Figure 16.3.)

In EV4, the system is held in inhalation, the phase where the groundswell is surging and potency is being expressed. Stillpoints in inhalation maintain the intention of the surge within the stillness. It helps the system enhance its fluid drive, as the imperative to surge intensifies while the system is in stillpoint. Potency manifests from the center out, longitudinal fluctuation of fluid is enhanced, and the resources of the system are more fully expressed. Many practitioners experience stillpoints in exhalation as an access into deeper depths of stillness and potentization, while stillpoints in inhalation mani- fest this potency. Thus in CV4 the system has a chance to deeply potentize, while in EV4, the system has the chance to manifest its potency more fully. Let's explore some processes that help the system express its potency as longitudinal fluctuation. (See Figure 16.4.)

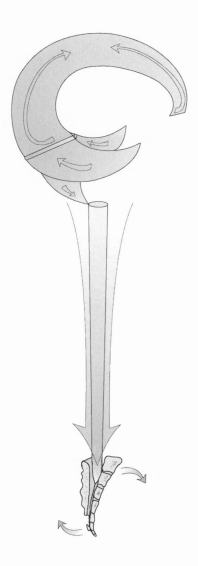

16.3 System in exhalation

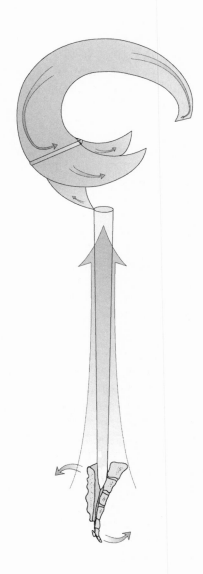

16.4 System in inhalation

Clinical Highlights

The intentions of both CV4 and EV4 can be constructively used in clinical practice. CV4 has the intention of contacting resources and repotentizing the system. It can bring the person to deeper stillness and actualize healing processes. EV4 has the intention of bringing potency from the core into the periphery and manifesting these resources. It can help clarify the fluid drive and longitudinal fluctuation of the system.

In hyperarousal states, CV4 can help down regulate the central nervous system and has an effect on the entire neuroendocrine axis. It can help shift the set point of the autonomic nervous system from fixity in hyperarousal to a more fluid response to the environment once again. It can also help the system discharge the shock affects of trauma in a resourced state, as the potency of the Breath of Life within the fluids resolves the traumatization. As this occurs the practitioner may sense perturbations within the fluids as the shock affects clear.

In hypoarousal states, where the system is running a different physiology, CV4 can help to build potency and vitality and again shift the system to a more resourced state. If either state is coupled with dissociation, then EV4s can help manifest the resources of the system from the center out and help in the reassociative process. In this expression of potency from the core to the periphery, the dissociated psyche is helped to find its way back to embodiment. This is a delicate process of a renegotiation of traumatization and its affects with the inherent biodynamic resources of the Breath of Life.

Clinical Application: EV4 via the Temporal Bones

In this section, you will learn to encourage stillpoint within the inhalation phase of the Tide. The focus will be to learn to negotiate this intention and to see if the experience of stillpoint accessed in inhalation has a different quality than that accessed in the exhalation phase. In this section you use the temporal bones as the way into this process. The use of the temporal bones to facilitate an inhalation stillpoint, or EV4, goes right back to the original work of Dr. Sutherland. In the following process you will be applying the principles in a gentle and negotiated way. One intention here will be to have a direct relationship to the potency within the fluids within the stillpoint process. EV4s can be used to encourage the expression of potency within the system, and this is best appreciated within the perceptual field of the biosphere and mid-tide.

1. Sit at the head of the treatment table with the patient in the supine position. As usual, negotiate your relationship with the patient's system. After establishing your relationship via the vault hold, contact the temporal bones in the ear canal hold as previously learned. (See Figure 16.5.)

2. Hold the biosphere and the mid-tide expression of tidal motion (2.5 cycles a minute) within your field of awareness. Let your hands float within fluid and extend your perceptual field to include the person's body and the field around him or her. Listen to the expression of the fluid tide. As you follow this, include the temporal bones within your field of awareness. Follow the temporal bones into their inhalation-external rotation motions. You may sense a welling up and widening apart as you listen. You may sense the motion of the bones within the larger context of the whole tissue-fluid matrix. Follow the temporal bones in their inhalation phase of expres-

sion. Suggest *wait* at the boundary of their excursion in inhalation-external rotation. The intention is not to force a stillpoint onto the system, but to negotiate its possibility.

3. Once you have established this perceptual field, you may sense the stillpoint deepening as the tidal potencies enter stillness. Sometimes a further intention of waiting, by subtly deepening your relationship to the boundary of exhalation, will help the stillpoint to deepen. Do not narrow your perceptual field as you do this.

4. Now, within the stillness, be especially aware of the interrelationship of fluid and potency. Be aware of the dorsal, fluid midline from the lumbosacral cistern to the midline of the ventricle system. Do not crowd the system as you do this. Let the fluid core come to you. With this awareness, simply listen within the stillness to the responses of the system.

5. The first thing you may perceive is a sense of building and welling up of potency within the area of the lumbosacral cistern. You may then sense a wavelike pulsation of potency arising through the fluids from below. This is an expression of the inhalation intention of surge within the stillness. This may at first be very sluggish, but you may sense a rapid release of potency from the sacral area. This may be sensed within the cerebrospinal fluid as an invisible force, or potency arising caudad to cephalad. You may sense a series of surges with greater and greater intensity within the fluid midline. You may also then be cast into a great depth of stillness.

6. Wait with this until the fluid tide is again perceived. Remember that it is the potency of the Breath of Life that makes the fluids move in a tide-like manner. As potency is expressed from the center out, the fluid tide will express a fuller and stronger longitudinal fluctuation.

7. Note the sense and the quality of potency within the system. You may sense an increase in its general potency, but even more, you may sense a clearer and stronger longitudinal fluctuation and a clearer manifestation of the potency within it.

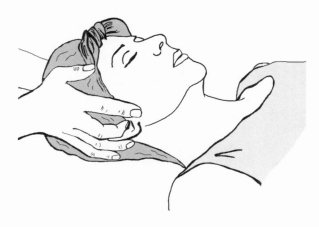

16.5 Temporal bone hold

Clinical Application: EV4 via the Sacrum

In this application you will again encourage a stillpoint within the inhalation phase, but this time you will use the sacrum as your place of contact. As you do this, again pay especial attention to the lumbar cistern and the sense of the dynamics within the dorsal, fluid midline. As above, you may sense a welling up of potency and wave-like expressions of potency cephalad. Remember the motion of the sacrum from previous palpation sessions. Read the section on sacral motility and motion in Chapter Eleven if it is not clear to you.

1. With the patient in the supine position, place your hand under the sacrum as you previously learned. (See Figure 16.6.) Synchronize your perceptual field with the biosphere and the mid-tide phenomena. Listen for the fluid tide and the expression of the motility of the sacrum within it.

2. Follow the sacrum into its inhalation phase and suggest *wait* at the boundary of its flexion excursion. Again, this is a negotiation, an inquiry into the possibility of stillness. Let your perceptual field hold the whole of the person and allow the tidal phenomena to settle into stillness. Again, a simple intention of *wait* in inhalation, as a back pressure at the furthest excursion of fluid and tissue motion, is all that is needed. This is again offered as an inquiry into stillness, not a demand on the system.

3. Once stillness is perceived, place your awareness within the lumbosacral cistern and dorsal midline. Do not narrow your perceptual field as you do this. You may first sense a building and welling up of potency under your hand at the sacrum. You may then sense a cephalad discharge of potency. It may be sensed as waves of potency arising cephalad through the fluids. You may then again sense the surge of the fluid tide, with a stronger fluid drive and clearer sense of longitudinal fluctuation cephalad.

Both of the clinical applications described above interface with the fluid system in subtle ways. By accessing stillpoint within the inhalation phase, the inhalation surge is intensified within the fluids. This is a surge of potency within the fluids, which carries the organizing imperative of the Breath of Life within its expression. This may manifest within the stillness of the stillpoint as waves of potency arising from the coccyx cephalad. You may also sense a movement of potency from the midline to the periphery of the body. It may feel like a fountain spray of life. Become aware of the potency within the fluid

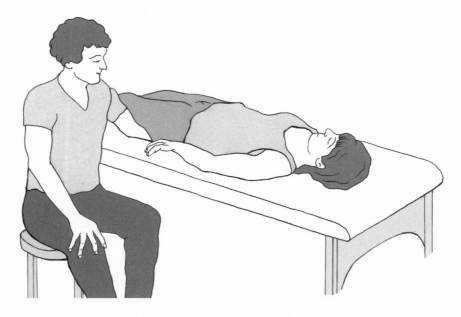

16.6 Sacral hold

as an invisible and potent force. It is this potency within the cerebrospinal fluid that is the driving force of the system and the carrier of the ordering principle. Remember that Dr. Sutherland stated that this potency is an Intelligence that helps maintain healing processes, homeostatic balance, and the ordered relationships of the human organism.

Stillpoint as the Mysterious Gateway

In the next clinical application, we are going to further explore the stillpoint process as the mysterious gateway into deeper stillness and even to the Dynamic Stillness itself. In this application, you will consciously be shifting your perceptual fields as the way into a deeper relationship to stillness. We started to do this above, but here we will move from the mid-tide to the Long Tide into deepening stillness. Think of the stillpoint process as the *eye of the needle*, or the *mysterious gateway* into deeper and deeper experiences of stillness and inherent Health.

You will discover that, within a relative experience of stillness, there is a sense of depth. If you are palpating within the CRI level, you may perceive a stilling of the CRI and different aspects of work being done physiologically. You may perceive fluid fluctuations, tissue reorganization, relaxation of tensions, and so forth. Within the mid-tide level, you may perceive a deepening potency, a greater availability of resources, a welling up of the potency within the system, and a clarity of healing forces at work. The inherent treatment plan may clarify as the forces of potency are expressed within the system. You may perceive a subtle processing of shock affect as fluid perturbations, tissue trembling, and resolution of autonomic affects. Within the Long Tide you may perceive a deepening relationship to the potency of the Breath of Life itself. A sense of the aliveness of the bioelectric field and its potency, a sense of vibrancy and of radiance may arise.

The inherent treatment plan may become obvious as the potency of the Breath of Life moves to resolve inertial issues. In the inherent treatment plan, the healing intentions of the Breath of Life manifest. Forces come into play, fluids and tissues respond, and specifics are attended to.[1] It is then simply a question of hearing this and serving its intentions as practitioner. Then the work is directed by a Presence deeper than any human mentality. Within stillness, patients may even experience archetypal forms and energies as the Original matrix unfolds. This can be an integrative experience. An inherent interconnection to life *as a whole* may be sensed and acknowledged here. Stillness is a gateway into Stillness. As one's mind and consciousness stills, another gateway into the Dynamic Stillness itself may open. Within the Dynamic Stillness, we are talking about a depth that is difficult to describe. It is about perception without a perceiver. More correctly, it is a state of "neither perception nor non-perception." I am afraid that words seem to elude me here. It is a depth of Stillness in which self-view is truly dropped, even for an instant. A state without subject-object relationship, a Whole. Healing can be instantaneous here, as can a spiritual resonance. It is, in essence, a state of grace within a clinical context. The practitioner and patient are totally within the depth of present time and something happens. It may even be said that they are beyond time, even for an instant. The practitioner may not realize the repercussions of the session work until returning to the world of form and relationship. Even in the most desperate situations, with impending death looming, fear may be dropped and life and death seen as a unified expression of the Whole.

Clinical Application: Stillpoint as the Mysterious Gateway

In this section you will use the stillpoint process as the "mysterious gateway" into deeper and deeper qualities of stillness. We introduced this idea in the chapter on the state of balanced tension. You may have perceived that, within a state of balanced tension, as you widen your perceptual field towards the horizon and deepen your relationship to the stillness within the heart of the fulcrum, a shift in both perception and healing process may occur. As you synchronize your perceptual field with the deeper unfoldments of the Breath of Life, deeper healing processes and forces become more evident.

In this section we will begin again within the mid-tide level of perception and action. You will initiate a CV4 process within the mid-tide as above and will then broaden and deepen your perceptual field using each tidal unfoldment as the mysterious gateway into a deepening stillness. This process can also be initiated from the CRI, but I find it more direct to begin this process within the mid-tide and then widen your perceptual field towards the horizon into a deepening stillness. The spectrum traveled will include the mid-tide, the Long Tide, and the possibility of entry into the Dynamic Stillness itself. Have patience. Do not expect anything and do not be disappointed because everything is perfect in its own right. All of this has its own timing, its own tone and tempo.

The most important thing here is the quality of the space you are holding for entrée into deeper healing processes. It is based upon your negotiated contact and the nature of the perceptual field you are holding. The nature of your stillness and listening is a call to the deeper forces at work within the human system. It is about resonance and humility. It is again really important here to establish a still clinical space. The quality of this space contains, initiates, and holds the process. It is a call, in the darkness of unknowing, for a relationship to the Breath of Life itself as its mysterious intentions unfold. Remember your practitioner fulcrums, come into breath and sensation, let your mind still and hold a wide and natural field of listening. Let this deepen. Again, this is a call to the deeper healing intentions within and beyond the conditional forces being centered. Much more important, it is a humbling entrée into a healing process that is a mutual journey for both therapist and patient.

1. With the patient in the supine position, again place your hands in the CV4 hold as described above. Synchronize your perceptual field to the mid-tide. Let your hands float within fluid and widen your perceptual field to the biosphere. Let the rhythm of the mid-tide come into your field of awareness.

2. Become aware of the motion of the fluid tide and include the tissues. Notice the boundary of excursion of the exhalation motion. As learned above, at this boundary, suggest "wait" through the occiput and the tissue-fluid field as a whole. Notice the unified dynamic between tissues and fluids and suggest a back pressure via your hand contact within the occiput and the fluids at the same time. This is a subtle suggestion, an inquiry into stillness. Again this is a negotiated intention, an exploration into the possibility of stillness. Listen for the settling into a stillpoint, a stillness within the midst of conditions. Settle into this stillness and listen for it to deepen. You can encourage this via deepening your hand contact in relationship to the fluids and tissues being palpated. Do not grab onto any of the three elements of potency, fluids, and tissues as you do this. Do not narrow your perceptual field as you do this.

3. When stillness is perceived to deepen, again widen your perceptual field, this time towards the horizon. Let your hands float within potency and widen your perceptual field towards the horizon. Do this very slowly and gently. Do not widen past your sense of safety and containment. With this intention, you are welcoming the Long Tide level of perception. You may again perceive a natural deepening of the stillness. Let your mind settle and still even more. Simply rest in a field of awareness. You may have a sense that your mind finds a balance in its sensory and motor function. You find that your mind is neither coming nor going. It sim-

ply listens within a wide field. A clarity arises within the stillness. At this level, it is not a matter of intending stillness or even suggesting it. It is simply a matter of accessing that depth within yourself and of recognizing it within the patient. You are both within the Tide and even may have an experience of being the Tide. This level of stillness can be a gateway into the Dynamic Stillness itself. The wide perceptual field and a mind that is neither coming nor going are the keys to this gateway. There is a further stilling, a further deepening, then unknowing, a darkness. Within the Dynamic Stillness, there is truly perception without a perceiver. Here the Originality opens itself to itself as subject and object fade away. It is in essence a state of wholeness. At this level there is deep interconnection and mutuality as life heals itself. There may be a merging into a silence. Within the darkness even time recedes.

4.   As you come out of this darkness, listen for the organizing winds of the Long Tide to manifest its potency. Listen for a sense of completion.

Very gently narrow your perceptual field to the biosphere and the embodied nature of the potencies and forces within the human system. You may notice tidal phenomena again being generated. This allows for integration and reentry into the embodied nature of experience. Give this process time. You are now back within space-time and embodied forces are at work. Let a process of realignment and reorientation occur. Wait for a clear sense of the fluid tide and for the tissue to complete any reorganization process occurring. Please understand that this process has vast clinical significance.

This chapter was a further exploration of the stillpoint process. In this there is a pointing to the depths of Stillness itself. It is up to each of us to journey into possibility and to know this territory for ourselves. In essence it cannot be taught. I can only give contexts and guidelines. As Dr. Becker counsels, it is a self-taught process.

1.   See the last chapter for a discussion of the inherent treatment plan.

287

17
....

Directing the Tide

In previous chapters, you learned to initiate certain kinds of conversations with potencies, fluids, and tissues. In this chapter, we will present a particular clinical approach to inertial fulcrums and the forces they contain, called *fluid direction*. We will initially concentrate on cranial sutures, but the work can be generalized to any site of inertia within the body. In this approach, you will learn to sense the inherent potency within the fluids and to direct that potency to sites of compression and rigidity. These are sites of inertial potencies and forces, which organize the resistance expressed within the suture. You will discover that the *direction of fluid* process helps activate these potencies and brings the whole field of potency to bear on inertial issues.

> ### In this chapter we will:
>
> - *Learn to further appreciate the Intelligence and healing power of the potency within the fluid tide.*
>
> - *Learn to direct that Intelligence to sites of sutural compression.*

Fluid Dynamics and the Fluid Tide

The fluctuation of cerebrospinal fluid is one of the most important principles in cranial work. As we

have seen, Dr. Sutherland considered the cerebrospinal fluid to be the initial recipient of the physiological potency of the Breath of Life.[1] He stressed that he considered the fluctuation of cerebrospinal fluid to be the fundamental principle in the cranial concept. He likened the cerebrospinal fluid to the sap in a tree. It is an essential life-giving fluid within the core of the body, imbued with Intelligence. This Intelligent principle is conveyed to all of the cells and tissues of the body via its fluids. The skilled practitioner can make use of the inherent potency within the cerebrospinal fluid and, indeed, within all the fluids in the body. Remember that the fluctuation of cerebrospinal fluid occurs along a natural longitudinal axis. This is organized within the dorsal or fluid midline of the system. This fluid midline is generated within the longitudinal axis of the neural tube of the embryo. In the adult, this midline is expressed within the spinal canal and ventricles of the brain. In the inhalation phase there is a rising of the fluid tide along this midline in a longitudinal fashion. Along with this longitudinal welling up, there is a transverse fluctuation within the lateral ventricles of the brain. There are also natural transverse expressions of potency all along the midline. In the following sections, you will learn to direct this potency via the fluids in ways that help access space and initiate the action of potency within specific inertial issues.

As we have seen, the potency of the Breath of Life is the vital invisible element carried within and conveyed by the fluids of the body. Imagine the salt in the sea. It is invisible, yet you can sense its taste. The potency of the Breath of Life is like that. Visualize this potency as an invisible factor, like the salt in the sea. Imagine that instead of salt, it is a biodynamic alive-ness that you can "taste." Remember that this force is an expression of the Intelligence of the system in action. It conveys the Original matrix, the expression of the Original intention of a human being, to all cells and tissues throughout life. This inherent potency is precise in its action. It is unerring in its intentions within the system. It can be directly used by practitioners to assist in the resolution of resistance and fixation. It is simply a matter of directing it to areas in need.[2] This begins a conversation with the inertial potencies that maintain and center the disturbance within the dynamics of the system. As you direct fluid and potency to sites of inertia, you will discover that you are initiating a conversation. The fluids and potency will tell you about the nature of the inertia held and the history of the trauma incurred. You will sense various kinds of phenomena, like fluid fluctuations, echoing of fluids and potencies, eccentric expressions of potency, and so on, all of which will give you clinical information. As you do this, you will learn that the work is both diagnostic and therapeutic all at once.

In previous chapters, you learned to access the state of balanced tension in relationship to an inertial fulcrum and pattern. The intention in that work was to allow the inertial potencies to express themselves within the organizing fulcrum. Sometimes, however, the forces and affects held within and around inertial fulcrums are very condensed. Inertial potencies may be coiled deeply, and the tissue and fluid affects, such as compression and congestion, may also be very dense. The inertia within the disturbance may be so deep that the inertial potencies may not have the space to express anything beyond the compensation that is being held. You may have perceived that, in some cases, the potencies did not seem to build or activate within the state of bal-ance. A "dullness" may have been sensed. The state of balance may have seemed dull; it may have lacked depth. Yet it is important to know that even within the most densely inertial relationship, there is always space in *potential*. There is always a kernel of life at work. There is always motion, even within the most inertial and dense fulcrums. There is always a kernel of Health in action. It is a matter of accessing it. As we shall see, it is possible to bring other skills into the relationship to access this expression of life and to initiate the expression of potency within the inertial fulcrum.

For instance, you may have noticed specific sutural compressions that seemed intransigent. Sutural compressions are the effects of the inertial forces of direct life experience. Birth trauma, accidents, and falls are common origins. They can also arise in compensation for other inertial issues within the system. Inertia anywhere in the body can be transferred to cranial sutures via the tensile membrane and connective tissue system. Indeed, inertial fulcrums anywhere in the body can effect the dynamics of any cranial suture. It is possible, via the process of fluid direction, to begin a conversation with the inertial forces organizing a sutural compression. This approach can also be generalized to other areas of the body, such as joints, and their inertial issues. You will first learn this skill within a mid-tide context. It is within the mid-tide field of action that the relationship among potency, fluids, and tissues is more easily discerned.

Directing the Fluid Tide

The following process will place you in direct relationship to the potency within the cerebrospinal fluid tide. In this process you will be directing cerebrospinal fluid, and the potency within it, to the site of the perceived inertia. This will initiate a conversation with fluids and potency and will yield both diagnostic and treatment information. Directing the fluid tide will initiate a conversation with the potency held within the inertial fulcrum. It will encourage the expression of its ordering principle within the sutural issue being explored. This process is really a manifestation of your attention and intention in action. The potency will respond to your intentions if they are offered within a framework of conversation and inquiry.

In this work, you will be placing a subtle compression into the fluid system with the intention of directing its potency to a specific relationship. You will have a "sending hand" and a "receiving hand." The receiving hand will be located over the inertial site and the sending hand will be located at the opposite side of the cranium. You will be offering a back pressure into the fluids via the sending hand in order to start a conversation about organization and history. Whenever you place compression into fluids, they will talk to you. They will show you the place and nature of the resistance and the relationship of the Health of the system to it. Dr. Sutherland initially hesitated to describe this process to practitioners. He initially considered the direction of the cerebrospinal fluid tide and its healing processes to be too uncanny to teach. He understood the importance of the work and eventually taught his associate faculty the process.[3]

Dr. Sutherland maintained that the cerebrospinal fluid tide has potency and Intelligence. He maintained that you can use it to work for you and, indeed, to help the patient's system do work for itself. *Potency* is the ability to do work. It is an inherent biodynamic force, which can restore order where disorder, rigidity, and fixation have become established. Dr Sutherland stressed that *directing the Tide* will give you direct clinical information. If practitioners were in doubt about their diagnosis, they were encouraged to direct the fluid tide and note the response within their receiving hand. If the area directed to is not inertial and resistant, then only a gentle yielding motion is sensed. It is like sea water gently washing upon a beach. If inertia is present, then an echoing or rebound of fluid and potency is perceived. It is like sea water clashing on the breakers on a beach. The quality and nature of this echo-

ing and rebounding convey much information to the skilled practitioner. When in doubt, direct the fluid tide and its potency and accurate clinical information will be conveyed to you. Direction of the fluid tide activates the inertial potencies involved and the whole field of potency will come into play.

The direction of the fluid tide is thus both diagnostic and therapeutic. As you will see, trusting the potency of the Tide as something you can depend on is one of the key healing principles within the cranial concept.[4] The response of the fluids and potency will tell you the exact quality and nature of the resistance that you are palpating. It will also show you the nature of the healing process needed to resolve the inertia being palpated. Once you have the ability to sense and understand this, then you can depend on the Tide to tell you the truth. In teaching this process, Dr Sutherland stated that the response is immediate from the directing hand to the area directed to. In other words, you are not directing a current of energy, but a unified field of potency.[5] It is a tidal phenomenon and is nonlinear in its expression.

The fluid tide is simply directed by a gentle pressure on the cranium towards the inertial site. In this, you are initiating a tidal intention, not a current flow. You are placing a subtle intention of compression into the fluids towards the inertial site. In this intention, the fluids will start to talk to you. It is a conversation about the life experience of that person and about the health centering that experience. As soon as the intention of a direction is placed upon the fluids, there is a volume shift of potency towards the receiving site. *The whole body of fluid and potency will respond all at once.* This is important. Dr. Sutherland was clear in stating that, in directing the fluid tide, you are not directing a current or flow. You direct the fluids from one area of the cranium and you sense an *immediate* response at the receiving hand in another area. The response is instantaneous. Potency and fluid will respond to your conversation by showing you the dynamics of the inertial site. Fluid rebounds and fluid fluctuations will

291

convey to you the nature of the inertial forces held within the inertial fulcrum, in this case a compressed suture.

Directing the Tide Is Not Directing Energy

In this process, you are not directing a current of energy. You are directing a tidal *intention* from one point to another. You are directing the tidal forces as a whole. Potency and fluid are a unit of function and their action is neither fragmented nor linear. When you place your intention into the fluids, there is a *tidal* response, which is nonlinear. It is not a current flow, it is tidal. It is a factor of the potency of the Breath of Life. If you are just directing a current of energy in a general way, there are many qualities and functions of energy that you may be in relationship to. A current will also have to pass through and relate to other structures besides the inertial site. It would be bound by time and space. The inherent healing potency of the Breath of Life is not bound by time and space; it simultaneously co-arises within all phenomena.

Thus, directing the fluid tide is *not* a general sending or directing of a current of energy to the site of resistance. It certainly is not about directing your own energy into someone else. It is very specific. Here we are tapping into the most primary life force, the potency of the Breath of Life in its most primal form. This is the neuter essence from which other phases of bioenergy derive. It is the inherent ordering principle within the human system. The Breath of Life and its potency is about the fundamental maintenance of order, integrity, and healing in the mind-body complex. It is about the universal blueprint made manifest. It is expressed within the fluids of the embryo, maintained in the fluids of the adult, and continues to maintain order through all stages of life. From the work of Mae-wan Ho, we can talk about this ordering principle manifesting as a quantum level biodynamic field of action, which is both coherent and whole.[6]

There are many other qualities and phases of bioenergy at work within the human system. For instance, there are the elemental energies of the chakras and of the acupuncture meridians. There are the electrodynamic relationships of physiology and chemical action; there are electrodynamic field phenomena present, and so forth. These all have different qualities and functions. They are all particular and discrete layers of the human energy system whose principles, if you are engaging with them, must be clearly understood. If you direct a *current* of energy, without understanding the nature of the energies you are directing, you may even aggravate a disturbance or traumatic fulcrum without realizing it.

It is the cerebrospinal fluid, and all the fluids in the body, that are potentized with the most primary life force or potency within the human system. Specific direction of the fluid tide and its inherent potency places you in direct relationship to the whole unified field of potency within the body. This is why it is important to stay within the fluid system when directing potency. We are interested in this fundamental biodynamic force or potency that maintains and reestablishes its inherent Intelligence within all of the tissues and cells of the human body. In this context, we are not interested in derivative energies. Thus, you are specifically directing the inherent potency and ordering principle of the primary respiratory system. To do this, you must be in direct relationship to the fluids that convey its potency throughout the body. Furthermore, I find that it is easier to do this if your perceptual field lies within the mid-tide field of action.

Clinical Intentions in Directing the Tide

The clinical intention of *directing the fluid tide* is to reestablish flow where there is fixity. It can initiate the action of potency within specific inertial issues, even within the density of an intransigent compression. Directing the tide can also help access space within the compressed relationship so that the state of balanced tension can be attained with depth. It can also call the whole field of potency into action and can initiate a permeation of potency within disoriented cells and tissues. It can help the cellular and tissue world reorient to the intentions of the Breath of Life as expressed through the action of its potency. Directing the fluid tide and understanding its relationships in the human system is a safe and extremely effective clinical process. You are interfacing with the potency and the ordering principles it expresses, and not derivative energies. Directing the fluid tide is a process whereby the total volume of potency held between your hands is directed to the inertial fulcrum *all at once*. The response will be immediate at the receiving hand. It is not bound in that sense by time or space. Again, imagine that the potency is like the salt in the sea, except that this salt is an inherent potency spread throughout the waters. It is *one thing*, a unity of function. It is this potency that drives the tidal dynamics of the fluctuation of cerebrospinal fluid and that generates tissue motility. When you direct fluid and potency towards a site of inertia, you are raising the energy economy of the area. You are bringing more potency to bear and the inertial potencies within the inertial fulcrum will be activated or intensified.

As you generate a back pressure on the fluid system with your gentle touch and clear intention, there is a shift in the direction of potency between your hands towards the receiving hand and the inertial fulcrum. This shift occurs all through the fluids between your hands as a unified response to your intention. Traditionally, because of this understanding, you would direct the fluid drive of the system as far away from the inertial site as possible. This is because, when there is a greater volume of fluid between the two sites, there is also a greater volume of potency to access within that fluid. Thus you might work diagonally across the cranium, rather than transversely. As you bring this intention to the fluids, you are initiating a conversation. Listen to the response and see if you can perceive what is being communicated.

Let's work with a clinical application of this principle, which can be used in many situations. In this process, you will be working with a specific application of directing fluids, called a V-spread. It is especially useful in sutural relationships that you can directly touch and palpate. Directing the tide can be used in more general ways, and we will introduce these as we relate to the various aspects of the system. In this process, you will first become aware of a compressed sutural relationship. Then, with one hand, you will make a gentle fingertip contact at the site of the compressed suture. You will place the other hand at the furthermost point on the cranium from that site. This may be diagonally across the cranium. For instance, if the fulcrum is located at the fronto-zygomatic suture, you might place your other hand at the diagonally opposite occipital squama. As the second step, you will learn to direct the fluid tide from the opposite area of the cranium back to the site of inertia.

Frontal, Parietal, and Temporal Bones: Common Sites of Compression

In the exploration below, you will be listening for inertial fulcrums located between the bones of the cranium. These will be expressed on a tissue level as sutural inertia and compression. A sutural compression is commonly generated by traumatic forces, or arises in compensation for them. They become sites of inertia around which the system must organize. Each cranial bone has specific sites that may be more vulnerable to the forces of trauma. Changes in the beveling of sutures are common sites. Complex sutural arrangements may also be sites where traumatic forces may cause compression and jamming. Remember that these are sites where both biodynamic and biokinetic forces have concentrated. *Biokinetic forces* are the traumatic forces that maintain the compression within the suture. The traumatically generated biokinetic force will effect the natural biokinetic motions of the tissues. These may be the traumatic forces of birth, of a blow or fall, or of an accident of some kind. Biodynamic potencies are the intrinsic forces that center the biokinetic forces in some way and hold the resultant fulcrums in the best possible compensation. In previous sections, you listened to the dynamics of the frontal, parietal, and temporal bones. Let's now look at some of their sutural dynamics.

The frontal bone has a number of areas to be mindful of. There is a change in beveling along the coronal suture lateral to bregma as it articulates with the parietal bone. The articulation with the ethmoid at the ethmoid notch is another relationship to be aware of. The articulation with the greater wings of the sphenoid have a triangular shape, and compressive forces can be transferred here. Finally, the frontal bone has a relationship with three other bones at pterion. At pterion the frontal, parietal, sphenoid, and temporal bones all overlap in alphabetical order with the frontal bone as the deepest in the relationship. This is also an area to be aware of. (See Figure 17.1.)

The parietal bone has similar vulnerabilities. Changes in beveling at the coronal suture are in common with the frontal bone. Pterion is also a vulnerable area, as is asterion where the parietal bone meets the occiput and temporal bones. The *parietal notch* is also a vulnerable area. The parietal notch is a classical fulcrum upon which the parietal bone moves in relationship to the temporal bone. It is where a peg-like projection from the parietal bone meets the temporal bone in a gomphosis (peg and socket) type of suture above the mastoid area. These are other areas to be aware of. (See Figure 17.2.)

The temporal bone also has vulnerabilities. Pterion, asterion, and the parietal notch are again areas to be aware of. Furthermore, the occipital mastoid suture is a common place for compressive issues to be found, as is the sphenopetrous suture, which will be discussed separately later. (See Figure 17.3.)

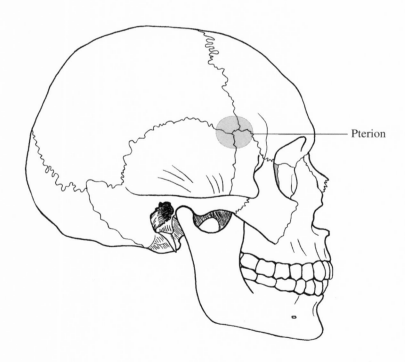

Pterion

17.1 Pterion

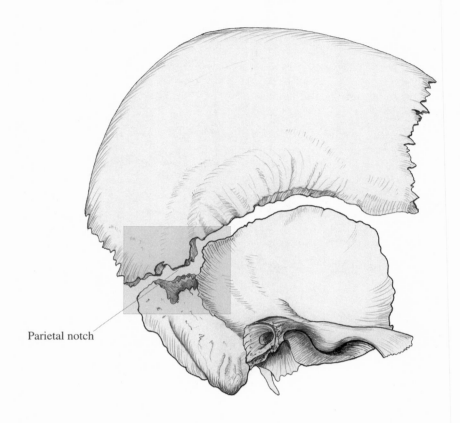

Parietal notch

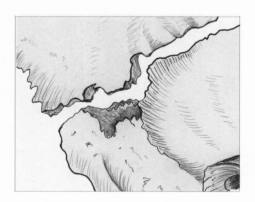

17.2 Parietal notch

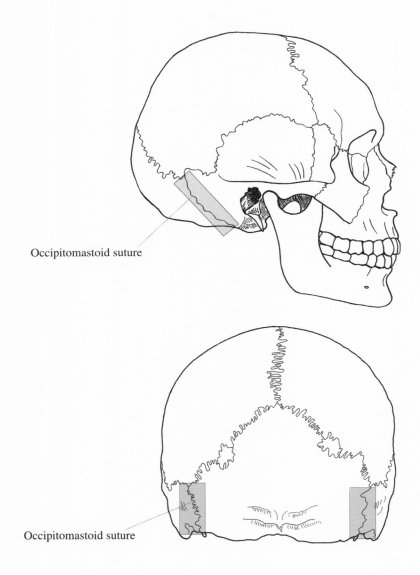

Occipitomastoid suture

Occipitomastoid suture

17.3   Occipitomastoid suture

The above vulnerabilities directly relate to the sphenoid bone, occiput, and SBJ. Their dynamics will obviously be effected by any inertial issue found within the relationships of the cranium. A last relationship to be aware of is the SBJ itself. Strong inertial forces can be directly fed into this relationship. Birth trauma is a common issue here, as are blows and falls. Furthermore, the SBJ can hold the traumatic forces generated by emotional shock as a protective compression within its dynamics. Lastly, the SBJ will be effected by compressive forces held anywhere along the vertebral midline and will reflect these in some manner. In other words, a compression found within the SBJ may be generated by an inertial fulcrum located elsewhere within the midline relationships of the body.

Perceptual Levels and Quality of Approach

In writing this piece, I have debated with myself and colleagues as to what level of work to present. Although this work is commonly taught at a CRI level, I would like to present it via the mid-tide level of perception. We will bring ourselves into the 2.5 cycles a minute tidal phenomenon to learn this specific approach. The fluid tide and the potency that moves it is most clear at this level of perception. I think that this is where most practitioners end up as they grapple with this process. In this exploration, you will learn to *direct the fluid tide*. You will start by dividing the process into a number of steps. In this learning exercise, you *could* begin within the CRI level of perception. At this level you would perceive the effects of the forces at work, the results of past experience. These may include tissue resistance such as compression, tissue density or dryness, and fluid congestion. As you palpate within the CRI, you might sense the tissue affects of the inertial forces as resistance and lack of mobility. This might be sensed to be a hinge-like or block-like motion around a compressed sutural relationship, or as a membranous pull into a specific area of articulation. You may simply notice motion organized around a sutural resistance.

Thus, at a CRI level of perception, you may notice a place of compression and rigid resistance within a sutural relationship. You might sense a sluggishness in the motion of the bone or relationship being palpated. You might sense a block-like quality to its motion. You might sense a hinge-like motion around the suture, or you might sense a strong pull into the inertial fulcrum. Basically, at a CRI level, you will sense a restriction in mobility. For instance, in palpating the frontal bone, you may notice a sense of hinging in its motion dynamic. Perhaps the frontal bone seemed to hinge off or to be pulled into the fronto-zygomatic suture. This might be a sutural relationship to which you could direct the fluid tide. Having listened via the CRI, you could then shift your perceptual field to the mid-tide level of perception. If you do this, you will gain experience as to how you receive information at each level. It is a useful learning exercise.

In clinical practice you might want to work exclusively via the mid-tide and experience its more precise communication of clinical information. That is the approach we are taking below. As you listen within the slower 2.5 cycles a minute tide, allow the tensile dynamics of the cranium as a whole to come to you. Notice the quality of motility and motion expressed at this slower rhythm. As you listen to this, you may again be drawn to a specific sutural fulcrum. You may sense this by being drawn into it by a tensile pull, or you may sense it as a tensile distortion around a particular site. It may seem that, as the tissues express their reciprocal tension motion dynamic, the whole tissue field distorts around a particular inertial fulcrum. Information may be communicated to you by the potencies, fluids, and tissues involved *as a whole pattern of distortion* within the cranium. This is a precise communication from the tissues through their whole field of action to you. As you perceive this, ask the question through your hands, "What organizes this?" Listen. You will be shown the inertial fulcrum that organizes the motion dynamic. This will be shown to you as you listen to the tissues as a whole, that is, as a unified tensile field. Furthermore, at this level of perception, the system will tend to express a particular inertial issue that needs attention, or that needs to be attended to before anything else can happen. As you listen over a number of sessions the *inherent treatment plan* will unfold as the system expresses its inherent resources and Intelligence.

Clinical Application: Directing the Fluid Tide with a V-Spread

In your practice sessions, you can palpate each major bone individually, as learned in previous chapters, to more directly sense their dynamics. This would include the frontal, parietals, and temporal bones, as well as the sphenoid and occiput. Again, you could do this at both a CRI level of perception and a mid-tide level. It is a useful exercise. Alternately, you could start at the vault hold and see which sutural relationship you are drawn to.

Here we will be introducing this work within the mid-tide perceptual level. You will initially meet the system via a vault hold and will synchronize your perceptual field with the mid-tide. Again, within this mid-tide awareness, as you palpate a specific bone or relationship, you may perceive how the entire tissue field responds as a tensile field of action. You may sense a tensile shift, distortion, or motion around a particular suture or a tensile pull into it. As this occurs, the system is showing you the particular suture to attend to. As you gain experience palpating within the mid-tide level of perception, you will notice how precise the information is as it is communicated to you. We will later discuss this precision in terms of the inherent treatment plan.[7] Let's use the fronto-zygomatic suture as an example to focus on. In the following application, it is assumed that you perceived an inertia site at this suture either from the vault hold or while palpating the frontal bone directly.

1. Listen from the vault hold previously learned.[8] Synchronize your perceptual field to the mid-tide level of perception. To do this, let your hands float on the tissues, immersed within fluid, and widen your perceptual field to include the biosphere (the person's body and the field around the person). Listen to the whole. Sense the motion of the fluid tide as you listen. Settle into this relationship and give the system time to clarify. Within your wide perceptual field, include an awareness of potency, fluid, and tissues as a tensile unit of function. As you settle into this, a particular inertial issue will come into the foreground. You may sense this as a distortion within the whole tensile field of bone and membrane or as a tensile pull into a relationship. For the sake of this explanation, we will assume that you perceived a pattern of distortion and an inertial fulcrum within the fronto-zygomatic suture.

2. Place the fingertips of one hand over the inertial site in a V-spread position. Be sure that you are clear about the anatomical relationship you are exploring. Make the V with your index and middle fingers. Place the V of your two fingers across the suture so that each finger is on opposite sides of the suture. In the example we are using, if you sense inertia within the fronto-zygomatic suture, you would place your V-spread across the suture, one finger on each bone. Your fingers are spread across the suture in a V-spread. (See Figure 17.4.)

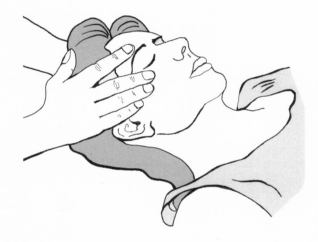

17.4 V-spread across
fronto-zygomatic suture

3. Place the fingertips or palm of the other hand on the cranium as far away from the inertial site as possible. In the cranium, this is commonly diagonally opposite the site. For instance, if you

sense the inertia to be within the fronto-zygomatic suture, you can place your fingertips or palm on the diagonally opposite occipital area.

4. Using the fingers of your V-spread, access the state of balanced tension across the suture. This is one approach to this process. It is always more effective to work within a state of balanced tension. It is here that you are in a more direct relationship to the inertial forces at work. You are seeking a neutral within the relationship. You may sense a tensile motion or rocking around the sutural relationship. All you need to do at most is to slow the motion down until there is a settling into a functional stillpoint. Remember that at the mid-tide level of perception, the state of balance can be perceived to be inherent within the inertial pattern being palpated. Listen for the settling of the tissues into stillness. This may be all you need to do. If there is enough space within the relationship, biodynamic forces will express themselves and you will sense a resolution at every level of function. By this I mean that the inertial potencies will be dissipated, the tissue and fluid affects will resolve, and fluids and tissues will realign to natural fulcrums and the midline.

5. However, it is not uncommon for the forces involved to be deeply inertial and for the tissue affects, such as compression, to be very dense. In this case, the direction of fluid process as now outlined can be of great benefit. It can help to facilitate something else to happen beyond the compensations held. Listen to the fluids between your hands. Maintain your wide perceptual field within the biosphere. The trick is to hold a wide perceptual field while appreciating the particulars within it. You still can be aware of the individual structures, but as part of a greater whole. Allow a perception of the fluid tide to come to you. Gently intend/suggest a back pressure or push against the fluids towards

the V-spread with your fingers. You are intending a subtle compression into the fluids towards the inertial suture. You may sense a shift in the action of the fluid tide as it expresses itself within the site of inertia. You are really sending an intention into the field of potency within the fluid. It is the potency within the fluid that is expressing action here. Potency can be directed to a site of density within its own field of action. You are simply directing attention to a site that needs attending to. (See Figure 17.5.)

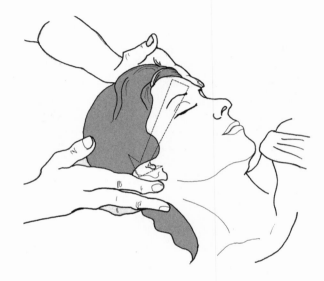

17.5 Direction of fluid process by V-spread

6. As you listen to the motion of the fluids, you may notice some interesting processes. Remember that anytime you place compression into the fluids, they will begin to talk to you. The fluids will convey precise information to you about the nature of the inertial fulcrum. If the inertia is very deep, you may sense an *echoing* back of the fluids and the potencies that move them towards your sending hand. This is like the tide of the ocean moving onto a beach and

hitting a stone breaker. On one level you are perceiving the motion of the water, but on a deeper level you are sensing the forces that move and organize that body of water. This echo can give you important information about the nature of the history you are meeting. You may also sense fluids and potencies swirling around the inertial fulcrum within the suture, or figure-eight-like motions of fluid and potency in relationship to it. These are like the eddies and swirls of water that form around a stone breaker as the tide meets it. Think of the inertial forces involved and the related tissue affects such as compression and density as these stone breakers. The difference here is that the stone breaker is not separate from the potency and fluids swirling around it, but is a density within this wider action. The fluctuations of fluid and potency, which seem to swirl around these affects or pulsate in relationship to them, are commonly called *lateral fluctuations*. They are very important to understand and to relate to in the healing process. We will go into detail about these fluctuations and how to relate to them in the next chapter. Listening to these fluctuant responses can give you much information about the nature of the inertial issue you are palpating. Dr. Sutherland called this listening process *reading the nuances of the Tide*.

7. Finally, at your receiving hand, you may start to notice a welling-up of fluid and potency within the suture under your V-spread. It will seem as if the rigid stone breaker on the beach is melting away and there is a welling-up of fluid and potency under your V-spread. This is really a welling up and permeation of potency within the inertial fulcrum. The whole tensile field of potency is brought to bear, and the inertial potencies within the suture respond. You may also sense heat and pulsation within and around the site as the biokinetic forces that were maintaining the inertia are dissipated back to the envi-

ronment. As this occurs you may sense expansion within the relationship.

8. When you sense the welling-up of potency under your receiving hand, you can then, if necessary, intend/suggest a spreading across the sutural relationship you are attending to. To do this, you use your index and middle fingers, which are on either side of the suture. You can suggest a very subtle spreading across the suture with these fingers when you sense the welling-up and spreading of the suture. This suggestion is in the nature of a conversation about space. In our example, you would intend this spreading across the fronto-zygomatic suture. Intend this spreading to the boundary of the space accessed and again seek the state of balanced tension. As you do this, you are initiating a further conversation with the tissues within the suture. What is the nature of this inertia? How much space can you give yourself? What is the potential here? Can you access the Health that is centering this?

9. You are waiting to sense a softening, spreading, and expansion within the sutural relationship. This is an expression of the resolution of the inertial forces within the suture. Notice how the potency, fluids, and tissue elements expand and realign to the midline and to natural fulcrums. Potency expands, fluids decongest, and tissues expand and disengage. When you sense this, return to your original vantage point and notice any changes in tissue motion. Do tissues reorient to the midline function and to the natural fulcrums of the system? In this case, you could return to the frontal hold and monitor its dynamics. Have they changed after the V-spread process? Does the frontal bone express a more balanced relationship to Sutherland's fulcrum?[9]

This process can be applied to any inertial fulcrum encountered within the body. The intention is essentially one of directing the inherent healing potency within the fluid system to the specific area in need of attention. This is the primary purpose of the process, to bring attention to a place that has become inertial and disordered. It is commonly used within states of balanced tension to help in the expression of potency within the inertial tissues being palpated.

Whole Body Fluid Direction

It is also important to remember that the fluid system in the body is an integrated unit of function. Potency is expressed within all fluids and functions within the fluids as an integrated whole. Furthermore, it is important to remember that tissues, fluids, and potency are a unit of function. Within this context, the fluid tide is expressed as a unified dynamic in the body. Traditional therapeutic approaches take advantage of this fact. There can be advantages, at times, to working in practitioner teams. For instance, in one process, one practitioner might palpate an inertial pattern and access a state of balanced tension in relationship to it. The other practitioner might then direct fluid and potency from the diagonally opposite foot, or from another part of the body remote to the inertial fulcrum being palpated by the first practitioner. The practitioners are taking advantage of the large volume of potency between their contacts.

In another application of this, a single practitioner can follow a pattern in the cranium or elsewhere in the body to its state of balanced tension. He or she can then ask the patient to dorsiflex the foot. If the inertial fulcrum is located on one side of the cranium, the practitioner may ask the patient to dorsiflex the diagonally opposite foot. If the fulcrum is centrally located, then the patient may be asked to dorsiflex both feet. In this process, the patient is generating a back pressure within his or her own tidal system, and it is naturally directed to the site being palpated, if the system is expressing a state of balanced tension around it.

Completions

As you become familiar with this process, you will learn to engage the tensile fields of potency, fluids, and tissues as a unit of function. This will be initiated via a conversation with fluids or more directly via the potencies. As you learn to sense the potency within the fluids as a palpable reality, the process really becomes one of directing the potency of the Breath of Life itself. Directing the tide is a powerful process and the subtlety of your listening skills will develop with it. The most important thing is to practice the principles in all the sutural relationships of the cranium over time. Do not work with more than one relationship in a session. Work simply and deeply and note the results! In the next chapter, you will approach another classical fluid skill, the use of lateral fluctuations of fluid and potency, in which you will learn to engage the fluids and potency in another kind of conversation.

1. See H. Magoun, *Osteopathy in the Cranial Field* (The Sutherland Teaching Foundation) and W. G. Sutherland, *Teachings in the Science of Osteopathy,* ed. Anne Wales (Rudra Press, 1990).

2. Ibid.

3. See W. G. Sutherland, *Teachings in the Science of Osteopathy,* ed. Anne Wales (Rudra Press, 1990).

4. See W. G. Sutherland, *Contributions of Thought* (The Sutherland Teaching Foundation).

5. See W. G. Sutherland, *Teachings in the Science of Osteopathy,* ed. Anne Wales (Rudra Press, 1990).

6. Mae-Wan Ho, *The Rainbow and the Worm, the Physics of Organisms* (World Scientific).

7. A term coined by Dr. Rollin Becker, D.O.

8. That is, either "Dr. Sutherland's hold" or "Dr. Becker's hold."

9. The primal midline is the midline that expresses the groundswell of the Breath of Life as an organizing principle within the human system.

18

Fluid Dynamics and Lateral Fluctuation

In this chapter, you will continue to explore perceptual skills related to fluids and potency. We will first discuss fluid dynamics and the state of balanced tension. Then we will introduce the concept of *lateral fluctuation* and related clinical skills.

In this chapter we will:

- *Discuss fluid dynamics, longitudinal fluctuation, and the state of balanced tension.*

- *Introduce the concept of lateral fluctuation.*

- *Discuss lateral fluctuations and their clinical importance.*

- *Learn appropriate clinical skills related to lateral fluctuation.*

Fluid Dynamics and the Breath of Life

In this section I would like to review some concepts about fluid fluctuation and fluid dynamics. As you have seen, the natural axis for the fluctuation of cerebrospinal fluid is longitudinal. As previously discussed, this longitudinal axis is embryologically derived. Within the primitive disc, the groundswell of the Tide is expressed via the primal midline and

notochord. From this midline a further *dorsal midline* is then generated. This is the midline of the neural axis within the embryo. It becomes an organizing axis for the fluctuation of cerebrospinal fluid and for the potency that moves it. I also call this the *fluid midline*. As described in Chapter Seven, the natural expression of cerebrospinal fluid fluctuation along this dorsal axis is called *longitudinal fluctuation*.

As you remember, three functions are discernible within the mid-tide: potency, fluid, and tissues. All three can be perceived as tensile fields in motion. Potency is expressed via transmutation within the fluids, and motion is generated within the system. In the inhalation surge, potency rises within the dorsal midline and fluids and tissues respond. The fluid component of this response is called the fluid tide. Tissue response is called motility. The fluid tide is an expression of the potency at work within the fluids of the body. This fluid surge can be perceived as an ascending longitudinal fluctuation of cerebrospinal fluid within the core of the body. As this occurs, there are also natural transverse fluctuations of fluid from the midline to the periphery. For instance, you may perceive a transverse fluctuation within the lateral ventricles of the brain during inhalation. This is all orchestrated by the Breath of Life and its potency. The potency within the fluids acts as an organizing ground for the fluid and tissue world. The blueprint of the creative intention is carried by the potency within the fluids as an active, embodied ordering force within the mind-body complex.

As we have seen, within states of balance, a phenomenon called *fluid drive* can be perceived. In this phenomenon, a drive of potency occurs within the fluids, which is directed through the fulcrum being attended to. It can be sensed to be a strong and sharp force that moves right through the fulcrum. You may also sense a softer permeation of potency through the area and the fulcrum being attended to. This has a different quality to it. It is more of a field phenomenon. You may sense the whole field of potency come into play. A building and welling up of potency may be perceived. As the system is poised within a state of balance around a particular fulcrum, the whole field of potency organizes around this particular inertial issue. A movement of potency throughout its field towards the inertial fulcrum may be sensed. As this occurs, a soft permeation of potency may be perceived within the area and fulcrum being palpated. It is like tidal water soaking through a dense knob of sand and melting it away. You may literally sense a welling up of potency and fluid within the whole tensile field, which moves right through the inertial fulcrum being attended to. Another fluid dynamic may also be perceived.

The inherent fluctuation of cerebrospinal fluid, and of fluids generally, is generated by the action of potency. As we have seen, unresolved inertial forces may affect these natural fluctuant phenomena. Unresolved forces are centered by the Breath of Life as its potency becomes inertial in order to contain and compensate for the disturbance within the system. This generates inertial fulcrums which become new organizing factors. The inherent longitudinal fluctuation of CSF may be effected by these inertial fulcrums in some way. When potency becomes inertial, so does the fluid and tissue world. These new fulcrums, which do not automatically shift with the Tide, will generate fluid congestion and eccentric fluid fluctuations. Fluids will begin to fluctuate in erratic ways around inertial fulcrums. These fluctuations are generically called *lateral fluctuations*. We will spend the rest of this chapter ex-

ploring this phenomenon. I will review these ideas in more depth and bring in some relatively new research that resonates with these concepts.

Potency and the Liquid Crystalline Matrix

According to Dr. Becker's concepts, at the heart of every disturbance there are inertial forces at work. Dr. Becker called the potency of the Breath of Life, in its physiological functioning, *biodynamic potency*. He called the environmental, genetic, and traumatic forces, which generate and maintain disturbances in the system, *biokinetic forces*. In the previous discussions on inertial fulcrums, we described their action within the system in terms of biodynamic potency and biokinetic forces. When biokinetic forces such as trauma, accidents, toxins, and so on, are introduced into the system, the biodynamic potencies of the Breath of Life will attempt to resolve them. If these biokinetic forces cannot be resolved, then the potency of the Breath of Life will become inertial in order to center and contain their disruptive influences. In essence, the potency of the Breath of Life becomes inertial within its own field of action in order to center the disturbance within the system.

These coalescences of potency become inertial sites, which will, in turn, organize tissue and fluid resistances within the system. Remember that it is the action of the potency that lays down the blueprint around which the cellular and tissue world organizes. As biodynamic potencies become inertial, the fluid and tissue world also becomes inertial. Fluid and tissue affects will result. The osteopathic lesion, a site of tissue, fluid, and neuroendocrine disruption, is the classic result of these deeper forces at work. Around these sites of inertia, fluctuant phenomena are generated. These eccentric fluctuations of both potency and fluid are direct manifestations of the inertial forces present.

One way to think about this is to look at the nature of connective tissues. There is now clear evidence that the unified connective tissue field within the body forms a *liquid crystalline matrix,* which is a true unit of function. All connective tissues form within a fluid ground matrix. This fluid matrix is a continuity of function. The fluids within the collagen fibers of connective tissues are bonded in ordered hydrogen bonds so that the fluid system literally forms one unified field throughout the body. This fluid field is continuous with the fluids within cells so that there is a true fluid unity of function throughout the body. I would postulate that it is the bioelectric potency that orders this fluid matrix. Furthermore, collagen fiber is made up of a triple helix of peptides that have charged amino acid side chains. These are, in turn, hydrogen bonded to the fluid matrix. In other words, water molecules are self-bonded in ordered and coherent ways, and the tissues are bonded to this fluid field to form a liquid crystalline matrix. Thus there truly is a unified fluid-tissue field. Furthermore, coherent quantum-level bioelectric field phenomena have been seen to be associated with this liquid crystalline matrix. A truly coherent and holistic quantum bioelectric field exists and co-arises with this liquid crystalline fluid-tissue matrix.[1]

When inertial forces are introduced into this bioelectric-fluid-tissue matrix, the liquid crystalline nature of the ground substance changes. Potency becomes inertial, fluids become dense, and tissues, likewise, densify, contract, and compress. Bony lesions and connective tissue adhesions result. If you bring more potency to bear within such an inertial site, the inertial potencies within the site will be activated or intensified. Again it is possible to initiate the action of potency within specific sites of inertia. When the potency within an inertial field is excited or activated in some way, the bioelectric-fluid-tissue matrix has a chance to resolve the inertial forces present and to realign to its original orientation. In other words, when the energy economy of the inertial area is raised, the liquid crystalline matrix has an opportunity to resolve the inertial forces being centered.[2] As you work with fluid processes, such as the direction of fluid discussed in the last chapter and lateral fluctuation in this chapter, you are raising the energy economy of the inertial area. Potency is activated and the liquid crystalline matrix will respond.

Lateral Fluctuations

Another way to picture this is to imagine a unified bioelectric field of potency within which fluids and tissues organize. Each aspect, that of potency, fluid, and tissue, is a function of increasing density. First there is a bioelectric field, then a fluid field, and then a more material field of cells and tissues. Each is a tensile field in its own right and all interact and manifest a unified dynamic. As biokinetic forces are introduced into this field, condensations or coalescences of potency will occur. Potency, within its unified field, condenses within the site of action of any disruptive force. In its natural expression of motility and motion, the whole field of potency must then express tensile motions around its own condensations. This, in turn, generates altered tensile dynamics within fluids and tissues. Eccentric tissue motion and altered fluid fluctuations result. Thus, eccentric fluctuations of potency generate eccentric fluctuations of fluid. The resultant fluid fluctuations are commonly called *lateral fluctuations.*

Although these motions of potency and fluid are called lateral fluctuations, they can take almost any shape or form depending on the nature of the inertial fulcrum that organizes them. This may be perceived by the sensitive practitioner as echoes against rigid restrictions, lateral pulsations of fluid, figure-eight pulsations, and swirlings and spiralings of potency around areas of inertia and congestion. Sometimes they can feel like vortices or spirals whose depth is located at the center of the inertia. An appreciation of fluctuant phenomena helps the practitioner become aware of the nature of the inertia in the system. It also helps to pinpoint areas of congestion, adhesion, resistance, and compression. (See Figure 18.1.)

It is also important to also remember that all expressions of potency are essentially expressions of Health at work. Lateral fluctuations of potency

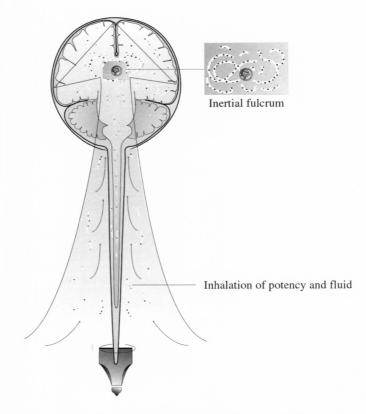

Inertial fulcrum

Inhalation of potency and fluid

18.1 Lateral fluctuations within fluid and potency dynamic

and fluid are found both within the natural fluctuation of fluid within the body and as a response to areas of inertia within the system. Lateral fluctuations generated by inertial fulcrums are expressions of the centering action of potency within its own tensile field. Lateral fluctuations are manifestations of the biodynamic potencies centering and containing the impact of unresolved biokinetic forces. Again, potency will coalesce to center the unresolved biokinetic forces held within the system. Eccentric fluctuations of potency and fluid will result. These are all manifestations of the Health at work acting to center the unresolved issues within the body-mind. An awareness of lateral fluctuation gives you entrée into clinical information about the interplay between universal and conditional forces within the system. Thus Health and history are a

unit of function within the unfoldment of our human condition.

Clinical Intentions and Lateral Fluctuation

Think of a site of inertia as a site of condensed potency, compressed fluid, and densified tissue. As we have seen, the bioelectric-fluid-tissue matrix is a liquid crystalline entity. When biokinetic forces are present, the liquid crystalline nature of this complex is compromised. Inertia arises within each of the three functions. The bioelectric potency condenses, the fluids densify, and the tissues contract and compress. The energy economy within the site of inertia lowers, and the ground matrix of the tissues densifies. In this work, the practitioner can either amplify or induce lateral fluctuations of potency within inertial patterns. This approach helps to raise or amplify the energy economy of the area. In other words, potency is stimulated to express motion and activity.

This approach can be used within states of balanced tension to stimulate the expression of the inertial potencies within the heart of an inertial fulcrum. When the practitioner helps the system access its state of balanced tension, there is a natural tendency for these inertial or condensed potencies to be expressed or to move in some way. In essence the energy economy within the inertial site is raised and inertial potencies are activated. Facilitating expressions of lateral fluctuation can help activate or intensify the motion and action of inertial potencies within the organizing fulcrum. An activation and permeation of potency may then occur within the inertial fulcrum and its fluid and tissue elements. In other words, the facilitation of lateral fluctuations can help the system express its inherent Health within inertial and disordered situations.

In the following sections, you will explore the use of lateral fluctuation in clinical work. This is of great benefit to understand, because an intelligent therapeutic relationship to lateral fluctuation deepens and enhances the work. In this work you will be intensifying the expression of eccentric fluctuation when it arises within an inertial pattern. This will, in essence, stimulate the expression of potency in the area and help the system express its healing resources within inertial sites more fully and effectively. You will be helping to reestablish the relationship of inertial and disordered tissues to the natural fulcrums of the system and to the Original intention of the potencies, fluids, and tissues involved. You will be, in essence, helping the system reestablish its relationship to the reference beam of the human hologram. Think of the potency within the fluids as maintaining an inherent blueprint principle around which the cellular and tissue world organizes. In essence, the work is about reconnecting to the creative intention of the divine as it unfolds the organization of a human being. Here I am not talking about genetics, but about a reconnection to

the inherent principle carried by the potency of the Breath of Life, which maintains this universal creative intention within each of us.

Clinical Applications

In the following clinical applications, you will first listen to the expression of lateral fluctuation within an inertial pattern in the system. You will simply let the system tell you its story via these fluctuations. You will then facilitate their expression. The intention will be to assist the system to do what it is naturally doing. Remember that lateral fluctuation is a natural expression of potency and fluid in relationship to sites of inertia within the system. It is an expression of Health and healing potency within inertial patterns. You will simply be encouraging and amplifying this manifestation of Health.

The first step is to cultivate a perceptual awareness of these phenomena. It is best to do this within the mid-tide field of action. Holding the biosphere, you will become aware of the fluid tide and listen for any fluctuant phenomena that are communicated to you. You may notice the tendency for potency and fluid to fluctuate in eccentric patterns in relationship to an inertial fulcrum. They may echo off rigid resistances, or spiral, or "figure-eight" around inertial fulcrums in some way. In the clinical application below, as you listen to the system, you may become aware of these lateral fluctuations of potency and fluid. An awareness of these phenomena can clarify the inertial pattern being expressed and can also lead you to the fulcrum that organizes it.

The second step is cultivating a clinical approach to these fluctuations. The clinical approaches I will share with you concentrate on enhancing or facilitating lateral fluctuations. Initially, you will simply listen. You will first monitor the system within the mid-tide and start to become aware of lateral fluctuations. Then you will initiate a *conversation* with the inertial potencies and fluctuations perceived. You will do this by simply amplifying the lateral fluctuations that you are sensing. The potencies will then begin to talk to you directly. This conversation initiates the expression of inertial potencies within inertial sites.

If the potencies are very dense and the related tissue affects very entrenched, then the inertial potencies within may not have enough space to express themselves. You may not sense any initiation of inertial potencies due to the density of the forces and affects involved. In these cases, you might *initiate* lateral fluctuations as a means of communicating to and stimulating the inertial potencies involved. In the first clinical application outlined below you will start in a vault hold, and work with whatever pattern the system shows you from that vantage point, and then go to another specific relationship for more practice.

Clinical Applications:
Awareness of Lateral Fluctuations

In this section, you will be simply tuning in to the sense of lateral fluctuation while palpating the system. The intention is to familiarize yourself with this phenomenon. It is already something that you may be aware of. The important thing is not to look for anything. Simply hold a wider perceptual field as described below and let the fluids and potencies speak to you. You may sense this conversation as pulsations, swirls, and fluctuations of fluid and potency. Please remember that these are communications. The system is showing you its history, its suffering, and the Health that is centering it.

1. In the vault hold, negotiate your contact and relationship with the patient's system. Then let your hands float within fluid and establish a wide perceptual field. Hold the whole of the person and the biosphere within your field of awareness. As you do this, include an awareness of the fluid tide. You are listening to the longitudinal fluctuation of fluid within the 2.5 cycles a minute mid-tide. Notice the surge and settling of its action in inhalation and exhalation. Within your wide perceptual field, allow an awareness

of the particular to come to you. Don't narrow your perceptual field as you do this. Notice the whole interplay of the fluid tide, including the cerebrospinal fluid fluctuation and the potency that moves it.

2. As you allow this awareness to build, bring in an awareness of the tissue elements. You may sense the tissues to express a whole tensile inhalation—exhalation motion within the cycles of the mid-tide. The tissues of the cranium may be sensed to be a true unit of function in their expression of tensile motion. Notice any eccentric motions or distortions in the tensile motion of fluids and tissues. Is tissue motion organized around natural automatically shifting fulcrums? How are they organized? Around what fulcrums are they organized? Stay with this inquiry for a while.

3. Now listen to fluid fluctuations that may arise as you listen to the dynamics of the system within the fluid tide. Do these fluctuations begin to speak to you? What is the story they are telling? Do they show the location of organizing fulcrums? Can you sense the "fluid within the fluid," the sense of the organizing force of the Breath of Life? Can you sense the drive of the potency within the fluids? Simply maintain your wide perceptual field and listen.

Clinical Application:
Amplification of Lateral Fluctuations

In this section, we will introduce clinical skills related to the amplification or intensification of lateral fluctuations. Enhancing the expression of lateral fluctuations can help the system express healing resources within an inertial pattern. Amplifying lateral fluctuations within an inertial pattern will intensify the expression of potency within its organizing fulcrum. You will facilitate the expression of lateral fluctuation within states of balanced tension. It is the natural tendency, within states of balanced tension, for potency to become expressed or stimulated within the organizing fulcrum. Let's look at this within the context of a clinical session.

1. From the vault hold, synchronize your field of awareness to the mid-tide level of perception. Let your hands be immersed within fluid. Holding the whole biosphere within your perceptual field, listen to the fluid tide and to the expression of potency within the system. Include the tissues and tissue motion within this perceptual field. Follow any particular inertial pattern that is communicated to you. See if you can sense the fulcrum that organizes it. Help access the state of balanced tension.

2. Notice any lateral fluctuations of fluid and potency that are expressed within the state of balance. Sense the motion of the fluctuations. Notice the pendulum-like expression of the fluctuations. You may notice that the fluctuations tend to move in a side-to-side or a figure-eight fashion. Even if they are sensed to move in spirals or swirls, there will be preferences within the swirls. While still within the state of balanced tension, you will encourage an amplification of their expression.

3. As you follow the lateral fluctuations, at the boundary to each of the pendulum swings, subtly suggest *push* in the opposite direction. Initially you may sense that you are pushing against the swings of fluid fluctuation. You may, however, also sense that you are in a more direct relationship to the potency within the fluid as you intend *push*. This will have a more electromagnetic or bioelectric feel to it. It is like pushing a children's swing just as it is about to swing away from you to amplify its motion. You will do this in both directions of the pendulum swing. Do this first in one direction and then in the other. With each push on the pendulum, the lateral fluctuations will become fuller, faster,

and the potency within its expression will be amplified. Continue to push back and forth until you sense a clear amplification of potency. Then stop pushing and listen to how the system uses the enhancement of potency in relationship to the inertial fulcrum. Notice how the potency is manifesting within the fulcrum that originally organized the pattern. (See Figure 18.2.)

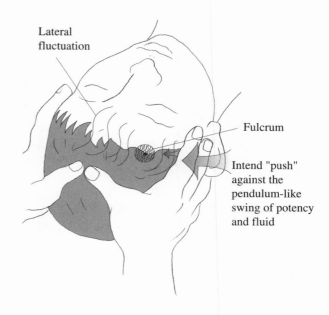

18.2 Facilitation of lateral fluctuation

4. Listen for expressions of Health. You may sense a permeation of potency within the area. You may sense the dissipation of biokinetic forces. Wait for a sense of expansion and for a reorganization of the tissues and fluids. You may notice that the resistant fulcrum has resolved. Remonitor the system from the vault hold as you simply listen to both the fluid tide and tissue motility. Note any changes that may have occurred. Has there been a reorientation to the primal midline and natural fulcrums?

Clinical Application:
Initiation of Lateral Fluctuation

Sometimes the potencies involved are so deeply inertial and the resultant fluid and tissue changes so dense that you do not notice any local expressions of lateral fluctuation within states of balance. There may be a general sense of inertia throughout the fluid system. This is commonly due to trauma and shock affects. The fluid matrix can become inertial due to potencies centering traumatization and shock affects throughout the system. In cases like these, you can *initiate* lateral fluctuations with the intention of stimulating the expression of lateral fluctuations and of the potency within the organizing fulcrum.

1. From the vault hold, synchronize your perceptual field with the mid-tide. Let your hands be immersed within fluids, and hold the whole biosphere within your perceptual field. Listen to particular inertial patterns as they are communicated to you. See if you can sense the fulcrum that organizes its motion. Help access the state of balanced tension. Sometimes, due to local compression, fluid congestion, and resistance, the state of balance is difficult to attain, or has a "flatness" to it. You might then want to stimulate an expression of lateral fluctuation by suggesting them within the pattern that you are palpating.

2. To do this, simply start a lateral fluctuation by suggesting push against the fluids and the potency within it, from one hand to the other. You are, in essence, generating a pendulum-like flux of potency between your hands. You can do this bioelectrically or electromagnetically by relating to the potency within the fluids and pushing potency from hand to hand. You may notice that a lateral fluctuation will be initiated between your hands. Keep pushing the potency back and forth between your hands. You will notice that the lateral fluctuations increase in

speed and intensity. As you push against the potency, the fluids will respond and lateral fluctuations of fluid will result. Remember that the potency moves the fluid, not the other way around. You are initiating the expression of the inertial potencies within the heart of the fulcrum being palpated.

3. Wait until the system begins to express these fluctuations on its own. You are essentially drawing more potency into relationship. As this occurs, you may perceive a permeation of potency within the inertial tissues and fluids. Once the system can express lateral fluctuations on its own within the pattern, you can stop pushing. Again help to access the state of balance. At this point, simply listen for expressions of Health and for a resolution of the inertia being palpated. You are stimulating the system to express its healing resources within the pattern where it originally could not. You are helping the innate healing resources of the system and its innate intelligence to be expressed in areas that have, in essence, become darkened.

4. Listen for the tissues to once again express motion and for a reorientation to the groundswell of the Breath of Life and the natural automatically shifting fulcrums of the system.

Clinical Application:
Working with Lateral Fluctuation
in Specific Relationships

The above intentions can be applied to any clinical situation. Let's apply this to the temporal bones. Imagine that you are perceiving an inertial pattern as you palpate the temporal bones.

1. Again listen within the mid-tide level of action, hold an awareness of the biosphere, and allow the 2.5 cycles a minute mid-tide to come to you. As this occurs, include the tissues within your

field of perception. Let the dynamics of the temporal bones come into your hands. Do not narrow your perceptual field down as you do this. Listen for the external and internal rotation motions of the bones. Notice their reciprocal tension motions within the mid-tide. Notice any eccentric patterns of motility and motion. As you notice this, you may also be aware of how these motions are part of a much wider dynamic. The temporal bones are part of the whole tensile tissue field of the body. Also remember that potency, fluid, and tissues are a unified dynamic. Listen for the tensile motions of the potency-fluid-tissue matrix. Notice how the temporal bones express their motion as part of a greater field of action. Listen for the sense of reciprocal tension surge and settling. You may perceive inertial tissue patterns as distortions within the entire tensile tissue field. You may sense the motion of the tissues of the cranium as a whole. Inertial patterns may be perceived as a reciprocal tension distortion throughout the whole osseous-membranous cranium. This will be especially clear within the inhalation phase of the Tide. Notice what this is organized around and help access the state of balanced tension directly. All that may be necessary is a slowing down of the motions being palpated. This is the level of perception where Dr. Becker's three-step healing awareness comes more directly into play.

2. As you become aware of lateral fluctuations within the state of balance, start to enhance them by pushing against their pendulum swings. Do this first in one direction and then in the other. Within the fluid tide, you may have a more direct sense of the action of the potency within the fluids. You may find yourself more directly encouraging lateral fluctuations of potency electromagnetically and the fluids will follow. You are following the pendulum swing to its furthermost excursion and subtly pushing it in the opposite direction, like a children's

swing, just as it is about to move in that direction. You are pushing first one way, then the other. Notice how the lateral fluctuations intensify and amplify. Notice the resultant initiation and amplification of potency within and around the fulcrum being palpated.

3. Remember that when you generate a lateral flux of potency and fluid within the state of balance, inertial potencies begin to express themselves beyond the compensations held. The whole unified field of potency comes into play.

4. Once the expression of fluctuation amplifies, you can stop pushing and simply listen. Listen for expressions of Health. Notice when the tissues again begin to express motion and be aware of their reorganization and reorientation to the midline and groundswell of the Breath of Life.

Further Examples of the Use of Lateral Fluctuation

You can use this principle in any situation. Let's say that you are palpating the frontal bone. You follow an inertial pattern and help access the state of balanced tension. You then notice lateral fluctuations arising. You can follow these and intensify them by pushing against the fluctuations at each lateral aspect of the frontal bone via the little and ring fingers of each hand.

Let's take another scenario. You have noticed a compressive pattern between the occiput and temporal bone at the occipitomastoid suture. You place your hands on each bone. You follow the perceived inertial pattern and help access the state of balanced tension. You then notice expressions of lateral fluctuation. You can intensify these by suggesting push against them between your palpating hands. If the compression and congestion in the area was so extreme that you could not sense any expression of lateral fluctuation, then you could stimulate them by intentionally pushing against the potencies between your hands. You would again wait for the system to express them in a stronger and more amplified way and then stop pushing and deeply appreciate what the system can do to heal itself. All you are doing is to help the system express its healing potency where this has, in some way, become inertial.

This can be applied in any situation when you are holding two poles of a relationship. You can even do this between the fingers of the same hand as you are listening to the system. For instance, you may be holding the sacrum and notice lateral fluctuations around a sacroiliac joint. You can enhance these by suggesting push against the fluctuations between the fingers of your hand under the sacrum. Remember that the fluids convey the potency of the Breath of Life to every cell of the body. You can, in Dr. Sutherland's terms, trust the inherent intelligence of the system. This Intelligence can be trusted and is the heart of clinical practice.

Look for the micromotions of fluctuation of potency and fluid within an inertial fulcrum. Even if it seems that no potency is being expressed, look for the *kernel* of expression within the pattern. There is always this aliveness present, even in the most seemingly intransigent situation. Remember that this kernel of aliveness is the system's attempt to express its Health and healing potency within any traumatic or disease process. Work with this kernel and it will build into a whirlpool of potency! Work with this whirlpool and the Tide itself will come into play. Remember that you can always initiate the fluctuation between your hands or fingers, and this may kick-start the expression of potency in the area. Sense the fluctuations, sense the potency, sense the life force, and trust the system!

1. See Mae-Wan Ho and David P. Knight, "Liquid Crystalline Meridians," *American Journal of Complementary Medicine.*

2. See Deane Juhan, *Job's Body* (Station Hill Press), for an excellent discussion of connective tissues.

19

Disengagement

This chapter introduces another skill that is important to understand and master in clinical practice. It is commonly taught as a technique or method. Here we will present it as a way to engage in various kinds of conversations with inertial fulcrums and the forces that organize them. This idea of *conversation* is essential to comprehend. In these approaches we learn to engage tissues, fluids, and potency in various kinds of conversations. These are about the Health of the system and about its history. They are ways to generate the conditions for reconnection and healing to occur. In this, we do not fix, unwind, or release anything. We simply engage in a depth of listening and conversation into the *how* of things. In this process we also learn to listen for expressions of Health within the system and for reorganization and reorientation to the midline function of the Breath of Life. The system has its resources; can we help liberate them? The system has its inherent treatment plan; it knows what needs to happen. Can we perceive and support this?

In this chapter you will learn a skill of conversation traditionally called *disengagement*. It is commonly used in relationship to sutural or joint compressions. In recent times, it has also become known as *decompression*. I like to use the classical term, disengagement. It gives the sense that something that has become coupled due to trauma or disease processes has become uncoupled. Within a

site of sutural resistance, it is important to remember that there are forces at work. Tissue compression is only one particular effect of these inertial forces and potencies. Sometimes the coiling and coupling of forces are so dense that there is no space within the state of balance for a dynamic equilibrium to occur. The potencies simply do not have the space to become activated beyond the compensations held. The intention of disengagement is not to decompress or disengage something, but to help access the *space* within which the inertial potencies can be accessed. This will, within a state of balanced tension, initiate the action of potency within the specific sutural issue. As the forces within the inertial fulcrum are resolved, the effected tissue structures will uncouple and disengage. In this uncoupling process, a reorganization and reorientation to natural fulcrums and a more ideal motility and motion dynamic may result.

In this chapter we will:

- *Introduce the clinical skill of disengagement.*

- *Give some clinical applications and examples of this skill.*

Adding the Conversation Skill of Disengagement

As we have seen, sometimes traumatic forces are so strong, and the resulting compression is so deep, that the inertial potencies involved do not have enough space to be expressed within states of balanced tension. The state of balanced tension may have a flat or dull quality to it. The tissues, fluids, and potencies involved may be deeply and intransigently inertial. Tissue and fluid changes may have occurred as a result. The *history* of the trauma may be deeply entrenched. There may be so much impaction between the structures involved that even within a state of balanced tension, the compressive forces are so intense that potencies within the fulcrum cannot be accessed. There is simply too much inertia to overcome. In these situations the skill of disengagement can help access the space needed to allow inertial potencies to be expressed. It is most commonly used in relationship to compression within sutures and joints. You will learn to use this skill within the context of a conversation with the potencies, forces, fluids, and tissues involved in the relationship. In other words, you will be conversing with the Health and with the history around which the system is organized.

The process will be explored in two stages. First you will simply listen, notice an inertial fulcrum within sutural dynamics, and help the system access a state of balanced tension. If the compressive forces are very condensed and the compression within tissue parts are also very dense, then further facilitation on your part may be useful. Here we will explore the skill of disengagement as a clinical conversation. In this work, you can make a direct relationship to the bones that make up the sutural relationship. You will place your hands on either side of the suture. As you listen to the dynamic expressed there, you will subtly intend a spreading apart of the bones. A subtle intention of *space* is offered to the inertial forces involved and to related tissue and fluid affects. You will intend-suggest this to the boundary accessed. This is the boundary of

the potential space within the relationship. There is always space in potential within any relationship, no matter how seemingly compressed. You will then help access the state of balanced tension at or near this edge. The intention is to initiate a conversation with the potencies, fluids, and tissues involved. When you intend space within the inertial relationship, the tissues and fluids will start to talk to you. You are asking the tissues various questions within this intention of space. How much space is there within this relationship? What is possible here? Once a sense of space is communicated to you, the conversation changes to that of Health. You now help the tissues access the state of balanced tension and, in that state, listen for expressions of Health. There is always a kernel of Health present within an inertial fulcrum, no matter how inertial and condensed the forces are. The intention is to help access potential space and to perceive this kernel of Health.

In this clinical application, you will be working with this intention. You will simply make a relationship to the two poles of the compressive pattern. For instance, if you sense compression within the squamosal suture, make a contact on the parietal bone above it and on the temporal bone below it. From this position, there are two approaches that you can take. In the first, you simply intend space by subtly tractioning the two bones away from each other. This is an intention, a conversation about space. It is not a technique to release anything. Once space is accessed within the relationship, then the intention will be to shift the conversation to Health. The intention now will be to access the state of balanced tension near the boundary of the space accessed. (See Figure 19.1.) In the second approach, you can stabilize one bone and subtly traction the other away from it, again to a boundary and state of balanced tension. Again, this is an intention of a very subtle traction to the boundary of the space accessed within the sutural relationship. At this boundary the state of balanced tension is then accessed. It is within the state of balanced tension that the Health within the resistance is accessed.

The intention in this clinical application is simply

to help access the potential space within the relationship. It is an exploration into the space that is potentially available within the inertial fulcrum. It is offered as a suggestion. It must not be a demand. It is an inquiry into what is possible. It is a conversation. The objective is to access enough space to allow the inertial potencies more room to express themselves within states of balanced tension. Once you do that, healing and disengagement occur from within. Dr. Sutherland emphasized that the intention within the cranial field is to facilitate the unerring forces from within. The Breath of Life and its Tide knows what needs to happen. The system is inherently organized. It is simply a matter of accessing and relating to that organizing and ordering function. This is a great gift to us all. Once accessed, the unerring potency does the work. Each phase is offered as a conversation. What space is possible for you here? Can you access a state of balance? Can

you access the Health within the inertial fulcrum? Can the inertial potencies be expressed? Can the inertial forces be resolved?

Clinical Applications: Disengagement

The skill of disengagement or decompression is commonly taught within the CRI level of perception. Within the mid-tide level, the skill is the same, but the experience of the intention is subtler. In clinical practice it is more efficient to focus on the deeper tidal phenomena of the mid-tide and Long Tide, rather than the CRI. The CRI can be an important way into relationship with the suffering held within a person's system, but the healing forces are found within the deeper and slower tidal expressions. Because many practitioners learn this process

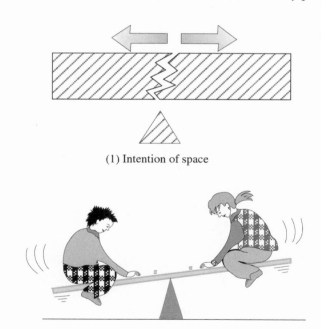

(1) Intention of space

(2) Acess the state of balanced tension, a state of dynamic equilibrium

19.1 Principle of disengagement

within the CRI level, I will first present this process from that level of perception. Once the point of balanced tension is obtained, the practitioner can learn to shift to the mid-tide level of action and begin to relate to the health within the disturbance being attended to. I will then describe the process from a mid-tide perspective, which is a more clinically effective, less tiring, and less activating starting point. I encourage you, if you are a practitioner and are used to working from a CRI level, to begin to explore the deeper tidal phenomena. If you are a student within a dynamically oriented course, I encourage you to learn this work from a mid-tide level of action and perspective.

I will outline this in two steps. In the first step you will access the point or state of balanced tension. In the second step you will assume that the inertia is very dense and change the conversation to the conversation of disengagement.

Disengagement within the CRI: Accessing the Point and State of Balanced Tension

In this first process, you will initially bring attention to the system via the CRI level of perception. Information here is obtained by listening to the relationship of individual parts, by analyzing, and by motion testing in various ways. In this perceptual exercise you are interested in the interplay of individual structures and will help access a point of balanced membranous tension within the tissue elements. You will then, within the point of balance, widen and deepen your perceptual field to the mid-tide level of awareness and shift or deepen into the state of balanced tension where you have more direct perceptual access to the forces at work.

1. Place your hands in either vault hold. Negotiate your relationship with the patient's system. Let's start from the CRI level of perception. Let your hands float on the tissues and narrow your perceptual field to the bones and membranes of the cranium. Get interested in how the individual structures are moving. Notice flexion and

extension at the SBJ. In inhalation the greater wings of the sphenoid and the occipital squama will be sensed to rotate caudad as the SBJ rises. The faster CRI level of action may then enter your narrowed perceptual field.

2. Stay with this awareness and notice how the different bones being palpated express their motion. See if you can notice any patterns of resistance, motion, membranous pulls, and so on. which may lead you to a particular sutural relationship. Alternately, for practice purposes, you may want to palpate each major bone and bony relationship already learned. So you might start off at the vault hold, move to a frontal hold, then a parietal hold, then to the temporal bones, and finally to an occipital hold. Note the reciprocal tension motions and patterns of inertia within each relationship. In practice situations take your time to get familiar with the motions of each structure and see if you are drawn to a particular suture. At a CRI level you might sense resistance between bones, eccentric reciprocal tension motions between structures, membranous pulls into sutural relationships, and so forth.

3. Choose a particular sutural relationship that is most prominent in its sense of resistance and inertia. Make a relationship with that particular suture. Let's say that you sensed an inertial fulcrum between the frontal bone and zygomatic bone. Move to the sutural relationship by making contact with the two bones involved. Let's say that you noticed a pattern of resistance at the fronto-zygomatic suture. In that case, place the fingertips of one hand over the frontal bone near the fronto-zygomatic suture and the fingers of the other hand over the zygomatic bone, also near the suture. You are now in relationship to the two poles of the sutural relationship. One hand is on the frontal bone, and the other is on the zygomatic bone. In this exercise you are free to choose any inertial relationship that

comes into your field of awareness. The main thing is that the fingers of each hand are placed on either side of the suture, on the two poles of the relationship. (See Figure 19.2.)

4. In this position, listen to the motion dynamic as it unfolds. How is motion organized around that suture? Is there any motion discernible at all? Follow the perceived dynamic. As you sense the reciprocal tension quality of the motion, help the tissues access the point of balanced membranous tension. This will be like helping a children's teeter-totter find the exact neutral point of balance around the fulcrum organizing its motion. You may sense the tension patterns around the suture finding a place of balance. Help the tissues find the precise neutral around which all membranous tensions are reconciled. Listen for the settling of the tissues into this point of balance.

5. Now, within this point of balance, shift your perceptual field to the mid-tide level of perception. Let your hands float within fluid and widen your perceptual field to the biosphere. Within this wider field, include potencies, fluids, and tissues in your awareness. As you do this, you may sense the point of balanced tension deepening into a state of balanced tension in which there is a deeper settling, and a neutral arises that includes all three functions (potency, fluids, and tissues). This state of balance has depth and can be, as we have already seen and will explore below, the gateway into even deeper levels of action.

Disengagement within the Mid-Tide

Step One: Accessing the State of Balanced Tension

In this approach, you will start your perceptual journey within the mid-tide. This is ideally where you would begin to listen from. You may sense how information is communicated to you differently at this level of perception. Here you are more in relation-

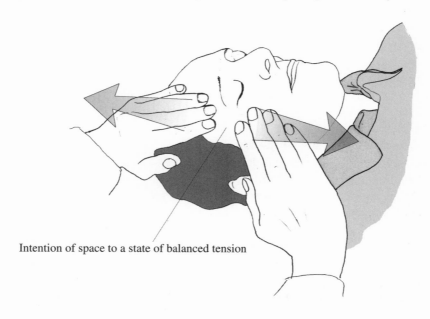

Intention of space to a state of balanced tension

19.2 Disengagement across the fronto-zygomatic suture

ship to the whole of the person and the biosphere, and rather than simply perceiving individual tissue motions, you may sense the tensile motions of structures as part of a wider whole. Thus, as the system communicates information about a particular inertial fulcrum to you, rather than just perceiving this as resistance between parts, you will more directly sense the organization of the whole tensile field around that inertial fulcrum. Information received this way is more precise and obtained with much less effort than at the CRI level. It is a matter of maintaining a wide perceptual field, listening, and allowing the system to clarify its intentions and communicate them to you.

1. Again start from the vault hold. Negotiate your contact with the client's system. Let your hands float within fluids and widen your perceptual field to the biosphere. You are holding the whole person and his or her field of environmental interchange within your perceptual field. Your attention is on the *whole* with an awareness of the particulars within that whole. It is important not to narrow your perceptual field as you become aware of particular structures and fulcrums within the wider field.

2. Settle into a relationship with the system within the mid-tide. You may start to sense the 2.5 cycles a minute tidal phenomenon as you listen to the wider field. You may sense the tissue being palpated expressing this rate of motion within a unified tensile field. You can still perceive individual motions, but an inner motility is more apparent and the structures are sensed to be part of a whole tensile field of action. You will sense the surge and settling of the tidal forces within this motion. Give the system time and space to communicate to you. Settle into this listening space. As you listen, the inherent treatment plan may begin to unfold and a specific within the system will begin to clarify.[1]

3. As you listen, specific inertial patterns may begin to clarify within your field of awareness. Listen to the tensile motion of these patterns. You may sense that the whole tissue field distorts around a particular inertial fulcrum within the cranium. See if a particular sutural relationship begins to clarify as the tissue field organizes around it. In clinical practice, you might help access the state of balance from this vantage point at the vault hold and then see what inertial issues are left. Here you will go directly to the sutural relationship discovered.

4. As above, place your fingers on either side of the suture being focused on. Let's again assume that you are drawn to the fronto-zygomatic suture. Place your fingers on either side of the suture. Reestablish your wider perceptual field. Again tune into the 2.5 cycles a minute mid-tide. Don't lose a sense of listening to the whole via the biosphere as you relate directly to the suture. Let the suture be a particular within the wider field. Don't narrow your perceptual field. Listen for Dr. Becker's three-step process. Notice the potency, fluids, and tissues moving towards a state of balanced tension. You may sense the whole tensile tissue field seeking a neutral in relationship to the specific inertial fulcrum being palpated. At most, simply slow the perceived motion dynamic down and listen for a settling into the state of balance and stillness.

Step Two: The Skill of Disengagement

Accessing the state of balanced tension as reviewed above may be all that is necessary for the inertial forces to be initiated and for the healing resources of the system to be expressed. However, if the suture is strongly compressed and deeply inertial, there may not be enough space within it to allow potencies to be expressed within the state of balance. Biodynamic potencies may be very condensed and deeply coiled in order to center strongly inertial forces. In this case, you can suggest an intention of space within the suture, which is classically called disengagement. This intention is about accessing the potential space, which is always available within even the deepest compressive issue. It is not about releasing anything.

Staying with the example above, let's say that you focused on the fronto-zygomatic suture. Perhaps you have facilitated the state of balanced tension, yet the inertial potencies are not expressing themselves. Don't hang out there if nothing is happening. It is important at this stage to engage in other kinds of conversations. You have already learned to direct fluids and potency to an inertial site and to intensify lateral fluctuations. Although either of these approaches can be useful here, our intention is to learn another skill to widen your clinical options. Let's now try the intention of disengagement as a new clinical skill. Your hand position is on either side of the fronto-zygomatic suture as above (or any other suture being attended to). You can use either of the following two options to initiate a conversation about space and disengagement. In both cases we will initiate this process within the mid-tide level of action.

Option One

1. Maintain a wide perceptual field. Listen through the 2.5 cycles a minute mid-tide. Hold this wide field as you become aware of the particular suture and the forces organizing its inertia. Don't narrow your field of listening. Subtly traction the two bones away from each other. This is offered as a *conversation* about potential space. This is an intention, an inquiry into space, not a demand to change or to release anything. This is as much intentional as physical. Do not narrow your perceptual field as you bring this conversation to the potency-fluid-tissue field. Maintain an awareness of the whole. Notice the response of the tissue elements as you intend this. This will have a tensile-fluidic quality to it. Listen. Remember that connective tissues are liquid crystalline in nature. You are always re-

lating to a unified fluid-tissue matrix. As you bring the intention of space to the relationship, you will sense potential space opening and a boundary to your intention as the tensile nature of the potencies, fluids, and tissues respond to your conversation and inquiry into space. This boundary is a communication about what is possible. Do not override what the dynamics can express. This is not a demand. This is not about decompressing anything. You are engaged in a conversation about the potential space that is already there. (See Figure 19.2.)

2. Help access the state of balanced tension near the boundary of your intention of space. This is the edge of the potential space allowable, given the compressive forces involved. If you override or push against this boundary, the system will respond to your touch as a force that needs to be contained and centered. You will lock up the potencies, fluids, and tissues involved, and the healing process will not unfold. Near this boundary, potencies, fluids, and tissues may naturally settle into a state of balanced tension. You may sense the tissue elements seeking this neutral as they rock and shift around the fulcrum that is organizing their dynamic. You can help them settle into stillness, if necessary, by subtly slowing these motions down, as you might with a children's seesaw, using the contacts you have made on both bones. This is very subtle, and you must not narrow your perceptual field as you intend this. Alternately, you can bring this intention of slowing down into the fluid and potency elements too.

Option Two

1. In the second approach, you can first stabilize one of the bones. For instance, in this case you might stabilize the frontal bone. Do this with a gentle intention within your palpating hand. Do not use pressure or force to do this. It is only an intention communicated via your gentle touch.

After stabilizing the frontal bone, gently and subtly intend the zygomatic bone away from it at the fronto-zygomatic suture. This is a gentle suggestion of space in the opposite direction to the stabilized bone. Intend this, as above, to the boundary of space allowed in that direction. Do not override what the system can allow. This is a conversation about space. It is not a demand. It is not about decompressing anything. At or near this boundary, help the tissue elements access the neutral, the state of balanced tension. (See Figure 19.3.)

Following On

1. In either case, once the state of balance is obtained listen for expressions of Health within the state of balance. Remember Dr. Becker's three-step process. The state of balance has been accessed, and you are now listening within the stillness. Within this state of balance, also allow an awareness of the midline to come to you.[2] This orients the field to its most primal ordering axis. Listen for expressions of Health. These may include fluid fluctuations, pulsations, and various expressions of potency. You may sense subtle permeations of potency within the inertial relationship and streaming of heat or energy as force vectors resolve. You may perceive many interesting things.

2. Pay close attention to the dynamics within the suture, but do not narrow your perceptual field as you do this. As you maintain your wider perceptual field, let these phenomena come to you. You may sense pulsation within the suture. This is an expression of the biodynamic and biokinetic forces that center and maintain the compression. They are initiated and expressed within the state of balance. As this occurs the

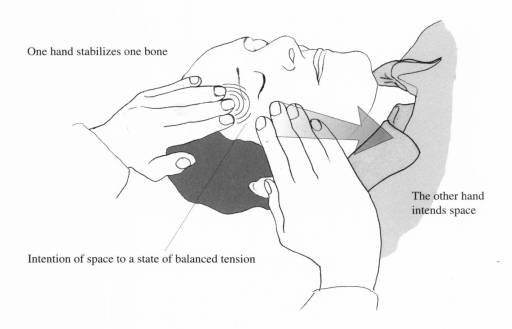

One hand stabilizes one bone

The other hand intends space

Intention of space to a state of balanced tension

19.3 Disengagement via stablilising one pole of the suture and intending space via the other

potency of the Breath of Life may well up within the inertial fulcrum. You may sense a permeation of potency into the inertial area. This is a field phenomenon. The whole tensile field of potency may come into play. It is important for the practitioner to recognize the expression of Health even in the most seemingly disordered circumstances. Remember that within even the most compressed relationship, there is always a kernel of Health centering the disturbance.

3. In stage three of Dr. Becker's process, the bio-electric, fluid, and tissue elements will again begin to move. This is not an unwinding of anything. It is a reorganization to natural fulcrums and to the primal midline itself. It is a remembering of an Original intention carried within the fluids of the embryo. Wait for a expansion of the sutural relationship and a greater ease in tensile motion. Finish by returning to the vault hold and notice if the tissues and tissue motion have reoriented to Sutherland's fulcrum and to the midline.

Disengagement from Within

Disengagement is a truly profound concept to grasp. It is really about the deeper intentions of the Breath of Life manifesting as the Original matrix is reestablished. It is about the intentions of the Breath of Life of life disengaging inertial forces from within. As you work with the intentions of disengagement and widen your perceptual field more and more, you will discover that disengagement is intrinsic to the function of the system as a whole. It is not a factor of your intervention, but is about a reconnection to the most primal organizing forces within the human body. These forces arise at the moment of conception, organize the developmental motions of cells within the embryo, and are with us until death. We have discussed the state of balance and stillpoint as entrées into the epigenetic forces and the Original

matrix itself. Here we will discuss disengagement in this same light.

On another level, disengagement is a concept that clarifies how bones and tissue structures move. In the inhalation surge of the Tide, an inner intraosseous motion is generated within bones and tissue structures. As this occurs, sutures and joints also expand. Space is generated within the suture or joint relationship. Within this space, there is a disengagement of the suture that allows an interosseous motion between structures to be expressed too. Here disengagement is seen to be a function of the ordering forces of the Breath of Life. Space allows disengagement, and disengagement allows motion. Disengagement is perceived to be one of the principles around which natural motility and motion occur. When inertial forces are present that do not allow the space to be accessed and the disengagement to occur, dysfunction arises. A loss of mobility results. Within a state of balance, the potency of the Breath of Life has the opportunity to resolve the inertial issue, and then a disengagement of the tissue relationship is again possible. Again, this occurs from within and is not a factor of your intervention. When the potency of the Breath of Life really comes through an inertial fulcrum, it is seen that disengagement truly comes from within. You may literally sense a drive or permeation of potency into the inertial fulcrum and the fluid-tissue elements all disengaging as a response to this action from within. It is a powerful and humbling process to witness.

Within the CRI level of perception, disengagement can be perceived to be a factor of practitioner intervention. "There is compression, I will decompress it." Disengagement can seem to be a factor of practitioner intention as resistance is perceived to be a problem to solve. At a mid-tide level of perception, disengagement may seem to be a factor of the potencies and forces at work within the system. The interplay between universal and conditional forces are perceived and, within the state of balance, the potency, as it acts within the fluids, is perceived to do the work. Within the Long Tide perceptual level, something else happens. There is a perception of potencies acting from the outside in. There can literally be an experience of the potency of the Breath of Life coming from space, entering the midline, and moving through the inertial fulcrum being explored. It is as if something gathers from the outside, wells up within the system, and moves right through the specific inertial fulcrum like wind through the eye of a hurricane. Then the experience is truly one of disengagement from within. Here there is a natural realignment to the Original intention of fluid, cellular, and tissue organization. The inherent potencies, within the depth of a stillness, bring you to the Original matrix itself as it unfolds its ordering function. It is about the nature of your presence, the stillness of your mind, and the natural balance of the sensory and motor functions of your awareness.

Clinical Application: Disengagement as the Mysterious Gateway

In the following process, you will use perceptual shifts to use the intentions of disengagement, the mysterious gateway or the eye of the needle, as an entrée into the deeper healing and ordering intentions of the Breath of Life. You will start from a perception of the biosphere and then shift to a much wider perceptual field. As you do this, the Long Tide may express itself. You may sense a much wider field of action, as if both you and the patient are within the same ocean, or greater field of organization. We will again use the fronto-zygomatic suture as an example.

Fundamentals Reviewed

It is really important here to establish a still clinical space. It contains, initiates, and holds the process. Remember your practitioner fulcrums, come into breath and sensation, let your mind still, and hold a wide and natural field of listening. This establishes a safe therapeutic space and is a call to the deeper healing resources within and beyond the conditional forces being centered. Much more important, it is a humbling entrée into a healing process, which is a mutual journey for both therapist and patient.

1. Again make contact with each bone on either side of the suture. In this exercise you will start at a mid-tide level of perception. Let your hands float on the bones and shift your perceptual field to the biosphere and the mid-tide. Let your hands be immersed within fluid and widen your perceptual field to the biosphere. Hold the whole body and the field around it within your field of awareness.

2. As you hold this whole within your perceptual field, you may sense the tissues as a unified tensile field of action. Notice the suture as a particular within that field. You may sense the whole tensile tissue field distort around the inertial forces held within the suture. Very subtly intend space across the suture. This is given in the sense of an offering. It is an inquiry into possibility and space. It is not a demand. Do not grab onto the tissues as you explore this. If you do, you will lock the tissues up and may unconsciously shift to the CRI.

3. As space is accessed, you may sense the inertial forces at work within the suture. Biodynamic and biokinetic forces have become coupled and an inertial fulcrum has resulted. In this process, biodynamic forces will attempt to center the inertial forces that are maintaining the disturbance in the system. Facilitate a state of balanced tension as outlined above. At most you may have to simply and subtly slow down the tissue, fluid, or potency elements involved. At this level of perception, you may experience that the state of balance is inherent within the inertial fulcrums being palpated.

4. Once the state of balance deepens, widen your perceptual field towards the horizon. Let your hands float within potency and shift your perceptual field towards the horizon. Widen your perceptual field to where it still feels safe and contained. As you do this, you may sense the deeper, slower tidal phenomenon of the Long Tide. The midline imperative generated by the Breath of Life may also become more obvious here.

5. Listen with an awareness of the intention of disengagement within the state of balance. The inherent biodynamic forces may begin to express their healing intentions. You may actually have an experience of the potency of the Breath of Life coming from "somewhere else," moving through the midline, through the tensile fields of the body, through the heart of the inertial fulcrums being attended to. As this occurs, you may have a direct perception of the biodynamic forces disengaging the sutural issue. The biokinetic forces resolve, and disengagement is perceived to truly occur from the inside out.

6. It may feel like intrinsic forces from within come through a mysterious gateway to disengage the sutural compression. Like the eye of the needle, the shift in your perceptual fields can bring you to the most formative organizing forces at work. The intention of disengagement and the state of balance can bring you, like the eye of a needle, to the Original matrix itself. The motion of the potency of the Breath of Life through the inertial fulcrums, like a fountain spray of life, is most clearly experienced here as the force that disengages and resolves the inertial issue. Even deeper, within this context, as you settle into an even deeper stillness, one in which your mind is truly neither coming nor going, the Dynamic Stillness may unfold. This ground of emergence is one where a mystery truly unfolds, and healing processes are impersonal, natural, and not about the centering of conditional forces. Here the question truly unfolds into its own answer.

I hope the process outlined above gives you a way into the intentions of disengagement. You will find that this intention is used over and over again within the cranial concept. It is about the accessing of space and potential. Explore this over and over again in your practice sessions until the intentions and responses of the system become clear to you. In this process, it is important not to impose your will upon the dynamics of the system. If you do, you will simply be chasing the system's reactions to your presence and intentions. You will end up chasing shadows. This learning process is truly part of your developing ability to converse with the system. If approached respectfully and intelligently, the potencies, fluids, and tissues of the system will be happy to tell you their story. Do you have the will and the ears to hear it? As this story is shared, you are in the privileged position of also listening to the Health at the heart of that story. We are always holding a balance of awareness between universal and conditional forces. The important thing within this process is to respect that dynamic and the inherent treatment plan that unfolds from this interplay.

1. See the last chapter in this volume for a discussion of the inherent treatment plan.

2. The primal midline is located within the axis defined by the notochord. It rises from the coccyx, through the centerline of the vertebral bodies, through the cranial base and ethmoid bone. Tissue motility and motion naturally orients to this midline. It is discussed in detail in *Volume Two*.

20 .... **Traction**

The last few chapters introduced some of the active conversation skills in the cranial concept. These included conversation skills related to the state of balanced tension, to fluid fluctuation, and to disengagement and space. In this chapter, we will continue with this exploration by introducing the conversation skill of *traction*. When you subtly introduce the intention of traction into the dynamics of tissues, they will begin to speak to you. They will relate their history, compensations, and defensive patterns to the respectful and skilled observer. They will tell their story. The principle of traction has a number of clinical uses. These include:

1. The engagement of membranes and connective tissues generally in a conversation about history and tensile dynamics.

2. The engagement of local fulcrums, such as compressed sutures, in a conversation about history, space, and Health.

3. The engagement, via membranes and connective tissues, of remote fulcrums in a conversation about history, space, and Health.

In this chapter we will unfold these various intentions via classical approaches to the membrane and connective tissue system.

In this chapter we will:

- *Introduce the conversation skill of traction.*

- *Use the frontal, parietal, and temporal bones as examples of the application of traction as a conversation skill.*

- *Use the SBJ as a further example.*

Connective Tissues and Liquid Light

I would like to review some concepts here. In this chapter, you will learn to generate a certain kind of intention within membranes and connective tissues. It is important to remember that connective tissues are fluid media. Connective tissues form within a fluidic ground matrix. Furthermore, collagen fibers are hollow and are filled with fluid. The fluid in collagen fibers has a similar composition to cerebrospinal fluid. Let's review some important research in relationship to fluids and tissues. It has been shown that the fluids within collagen fibers are an ordered network of water molecules, connected by hydrogen bonds, which create a unified and cohesive fluid field. Collagen fiber itself is made up of triple helix tripeptides. The peptides are wound around each other in a helical manner. There is clear evidence that the fluid within the collagen fibers forms coherent molecular bonds with these peptides. The fluid-cellular matrix that results forms a unified and ordered field throughout the body. Collagen fiber, and its ordered fluid field have been likened to *liquid crystal*. The fibers assemble into coherent sheets, which form an open, liquid crystalline meshwork of molecules throughout the body. This meshwork has been found to be a unit of function, that is, a *whole*. Furthermore, this unified fluid-tissue field is malleable and responsive to stresses and environmental inputs. A stress anywhere within the field will effect the whole field. In others words, scientists are discovering that the fluid and tissue system within the body is truly whole and responds to internal and environmental inputs as a whole. There is further evidence that this fluid-tissue matrix is a field of rapid communication, much faster than the nervous system, and that this occurs within a coherent, quantum-level bioelectric field of action. Communication throughout this field is organized as a *whole* in coherent quantum wave forms, perhaps at near the speed of light!

There is also evidence that cerebrospinal fluid contains a high charge of light photons generated by the DNA from the cells that line the ventricles of the brain. Russian scientists have discovered that light photons are concentrated within the cerebrospinal fluid and move in coherent wave forms throughout the fluid system. Due to these discoveries, an even faster system of communication has been postulated, that of coherent wave forms of "liquid light" within the cerebrospinal fluid and collagen fibers of the body! Here Dr. Sutherland's intuition is being borne out by scientific inquiry.[1]

There is thus a unified liquid crystal matrix expressed as a whole throughout the body. This matrix is a unified field of communication. Furthermore, it has been postulated that this system is one whereby states of consciousness are quickly communicated throughout the body as bioelectrical inputs, which mobilize the cells for various kinds of activity. Thus

we have a unified and coherent bioelectric, fluid and tissue field, a true unit of function. We now have the three functions of potency, fluids, and tissues, which are appreciated in the practice of craniosacral biodynamics, being discussed within scientific circles as a unified field of action!

These three unified functions are:

- the potency of the Breath of Life, which is expressed as a subtle bioelectric field,

- the fluid matrix,

- and the tensile tissue field; all three of which form a unified field of action as described above.

All of this has huge implications for the healing arts, no matter in what framework they are practiced. In the cranial concept we consciously work with this unified bioelectric, fluid, and cellular matrix and this is, perhaps, one of the strengths of our work. Here we are seeing scientific input that supports some of the foundations of work in this field, even Dr. Sutherland's insight when he spoke of *liquid light*.

Connective Tissues and Stress

Connective tissues all have tensile capacity. Even bone and membrane, which are relatively inelastic, have this ability. As stated in the chapter on inertial fulcrums, tissues under stress will contract to protect the organism. Membranes, fascia, ligaments, and tendons will all contract when placed under stress. This ability to contract is critical to understand. It can even be seen at a cellular level as the microtubules within the cell also have the ability to contract. Here we can see that the microcosm and macrocosm are reflections of each other. Connective tissues respond to stress as a whole field of action. As we have seen, a stress anywhere within the field will be expressed throughout the field. There is now much scientific evidence for this assertion.

There is even evidence for a "crystal memory," which is based in the continuity of the bioelectric matrix with the fluid and tissue field. Perhaps it can be said that the bioelectric matrix is what originates and maintains the order of the collagen-fluid matrix. Dr. Mae-Wan Ho and Dr. David Knight write about what they call "crystal memory," that is, memory based upon the crystalline nature of the fluid-collagen matrix:

> As the collagens and bound water form a global network, there will be a certain degree of stability, or resistance to change. This constitutes a memory, which may be further stabilized by cross-linking and other chemical modifications of the collagens. The network will retain tissue memory of previous experiences, but it will also have the capacity to register new experiences, as all connective tissues, including bones, are not only constantly intercommunicating and responsive, but also undergo metabolic turnover like the rest of our body. Memory is thus dynamically distributed in the structured network [e.g., the bioelectric, fluid-collagen field—Ed.] and the associated, self-reinforcing circuits of proton currents, the sum total of which will be expected to make up the DC (direct current) body field itself.[2]

In the terms of craniosacral biodynamics, tissue memory is a function of the bioelectric potency of the Breath of Life. In our terms, it is the potency, as a unified field of action, which maintains the organization of the unified fluid-tissue field. As we have seen, when traumatic forces are introduced into the body, the potency of the Breath of Life will condense, or coalesce, to protect the organism within its unified field of action. This can be likened to a quantum-level bioelectric field of action in which the bioelectric field acts as a whole to meet forces that enter its domain. The very nature of the field is to be responsive. As inertial forces enter the field, the potencies that make it up naturally track the motion and force of the traumatic impact. Potencies will coalesce and compress in order to contain the biokinetic forces introduced to the system. Fluids and tissues will follow this imperative. Fluids will densify under stress and tissues will contract and compress. When tissues are exposed to traumatic forces and inertial potencies, they will contract to protect their integrity. If these inertial forces cannot be processed within the immediacy of the experience, then this protective tissue contraction may be retained by the system. This is because the biokinetic forces that originally generated the contraction have not been resolved. Inertial fulcrums will result and the tissues will continue to organize around them. *This is important.* Tissue memory is not about the past. It is about unresolved forces that are maintaining the disturbance in the present. It is about current origins, not past history per se. There is a history, a context, but the forces originating the disturbances within the field are still present. Patterns of tensile and compressive distress will be retained by the system as a whole and will not resolve until the biokinetic forces that originate and organize them are processed in present time.

The tendency for connective tissues to maintain a tensile pattern of contraction is sometimes called *tissue memory*. As we have seen, it is not so much that tissues are remembering a past experience, it is more that the forces around which they had to organize during the trauma or environmental insult have not been resolved. They still must organize around them. One of the intentions of the work is to help the system resolve these forces. When inertial forces resolve, tissues are again free to reorient to their natural fulcrums and the primal midline. They can return to their original intention and natural motility. When a practitioner introduces *traction* into the tissue system, he or she is initiating a conversation with the tensile forces that organize the inertial pattern. This is a conversation with the biodynamic potency and biokinetic forces found within the heart of the inertial fulcrums and with the related strain patterns organized by their action. During this conversation, the history, conditioning, and suffering of that person may be communicated and the Health accessed. In the following exercises, the intention will be to engage in an active conversation with tissues via traction.

The intention will be:

1. to start a conversation with tensile patterns of conditioning held within the tissues,

2. to start a conversation with the fulcrums and forces that are organizing that pattern, and

3. to access the Health that is centering it.

Engaging in the Conversation of Traction

In this section, you will learn to directly relate to inertial fulcrums via the skill of *traction*. Here we will be focusing on the membrane system within the cranium. In the second volume of this book, we will extend this concept to the dural tube and to connective tissues throughout the body. We will also look at this process in terms of the major joints of the body. Here we are focusing on the reciprocal tension membrane within the cranium. You will again be offering this work as a conversation with tissues and inertial fulcrums. You will learn to use various structures as "handles" into the membrane-connective tissue system. Many of these approaches have classical names, such as "frontal lift" or "parietal lift." Here we are introducing the process more as a skill of conversation than as a means to release resistance related to specific bones, although this will also happen. The conversation will initially be about the tensile patterns within the tissues and the fulcrums that organize these patterns.

Once an inertial fulcrum is engaged via the intention of traction, then the conversation will change in its intention. It will shift to an exploration of the state of balance and an exploration of the Health found within the heart of the fulcrum. When

you introduce traction into the tissue system, you are really initiating a conversation with the unified bioelectric, fluid-tissue matrix discussed above. Within this field there is condensed potency, congested fluid, and compressed tissue. As you introduce traction into the field, you are engaging the whole of this, which is organized in some way by current inertial forces. The biokinetic forces found within the inertial fulcrums may be of traumatic, environmental, or pathogenic origin. They may even be factors of mutation and genetic process. In the conversation with the unified field, the intention is to help generate a communication between these conditional forces and the potency of the Breath of Life and the Original matrix it carries. Let's see where we get with this in terms of your perceptual processes.

As you palpate a particular cranial structure, you may perceive a pattern of motion that is organized around an inertial fulcrum of some kind. Thus, the motion palpated may not only be organized around the natural automatically shifting fulcrum ideally located within the straight sinus, but may also be organized around an inertial fulcrum. Remember that natural fulcrums automatically shift with the intentions of the Tide, while inertial fulcrums do not. You may perceive this as a place of inertia, a distortion within the tissue, fluid, or potency field, or as a membranous or connective tissue strain or pull. The inertial fulcrum may or may not be located directly around or within that structure. It may be local to the structure, like a suture, or remote, like another joint relationship. Remember that the tissue system is *one thing*. As seen above, not only are connective tissue relationships within the body continuous, but they are truly one unified tensile field. Remember that the whole tissue system will express and compensate for any unresolved inertial forces and potencies present. The strain or inertial pattern generated by an organizing fulcrum will take shape within the tissue system as a whole. Compensatory fulcrums will also arise because of this continuity of function. Compensations and eccentric motion dynamics will result. Thus a compressive fulcrum within the SI joint may give rise to a related compensatory fulcrum within the O/A area, and so on.

Thus, as you palpate a structure, you may sense a particular motion dynamic whose fulcrum seems to be remote to it. Trust your perception and intuition as you notice this. For instance, as you palpate the frontal bone, you may sense that its motion is organized around somewhere else in the body. Be open to this possibility. Perhaps you noticed a pull posterior towards the occiput, or even noticed a pattern of motion organized around a fulcrum below the cranium. For instance, unresolved biokinetic forces may give rise to a place of vertebral fixation. Let's say that this fulcrum is located within the dynamics of T4. This may give rise to dural adhesion, which may be expressed at the anterior pole of the falx in some way. This may, in turn, effect the frontal and ethmoid bones and their motility and mobility. It may even generate compression within the ethmoid notch of the frontal bone, or within any of its sutural dynamics. Think of the connective tissue field as one thing, with bones being compression structures and membranes, connective tissues, and muscles being tension structures which are all continuous. Strains will be expressed throughout this unified field as a whole.

When you a access a *state of balanced tension* within a particular tissue relationship or pattern, its organizing fulcrum may be remote to its local dynamics. Sometimes accessing the state of balanced tension is all that is needed. The inherent intelligence of the system will express its potency within a state of balance within the organizing fulcrum. For instance, as you work with the frontal bone and help access the state of balanced tension, your patient may become aware of motion, heat, and pulsation somewhere remote to it. Perhaps its motion is organized around a sacroiliac joint, or a hip joint, or a vertebral relationship. The patient may notice the remote area pulsating and its inertia resolving. The dynamic at the frontal bone would then also tend to resolve. Sometimes, however, you will find that it is useful to engage the inertial fulcrum more directly from your vantage point. In the following sections,

we will introduce some ways of doing this via traction. We will describe this process at the frontal bone, the parietal bone, the temporal bones, and at the SBJ. We will first use the frontal bone as an example of the principle.

The Principle of Traction via the Frontal Bone

In this section we will be exploring a process in which you will learn to introduce a subtle traction into the reciprocal tension membranes via the frontal bone. The following process will allow you, as practitioner, to be in a more direct relationship to inertial fulcrums, and to engage these fulcrums in a conversation via the tissues. For instance, as you listen to the motion dynamics of the frontal bone, you may become aware of a membranous pull or sutural inertia effecting it. Alternately, you may sense a tensile motion via the frontal bone organized around a fulcrum remote to its local sutural dynamics. The intention of traction can begin a conversation with the inertial fulcrum and the forces that organize it.

In this process, you will be introducing a subtle suggestion of traction into the membrane system via the frontal bone. As you do this, you will sense through the membrane system until you encounter an inertial fulcrum. You will know that you have engaged the fulcrum when you come to the boundary of your intention of traction. Engaging the boundary of your intention of traction begins to engage the inertial forces within a particular inertial fulcrum. In this, you are starting a conversation with the inertial forces and potencies that are maintaining and centering the pattern. In this conversation, you are also engaging the whole of the membranous articular strain pattern affecting the dynamics of the frontal bone.

When applied at the frontal bone, this process is classically called a *frontal lift*. As you palpate the frontal bone, a particular inertial pattern or issue may present itself. You can use the intention of traction to engage in a conversation with the tissues about a tensile pattern and its organizing fulcrum. As you sense into the membrane system via the frontal lift, you may become especially aware of the vertical aspect of the membrane system, the falx cerebri and cerebelli and the dural tube. You may sense an inertial fulcrum anywhere within these relationships, or elsewhere within the body. It may be a local fulcrum located within a suture, like the frontozygomatic suture, or a fulcrum more remote to the frontal bone. The intention will be to sense into the membrane system via the suggestion of traction to the boundary encountered. Accessing the boundary helps to access the fulcrum and the inertial forces, that are organizing the inertial pattern. The intention will then be to help the system access the state of balanced tension within the organizing fulcrum. It is thus a dual conversation, first a conversation with the membranes in order to discover what organizes their reciprocal tension motion, then a more direct conversation with the inertial fulcrum and the Health centering it. In the first aspect, the conversation is, "What organizes this pattern?" In the second, the conversation changes into a direct inquiry into the Health found at the heart of the inertial fulcrum itself. The conversation then becomes, "How can you express your Health here?"

Clinical Application: The Principle of Traction

The Frontal Lift

1. In the vault hold, access your practitioner neutral and negotiate your contact with the patient's system. Widen your perceptual field to the biosphere. First sense the fluid tide and the expression of potency within it. Note the quality of this. Then include the tensile tissue field within your awareness. Let the tissues begin to speak to you within the mid-tide and its 2.5 cycles a minute rhythm. Do you sense any tensile patterns that seem to relate to the frontal bone from this vantage point? You may sense a mo-

tion pattern organized around the frontal bone, or a membranous pull into its relationships. You may sense the tissue field literally distorting around an inertial site. It may seem as if the bones and membranes of the cranium are literally distorting around a particular issue within its dynamics.

2. Then move to the frontal hold as learned earlier. (See Figure 20.1.) Again widen your perceptual field to the biosphere. Let the mid-tide (2.5 cycles a minute rhythm) again come into your awareness. Do not lose awareness of the frontal bone and of the tissues as you do this. Do not narrow your perceptual field down as you do this. Listen to the reciprocal tension motion of the frontal bone and the tissue field as a whole. Listen for the dynamics of the frontal bone as you hold the whole body, and the field around it, within your awareness. Can you sense the frontal bone as you listen to the whole biosphere? What is its expression of motility and mobility like? Does it relate to Sutherland's fulcrum in a balanced way? Is there a sense of an inertial fulcrum organizing its dynamic?

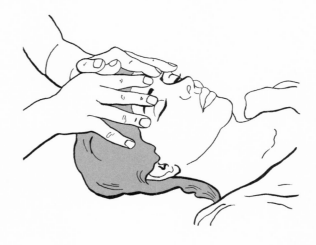

20.1 Frontal hold

3. Again, an inertial fulcrum may be sensed via an eccentric motion at the frontal bone, a subtle membranous strain or pull posterior through the falx, or through a sense that the motion of the frontal bone is organized around someplace remote to its immediate dynamics. You may even sense a distortion within the whole tissue field as you listen to its motility and motion. If you become aware of tensile distortions, the information received can be very precise. For instance, as you palpate the frontal bone, you may sense its continuity with the whole tissue field. You may sense a unified reciprocal tension motion expressed as a tensile action through all of the tissues at once. While palpating the frontal bone, you may then sense the tissues expressing a motion like a distortion within the whole field. If you sense a tensile distortion being communicated, bring the question, "What organizes this?" to your hands. In clinical practice, all that may be needed here is to acknowledge or facilitate a *state of balanced tension*. The inertial potencies may be initiated within that intention. Here we will, however, practice the intention of

traction via the frontal bone in order to learn a new conversation skill and more directly engage an inertial fulcrum in a conversation about history and Health.

4. With your hands in the frontal hold position, suggest/intend traction in an *anterior* direction (with the patient in the supine position, towards the ceiling). Initially, the intention is to very subtly engage the frontal bone and its tissues. Use the lateral aspects of the frontal bone as contact points for transferring the intention to the membranes. This is just a *suggestion;* do not apply any physical pressure, just an intention. First begin by bringing the intention to your fingers. Then extend the intention to the patient's skin and flesh covering the bone. Then extend the intention of anterior traction into the bone and then into the membrane system. It is an increasing intensification of your intention of traction into the tissue layers until you have engaged the osseous/membranous system. (See Figure 20.2.) If, when you do this, you sense any local sutural resistances, you can use the

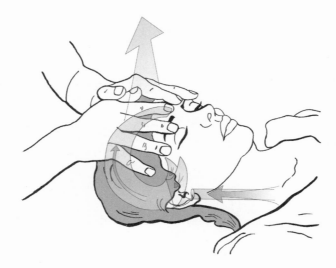

20.2 Frontal lift (frontal hold showing direction of traction)

331

V-spread process to help the system resolve them. Then return to your intention of traction as you engage the membranes. This is just a *suggestion;* do not apply any physical pressure, just an intention through your fingers.

5. You are encouraging a subtle traction within the membrane system via its relationship to the frontal bone. You may sense the frontal bone lifting subtly anterior. As you intend anterior traction, sense posteriorly through the reciprocal tension membranes. As you do this, you may sense a boundary to this intention. Engage the tissues with the intention of traction to this boundary. If there was no membranous articular strain effecting the frontal bone, you would sense a membranous fluidity in which the frontal bone is allowed to subtly float towards the ceiling with a sense of ease. The boundary accessed may relate to a local fulcrum around the frontal bone, or to a more remote fulcrum. As you do this, you are starting a conversation with the tissues about their history and about what organizes their motion dynamics. Do this very slowly and subtly. The tissues will show you their tension dynamic and the fulcrum that organizes it.

6. At the boundary to your intention, notice if you can sense the location of the inertial fulcrum that organizes the strain pattern. Once you have engaged the boundary, you have engaged the fulcrum that is organizing the pattern being palpated. This may be expressed at a tissue level as a place of sutural compression or tissue adhesion or as a site of tissue inertia located literally anywhere in the body. Remember that the tissue system is one thing and an inertial issue located anywhere affects the *whole*. You are initiating a conversation with membranes and tissues and with the inertial fulcrum that organizes their motion and motility. You may sense this fulcrum anywhere from the most an-terior aspect of the falx to the most inferior aspect of the dural membrane system at the coccyx or beyond.

7. At the boundary to your intention, help the system access its state of balanced tension just as you have practiced. Do not lose the intention of engagement via traction as you do this. Seek a neutral within the motion dynamic or tension pattern engaged. Remember Dr. Becker's three-step awareness of the healing process. Listen as the system expresses its self-healing processes within the stillness. Again, within the state of balanced tension, you may notice various self-healing processes coming into play. These may include expressions of potency and fluid fluctuations. Just listen to the dynamics within the stillness and sense how the Health of the system is expressed. When the inertial forces have resolved, you may sense a reorganization of the tissue system and the frontal bone may seem to float towards the ceiling.

8. When the inertial fulcrum has resolved or moved towards resolution, again listen to the motility and motion of the frontal bone. Is this more balanced? Is it expressed with more balance around Sutherland's fulcrum? Also notice the expression of the fluid tide. Is the fluid drive of the system stronger? Is there a clearer sense of longitudinal fluctuation?

Applying the Principle of Traction: The Parietal Bones

Let's apply this same principle to the parietal bone and its relationships. As you earlier listened to the dynamics of the parietal bones, you may have noticed eccentric or conditioned motion patterns of some kind. These might have included patterns of motility and of eccentric reciprocal tension motion. These motion patterns would not be organized purely around the action of Sutherland's fulcrum. They may have been organized around local fulcrums, like a sutural compression, or around a more remote fulcrum. You may, for instance, have sensed a membranous pull along the falx. This might have been transferred to the parietals from almost anywhere in the body. For instance, a compression in the occipitomastoid suture may have organized the motion of the parietals. Likewise, a vertebral fixation, or connective tissue adhesion remote to them, may have affected their dynamics. Alternately, you may have sensed an eccentric pattern of motion organized around a fulcrum remote to local dynamics. For instance, you may have been tracking a particular motion dynamic at the parietals and sensed it to be organized around a sacroiliac joint or other remote location.

In this clinical application, you will again use the principle of traction to engage an inertial fulcrum in conversation. This process is classically called a "parietal lift." Its intention is similar to the frontal lift explored above. It is best, however, to think of this as another application of the principle of traction, rather than as a technique. The intention of this work is to again sense into the membrane system via a subtle suggestion of traction and to follow the sense of the traction to any inertial fulcrums that may effect the dynamic at the parietal bones. At the boundary to your intention of traction, you will again help the system access its state of balanced tension. Here we are presenting this as another opportunity to practice the principle of traction in order to engage the membranes in a conversation. The parietal lift is commonly taught as a two-stage process. First a compression is applied to the parietals to disengage them from the squamosal suture. Secone, there is a superior or cephalad traction into the membranes. The first step is really unnecessary if the major sutural resistances around the parietals have been resolved. If they haven't, then the direction of fluid or disengagement processes described earlier can be used to resolve the local sutural issue effecting the parietals. In the following clinical ap-

plication you will be listening to the dynamics of the parietals and will then engage the membrane system directly via traction by using the parietals as the contact points.

Clinical Application: Traction via the Parietal Bones

The Parietal Lift

Again, hold the biosphere within the field of your awareness. With your hands in the parietal hold, sense the dynamics of the parietal bones. (See Figure 20.3.) Be sure to establish elbow fulcrums and to be comfortable as you do this. Do not narrow your perceptual field as you listen to the dynamics via the parietal bones. Listen to the particulars within this wider field of awareness. Sense how the parietal bones express their motility and motion within the 2.5 cycles a minute mid-tide. Also sense the quality of the fluid tide, its drive and potency. Again, allow your hands to just float on the tissues within fluid and notice how they are moved by the unified action of potency, fluid, and tissue. Be

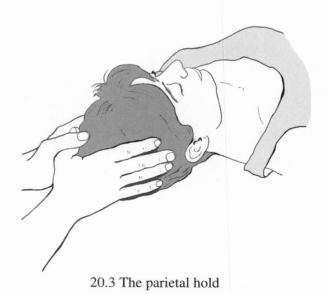

20.3 The parietal hold

333

sure that your finger contacts lie directly on the parietal bones and not on the squamosal sutures. In a clinical situation you might first follow the dynamics of the bones to their state of balanced tension. That is all that may be needed to elicit healing processes beyond the compensations held. Here we will go directly to the principle of traction for practice purposes.

1. From your parietal hold, very subtly suggest a cephalad traction (with the practitioner at the head of the table and the patient in the supine position, the cephalad lift is towards the practitioner). The intention of this is to introduce a subtle traction into the membrane system. Use the lateral aspects of the parietal bones, just above the squamosal suture, to engage the membranes in this intention. If, when you do this, you sense any local sutural resistances around the parietal bones, first use the V-spread process to help the system resolve them. Then return to your intention of traction as you engage the membranes. This is just a *suggestion;* do not apply any physical pressure, just an intention through your fingers. (See Figure 20.4.)

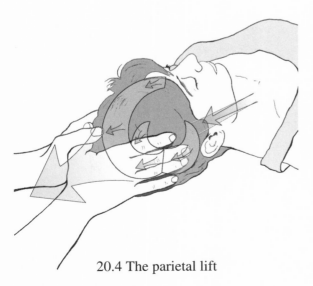

20.4 The parietal lift

2. First begin by bringing the intention to your fingers. Then extend the intention to the patient's skin and flesh covering the bone. Then extend the intention of cephalad traction into the bone and then into the membrane system. It is an increasing intensification of your intention of traction into the tissue layers until you have engaged the membrane system. Remember that bone is a connective tissue and all connective tissues are unified in their structure and function. As you do this, you may be able to feel/sense your way through the membrane system via the falx and dural tube. You are now, in a sense, using the parietal bones as windows into the membrane system. *Remember, you are using this process to initiate a conversation with the tissues about their experience.* Suggest this subtle traction into the membrane system to the boundary to your suggestion. The intention is to engage an inertial fulcrum in a conversation about history and Health via the intention of traction.

3. Near the boundary to your intention of traction, help the system access the state of balanced tension. Remember Dr. Becker's three-step awareness of the healing process. Listen as the system expresses its self-healing processes within the stillness. Listen for expressions of Health within the functional stillpoint within the state of balance. You sense may pulsation, various expressions of potency, fluid fluctuations, heat and force vector resolutions, and so on. You may sense a permeation of potency into the inertial area. Wait until you sense a softening and reorganization of the tissues. You may sense the parietal bones floating cephalad as the biokinetic forces that originally organized their inertial pattern are resolved.

4. Finally, listen again to the quality of the membranous articular motion. How do bone and membrane now express their dynamic as a unit of function? How do they relate to Sutherland's

fulcrum? Are the parietal bones expressing the potency of the Breath of Life as an inner motility in a more full and balanced way? Has the sense of fluid drive in the system increased, and are you sensing a clearer, stronger longitudinal fluctuation?

The Tentorium, the Three Diaphragms, and Structural Issues

In this section we will talk about the tentorium cerebelli in more detail. The tentorium cerebelli is a more or less transversely oriented membrane, which is "tentlike" in its position within the cranial bowl. It can be thought of as the transverse diaphragm of the cranium. Over the years, practitioners have noted a direct relationship between its dynamics and the dynamics of the other major transverse diaphragms of the body, the respiratory diaphragm and the pelvic diaphragm, or perineal floor. These three are sometimes called the "three diaphragms." These three express a triad of interrelated structural and homeostatic balance. Inertial issues located in any of the three diaphragms will be transferred to the others and resolution of inertia in any will, in turn, help resolve tension patterns in the others. They are thus in a reciprocal relationship and function as a triad unit of function. (See Figure 20.5.)

Structural issues effecting the horizontal balance of the body will be directly expressed within their transverse dynamics. For instance, torsion in pelvic dynamics will generate strain patterns in the transverse relationships of the three diaphragms and will also affect their direct structural relationships. Thus imbalance in the relationships of the hip joints and the sacroiliac joints will yield subsequent strain patterns in the pelvic diaphragm, the respiratory diaphragm, and the tentorium. Their structural relationships will also express this dynamic in some way. Hence the rib cage and its vertebral relationships may be compromised, as well as the position and function of the temporal bones and the cranial base in general.

The temporal bones and the tentorium are unified dynamic and are very sensitive to issues of structural balance. They will, as a unit of function, reflect the patterns of all the horizontal relationships in the body. Thus the temporal bones will express whatever compensations the body has had to make in order to maintain a balanced relationship to the earth. The temporal bones will express motions and positions relative to the other horizontal relationships in the body such as the thoracic inlet, the shoulder girdle generally, the diaphragm, the sacroiliac joints, and the hip joints, to name just a few.

As we have seen above, all connective tissues can be thought of as one thing, that is, a continuous and unified system. When you are in direct relationship to the tentorium, you are therefore also in relation-

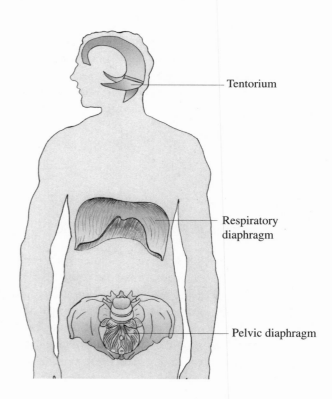

Tentorium

Respiratory diaphragm

Pelvic diaphragm

20.5 The three diaphragms

335

ship to all of the horizontal structural dynamics of the entire body. Structural compensations that arise in order to maintain homeostatic balance will affect the dynamics of the tentorium and will, in turn be affected by it. Thus the balance and integrity of the reciprocal tension membrane system is an expression of the balance and integrity of the whole body. As we have seen, the natural fulcrum of the reciprocal tension membranes is called Sutherland's fulcrum and is located within the straight sinus. This can also be thought of the natural fulcrum for all of the connective tissue dynamics in the whole body as membrane, fascia, and connective tissues form a *whole body reciprocal tension structure*. Thus accessing the state of balanced membranous tension, as learned earlier, has far-reaching implications within the whole body.

In the following exploration, we will be looking at the dynamics of the temporal bones in relationship to the tentorium and the reciprocal tension membranes in general. In this, it must not be forgotten that these dynamics have repercussions throughout the body, and a delicate homeostatic balance exists between all of the structures in the human system. Because structure and function are interrelated, the homeostatic balance of the structures of the body is crucial in its functioning.

Temporal Bones:
Medial Compression

In previous palpation sessions, you have listened to the dynamics of the temporal bones and their expression of motility and mobility. In these palpation sessions, you may have also noticed eccentric dynamics. Perhaps you noticed very little motility or motion, eccentric motions, or strong membranous pulls. It is not uncommon to perceive very little motion within the dynamics of the temporal bones. This may be an indication of compressive forces present within their relationship to the cranial base. The temporal bone may have become medially compressed between other cranial base structures.

Commonly, you may perceive compressive forces at work between the temporal bones and the occiput and/or sphenoid bone. If a compressive fulcrum is very intense, then you may not be able to sense much motion at all. The compressive pattern might be either unilateral, involving only one temporal bone, or bilateral, involving both. Medial compressions of bony relationships will obviously have membranous strains or tensions related to them. Remember that bone and membrane are a unit of function, and that patterns of inertia have classically been called *membranous articular strain patterns*.

In previous palpation sessions, as you worked with states of balanced tension, you were in direct relationship to the whole of a membranous articular strain pattern. Usually the state of balance allows the potencies within the inertial fulcrum to manifest in some way, and this is enough to resolve the inertial issue. However, it is important to learn to directly and appropriately relate to the specific type of inertia involved, because it may be critical in a treatment process to do so. In this case there might be both local and remote fulcrums effecting the dynamics of the temporal bones. There may be sutural resistances around the temporal bone, and there may be membranous strains transferred to it via the tentorium and connective tissues. If the local sutural compression was the primary fulcrum, then any membranous component would tend to resolve when the sutural issue resolved. However, there may be a remote fulcrum whose forces are transferred to the temporal bones via the membranes, and you might want to relate to these in a more direct way. Again, the principle of traction may allow you this more direct relationship.

As you palpated the temporal bones, you have sensed a membranous pull medially. This may relate to the strain patterns held within the dural membrane system and to a remote fulcrum. For instance, you might have been able to track this sense of membranous strain along the petrous ridge towards the SBJ or to somewhere else in the body. This remote fulcrum creates a membranous strain, which is transferred to the tentorium and then to the related temporal bone. A membranous strain or contraction within the tentorium cerebelli can cause a persistent medial compression of the temporal bone and cranial base. (See Figure 20.6.)

In this section, you will learn a new hold that will help you make a more specific relationship to the medially compressive forces affecting the temporal bones. It is called the *temporal ear hold*. The tem-

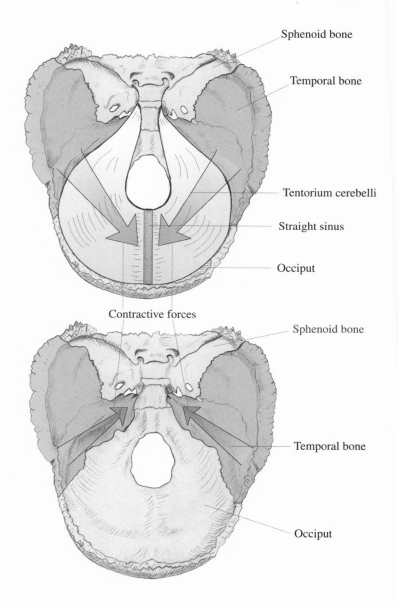

Sphenoid bone

Temporal bone

Tentorium cerebelli

Straight sinus

Occiput

Contractive forces

Sphenoid bone

Temporal bone

Occiput

20.6 Contraction in tentorium
(chronic contraction in tentorium can generate
medial compression issues within the cranial base)

poral ear hold can place you in a more direct relationship to medial compression of a temporal bone and to the membranous strains relating to them. Medial compression of the cranial base will commonly involve: (1) medial sutural compression of one or both temporal bones and (2) membranous strains transferred to the temporal bones via the tentorium.

Clinical Applications

Let's review some approaches to temporal bone patterns and the inertial forces that organize them. In the following clinical applications, you will be applying two of the principles you have already learned, the *state of balanced tension* and *traction*. We will first review the process of accessing a state of balanced tension within the mid-tide level of perception. Review is always useful.

(A) The State of Balanced Tension

1. In your original *temporal bone hold*, listen to the motility and motion of the temporal bones. Again hold a perceptual field that includes the whole of the biosphere and allow the mid-tide to come to you (the 2.5 cycles a minute tide). Notice any inertial issues, such as poor motility, lack of motion, or eccentric motion. Notice any sense of medial pull, or a sense of compression between the temporal bones and sphenoid and occiput. Do not narrow your perceptual field to do this. These issues may be perceived as a lack of motion, which exhibits a dense or congested quality. You may sense an anterior, medial pull towards the SBJ. Compressive pulls, if present, are commonly sensed along an approximately 45-degree angle from the horizontal of the treatment table, formed as the temporal bones rest within the wedge-shaped space between the occiput and sphenoid bones. The petrous ridge of the temporal bone follows this angle. As you listen within the mid-tide level of perception, you may sense a distortion within the

whole tissue field. If you do, again ask the question, "What organizes this?" (See Figure 20.7.)

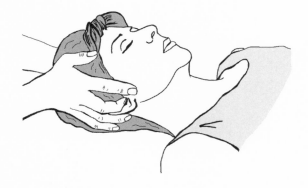

20.7 Temporal bone hold

2. Listen to the story that the temporal bones have to tell. As you palpate these dynamics, help access the state of balanced tension. Remember Dr. Rollin Becker's three-step awareness of the healing process. As you *seek the neutral*, you will discover that you are engaged in a delicate conversation with the tissues. Let them show you their history. Do not *do* anything. Simply listen and follow. Delicately *seek the neutral*. Subtly, using your finger contacts, help the tissues access their state of balanced tension. This may simply involve slowing the motion down, or more actively accessing a balanced state within the membranous articular tension dynamics. In this process, you will sense the reciprocal tension motion of the tissues. Via palpation, seek the *precise neutral* in this reciprocal tension motion. Seek the point where the tissues settle and access stillness, the functional stillpoint. This is a subtle process. It is a factor of your *attention* and *intention*. Let your hands float within fluid, sense the reciprocal tissue tensions, and subtly

adjust your relationship to these tension motions until a settling into stillness is perceived.

3. The state of balanced tension allows a direct relationship to the inertial forces that maintain and center the tissue compression. Accessing the state of balanced tension is the key to a healing relationship with these inertial forces. Within the state of balanced tension, the potency of the Breath of Life will be expressed within the inertial site. Over time, you will become very sensitive to the nature of compression and compressive forces and will be able to sense their precise location.

4. Listen within the stillness of the state of balanced tension. You are waiting to hear expressions of Health. You may sense the initiation of the inertial potencies involved. You may perceive expressions of potency as pulsation, fluid fluctuations, and heat release. You may even sense a permeation of potency within and around the inertial site. Sometimes this can be perceived to occur throughout the system as the potency wells up within the body. This occurs as the biodynamic and biokinetic potencies are expressed within the compression and the whole unified field of potency responds.[3] Remember that inertial potency is part of a greater whole and it is this whole that responds in a depth of healing process.

5. As you listen for expressions of Health, you may perceive these potencies at work. Part of this process will be the resolution of the biokinetic forces that maintained the inertial or compressive issue. As these forces are resolved, you may then perceive a sense of expansion and reorganization within the fluid and tissue relationships. As inertial forces and potencies resolve, fluids and tissues will resolve their compressions and contractions. Tissues will reorganize to natural fulcrums and the temporal bones may be sensed to disengage from compressed sutural relationships. You may even sense that the temporal bones float freely along the 45-degree angle they occupy within the cranial base. As the inertial forces are resolved, the tissues will have the opportunity to express their Original intention. You may also sense a better expression of motility and motion around Sutherland's fulcrum.

(B) The Temporal Bones and the Principle of Traction

In this section, you will be exploring the relationship of the temporal bones to the sutures around them and, most importantly, to the tentorium cerebelli and the membrane system more generally. To do this, you will be initiating a conversation with the tissues via traction. The tentorium stretches transversely between the two temporal bones. As you bring an intention of traction to the tissues, you will engage this transverse relationship. You will use a hold that will help you make a more specific relationship to medial compression and membranous strains relating to the temporal bones. It is called the *temporal ear hold*. Medial compression of the cranium may involve two related issues: (1) medial sutural compression of one or both temporal bones, and (2) the related membranous strains or tensions transferred to the temporal bones via the tentorium. When approaching these issues, it is important to remember that our intention is to make a relationship to the *forces* at work, not just to the resultant tissue resistances.

1. With the patient in the supine position, from the original temporal bone hold, place your hands in a *temporal ear hold* position. To do this, place your fingers posterior behind and around the ears with fingertips at the temporal bones and thumbs over the ear canal. You are basically cupping the ears posterior with your fingertips where the ears meet the cranium, while you place your thumbs over the ear canals. (See Figure 20.8.)

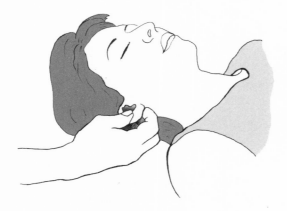

20.8 Temporal bone ear hold

Via your *temporal ear hold*, you first subtly engage the tissues of the ears, then the temporal bones, and then the tentorium. As you do this, you are engaging the unit of function of the two temporal bones and the tentorium. As you bring the intention of traction into the tissues, you may also sense the location of any inertial fulcrum that effects temporal bone dynamics. See if you can follow your intention of traction to the location of any inertial fulcrums effecting temporal bone mobility. (See Figure 20.9.)

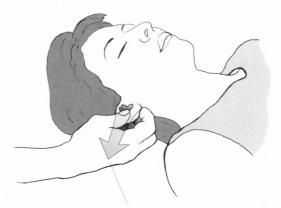

45° Intention towards the table

20.9 Intention of traction
via ear hold

2. If, after accessing the state of balanced tension, you do not sense a natural disengagement of the temporal bones, you can use this hold to engage in a different conversation with the tissues involved. This will entail intending using traction to engage in a conversation with the organizing forces involved. You can do this by placing a subtle suggestion of traction into the tissues being palpated. When you place a subtle traction into the membranes, a conversation is started. Remember that the intention of traction is not to impose your will on the system, but to begin a negotiated conversation. The tissues will tell you their story, and it can be deeply acknowledged.

3. Intend traction along a 45-degree angle away from the cranial base towards the treatment table. The direction of your intention of traction is along the 45-degree angle of the axis of the wedge-shaped space in which the temporal bones rest. This is along the axis of the petrous ridges of the temporal bones. This must be an intention or suggestion; you are not exerting any physical force. It is initiating a conversation.

4. As previously learned, the intention of traction is a subtle suggestion. Here, you are not pulling on someone's ears. In intending traction, you are first beginning a conversation about space within the sutural relationships around the temporal bones. You are also directly engaging the tentorium cerebelli and thus any membranous strains that relate to them. Finally, you are beginning a conversation with the inertial fulcrum, or fulcrums, which organize the inertia being palpated. The basic conversation is,

"What organizes this?" As you intend traction, you may sense a boundary to your intention. Do not override this. The tissues are communicating the location of the inertial fulcrums.

5. Help the system access its *state of balanced tension* near the boundary to your intention of traction. Now the conversation changes from, "What organizes this?" to " How can you express your Health here?" Again, this is a delicate exploration of the reciprocal tensions held within the membranous articular patterns that you have engaged. Sense the membranes seeking this neutral and assist the tissues to settle into a state of stillness. Within a wider contest, you are assisting reciprocal states of balance within the potency, the fluids, and the tissues as a unit of function. See the chapter on the state of balanced tension to review these concepts. Within the state of balanced tension, you may sense the action of the biodynamic potencies and biokinetic forces held within the inertial fulcrum.

6. As inertial forces are resolved, you may then sense the temporal bones and their dural relationships softening and reorganizing. Wait for a sense of softening and disengagement within the relationships of the temporal bones. If the inertial forces involved have fully resolved, the temporal bones may be sensed to float with ease laterally along the oblique angle of their petrous ridges. If the forces have not been fully resolved, you will still feel inertia within the relationship. This still may take the form of membranous resistance and fluid congestion. You may thus sense a partial resolution to a new boundary. If this is the case, then again access the state of balanced tension at the new boundary. Again wait for another cycle of resolution until there is a sense of the temporal bones literally floating away from the cranial base with ease. Do not apply any outside force to do this. Allow the inherent forces to do the work. Return to your original temporal bone hold and notice how the temporal bones now express their motility and mobility.

Clinical Highlights

Medial compression of the cranial base can be a factor in diverse symptomology. It is commonly a factor in vertigo and tinnitus and has been indicated as a factor in childhood learning difficulties. Intraosseous lesions of the temporal bone, compressions within its bony tissue, are also commonly involved. These inertial patterns commonly arise due to birth trauma. We will explore intraosseous lesions in *Volume Two*.

A number of years ago an architect came to see me. He had developed vertigo over a number of months, and it had become so acute that he could not work at his drafting table. Upon examination, it was found that there were strong intraosseous forces at work within both temporal bones and strong transverse force vectors affecting their dynamic. These forces related to unresolved birth dynamics within his system. Stress at work had shifted his system away from its compensations, and it gave at its weakest point. His symptoms disappeared after two treatments. He had follow-up sessions because he wanted to go deeper into historical patterning. Over a number of subsequent sessions his system was able to shift to a much more potent and fluid expression, and he experienced greater energy and drive. He also took up Taiji Quan (T'ai Chi Ch'uan) for relaxation purposes, which helped maintain his system at this new point of balance.

Sphenoid and Occiput

In this section, you will continue your exploration into the relationship between the reciprocal tension membranes and the cranial bones. We will again be using an intention of traction to do this. In the work with the temporal bones above, you were exploring the relationship between them, the tentorium cerebelli, and the membrane and connective tissue system as a whole. In this section you will continue this journey and again tune in to the motion of the sphenoid and occiput with the intention of sensing the continuity of their relationship with the tentorium cerebelli.

The sphenoid bone is classically considered to be the bony keystone of the cranial bowl. As we have seen, the relationship of the sphenoid and occiput is of critical importance in the cranial concept. They form the heart of the cranial base and their meeting point, the sphenobasilar junction, is considered by many to be a fulcrum for bony motion within the cranium and the body as a whole. All bony-membranous patterns and compensations within the body will be expressed in some kind of dynamic

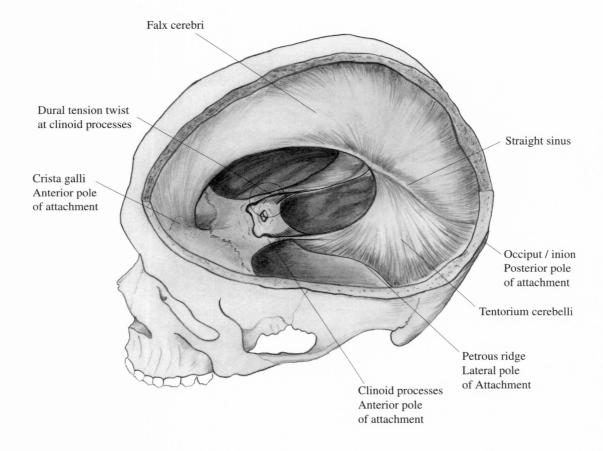

Falx cerebri

Dural tension twist at clinoid processes

Straight sinus

Crista galli
Anterior pole
of attachment

Occiput / inion
Posterior pole
of attachment

Tentorium cerebelli

Petrous ridge
Lateral pole
of Attachment

Clinoid processes
Anterior pole
of attachment

20.10 Reciprocal tension membrane and dural twist

within the sphenobasilar junction (SBJ). And any inertial fulcrums within the SBJ will be likewise be reflected in the body as a whole. The tentorium cerebelli stretches anterior from the occiput to the clinoid processes of the sphenoid. The superior leaves of the tentorium attach to the anterior clinoid processes of the sphenoid, and the lower leaves attach to its posterior clinoid processes. There is a tension twist within the tentorium as it meets the clinoid processes of the sphenoid bone (see below).

As you listen to the dynamics of the sphenoid and occiput, you will also be in direct relationship to the tentorium, especially in an anterior to posterior direction. As you tune in to motility and motion, various inertial fulcrums and their related patterns may be shown to you. These always involve both bone and membrane. Thus you are always in relationship to *membranous articular* patterns, and the continuity of bone and membrane must be appreciated. As you explore the relationship between the sphenoid and occiput, you will become aware of this continuity.

The Sphenobasilar Junction and the Tentorium Cerebelli

In the section above, you explored the relationship of the temporal bones to the tentorium. This is basically a transverse relationship across the cranial base. The intention of the following section is to enhance your sensitivity to the continuity between the sphenoid bone, tentorium cerebelli, and the occiput, which is basically an anterior-posterior relationship. The tentorium stretches like a taut tent between the occipital squama and the clinoid processes of the sphenoid bone. The superior leaf of the tentorium attaches to the anterior clinoid processes, while the inferior leaf attaches to the posterior clinoid processes. The tentorium stretches from occiput to sphenoid and meets the clinoid process in a twisted, tensioned manner. (See Figure 20.10.) The twist is an expression of the reciprocal tensioning of the membranes across the cranium.

Previously, you learned to tune in to the motion between the sphenoid and occiput at the SBJ and their reciprocal tension motion. You also learned to relate to inertial fulcrums via the state of balanced tension. In this section you will become more aware of the continuity of bone and membrane across the SBJ. The intention of the following section will be to deepen your appreciation of this continuity. In this process of exploration you will use *Dr. Becker's vault hold,* which will help you focus your attention within the tentorium as it stretches between the sphenoid and occiput. It will also help to focus attention at the SBJ.

In the following clinical application you will:

1. Tune in to the motion around the SBJ with an added awareness of the tentorium,

2. access the state of balanced tension,

3. further appreciate the continuity of the relationship among the sphenoid, occiput, and tentorium, and

4. more directly engage the tentorium and membranes in a conversation via the intention of traction.

Clinical Application: The Sphenoid, Occiput and Traction

(A) Accessing the State of Balanced Tension

1. Using Dr. Becker's hold, negotiate your contact with the patient's system. Place the thumb of each hand at the greater wings of the sphenoid. Place your other fingers along the posterior aspect of the occiput and temporal bones. Your little fingers are on the squama of the occiput.

(See Figure 20.11.) Hold an awareness of the biosphere within your perceptual field. From this relationship, first tune in to mid-tide and the sense of tissue motility and motion. Do not narrow your perceptual field as you do this.

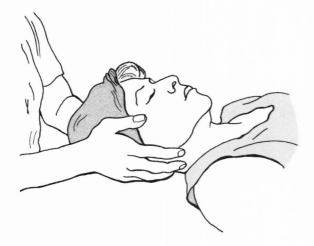

20.11 Dr. Becker's hold

2. Notice how the sphenoid and the occiput express motility and mobility. As you are listening, you may notice that the motion between the two bones may be expressed in various ways. There may be motions like rotations, pulls in various directions, twisting sensations, and so on (we will explore these kinds of motions in detail in *Volume Two.*). As you sense this, notice how the motion is a continuity of relationship among the sphenoid, occiput, and membranes. Listen to the reciprocal tension motion of the tissues. You may sense distortions within the tissue field you are palpating. Bring the question, "What organizes this?" to your hands.

3. As learned previously, follow the predominant dynamic, see if you can sense the inertial fulcrum that organizes it, and help access the state of balanced tension within its dynamic. It may

simply be a matter of listening to the motion dynamic as it seeks and attains its state of balance, or it may be a process in which you subtly slow it as it expresses its dynamic. Once the state of balance is attained, listen for expressions of Health within the stillness. The biodynamic potencies of the Breath of Life may be expressed within the neutral, and the biokinetic forces maintaining the strain may be processed. Listen for pulsations, fluid fluctuations, heat and force vector resolution.

4. Biokinetic forces may resolve, fluids may decompress, and tissues may release their contractions. Wait for a sense of softening and reorganization of the tissues in relationship to Sutherland's fulcrum. Do the reciprocal motion and the reciprocal tension among the sphenoid, occiput, and membrane system feel more balanced in relationship to Sutherland's fulcrum?

(B) The Sphenoid, Occiput, and the Principle of Traction

In this section, you will use the principle of traction to initiate a conversation with the tissues via your relationship with the sphenoid bone and occiput. In the session above, you may have noticed particular inertial fulcrums that effected their dynamics. One common location of inertial forces and fulcrums is directly within the dynamics of the SBJ. These commonly arise due to trauma, such as birth trauma, blows, and emotional shock. Under these extreme conditions, potencies will coalesce and compress to protect the system, and fluids and tissues will follow. Because of the important position of the SBJ relative to the system as a whole, compressive forces held within its dynamics can generate strong inertial patterns throughout the body. Inertia within SBJ dynamics can strongly influence *and* reflect the quality of motility and mobility throughout the body.

Using the principle of traction can help access the potential space within the compressive forces involved. The conversation will thus initially be about space. In this clinical application, you will also be using this principle to engage the membrane system and any fulcrums affecting the dynamics at the SBJ. If there is a strong compressive issue within the SBJ, this may be the clearest pattern that you sense. There may be a sense of a "dampening down" of the motility of the structures being palpated, or of fluid density, and so on. There may also be a sense of a locking or jamming between the occiput and the sphenoid bone within the overall tensile motion of the tissue field.

As you use traction to start a conversation with the tissues, there will be a number of avenues of inquiry. The first inquiry is, "Are there patterns of distress here?" and, if so, then "What organizes this?" In this process the conversation is about the history of the tissues and the resultant organizing fulcrums. If there are compressive issues within the SBJ itself, the conversation shifts to, "Can you allow yourself space here?" Once a fulcrum is engaged, the conversation changes to, "Can you access Health here?" This becomes a conversation about states of balance and potency. It is about the "neutral" and the expression of healing resources.

Conversations with the tissues via traction:

- Are there patterns of distress here?

- What organizes this?

- Can you allow yourself space here?

- Can you access Health here?

---

1. Staying in Dr. Becker's hold as described above, again listen to the dynamics of the sphenoid and occiput as they express motility and motion. Widen your perceptual field to the biosphere as you listen to the dynamics of potency, fluids, and

tissues. Listen for the mid-tide phenomenon. Once you have a clear relationship to the system, very subtly suggest traction at the greater wings of the sphenoid in an *anterior* direction (anterior to the patient's body, towards the ceiling in the supine position). Do not narrow your perceptual field as you do this. This is exactly like your previous session work when you used this principle at the frontal, parietal, and temporal bones.

2. First bring the *intention* of anterior traction to your thumbs, then *very subtly* engage the skin over the greater wings with this intention. Subtly transfer the intention of traction to the greater wings and then to the tentorium. *Do not create any medial pressure on the greater wings as you do this.* You are simply bringing an intention, a suggestion, to your thumbs in an anterior direction. As you intend this, be aware of the quality of motility and motion at the SBJ. In this intention, you are again engaging the tissues in conversation. "How is this? What's important here? What organizes this?" (See Figure 20.12.)

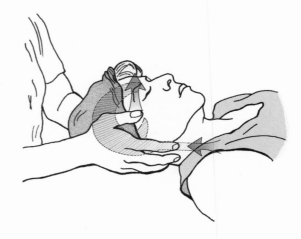

20.12 Traction via the sphenoid
(Dr. Becker's hold)

3. Follow this suggestion of traction through the membranes and, at the boundary to what is allowed, notice the location of the organizing fulcrum. At or near this boundary, help the system access its neutral, the state of balanced tension. Again, sense for expressions of Health. Do you notice expressions of *variant potencies* within the inertial fulcrum that is affecting the SBJ? What expressions of Health do you notice as the self healing forces come into play? You are waiting for a sense that the biokinetic forces involved are being resolved. You may sense heat and expansion as this occurs. As the forces resolve and the tissues reorganize and realign to their natural fulcrums, the sphenoid may be sensed to float freely in an anterior direction. Give this process the time and space it needs.

4. Listen for the new organization of fluids and tissues. Does the fluid tide express more potency? Do the tissues express a more balanced motion in relationship to Sutherland's fulcrum and the midline?

In this chapter we explored one of the classical conversation skills of the cranial concept. This skill can be applied to any tissue relationship. It is a principle of conversation, not a technique per se. This skill is especially useful when you want to initiate a conversation with the tissue field about the history of the fluid-collagen matrix and its "crystal memory," described above. In this process, as you hold an awareness of mid-tide dynamics, you are really conversing with the unified dynamic of potency, fluids, and tissues. Remember that, under stress, potencies will coalesce and condense, fluids will densify, and tissues will contract and compress. This is an expression of inertial forces at work and the need to center and contain their effects on the system. When these forces resolve within states of balance, you will commonly perceive expansion and reorganization to natural fulcrums and midline phenomena. It is important to give the system time to reorganize and to listen for the new shape and quality of organization expressed within the system.

1. Mae-Wan Ho and David P. Knight, "Liquid Crystalline Meridians," *American Journal of Complementary Medicine;* also, Mae-Wan Ho, *The Rainbow and the Worm, the Physics of Organisms,* (World Scientific).

2. Ibid.

3. See Chapter Fifteen.

21 Trauma and Trauma Skills I

In the next two chapters I will address some important issues that are certainly not unique to the cranial concept. These involve life processes and experiences that are traumatic and potentially traumatizing. Within any therapeutic setting, when practitioner and patient are investigating the roots of suffering, be they physical, emotional, or psychological, issues of past traumatization will arise. It is essential for practitioners to appreciate the nature of traumatic process. They must have a clear sense of appropriate clinical approaches to traumatization, especially when shock affects arise within the context of session work. It is not uncommon for patients to encounter overwhelming sensations and feelings within the context of session. These commonly take the form of emotional flooding and/or freezing states. Sometimes emotional flooding may be mistaken for a true emotional completion. The patient, if encouraged to continue emoting, may actually be engaged in a retraumatizing experience.

We will look at these issues in some depth here. This chapter draws heavily upon the work of Dr. Peter Levine, a recognized expert in the field of trauma resolution. I met Dr. Levine many years ago at a conference in which we were both presenting. I thank him for his kind answers to my many questions. I appreciate the encounters I have had with some of his students and co-workers, which have been very illuminating. I also appreciate the work of Dr. Angwynn St. Just, an associate of Dr. Levine,

who has presented work at the Karuna Institute. In training courses I also draw upon the work of a British psychiatrist, Dr. Frank Lake, who, along with Dr. William Emerson, developed what is known as the Transmarginal Stress Model. The work of Dr. Stanislov Grof is also extremely useful. His clear elucidation of the COEX matrix, matrices of condensed experience, is important to understand in any clinical context. Finally, my understanding of work in the trauma field has also been strongly influenced by my wife, Maura Sills, the founder of Core Process Psychotherapy.

In these two chapters I will focus on the stress response in a general way with an emphasis on clinical skills. In *Volume Two* of this text, I will present some of the important physiology to be aware of

---

In this chapter we will:

- *Review the physiological processes of the stress or trauma response.*

- *Discuss trauma, shock, and traumatization.*

- *Discuss the trauma process within the context of the work of Dr. Peter Levine and within a cranial context.*

- *Discuss the trauma and healing vortices.*

- *Discuss over- and undercoupling.*

and how to directly relate to physiological stress responses within the cranial field.

The Mammalian Stress Response

As a cranial practitioner, it is important to appreciate the physiological aspects of trauma. If you don't understand these processes, you might find yourself generating, or colluding in situations where your patients, rather than moving towards greater health, are actually being retraumatized. For instance, in a session, it may look and feel as if a lot is happening, perhaps a really powerful emotional release, when in fact the patient may actually be reinforcing the trauma or even experiencing a retraumatization. The first thing we have to understand is something quite basic. We have to understand that we are all mammals. As much as we might like to deny that, we are all in this body, a mammalian body. Furthermore, we respond physiologically to traumatic situations as any mammal would. The physiology of shock is largely mediated by the limbic system, specifically the amygdala and hippocampus, the hypothalamus, and the autonomic nuclei of the brain stem. The hypothalamus-pituitary-adrenal axis is also pivotal in stress mechanisms. Our thinking brain, the neocortex, is only indirectly part of this process, although it can influence it strongly. Again, I will discuss the physiology of stress responses in much more detail in a chapter in Volume Two. Stress responses are a primal, almost primeval aspect of our central nervous system. They are an expression of the deep survival drive of the species and the individual survival responses of human beings. The physiology of that is a mammalian physiology. So to start to discuss shock and trauma, it is useful to talk about the process of trauma response and shock as a basic mammalian survival process.

The Trauma Response

Let's look at the body's response to danger and traumatic experiences. We human beings are mammals, and we share in the response to trauma that all mammals have in common. In the following discussion we will look at the "fight or flight" process, which was originally described by Dr. Hans Selye. "Fight or flight" is a term that was coined by Dr. Selye in his work on stress in the human system. The fight or flight response is the response that arises within the system in dangerous or threatening situations. This is the process in which the animal mobilizes itself for perceived danger or threat. Let's look at some basic responses to danger by looking at an antelope on the African plains. By understanding the antelope's response to traumatic situation, we may start to understand our own trauma responses.

Scenario One

Let's imagine an antelope grazing on the African plains. I'm sure that you have seen scenes like this in television documentaries. In our visualization, it is grazing at a short distance from the rest of the herd. At first there is no sign of danger, and it is grazing in a relaxed fashion with no obvious tension or fear. This relaxed state is sometimes called the *ideal state*. The antelope is grazing in a fully present state, without any neurotic tensions held over from past experiences of trauma or stress. The antelope suddenly smells a micro-amount of lion spoor on the wind. "Hint of lion" on the wind! The first thing that will occur is sometimes called the *active alert* stage of the flight or fight mechanism. Certain neurohormones will be instantly released within its central nervous system. The antelope will stop grazing and become actively alert. It will stop its current activity and go into the active alert stage of heightened awareness. It will express what is called *orienting responses*. It will try to orient to the environment to detect sources of possible danger. It will scan the environment for clues. If the environment gives no further clues that there is danger, let's say that the lion is not in the area and the lion spoor is not obvious, then the antelope will come out of the active alert stage and return to relaxed grazing. It returns to its ideal state and is not traumatized by the process.

Scenario Two

Let's imagine another scenario. The lion *is* in the area and is stalking the antelope. The lion is hiding behind a bush, and the danger is clearly present. The antelope smells lion spoor and goes into its active alert state. This time, let's say that the lion jumps out of hiding and runs towards the antelope. The antelope will instantly and dramatically engage its flight or fight response. The sympathetic nervous system will become highly charged. The sympathetic response is immediate and powerful in these circumstances. The nervous system becomes highly charged, metabolism dramatically increases, blood is directed to the periphery for muscular use, and the neuroendocrine system floods the body with stress hormones such as adrenaline, cortisol, and endorphins. This is an attempt by the antelope's system to *mobilize* its resources and to flee the lion. This is an important point. The flight or fight response is directly tied into predator-prey issues. In the animal kingdom, each animal knows how it fits into the scheme of things. Predators know that they are predators and prey know that they are prey. It is not ambiguous. The antelope knows that it cannot fight the lion. Its survival rests on its ability to run faster than the lion. It will flee. In this case, let's first imagine that this survival flight is successful. The antelope mobilizes its flight response, and it successfully flees the lion. The antelope runs, jumps, and soars through the bush and the lion is left in the dust. The neuroendocrine system is strongly engaged as, during its successful flight response, adrenaline and other neuroactive substances pour into its system.

In this case, there will be a point when the lion knows that it is not successful. It will stop the chase and even may express what, looking at the lion, may be called dejection. When the antelope knows it is successful, other hormones, such as endorphins, may flood the system. The antelope may experience exhilaration, euphoria, and even altered states of near ecstasy in its successful flight. When the antelope is free from danger, it will slow down, come to a stop, return to its alert state, and re-orient itself to the environment. If no further signs of danger are present, then it will naturally return to the relaxed, ideal state and may continue grazing. The important thing to note here is that the antelope successfully expressed its response to danger, successfully fled, and *was not traumatized by the experience*. It had the *resources* to meet the experience and could *mobilize* those resources with success. It was not overwhelmed by the experience; it was able to return to its relaxed state. How many humans can do that?

Scenario Three

Let's look at a different scenario. Let's say that the lion has managed to stalk the antelope successfully and is quite close. The antelope has gone into its active alert phase and now engages its fight or flight response. It flees. This time, however, the lion is more successful. Perhaps there are a number of lions involved in the chase. Lions commonly hunt as a pride, or pack of hunters. Now the antelope's flight response will not be successful. It is surrounded and trapped. It knows this very deeply within its autonomic nervous system. Its flight or fight response has been overridden and *overwhelmed* by the lions. In other words, it cannot express the energy of mobilization in successful flight. If the fight or fight response is thwarted, the system will still try to protect itself. It does this by going into *shock*. The next thing that happens is that the antelope will go into a shock response. If the antelope is really successful in its shock response, it may occur before the antelope is even touched by any lion. The parasympathetic system will charge and other neurohormones will be released. The antelope will suddenly collapse. This is a critical survival ploy to understand. Shock is part of our natural survival mechanism; it is a natural response to an overwhelming situation. The antelope will collapse, and a number of things will occur that are of critical importance to understand.

First of all, the antelope will go into a *dissociative* state. It will dissociate from the sensations in its body. In effect, its psyche will dissociate from its soma and its sensations. This dissociative process is of extreme importance to understand in the therapeutic setting. Along with dissociation, the body will also go into an immobilized or *frozen* state. Its vital signs may become almost impossible to detect from the outside. It becomes *immobilized* and *frozen*. The important thing to realize here is that this frozen state is a highly charged state. In the shock response, the normal balance between the sympathetic and parasympathetic systems is upset. As the sympathetic charge is thwarted, the parasympathetic system comes strongly into play. The parasympathetic charge overrides the original sympathetic surge and the animal is catapulted into a catatonic state. Now both systems are charged, that is, are expressing greatly heightened activity. The huge charge within the sympathetic nervous system cannot be discharged in physical flight from the lions. This charge has to go some where. In this case, when the animal goes into shock, it literally implodes inward. The sympathetic charge, rather than being expressed and discharged in action, implodes and keeps cycling. So now the antelope has gone into shock. It is dissociated and immobilized. Its parasympathetic system has surged, new neurohormones are released, and its sympathetic charge is overridden. If the shock response is successful and the antelope is deeply in shock, then, from the outside, it will seem as though all vital signs cease and the antelope may seem to be dead. *This is all part of the antelope's survival mechanism.*

The lions, when they reach the antelope in its shock state, will find an animal in a catatonic and frozen state. If the antelope is fortunate, the lions may think that it is dead. They may smell the antelope, nudge it, and then, amazingly, leave it alone! Lions have learned in their own evolution that eating dead animals may leave them very sick and is dangerous. The shock mechanism may have actually saved the antelope's life! If the lions do eat the antelope, it is spared the pain of its death because it is dissociated from its sensations and is basically in a frozen, catatonic state. It is again important to note that from the outside the antelope may seem frozen or dead, but inside, its central nervous system is in a highly charged state.

Let's look at what happens to the antelope's system if the lions go away and it is not eaten. The antelope will gradual come out of the shock response. It reassociates with its body and sensations. Its energies begin to shift and move as it comes out of shock. Its parasympathetic system down-regulates and the sympathetic system discharges its energies. The imploded, or cycling charge of the sympathetic nervous system begins to manifest. You may note color and size changes in its lips, and its pupils may rapidly change size. The antelope then does something that is again important to note. It discharges the energy that was imploded in its shock response. Its body may tremble and then shake as the central nervous system discharges its cycling energies. It may then shift into expressing this discharge by bucking, running, or jumping. In other words, it further discharges its energy by again mobilizing its fight or flight response. In this process it discharges its cycling sympathetic energy and related stress hormones in action. It shifts from a frozen state to an expression of its defensive energies. It may then return to an active alert phase, reorient itself to its environment and to possible danger, and if none is perceived, it will then go back to its relaxed, ideal state. The powerful thing to point out here is that the antelope has survived, has successfully come out of shock, has discharged its imploded energies, and *was not traumatized by the experience!* It went through the stages of its defensive strategies and, although it had a traumatic experience, it was not left traumatized by it. *Traumatization occurs when the antelope cannot, for whatever reason, process the cycling energies of its shock response.*

Scenario Four

Let's look at different possible ending for the above scenario. Let's say, for instance, that you are sitting in a Land Rover and have witnessed the whole event. You have seen the chase and have seen the antelope go into shock. You feel sorry for the antelope. The lions have left, and you rush over to the animal while it is still in shock. The antelope starts to come out of its shock response and begins to tremble. It is starting to express its natural discharge of the imploded energies of shock. But in this case, you feel so sorry for the antelope that you begin to comfort it and stroke it. This seemingly compassionate act may actually stop the antelope from processing its shock. You may have prevented its cycling energies from being discharged in trembling, shaking, and running. In other words, you have prevented it from negotiating its way out of its shock response. It is now inappropriately running both parasympathetic and sympathetic energies. Its hormonal system is also unbalanced, and a high volume of stress hormones may be found within its system. Dr. Levine calls the inappropriate cycling of these stress-related energies and hormones *trauma-bound energy*.

As the antelope tries to come out of its shock, it will be very shaky and wobbly and will take a longer time to come back to consciousness and present time. The antelope may now be left with all or some of the energies of its fight and flight and shock responses still cycling. It may be left *traumatized* by the experience. That is, the energies of its shock response have not been processed by the system, and the animal is left traumatized. This state is called *shock traumatization*. Due to the heightened states of the sympathetic nervous system and the cycling of stress hormones, it might even be left in what we might call anxiety or depressive states. When it next meets a lion, due to these cycling energies, it may not be able to express its flight or shock response with as much efficiency. Because it is still cycling sympathetic stress responses, and the hormones re-lated to the freezing response are also still cycling, its flight response may not be as fast as it should be. It may even freeze when it sees the lion. Hence, its survival mechanisms are now compromised, its resources are lowered, and its ability to meet traumatic or stressful situations has also been compromised. This is a very dangerous situation for an antelope. The antelope may become more easily overwhelmed by a dangerous situation and may not be able to mobilize its resources as quickly or efficiently as before. Thus, *traumatization* occurs when the system cannot process its fight or flight and shock responses within the immediacy of the experience. The cycling energies and the experience itself become frozen within the body physiology. It is almost as if the system becomes frozen in time and has to react to present situations from past time. This may occur for many reasons, but the bottom line is that the shock and the experience that it relates to has become locked or frozen into the system. The powerful energies of the flight or fight response continue to cycle, and frozen and immobilized states may more easily be expressed by in the system in inappropriate ways. A similar process occurs in humans, as we shall see later.

Scenario Five

Another aspect of this process is that the antelope's emotional system may also become actively engaged in the process. Let's imagine that the antelope is again grazing on the plain. The lions attack, and the antelope engages its flight or fight response. As above, in this scenario, the lions are hunting in a pride and have the antelope surrounded. In this case the antelope is surrounded, is deeply in its flight response and is cornered, yet there is still escape possibility. In this scenario, the antelope may express strong emotions like anger or fear. There may be survival value in this. In certain circumstances anger may give an added spur to the system to further engage its flight response. The added energy can be instantly channeled into the flight response. Likewise, in a resourceful antelope, fear may spur the animal into intensified flight. This is, however, a strategy of desperation. This is a risky strategy on two counts. In this case, there will be a emotional charge experienced along with the fight or flight response. If the antelope is cornered and its system is overwhelmed by the traumatic experience, and it then goes into the shock response, these emotional energies may also become imploded along with the sympathetic charge. This may make its freezing response less effective and be dangerous to the organism. If it survives, when it comes out of the shock response, the

---

Summary of Stress Response

Ideal state
Fully resourced
relaxed, resourced, and present.
↓
Sense of danger
↓
Active alert state
Orienting response, heightened alertness, orienting to danger.
↓
Fight or flight response
Highly aroused state, highly charged mobilization of defensive energies.
↓
Overwhelm
Resources overwhelmed because they cannot be expressed.
↓
Shock response
Dissociation and freezing.
Cycling of aroused central nervous system energies.
Fight or flight response is overwhelmed.
Shock is a highly charged state of cycling energy and hormones,
immobilization and dissociation, separation
of psyche from soma. Catatonia results.

Movement out of shock response
Re-association and re-integration of psyche
and discharge of cycling energy through the body,
trembling, shaking, etc.
↓
Further discharge of energy via mobilization of fight or flight response.
↓
Return to active alert and to orienting movements.
Return to relaxed ideal state.

---

antelope may discharge its emotional energies by bucking and shaking. If the charge is not fully dissipated, the antelope may again be left traumatized and its resources will not be as strong or available in its next encounter with a traumatic experience. When it sees a lion, it may more quickly express a freezing response along with strong emotions, again not an optimum strategy. Emotions like rage or terror may arise, but they will have no survival value. They are inappropriate to its initial flight response and will get in its way. Fear may cause it to go into an immobilized state while it is still trying to mobilize its flight response. Anger may make it inappropriately defend itself, a sure nonstarter against the lions. Thus traumatization can lead to inappropriate emotional responses in times of stress or overwhelm.

The Human Dilemma

Peter Levine points out that human beings aren't as successful in processing their shock trauma as other mammals tend to be. This is due to a number of factors. One is the complexity of our nervous system and the tendency for our higher cortex to kick in with its cultural and familial conditioning. When stress or threat is perceived by the senses, the information goes from the sense organ to the thalamus. Then both to the cortex and to the amygdala. The circuit to the amygdala is much faster than that to the cortex. The amygdala circumvents cortical processing for quicker response to danger. The system gears up for action without having to think about it. (See Figure 21.1.) If the cortex kicks in inappropriately, the mobilization can be overridden

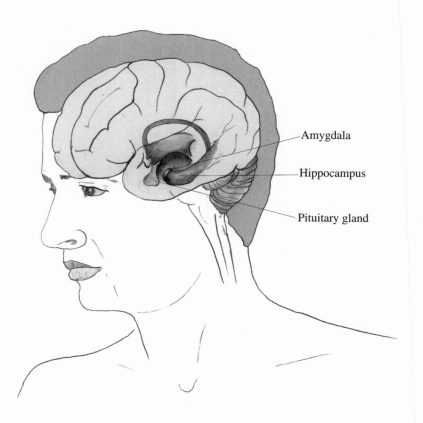

Amygdala

Hippocampus

Pituitary gland

21.1 The Amygdala

and the fight or flight energies will be expressed less easily or incompletely.[1] We are conditioned from an early age not to show our shock and/or our feelings during or after a traumatic process. "You should be able to handle that" or "Pull out of it" are common imperatives. We also tend to stop people processing their shock by interfering with their attempt to discharge it by shaking and trembling. Furthermore, as human beings, we have an ambiguous relationship to our flight or fight processes. We are both predator and prey. The lion knows that it is a predator, and the antelope knows that it is prey, and they act out their parts of the drama clearly. Humans are both predator and prey. We humans have ambiguous responses to danger and our neocortex seems to kick in much faster than in other animals. This is perhaps a major aspect of our difficulty in processing our shock trauma.

Another important aspect of this process is the strong relationship among fear, rage, and the dissociative process. In stressful or dangerous situations, a strong emotional charge of fear and/or rage can become coupled with processes of dissociation and immobilization. Just before the person enters a shocked state, strong feelings of fear or rage may arise as part of the natural mobilization response to the traumatic situation. This is a limbic response mediated by the amygdala in the stress response. The amygdala, when threat is perceived, mobilizes the system for action. It also orchestrates strong emotions, such as fear and anger, which may also arise during the process. During traumatization, if the fight or flight response is thwarted, a strong charge of rage or fear may implode and cycle in the system. Commonly, a mixture of rage and fear may become associated or coupled with the charge held in the central nervous system due to traumatization. When the person's trauma process becomes restimulated in some way, the cycling energies within the central nervous system may become expressed as inappropriate rage or terror. You may have experienced this in your own life, or noticed people inappropriately freezing or expressing anger in stressful situations. For instance a colleague at work may "fly off the handle" for seemingly little cause; or a friend may suddenly freeze while driving a car for no obvious reason. In the following paragraphs we will introduce some concepts and processes that more directly discuss these ideas within the context of our human condition and clinical practice.

Resources Revisited

Peter Levine stresses the understanding of resources in his work. We have introduced this concept in Chapter Eight and elsewhere. See Chapter Eight for an introductory discussion of resources and for some related perceptual exercises. Resources are the spiritual, psychoemotional, and physical aspects of a person's makeup, which support and nurture being in the world. They are the strengths that a person can draw upon when in stressful or threatening circumstances. It is important to realize that it is *how* a person perceives and experiences stressful circumstances that is important, not just the situation itself. To an outside observer, the circumstances may not look or feel threatening, but if the person perceives and experiences that they are, the system will respond to the situation as a present threat. We, like all mammals, respond to stress in the same physiological way as outlined above. In a stressful situation the whole cascade of processes leading to the fight and flight state and/or the shock state can be set off when stress is experienced.

Resources allow a person to meet these life experiences in ways that are appropriate and skillful. Resources can be anything that gives strength and ground to the person's ability to move through life in ways that are fulfilling and satisfying. Most of all, in this context, they are all of the physical, constitutional, and psychoemotional processes that enable a person to meet stress and danger in appropriate ways. They ensure that he or she can meet life and not be traumatized or retraumatized by the experience. Within the cranial concept, the most inherent resource is seen to be the potency of the Breath of Life and its ordering and healing functions.

Mobilization and Resources

In the mobilization response, the sympathetic nervous system will gear up to express the fight or flight response as outlined above. Basically, the system will try to mobilize its resources to deal with the perceived threat or stress. If this mobilization cannot be expressed, or if there are no resources to express them, then the system may go into a shock response. Furthermore, the system's response may already be depressed or facilitated inappropriately due to past trauma. The more traumatized our system is, the more our resources are bound up, and the more difficult it is to express them. If we are already inappropriately cycling flight or flight energies within the system, then its efficiency is compromised, and it can't respond to stress as effectively as it should.

In the therapeutic context, these concepts of *mobilization* and *resources* are important to grasp. The system will try to respond to stress by mobilizing itself to react and deal with a situation. How successful a person is in this response depends on his or her resources. It is important to realize that an experience that may be strongly traumatizing to one person may not be so traumatizing to another. It depends on the *resources* that a person has and if these resources can be *mobilized* within the context of the trauma. Resources may be psychological, emotional, and physical. One person may have the psychological and emotional resources to process a traumatic event like a car accident, while another person may not. Another person may have strong constitutional resources and another may not. One may be severely traumatized by the event and the other may be able to process the trauma of the incident relatively quickly.

Immobilization and the Frozen State

As we have seen, in shock traumatization, the system can become frozen and immobilized. The heightened energies of the fight or flight response implode, keep cycling, and a dissociative and frozen state may result. Vital signs may become erratic or be drastically reduced, and the natural pain response of the system may be undermined. In physical trauma, an accident for instance, the person in shock may not be able to sense that the body is bleeding and is badly damaged. To the person in shock, everything may seem to be okay when, in fact, drastic circumstances are occurring. The person may even experience euphoria as adrenaline and endorphins flood the system. This is part of the body's natural self-protection mechanism. It cuts the person off from the immediacy of the sensations and the pain of the event. If we are still cycling these energies due to past traumatization, then we are more likely to go into dissociation and freezing, or to experience anxiety states, as we experience challenging and stressful new experiences.

It is thus essential that the practitioner be aware of the nature of traumatic experiencing and shock responses in relationship to the patient's system. When patients enter shocked and traumatized states, it is essential to recognize these and to know how to relate to them. Within this context, there may also be unresolved emotional affects related to the trauma, such as fear and anger. Due to the process of shock and related emotional affects, protective connective tissue and muscular contractions may also tend to become fixed in the system and will be retained as chronic tension patterns within the tissue field. Within a cranial context, potency will become inertial in order to center the cycling energies as best as possible. The fluid and tissue world will follow and respond, as we have seen, as a unified field of action.

The Overwhelm: Traumatic Experience and Traumatization

As noted above, it's really important to understand that a person may or may not be traumatized by the circumstances of a traumatic experience. As I said above, whether or not a person is traumatized by an experience depends on the resources that he or she can bring to bear in relationship to it and whether or not these resources can be mobilized at the time of the experience. Within a cranial context, the basic resource of the system is its expression of the potency of the Breath of Life. Organization is a function of its ordering matrix. If much potency is bound in the centering of trauma-bound energy and shock affects within the system, then the expression of this most vital resource is compromised. A person's resources also include the physiological, constitutional, and psychoemotional processes that a person can bring to bear in traumatic situations.

There are two important factors in stressful situations:

- A person may or may not have the resources to deal with the situation.

- A person may or may not be able to express or mobilize them.

An experience may be potentially traumatizing if:

- The person hasn't the resources to deal with the circumstances.

- The resources become overwhelmed by the nature of the experience.

- shock affects of past traumatization arise and override the natural expression of fight or flight energies; these may include emotional affects like rage or fear and dissociation and freezing states.

- If the person goes into shock and can't discharge and process its charge.

Trauma, Shock, and Traumatization

There are three totally interrelated aspects of the stress, fight or flight, and traumatization process: *trauma, shock, and traumatization*. A *traumatic experience* arises due to a situation or event that is physically and/or emotionally stressful, threatening or dangerous to the integrity of a person. The experience is a *trauma* and is potentially traumatizing. *Shock* occurs when that traumatic experience *overwhelms* the resources of the person, and *traumatization* occurs when the fight or flight and shock energies cannot be processed by the system. The person ends up cycling both sympathetic and parasympathetic energies with a high volume of stress-related hormones in the system. (We will discuss this in more detail in *Volume Two* of this text.) This charge is held within the central nervous system and within the fluids and tissues of the body. These fight or flight and shock energies, in the form of neuroendocrine-immune processes, continue to cycle until they are resolved in some way. Psychological, emotional, and pathological processes will become coupled with these energies.

A person may become traumatized by an event if resources become overwhelmed or cannot be expressed. The concept of a person's resources being *overwhelmed* is extremely important to grasp. If a person's resources are overwhelmed by an experience, he or she won't be able to appropriately respond to the situation. Furthermore, past shock traumatization may be activated, or restimulated, and the person may respond to present circumstances inappropriately. This is especially true if there was a strong survival emotion, such as rage or fear, coupled with the fight or flight process.

Thus, if a person's resources are overwhelmed, he or she may end up traumatized by the new experience, and layers of past traumatization may be restimulated and will become coupled to the new traumatization. As an example of this, a number of years ago, a friend of mine had a motorcycle accident. He was thrown off his motorcycle, and his body slid along the road until his clavicle struck the pavement and was fractured. This was a very traumatic event. Fortunately he was not badly injured beyond the fracture, but many processes were touched off for him. There was the immediacy of the present trauma. He had knowledge of trauma work and processed the immediate experience quite well. Then something happened. He started to feel anxious and depressed. He experienced low energy and anger at the same time. He felt stuck. He was wise enough to pay attention and discovered that unresolved birth trauma had been touched off by the event. The nature of the accident, when he slid along the road and was suddenly stopped, echoed his own birth process. He was able to work through this and learned a lot in the process. A recent trauma had activated a very early traumatic process, and he was able to skillfully take advantage of it.

Shock Affects and the Cranial Context

Within the context of cranial work, it is not unusual for shock or trauma affects to be expressed within a session. Commonly the term "affect" is applied solely to the emotional aspects of a process, but I am using it in a wider sense. When I use the term "shock affect," I mean *any* process of activation that may arise within the system due to past traumatization. This might include things like emotional flooding, freezing states, and dissociative states. They will take different forms depending on the nature of the original trauma, how it is being centered within the system, and how the system manifests its shock affects. Within a cranial context, you, as practitioner, are in an intimate relationship to the patient's patterns of suffering and past history. As you work with inertia fulcrums, you come into direct relationship to the unresolved traumatic forces still being centered in some way by the system. These traumatic forces hold the power to organize, and it is not uncommon for people to organize their whole life around unresolved trauma. This must be appreciated and understood.

As a practitioner, when trauma affects arise within a session, you may sense various processes that let you know what is occurring. Within the tissues, you may sense very subtle tremblings and oscillations. These may feel disorganized and chaotic. They can be very subtle or quite obvious. The client may even begin to shake as the system attempts to discharge the affects. Trembling and shaking are natural attempts by the system to process the shock affect. If it occurs within the patient's resources, then there may be a real opportunity for resolution here. We will discuss this in the next chapter. On a nervous system level, you sense a kind of electric discharge throughout the fluids and tissues. The patient may remark about this. Again, if this occurs within the patient's resources, the cycling of the nervous system has the potential to resolve, and it may even be experienced as a pleasant relief by the patient.

On a fluid level, you may sense perturbations within the cerebrospinal fluid as nervous system shock affects release. This can again be very subtle or more obvious in expression. Fluid perturbation is not the same as fluid fluctuation. It has a more chaotic quality and is not an expression of the natural longitudinal or lateral fluctuations organized around midlines and fulcrums. Perturbations may be sensed within the fluid system as a whole. Fluid perturbation can be a sign that the system is attempting to resolve the shock affects held within the neuroendocrine and autonomic nervous systems. If they occur within the person's resources, as an expression of potency acting to resolve the shock being centered, there is much potential for healing here. A practitioner should become very sensitive to these expressions of shock release in the system.

On the level of the potencies you may also sense various qualities of motion and perturbation. You may even sense that the potency is "locked up" centering the traumatic affects involved. This might be perceived as a quality of inertia that seems to infuse the cerebrospinal fluid system. The fluids may seem dense, and you may not sense much expression of potency within the system. I have even seen this in newborn babies due to the centering of traumatic birth forces. Caesarean sections, traumatic births, and medical interventions can generate inertial potency throughout the fluid system as the baby attempts to deal with the traumatic forces and toxins encountered. This will in turn prevent a complete ignition of the fluid system at birth and will lock potency and fluid up in centering the traumatic forces. Other processes, which can generate more global shock affects, are strong emotional shocks and overwhelming experiences such as accidents and recurring physical or sexual abuse. When you sense shock affect via the potencies, you may also perceive perturbations of potency, similar to the fluid perturbations that they generate, and electric qualities, similar to central nervous system discharge. These are similar but subtler. Here it is the potency within the fluids that is perturbating due to the centering and release of the shock affect.

When working within the CRI, it is not uncommon for shock affects to be activated as the practitioner works with patterns of resistance in the system. This is because, within the CRI, you are in relationship to the *results* and *affects* of past experience. The potencies and forces at work, and the Health within the system, are not as obvious at this level of perception and work. Here you tend to access the affects of past suffering. On a psychological level these may include various defensive mechanisms such as withdrawal or aggression. On an emotional level these may include processes of emotional flooding and/or states of anxiety and depression. On a fluid level you may perceive congestion and various fluctuant phenomena. Finally, on a tissue level you may perceive tissue affects such as resistance, changes in density and quality, adhesion, compression, and contraction. It is not uncommon for strong emotions to be released within CRI level work. If this occurs, it is important for the practitioner to have the skills to help the patient safely resolve the traumatic fulcrum being accessed. The patient may experience strong emotions and freezing states and may also experience dissociative states. We will talk about these states in the next chapter and introduce some clinical skills to help the patient process them.

When working within the mid-tide level of perception, shock affects tend to manifest in relationship to the inertial potencies involved and are processed in a more resourced way. They tend to be more subtly expressed in streamings of energies and expansive sensations. The quality of perturbation of potency and fluid is finer here and clearly coupled with the resolution of trauma and its inertial forces. Practitioners may sense expansion within the fluids and tissues and a realignment to the midline and natural fulcrums as the affects are processed. Within the mid-tide, you will commonly perceive the potencies and fluids processing the shock affects in resourced and manageable ways. Patients will tend to sense the processing of shock affects as a pleasant and supportive experience. When accessing shock affects within the mid-tide level of work, patients tend not to be overwhelmed by the process. However, if the system cannot access or manifest its potencies here, there may be a tendency to shift to the CRI and its more acute expressions of traumatization. We will discuss the management of traumatic overwhelm within a cranial context in the next chapter.

The Trauma Vortex

Peter Levine has created language and images around the processing of trauma, which I find very useful. He uses the image of a vortex within a stream of water to image the nature of traumatization and its cycling energies. He likens life to a free-flowing stream. A traumatization occurs when the wall or bank of the stream has been breached and a vortex of spiraling water forms outside the flow of the stream. (See Figure 21.2.) It is as if life energy has become captured in a vortex outside the natural stream of life. This vortex begins to generate its own energy and takes on its own identity. It becomes a fulcrum that will organize life experience. A vortex is a very stable system. Once it forms, it sucks the moving water, or energy, of the stream into itself and is maintained as a relatively stable structure. Its energies continue to cycle until they are resolved in some way. It becomes an entity unto itself and sucks in and entraps the natural energies of the system. Remember that shock is a highly charged state, which cycles a huge amount of energy. This energy is then unavailable for natural life processes. Peter Levine calls this a *trauma vortex*. The trauma vortex cycles energies outside the stream of life, and these energies become unavailable for normal functions. He says that if a person enters the trauma vortex in an unresourced state, he or she may become overwhelmed by the experience. The person may enter dissociative states, express shock affects such as emotional flooding, and experience the process as a new or reinforced trauma. Hence the person may be retraumatized by the experience. When a person encounters shock affects, it can literally feel like being sucked into a vortex of overwhelming proportions.

Dr. Levine takes this image a further step. He says that it is the natural tendency of the system to generate what he calls a *countervortex*. He also calls this a *healing vortex*. As we see in the cranial field, it is the natural tendency of the system to move towards healing and balance. Health is never lost. The healing vortex is the system's attempt to balance and contain the trauma vortex. It is important that both are acknowledged as traumatization is activated within in a person's system. The healing vortex is the conglomerate of energies, mental states, sensations, and processes that attempt to move the system back to its ideal state. A tension develops between the healing vortex and the trauma vortex. The healing vortex attempts to contain and compensate for the presence of the trauma vortex. It is a very similar concept to the inertial fulcrum in which both the potencies of the Breath of Life and the forces of trauma are present. The potencies of Health attempt to contain and compensate for the unresolved traumatic forces. Within the cranial concept, it is within the state of balanced tension that the tension between the two vortices enters a balanced state, and something else can happen beyond the traumatic forces and compensations being centered.

In this context it is important to help the patient establish resources and develop an awareness of

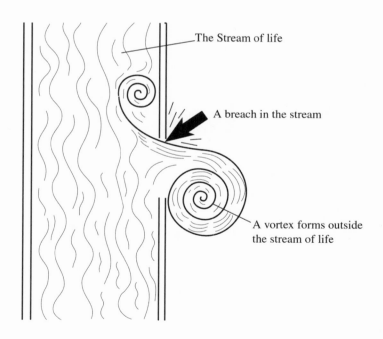

The Stream of life

A breach in the stream

A vortex forms outside the stream of life

21.2 The stream of life

resourced sensations. We introduced this idea in previous chapters and will further develop it below. Within a cranial context stillpoints (CV4 and EV4), stillness, and states of balance within inertial issues also help encourage the expression of resources. Here we are encouraging the most fundamental resource to express itself, the potency generated by the intentions of the Breath of Life. Within the cranial context, accessing a state of balanced tension within a specific inertial pattern helps to uncouple that particular pattern from all others held within the system. The system can then attend to one thing at a time and will not be overwhelmed by the activation of many fulcrums at once. Establishing resources will give a person a "place to come from" as he or she encounters the push and pull of the trauma and healing vortices. Once resources are established, your patient may gradually gain the ability to be in relationship to the trauma vortex without becoming sucked into its energies. It is important to approach trauma vortices slowly, from a resourced place in ourselves, and it is important to learn to stay on the "edge" of the vortex and its potentially overwhelming sensations. This again is a skill that people can gradually develop. For instance, let's say that a person begins to experience a flooding of fear. As he or she builds resources, he or she may be able to slow the process down and to have a relationship to the arising sensations and feelings,

rather than becoming overwhelmed by them. As the person does this, he or she is meeting the "edges" of the traumatization, rather than becoming sucked into the center of its cycling energies. This is very empowering.

As your patient brings attention to the *edges* of the trauma vortex and its sensations and feeling tones in the body in a resourced state, you may perceive various kinds of phenomena as the cycling energies discharge. The person may begin to tremble or shake, emotions may resolve as streamings of energy, and true emotional completions may occur. Gentle experiences of electric-like discharges and expansive sensations may also be felt. When this occurs you may notice that the patient takes a big sigh or deep breath as more spacious sensations arise. You may then notice the person moving back and forth between the sensations of trauma affects and resourced, spacious sensations (i.e., between the trauma vortex and the countervortex). Peter Levine likens this movement to a figure-eight or infinity sign. One side of the figure-eight represents the trauma vortex and the other side represents the countervortex. (See Figure 21.3.) The skill of assisting in the resolution of traumatization is to help the person stay in touch with resources and to move around the edges of both vortices, first touching one, then the other. The person learns to resolve and process the shock af-

Trauma vortex   Counter vortex

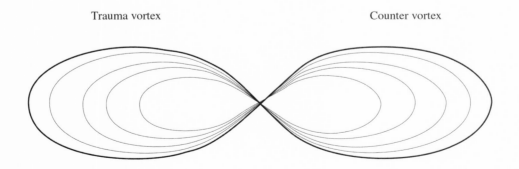

21.3 The trauma vortex

fects a little bit at a time. This gradual process of resolution has been called *titration*.

Activation and Titration

Peter Levine calls the process of pacing and processing trauma *titration,* a term that comes from chemistry. Titration is a process of determining the concentration of a substance in terms of the smallest amount of a reagent required to bring about an effect in a reaction. In other words it is about finding the smallest amount of a substance to produce a change, In trauma terms, titration is about pacing a process so that it is not overwhelming to the patient and an "explosion" into a traumatized state does not occur. Within the cranial context, it is about the state of balanced tension. It is within the state of balance that a dynamic equilibrium is attained between the tensions of the traumatic forces that maintain the pattern and the biodynamic potencies of the Breath of Life.

It is in the stillness of this state that something else can happen beyond the conditions being centered. Within the context of the patient's experience, it is about being with the arising process in *present time* with a witness consciousness so that a transformation, rather than an explosion, can occur. In this process it is important to help a patient bring resources into relationship to their arising process. It is important to pace the session work so that traumatization is processed in manageable pieces in a contained and resourced way. It is also about empowerment and reowning possibilities and options. It may be about slowing a process down and helping the patient to contain its potentially overwhelming nature. It is about slowly uncoupling aspects of the process that have become overcoupled and compressed, as outlined below.

It is important to understand the nature of activation. When a trauma-bound process is activated, the forces of the trauma begin to surface in an attempt to heal them. In a resourced processing of these forces, the patient enters what Peter Levine calls the *zone of activation*. In this zone, the patient's trauma-bound energies are *activated* within resources and appropriate pacing. The experience is titrated in manageable chunks, and the system moves to resolve traumatic energies in a resourced manner. In this, the cycling trauma-bound energies can be discharged more safely within the present. In this process the person does not plunge into the trauma vortex, but stays on its edges until he or she can bring more and more resources to its resolution. It is a gradual process of "touch and go," in which a person touches on the traumatic cycling of energies and their related sensations and images, within the context of resources. The person learns to touch the overwhelming nature of these energies and shuttle back and forth between them and the resources. Again, it is initially about staying on the edges of both the trauma and healing vortices, letting energies resolve a little bit at a time. If a process is not titrated, that is, if things move too fast, or if the therapist encourages emotional releases without an awareness of the person's resources, then the patient may dive into the center of the trauma vortex. He or she may then experience its related shock affects, sensations, and images in an overwhelming way.

There is also a danger that a person may not stay on the edge of the *healing vortex* and may also plunge into that in an unresourced state. You may then see a patient enter euphoric or manic states in which he or she is dissociated and very "high." These states may seem to be comfortable and pleasurable. However, they may be dissociative states. Dissociation is one of the protective mechanisms of the body-mind. As we have seen, in this process the psyche dissociates from the soma, from overwhelming sensations, and from the danger perceived. Dissociation can feel good as the defensive mechanisms of the system kick in. This can be very subtle. A person may seem to be having a healing experience, but it may really just be a cycling of unresolved trauma. The process may then reinforce the cycling energies of the trauma vortex.

A patient may have altered states of consciousness and what seems to be spiritual experiences. But again, if they are dissociated and not really resourced within the process, these experiences are more likely an expression of the response to shock affects within the system. They are not the transpersonal or spiritual experiences that they seem. Spiritual experiences feel grounded, not spaced out or dissociated. When these really do arise within the context of a session, they are a function of grace and are a true blessing. If a person plunges into the healing vortex in an unresourced state, he or she will soon be thrust back into the trauma vortex with a vengeance.

As a practitioner, you may see similar processes in your patients when they experience traumatic forces, sensations and images, yet feel euphoric and even ecstatic. Perhaps they experience strong emotional releases, even a flooding of emotions, but if they are not well resourced, they will likely enter dissociated states. In this state, the mind-body system may experience the emotional release as a new trauma, and the traumatization may actually be reinforced. Remember that dissociation may feel euphoric and "good." Hormones that give rise to euphoric feelings may flood the system. I have seen people make very unwise decisions while in these states, such as precipitously leaving their wives, husbands, work, and so on. It is always important to be in the present, in the embodied process, aware of sensations and feeling tones, with options and skills in relationship to the arising process. Most of all, go slowly! Over a period of time, as the patient builds up resources, he or she may indeed be able to go to the heart of the trauma vortex in a resourced and present state, but it is important always to work slowly and gently.

SIBAM

Peter Levine talks about the components of the mind-body process as the SIBAM. SIBAM stands for *Sensations*, *Images*, *Behavior*, *Affects* (emotional affects), and *Meaning*. The SIBAM holds and expresses the content of our experience and our responses to that experience within present time.

Sensations, images, behaviors, emotional affects, and meaning are all interrelated and naturally co-arise as a unit of function.

SIBAM

- *Sensations*—the sensations contained, generated, and perceived within the body.

- *Images*—the images that arise within conscious awareness; they represent the mental aspect of the meaning and experience of life.

- *Behavior*—the behaviors we express relate to our experience of life.

- *Affects*—the emotional affects held in relationship to past experience and traumatization; ideally emotions arise in relationship to present experience and are appropriate responses to that experience.

- *Meaning*—the meaning we give to our experience; again meaning ideally arises directly in relationship to present experience.

The SIBAM is a naturally flowing and unified process. The aspects of the SIBAM inter-be. Thus, in an untraumatized system, the SIBAM is experienced and expressed fluidly as an integrated and interpenetrating process. Our sensations, images, behavior, emotions, and the meanings we give to life are ideally based on a fluid response to our present experience. The SIBAM should be a natural and integrated arising of life process in relationship to the immediacy of the present moment. Ideally, its expression is not based on the past conditions of our life. It is a response to experience as a spontaneous arising in relationship to current and present life circumstance. Thus the SIBAM should be a fluid, spontaneous and integrated process of experience and response to experience. In Peter Levine's words,

> In a self experience that is complete and whole, these five components (SIBAM) are linked coherently. They encode information about the environment that is meaningful to the organism in the moment; information which helps it to map internally the "out there" world in an adaptive purposeful way. . . . It is the ability to transduce and organize information that gives us a sense of continuity and orientation in space and time.[2]

Becoming aware of the SIBAM can give us a real handle on the nature of our life process. An awareness of the sensations, images, and emotions within us, of the meanings we give to life, and of the behaviors we generate can give us enough space to heal the splits and fragments they may represent. Healing is really about *awareness* within the present moment. An awareness of our present experience and how we organize our responses to that experience is an essential part of the healing process.

We see similar concepts in classical Buddhism. The SIBAM is very similar in concept to the Buddhist *skandhas*. The *skandhas* are considered to be the mind-body aggregate that relates to the processing of our experience and upon which our sense of selfhood rests. The Buddha described five interrelated mind-body processes that tend to generate a sense of self: *form, perception, feeling tones, predispositions and consciousness.*

I perceive the skandhas to be a level of organization beneath or deeper than the SIBAM. They seem to be a subtler energetic level of organization that underlies the SIBAM. They, like the SIBAM, are ideally a fluid process, and all five aspects are enfolded within one another. The Buddha said that the first step in any spiritual awakening is to become aware of the skandhas and the self-constructs we generate from them. We are not the skandhas, but we become very identified with them. It feels as if we are our perceptions, our sensations, and so on. Our seemingly solid sense of "me" is derived from the interactions of the skandhas. The Buddha had some very astute things to say about the skandhas in terms of trauma and traumatization. He directed us, in a very particular way, to become aware of the interactions of the skandhas within our body-mind. He said to be aware of the body within the body, to be aware of feelings within the feelings, to be aware of mental processes within the processes. That is, 2,500 years ago, he counseled us to create a nondissociated relationship to our experience![3] To bring awareness to the experience *within* the experience. He said that the ability to do this is an essential part of healing and spiritual practice. Within trauma work we see similar principles at work. No matter how we talk about it, awareness within the present moment is a key to healing traumatization.

The Skandhas

- *Form* is the physical body and all of the forms we generate due to our tendencies and experiences (like thought forms and feeling forms).

- *Feeling tones* are the push-pull of our response to experience, the subtler feeling qualities that underlie our sensations.

- *Perception* is the conditioned process of identifying objects, that is, our process of identification and naming.

- *Predispositions* are all of our conditioned tendencies; these relate especially to our volitional and mental processes.

- *Consciousness* is the immediate arising of conscious experience via the five senses and the mind.

SIBAM and Traumatic Coupling

A final thing that is essential to discuss is what Peter Levine calls *coupling*. Coupling processes relate to how aspects of our experience and behavior become either coupled or disconnected due to traumatization. When a person becomes traumatized, as discussed above, a number of things occur within the mind-body complex. The most important aspect is that the elements of the SIBAM become incoherent. Peter Levine calls what occurs overcoupling and undercoupling. Maura Sills calls the same phenomena compression and fragmentation. Due to this process, the spontaneity and integration of our mind-body system is lost. The elements of SIBAM become both compressed together and fragmented at the same time. In essence, the relationships of the SIBAM, which are ideally integrated and fluid, lose coherence. Again in Peter Levine's words,

> In traumatic shock . . . this organization [of SIBAM] breaks down leaving the individual in a state of disorientation. Rather than an overall sense of information relating external and internal environment, trauma fragments the person into a number of relatively unrelated information sources. Consciousness loses its overall sense of continuity and wholeness.[4]

Basically the components of the SIBAM lose their interrelatedness and the person loses the ability to function in an integrated way in relationship to the experience. Over- and undercoupling are totally related processes. During traumatization, aspects of the SIBAM will become overcoupled or compressed together. For instance, certain sensations may become coupled with certain emotions and behaviors; or certain emotions may become coupled with certain images and behaviors, and so on. Whenever one aspect of the overcoupled matrix arises, *all* of the coupled elements also arise. For instance, whenever a particular image arises within someone's consciousness, the person also experiences overwhelming sensations and emotions; or

whenever anxiety arises, the person immediately experiences a need to run away, and is flooded by a sense of doom. Basically, what is happening is that the activation of past traumatization overrides the natural responses of the mind-body system. The ability to orient and explore is compromised. The fluid feelings and behaviors of life, like the ability to nurture and be nurtured, to orient to present experience, sexuality, appropriate modes of defense and protection, and so forth, are overridden and overwhelmed. The basic idea is that aspects of the SIBAM become rigidified and coupled together. The range of response is lessened and options are narrowed.

For instance, a state of anxiety or fear may become associated with a belief that "I may die here," or "I'll be abandoned here," which may become further coupled with a behavior pattern of running away, leaving relationships, quitting jobs, and so on. What may then happen is that as soon as the sensation of anxiety is felt, the overcoupled elements also arise and an automatic process and inappropriate reaction occurs. The dissociated fragments of the SIBAM become coupled or condensed together and lose their fluidity. The openness and fluidity of the relationships of SIBAM are lost and options of response to present circumstances are reduced. The traumatized person loses the ability to *respond* spontaneously to present situations and instead meets them with *activation* and *reaction*. The overcoupled elements arise all at once as a reaction to perceived threat or stress, and it seems, to the traumatized person, that no other options are possible.

These overcoupled elements may become activated by new trauma, by internal sensations that resonate with the traumatic event, by images that arise and touch off the coupled sensations, or, indeed, by any stress factor that overwhelms the system. The important point here is that once the traumatic energies are activated, the whole matrix of the traumatically coupled elements arise at once and the coping resources of the system are more easily overwhelmed. In this state, the behaviors associated with the coupled elements automatically arise and the person has lost the potential for a spontaneous and free-flowing experience of life. He or she is trapped in an activation of trauma-bound energies in which any sense of control over the person's own process is lost. Options have been reduced by the process of traumatic coupling. A sense of disempowerment commonly results.

Let's take another example. Let's imagine that a person is in a stressful situation. Perhaps he works in a shop and is being berated by a customer. As he senses the customer's anger, maybe he feels spacey and starts to sweat. Perhaps an urge to run away overcomes him and it feels as if he is about to be attacked and will die. All of this is disconnected from the current situation and will prevent appropriate responses. The overcoupled elements are undercoupled from other potential sensations, images, behaviors, feelings and meanings. They are also undercoupled, or disconnected, from present reality. Here dissociative sensations arise coupled with autonomic responses, feelings of dread, and a behavior flight pattern of running away. All of these are expressions of aspects of the SIBAM that have become overcoupled, that is, they arise together as the person meets stress or threat. Moreover, this particular matrix of overcoupled elements have also become undercoupled from other qualities of sensations, feelings, and responses, and from the present reality of the experience. In over- and undercoupling the coherence and connectedness of the SIBAM is lost.

Another way to look at this is in terms of shape and fulcrums. Ideally the psyche and the mind-body complex should function as an integrated whole. The system should basically be one unified shape. The SIBAM should function as a pulsating tensile field in response to the present experience of life. In an untraumatized person, the movement of SIBAM relates directly to present experience. It is an arising and passing of interrelated process that is directly responsive to the present circumstances. Hence, sensations, images, behavior, emotions, and meaning all arise in relationship to present experience as a single gestalt (i.e., a whole, unified shape).

As we have seen above, when a system becomes traumatized, this wholeness breaks down. The SIBAM splits into fragments, breaks down, and rigidifies into fragmented shapes and fixed patterns. What is naturally a fluid, unified process loses its coherency and becomes fragmented. The person now has a series of under- and overcoupled SIBAM fragments (i.e., trauma shapes made up of the fragmented and overcoupled elements of the SIBAM). These trauma shapes do not and cannot relate to each other. They move around separate fulcrums of experience and have become rigidified into separate, fragmented shapes. The cycling of trauma-bound energies keeps the overcoupling processes and the trauma vortex spinning. These trauma fragments, or overcoupled aspects of the SIBAM, now take on a life of their own separate from the natural movement of the SIBAM. They become expressions of trauma vortices outside the natural stream of life.

Thus, along with overcoupling, comes undercoupling. The overcoupled elements become dissociated from the rest of the person's experience. The coherence of the SIBAM as a life process is lost. Sensations become dissociated from emotions, from meaning, from behavior, and so on. Under stress, only certain sensations, emotions, images, and mental states tend to arise. Likewise, only certain meanings are given to experience, especially stressful experience. Along with this, certain behaviors become fixed and fluidity is lost. The unity and fluidity of the interrelatedness of the SIBAM becomes fragmented. Processes that would normally be linked with each other in one's awareness may become dissociated. A person hears a noise while walking down the street and immediately feels threatened, freezes, and is overcome by feelings of dread. This is a conditioned fear, or stress response, and is mediated by ancient parts of the brain that relate to survival and responses to danger. Once conditioned, these responses become deeply compressed together and automatic. The overcoupled elements immediately arise *together* as a response to the noise. These elements are, in turn, undercoupled from all other potential sensations and responses, and from the present experience of life.

During treatments, as the cycling of trauma-bound energies resolves, these seemingly overcoupled elements have a chance to resolve their linkage, and the person has the opportunity to once again experience the process as a fluid and integrated whole. The person has the opportunity to allow the system to process the trauma, to reintegrate and heal its fragmentation, and to allow trauma-bound processes to complete. In other words, during the resolution of traumatic forces and processes within the body-mind, the SIBAM has the opportunity to once again become coherent and fluid. The important thing is that this healing process proceeds in a gradual, titrated fashion with awareness and resource. In the next chapter, we will further discuss these concepts and will attempt to describe, in a very basic way, the kinds of trauma skills that are important to develop in your clinical practice.

1. See LeDoux, *The Emotional Brain* (Weidenfeld & Nicholson); and *Craniosacral Biodynamics,* vol. 2 for physiological discussions of this process.

2. Peter Levine, *Waking the Tiger: How the Body Heals Trauma* (North Atlantic Books).

3. See the Maha Satipatthana Sutta, Majjhima Nikaya, Pali Canon.

4. Peter Levine, *Waking the Tiger: How the Body Heals Trauma* (North Atlantic Books).

22

Trauma and Trauma Skills II

In this chapter we will expand upon the concepts introduced in Chapter Twenty-One and in earlier chapters. We will discuss the kind of skills needed to safely help patients process shock affects should they arise within sessions. These affects commonly include emotional flooding, freezing states, and dissociation. They commonly arise in overwhelming fashion in a CRI context. We will discuss these approaches both from the perspective of verbal and perceptual skills and in a more classical cranial context. This chapter again relies heavily upon the work of Dr. Peter Levine. I humbly apologize for any misinterpretations. We will introduce Dr. Levine's concept of the trauma vortex and of titration. I will also

introduce the *focusing* process developed by Dr. Eugene Gendlin. *Focusing* helps patients access the subtler feeling tones of a process and the meaning it holds for them. I have found focusing to be an invaluable aid in the exploration of traumatic patterns as they arise in sessions. I teach the focusing process to patients who are open to exploring their inner world. I have found that these skills give practitioners a ground to come from when patients express traumatic processes or go into overwhelmed states. They help both practitioner and patient feel safer in the context of session work.

Resources within the Cranial Context

As you know, within the cranial field, there are very powerful processes that encourage the expression of inherent resources. We have described these in some detail in earlier chapters. I will simply remind you of them here. The foremost resource is stillness. Stillness is the ground of our being, and the same Stillness that permeates my being permeates yours. Processes that bring us into a deeper and more immediate relationship to Stillness will encourage the resources of the system to be expressed. We introduced some processes in Chapters Eight and Sixteen to help patients contact their inner resources. These were called stillpoint processes. Stillpoints are really about a deepening stillness. Stillness is the ground of emergence from which

---

In this chapter we will:

- *Discuss resources within a cranial and a general context.*

- *Work with some perceptual exercises around resources.*

- *Introduce the focusing process.*

- *Discuss dissociation.*

- *Further discuss trauma theory.*

- *Introduce particular trauma skills related to hyperarousal and hypoarousal states.*

---

potency arises. Stillpoints and a deepening into a Stillness help potency to manifest and express the ordering principle from within. The exercise we introduced in Chapter Sixteen with the CV4 process, the "eye of the needle" or the "mysterious gateway," is a key process to explore here. As the practitioner shifts the perceptual field to the deeper unfoldments generated by the intentions of the Breath of Life, an entry into the Dynamic Stillness may become possible. This is really about letting go and allowing a deepening relationship to the unknown. Within the Dynamic Stillness, the potential for order and a sense of great peace can be accessed. It is a state in which potential is again appreciated. Here resources are accessed at a very primary level of process.

Another important process that helps access and liberate potency is the *state of balanced tension*. We introduced this concept in Chapter Fifteen. It is within states of balance that "something happens" beyond the compensations and inertial forces present. The state of balance is a state in which a *dynamic equilibrium* is attained between the inherent potencies centering the disturbance and the inertial forces maintaining it. In Peter Levine's terms, it is when a dynamic equilibrium is attained between the forces within the trauma and healing vortices. A stillness is attained in which potential and fluidity are again possible. Within the state of balance a precise neutral is accessed in which a particular inertial fulcrum is uncoupled from others in the system. A specific fulcrum can be focused upon without initiating the forces found in other fulcrums. The stillness accessed within the state of balance functions to allow inertial potencies to be expressed beyond the forces being centered and the compensations being maintained. It also allows the unified field of potency, as a tensile field of action, to come into play. The state of balance can initiate the whole field of potency to express its inherent healing function. A permeation of potency into disordered and chaotic cells and tissues will result. In other words, resources are activated and expressed within a wide field of action.

The awareness of these processes occurs within the mid-tide level of action and within the deeper action of the Long Tide and the Dynamic Stillness itself. As you deepen and widen your perceptual fields, these deeper intrinsic forces and ordering intentions will also begin to manifest. The biodynamic potency is epigenetic and carries the ordering matrix to all cells and tissues. You may sense the potency of the Breath of Life rising within the midline and manifesting within inertial fulcrums as the inherent treatment plan unfolds. We called this idea the "eye of the needle" or the "mysterious gateway" in which the stilling, deepening, and widening of your field of perception initiates a relationship to potency and the ordering matrix it carries in its purest form.

Working with Resources and Sensations

We have introduced the idea of resources both in the last chapter and in Chapter Eight. Here we will further discuss the importance of resources and resourced sensations within a clinical context. The establishment of resources is an essential part of the titration process, which was introduced in the last chapter. It is very useful for a person to have a *felt awareness* of his or her resources. By this I mean an awareness of resources as sensations and feeling tones within the body. Sensations are the physical sensations that give you clues to your current state. Feeling tones, or felt senses, are more global. They are commonly unclear feelings "about" the process or issue being addressed. They are a mixture of physical sensation, subtler feelings, and even psychological process and mental images. It is commonly hard to name them, but they hold essential information about the nature of the process being explored. It is like the feeling you might wake up with after a deep sleep with dreams. It may leave you with a subtle feeling tone that you struggle to name, but if you do, an "ah ha!" experience ensues.

We will discuss the *felt sense* in more detail below when we introduce the focusing process.

The quality of sensation and feeling tone that a person is experiencing can be a real resource. If a person is only aware of "bad" and uncomfortable sensations, then he or she can be more easily overwhelmed by the activation of shock affect. Within this context, the concept of *space* is important to understand. If a person is only aware of bad or uncomfortable sensations, then there may not be any space within his or her experience to allow the affects to process without overwhelm. One aspect of the *experience* of space relates to a person's ability to perceive spacious, warm, open, and expansive sensations within the body. The experience of space may also be linked to resourcing images and memories that generate the felt experience of space. These can balance the uncomfortable and many times terrifying sensations that may be experienced as the system expresses its shock affect. If a patient can also access the felt sense of the fluid tide and the Long Tide, this can be an extremely resourcing ability. There may even be times when a patient can settle into the Dynamic Stillness and truly let go of self-view and fear, even for a moment. These kinds of experiences can be transforming.

Spacious and resourced sensations also allow a person to approach the edges of the difficult or frightening sensations without being sucked into the vortex of the trauma. If overwhelming sensations or processes arise, the ability to be on the edge of these traumatic affects without being overwhelmed by them is an essential personal skill in the resolution of trauma. Being on the "edge" of the process allows a person to stay with uncomfortable or frightening activation without becoming overwhelmed by it and without entering dissociated states. An ability to bring awareness to the sensations and feeling tones within the body and to stay on the edge of them without being overwhelmed can be an essential aspect of the healing process. In order to help this process, it is important to be sure that the patient can experience the resolution of shock affect with a sense of space and resource. By this I mean that the patient can be with the sensations and feeling tones of the experience without totally identifying and being overwhelmed by them. There is the space to be with the process and not be swept away by it. The person has an inner witness to the arising sensations and feelings and can relate to them with some space and curiosity. With space, a person can witness the activation of shock affects without experiencing them as though the trauma is happening again. Being in the present, with an awareness of arising sensations and feeling tones, can be a great benefit.

The most important aspect of this process is a developing ability to inquire into the nature of our human condition. Stillness lies at the heart of this inquiry. Inquiry within the present arising of life process is essential. When difficult processes arise, the ability to inquire into them, and to help the patient begin a journey of inquiry, is the key to success. There are some simple things that can help ground your patient in the present and bring him or her into relationship to sensations and feeling tones. One approach is to maintain verbal contact and start an inquiry into the quality of what is arising. An inquiry into sensations and feeling tones can help set up a witness consciousness and encourage space within the person's experience. Questions like, "Where do you sense that in your body? What tells you are afraid (or sad or angry etc.)? What sensations tell you that? Can you describe the feeling tone of that?" can be useful to initiate an inquiry. A useful structure for this is described in the focusing process below.

Another thing that is useful is to help a person find the way back into an awareness of the body. It is not about demanding that the person be present, or "be in the body," but it is about setting up an inquiry into where the person senses himself or herself to be and creating a relationship to the present experience. Simple processes like bringing awareness to breath and breathing can help slow a process down and start to bring a person into relationship to the present sensations of whatever is arising. As we sense and build our resources, we can develop options and choice in our responses to stress and danger. Helping a person establish options in the response to stress is an important aspect of being able to safely be with shock release. Never make a person stay with something that is overwhelming when he or she doesn't have the resources to do so. We will expand upon these ideas below.

Resources: Clinical Discussion

Resources is an extremely important concept to grasp within the cranial field and, indeed, within the context of any therapeutic or clinical work. Any deep exploration into the human condition and its suffering will touch upon past experience and trauma. Helping people recognize how they already resource themselves can be very empowering. In a traumatic experience people's resources are overwhelmed and in the process of trauma resolution, these resources must be again felt and deepened. Notice simple things, like the clothes they wear or a particular piece of jewelry they tend to use. Bringing their attention to these, and to the sensations and feelings associated with them, can help them get in touch with a sense of inner resource. Let's review a simple exercise from Chapter Eight that usually helps access resourced and spacious sensations. In this process you work with both imagery and sensation. Sit in a comfortable position and take a deep breath. The first thing to do is to find your way into a relationship to the sensations within your body. To do this, you might first become aware of your breathing. Follow your breath into your body and then notice the sensations you encounter. Use the breath to anchor your awareness within sensations and then simply notice the arising sensations and feeling tones. Take a few minutes to simply become aware of your inner sensations.

Once you have a relationship to these sensations, imagine a person, place, activity or thing that you really like, that really resources you. If it is a person, choose a person who truly represents a re-

source to you. You may find that your relationships hold a lot of ambiguity and it may be better to use a place, an activity, or an object the first time you try this exercise. Bring the image of this resource into your mind's eye. Then notice the quality of the sensations that arise within your body. Where in the body do you sense these? Describe them. Are the sensations/feeling tones familiar? Do you sense anything telling you that you are okay? Can you find some words to describe them? Once you sense the resourced sensations and have described them, try to remember them. You can later use the image to access these sensations within the clinical context. This is not as artificial as it sounds. All that is happening is that you are accessing sensations that you already know. The intention is to have them readily available. It is just a matter of becoming skillful in sensing and allowing them. Within sessions, if overwhelming sensations arise, this process can be a godsend. Once this is established, the patient may be able to meet the shocked, frozen, and emotionally charged sensations with more space and some sense of control and containment.

Resources can be sensed and cultivated in many ways. For instance, it may be important to notice how a person protects himself or herself psychologically and emotionally. If a person habitually reacts to stress by withdrawing or running away, this behavior can be experienced more consciously and used as a skilful option in circumstances that may feel overwhelming. What was a habitual reaction can become a conscious choice and a resource. If a person reacts to stress by dissociating, he or she can explore that state too. Once a person has a relationship to the dissociative process, even this can be a resource. For instance, in my own case, until I was thirty-two years old, I tended to go into dissociative states very easily. I was not consciously aware of this process. It was a manifestation of very early trauma and dissociation. Other layers of trauma were coupled with it. As I became aware of my dissociative state within the context of psychotherapy sessions, I was able to form a relationship to the present sensations within my body. From this base, I was then able to come back into relationship to my present experience. When dissociation arises now, I am usually aware of it. It is like the red warning light on the dashboard of a car. It warns me to *pay attention* to what is going on. It tells me, "Something important is happening here." Thus the dissociative process itself can become a resource! It is important to help patients sense both the uncomfortable or potentially overwhelming sensations, if these arise within sessions, *and* their resources. As they learn to do this, they may find themselves moving back and forth between their trauma and healing vortices as their system moves to resolve the trauma. For instance, you might notice that your patient begins to tremble, some shock affects are expressed, and then there is a great sigh and deep breath as more space is felt. A movement from the expression of traumatic energies and their affects to a sense of greater space occurs. A useful process to work with in this context is called *shuttling*.

Resources and Shuttling: Clinical Discussion

Shuttling is a term that originally comes from Gestalt therapy. It denotes the ability to *not* be with something. By this, I mean that a person has the resources to notice the activation of a trauma-related process and can decide not to enter it. In other words, the person has the option of exploring it or not. The person can shuttle into the process and shuttle out of it. The ability to do this is very empowering. The person does not "become" the process and is not swept away by it. If you totally identify with and become an arising process, you cannot have a spacious relationship to it. Processes that may commonly arise include experiences of overwhelming emotions, anxiety, freezing states like numbness, coldness, or even immobility, and dissociative processes. Related kinds of processes may be more psychological in nature, like projected fear or anger. It *is* possible to be swept away by an overwhelming process and to come out the other side.

However, over the years I have seen too much reinforcement and reenactment of trauma in these circumstances to trust this. It is better to slowly build resources and to meet arising trauma processes within the context of an inquiry into their nature, rather than becoming totally identified with them. Indeed, the ability to have space from a trauma-bound process is an essential part of its resolution.

The process of shuttling can help a patient gain some experience of the possibilities of an inquiry into his or her state. For instance, the work is not necessarily about expressing emotions or feelings, although this may happen, but is more about exploring and inquiring into them with space and resources.

Let's again use a perceptual exercise to explore these ideas. Again sit in a comfortable position. Become aware of resourced sensations and feeling tones as described above. Start an inquiry into these. Where do you feel these in your body? What is your experience of them? Can you find some words that describe them? Stay with these sensations for a while. See if you can bring awareness to the body area in which you sense the resourced feelings.

Now, as you sit with this, notice anything in your body that feels uncomfortable. "Look" at it, or listen to it, from the area of your body that has the more resourced sensations. For instance, if you sense a warmth within your belly telling you that you are okay, see if you can rest your awareness within that area. Let's say, as you rest within your belly, you also notice a tightness and heaviness in your chest area. Very slowly move your attention from your belly and its more resourced feelings to the edge of where you sense the heaviness. Don't go into it, just to the edge. Notice the sensation or feelings that arise as you do this. Now shuttle back to your belly and its more resourced sensations. Again stay with this for a while and then move back to the edge of the discomfort. Practice shuttling back and forth, giving yourself time to experience the sensations generated by the process. Do you sense anything changing? Are there sensation of movement from the area of discomfort? Are there any tremblings or sensations of energy moving? Stay with this shuttling process for a while and finish by again acknowledging the resourced sensations within your belly, or any other perception of resources that arises. Some people are more comfortable working with this process in other ways. For instance, a person may find that he or she can take the resources into the area of discomfort rather than stay on the edge of it. See what works for you and keep exploring these ideas. In the above example we worked with a discomfort within the body. As you did this other, related sensations and feelings may have arisen. These may have included sensations related to the processing of some shock affect in the system, or emotional tones or releases, or energy releases. As you get familiar with the shuttling process, you will find that it can be applied to any arising process including emotional releases, unclear feeling tones within the body, and even arising images and memories. It is a very useful process to practice and to lead patients through when appropriate.

Focusing

Focusing is a therapeutic inquiry developed by Dr. Eugene Gendlin and his staff at Chicago University. While working in the student counseling center some important things became apparent to him. There were many kinds of psychotherapists working at the center. They practiced the whole gamut of approaches and theories from classical psychodynamic therapies, to humanistic therapies like Gestalt, to Transpersonal therapies. In consultation with colleagues, Dr. Gendlin noticed something important. It did not seem to matter what kind of therapy was offered, or even the theories involved. Students got better not because of the therapy or belief system employed, but because of something that they were doing internally. It seemed that certain students were able to internally process their experiences within the sessions better than others. Dr. Gendlin headed a research project that set out to discover if this was true and, if it was, if the skill could be taught to others. The *focusing* process de-

veloped out of that research. Focusing has helped a multitude of people over the last thirty years. It is a skill that can be used within any kind of therapeutic context and is really a life skill rather than a specific therapy process.

Focusing makes important inner skills available to both practitioner and client. Focusing focuses on what Dr. Gendlin called the *felt sense*. A felt sense is a global sense of something. It is not just physical, but is composed of sensations, emotional tones, feeling senses, and even images. It is the unclear, whole *bodily* sense of something. It is an expression of how we embody our experience. It is a realm within, which allows access to how we hold meaning in an embodied way. One important thing about the felt sense is that, initially, it is usually unclear. It is like waking up from sleep and sensing a feeling tone of something left over from a dream. You might at first struggle to name it, but when you do there is an "ah ha!" experience. The following is a brief summary of the process. I must refer you to Dr. Gendlin's book, *Focusing,* for a much more complete description. The focusing process entails learning six movements or steps. Once internalized, they become one fluid process.

Some suggestions to help you enter your body space:

- Try following your breath into your body and its sensations. As you inhale, follow the feeling sense of your breathing into your body space.

- An alternative is to "inhale" your way into your body from the bottom up. To do this, imagine that you have nostrils on the soles of your feet and as you inhale, imagine/sense that you are drawing your breath from the soles of your feet, up your legs, into your abdomen.

Entering Your Body Space

The first thing you do in the focusing process is to find your way into your *body space*. The intention is to be inside your body with awareness from the top of your neck to your pelvic floor. *This is the embodied realm of the felt sense.* It is within this body space that access to the embodied meaning of our experience can be accessed. The focusing process will only work if you have a relationship to the feeling tones held within this body space. It is where the "all-about-ness" or the "whole of something" is held and experienced. To paraphrase the Buddha, when your awareness is held *within* your body space, you can be with the feeling tone *within* the feeling tone (i.e., not dissociated from it)

Accessing a Felt Sense

I use a number of perceptual exercises to help a person gain access to the realm of the felt sense. Let's explore one here. Sit in a comfortable position. Bring awareness to your body space. Use one of the suggestions above if that is helpful. Now bring an image of a person, a memory, or a place or activity that you find *totally resourcing and positive*. Be a lit-

---

The Felt Sense Is:

- a global sense of something.

- not just physical, but is composed of sensations, emotional tones, feeling senses and even images.

- accessed within our body space.

- the unclear, whole bodily sense of something.

- an expression of how we embody and give meaning to our experience.

- usually unclear, hard to grasp or name.

---

tle wary about choosing a person, because we commonly have mixed feelings about people. Bring this image to your body space. What do you notice as you do this? What are the qualities of feeling tone that arise? Where in your body do you sense them? Can you describe them? Now shift the image. Bring an image of someone or something that you definitely do not like. You may have a strong aversion to this person, place, activity, or thing. It can even be a historical figure. Notice the change within your body space. Does the sense of the feeling tone change? What is the quality of the new feeling tones? Can you describe them? Now, staying within your body space, again shift to the totally resourcing image. Can you again sense the shift in feeling tone? What is this like now?

The Focusing Movements

- *Movement One: Clearing Space*

The intention of the first movement is to bring attention to your inner sense of significance, concern, or disquiet. It is about sensing the inner issues held as bodily tones or senses within your mind-body matrix. Bring attention to your inner body space as suggested above. Bring an inquiry to your mind-body system by floating the question, "What's important here?" or, "What is of concern here?" As a concern arises, do not go inside it, simply note that it is there. See if you can create space between you and the concern. As concern, disquiet, issues, and so forth, arise, perhaps imagine/sense that you are putting them aside or outside of yourself. Perhaps put them on an imaginary shelf from which you can retrieve them later, or place them in a bubble and let them float away. Perhaps the simple act of acknowledgment is enough. Sometimes it helps to make a list of them in order to clear your inner space. As each concern arises make space, ask the question again, and then wait awhile to see what else arises. Follow this process as many times as necessary as you allow space to arise. The intention is to *clear inner space* so that you can engage in an inquiry into *one* specific issue or concern. This helps uncouple it from others and allows a specific inquiry into the felt sense of a particular concern. This is also a great process to use on its own. It helps you access a sense of inner spaciousness.

- *Movement Two: Accessing the Felt Sense*

The felt sense is the realm of the unclear, whole bodily sense of our mind-body process. It is a realm of meaning. It is the whole sense of something, which includes *meaning* and the felt energies of experience. It is also a realm where intuitive, holistic information is available and accessible. It is a realm where the co-arising nature of reality can be appreciated. Unresolved issues, concerns, and qualities of disquiet will be held within the body as feeling tones or felt senses that contain the meaning of the issue or concern. They will be experienced within the felt sense realm as unclear feeling tones. The felt sense realm also contains all the information necessary to resolve the inner conflict or concern. Thus as you bring awareness to this realm, it is seen that the concern or problem unfolds into its own answer. Thus the felt sense is not necessarily about something difficult or traumatic. It is a *feeling realm,* which holds meaning and can be accessed via a natural movement of awareness. Personal issues and/or felt senses will arise spontaneously within sessions as part of a person's process. When they do, focusing becomes incredibly useful. Here we will choose a particular issue or concern in order to learn the process.

One way to access the felt sense is to bring a particular concern or issue into your body space. Select one of the concerns discovered in the first movement. Bring it to your body as an image, memory, or sensation. Let yourself soften into the issue as you become aware of its *felt sense* within your inner body space. Allow an unclear sense of "all of that" to arise. This will be a tonal quality within the body, but not just physical. It is a combination of body, mind, and feeling states, which are the *embodied* sense of the issue you are exploring. See if an unclear feeling sense arises. Remember that even feeling tones that seem empty and blank, or sensations of numbness and immobility, may be part of the overall felt sense of something. The next step is to try to get a handle on this often nebulous quality.

- *Movement Three: Getting A Handle*

Felt senses are commonly unclear, nebulous, and difficult to grasp. As we have seen, the felt sense is not just physical, but is a matrix of feelings, mental tones, and physical sensations. The process of *getting a handle* helps to clarify the felt sense and invites its meaning to speak to you directly. As you become aware of the tonal qualities arising in relationship to the issue being explored, see if you can find a word, phrase, or image that gives you a handle on the felt sense. Don't try to find a handle; don't look for a handle. *See if the handle arises from the bodily sense of the concern.* Let the body speak to you; let the felt sense clarify itself to you. See if you can allow the *embodied* sense of the concern to speak to you. The handle helps you access the *meaning* of the felt sense or feeling tone that arises in relationship to the concern being explored.

- *Movement Four: Resonating*

See if the word, phrase, or image *resonates* with the felt sense. Bring the handle to it within the body and see if it fits, or resonates. This is like an "ah ha!" kind of experience. If the handle fits the felt sense, it will feel right; it will resonate with it. Once you access this handle and have a sense of its resonance with the felt sense, simply be aware of it within your body space.

- *Movement Five: Asking*

Once you have a handle, the next step is to inquire into it. This is the step of *asking*. It is basically an act of awareness. It is about actively bringing awareness to the handle and the felt sense. It is an inquiry. "What is this for me? What is important here? Is this the whole of it?", "Is this the worst of it?" Let whatever arises enter your body space and see how the felt sense of the concern or issue speaks to you. As this inquiry continues you may sense a *felt shift*, a change in the felt sense that tells you something has been processed. You may experience expansion, relief, insight, as the energies of the felt sense shift. They may even fully resolve or evolve into something else. You can check if the felt sense has shifted by simply bringing the handle back to it. If there has been a shift, the handle will not fit anymore. It will not resonate with the felt sense.

- *Movement Six: Receiving*

Receiving is really not so much a final step, but a chance to acknowledge the process that has occurred, a time to put a hold on things for now, like a punctuation mark in a longer story. It is also a time to fully take in and integrate the insights or shifts that may have arisen within the focusing process. This last movement allows recognition and acknowledgement of the process. Let yourself receive and acknowledge the process as it is. Receive anything that the felt sense and the process of inquiry have offered you. Acknowledge any felt shifts. You can also go back to the *clearing space* step above to set aside any unresolved issues, feeling tones, and concerns.

Working with the Felt Sense

I find the focusing process very useful in session work. When patients encounter feeling tones and sensations that either call to their awareness or are uncomfortable and challenging, the focusing process can be extremely useful. I generally don't teach the process to patients in a formal way, but introduce the focusing movements as they become appropriate within the sessions. It is truly magical to be in the presence of a person who connects with the inner meaning of a seemingly difficult or challenging feeling, sensation, or mental process. It liberates the potencies that have become inertial in order to center the unresolved issue. As in all the work we do, when inertial potencies are liberated, expansion and realignment to natural fulcrums will occur. Thus, even in a habitual mental or psychological process, once the energies of that are resolved, the mind is freer to access states of balance and stillness. If you want to learn more about focusing, I recommend finding a focusing teacher or group to work with. Focusing tuition is available in North America and Europe and, I expect, in many other locations.

Resources and Tracking Sensations

Another important skill for patients to develop is the ability to be with and to track sensations and feeling tones within the body. Tracking these can help the person come into direct relationship to the feeling tones and sensations of the trauma as they are held in the body. A patient's resources must first be established, and his or her ability to be aware of sensations with clear psychological and felt space is essential. Again the establishment of resources becomes the ground for the processing of any shock affects within the system. Once these resourcing skills are developed, the work encompasses (1) an awareness of the sensations and felt senses in the body, (2) the ability to notice their qualities, (3) the ability to notice how and where they move, and (4) the ability to not be overwhelmed by them. A useful approach within this tracking process is to track these sensations to their focus in the body.

For instance, a sensation may arise in a patient's arm; you might notice this as a motion or twitch, or

> ### Tracking Sensations Encompass:
>
> - *the establishment of resources,*
>
> - *the ability to generate psychological and felt space,*
>
> - *an awareness of the sensations in the body,*
>
> - *the ability to notice their qualities,*
>
> - *the ability to notice how and where they move, and*
>
> - *the ability to not be overwhelmed by them.*
>
>   It is the ability to track sensations to their focus in the body and to stay with that without becoming overwhelmed.

the patient may comment on it. You might ask the person to notice that sensation and to stay with it with awareness. You might ask if it has a particular focus within the body. Or ask a question like, "Where does that seem to come from within your body?" The patient may then track some sensations into the chest and heart area. You may help them stay on the *edge* of these sensations without becoming overwhelmed by them. In this process you might also help initiate an inquiry into the qualities and the nature of the sensations the patient is tracking. In this process of inquiry, you might also help him or her access the *felt sense*, the "all-about-ness" of the process, as described above. Finally, the practitioner can help the patient to allow any related shock affects, such as emotional qualities, electric-like streaming of energies, tremblings, and so on, to process and be expressed through the body within its resources. As the patient stays with the sensations and with the process of inquiry, the tissues and the body may tremble and shake as the cycling of energies within the system is processed throughout the body. Remember the antelop. Its body shook and trembled as it came out of the shock and processed it. As noted in the last chapter, if your patients are resourced, you will see them moving between their trauma vortex and their healing vortex; first processing some shock, then breathing deeply and sensing more space and lightness in their system. Remember to always give your patients the option of not staying with overwhelming sensations and of pulling themselves out of any sensations or discharges that are overwhelming.

The Warble

Another aspect of this process is what Peter Levine calls the *warble*. A person holding shock affects in the system is also holding a huge amount of cycling energy. These cycling energies have not been able to complete and discharge. This "charge" is especially held in the neuroendocrine system. You will perceive it with your sensitive palpation skills, within the tissues and fluids of the body, even perhaps on a cellular level. Remember that this charge becomes frozen within the system as it goes into the immobilized state of the shock response. Stress responses start to cycle and, if not resolved in some way, will keep cycling. When a person builds resources and can stay on the edge of these cycling energies, they will start to move in some way. The first thing you might perceive are subtle motions, or "micromotions," within the body. You may also sense perturbations of fluid and potency within the cerebrospinal fluid. This is a sign that the person is shifting from a cycling of the energies to a discharge and processing of them. They start to express this as motion. You may also note other signs that the person is shifting from a cycling of trauma-bound energies to a discharge of them. This may include temperature changes, skin color changes, rapid eye motions and pupil changes, sweating, and so on. Peter Levine calls these expressions of motion and autonomic discharge, the "warble." This is a very visually descriptive word for these kinds of motions and discharges of energy.

A person will warble as he or she starts to manifest the cycling energies of traumatization. If your patients start to warble, make sure they are resourced; ask questions like, "Can you stay with this?" Slow their process down if necessary. Reassure them and have them slow their breath down. Bring their attention to the motions and sensations expressed. Start an inquiry. This sets up a witness consciousness, which is essential in trauma resolution. "Where do you sense that in your body? What is the quality of that?" Help them track the quality and motion of the sensations that arise. Use the focusing process, as outlined above, to allow access to the space to explore the deeper felt sense of the process. Here an inner, visceral meaning can be appreciated and can be transformative. All of this needs practice and confidence on the part of the practitioner. Do your own work. Explore your own layers of traumatization in a resourced way. *Do not* go for cathartic releases. Explore the arising process with space in present time. Remember that there *is* a process, but you are *not* the process. You are much more than that. Take trauma resolution courses, within the context of Peter Levine's work, if possible and appropriate.

Within the cranial context, see if the cycling energies of traumatization are discharging in relationship to available potency. Is there a sense that the shock affect is clearing through the action of the potency within the fluids? If it is, you will sense a discharge of autonomic energies via subtle electric-like clearing through the fluids. You may sense the fluids, especially cerebrospinal fluid, perturbing as the shock affect is clearing. The body may also tremble and discharge the energy like the antelope described earlier. Be sure that this is expressed in a paced and resourced space. Reassure the patient and help keep the session paced by slowing things down if necessary. The process is similar to the one described in the last chapter. The person is processing the charge like the antelope who comes out of the death-feigning, frozen state. He or she will move from cycling the energies to expressing them in some way. If this occurs, help the person express and process the shock affects as trembling and body motions in a paced and resourced way. The electric-like discharges and tremblings of the body arise as the person comes out of the shocked state and dis-

charges the fight or flight energies that were cycling within their system.

A final thing to note are the kinds of movements that a person's system may express as he or she moves from the shock towards fight and flight and orienting motions. You may see patients move their arms, legs, head, or body in ways that appear to be about protecting themselves from danger or about orienting to the danger in some way. For instance, you may notice them starting to push out with a hand or arm or use an arm to protect their body. Or you may notice their legs moving as though to push out or run; or you may notice their head moving towards a particular direction. These are expressions of the system moving towards fight and flight and orientation responses. Remember how the antelope did this as it came out of shock? It is really important here to slow things down, to "titrate" in Peter Levine's terms, and to bring the patient's attention to these movements. If the motions and the charge related to them move too fast, the patient may go into a dissociative state. He or she may express strong emotions or powerful movements such as hitting out and kicking, but if the person enters a dissociative state, then the process may become overwhelming and possibly retraumatizing. Slowing the process down and bringing the patient's attention to the mobilizing or orienting motions helps to move the frozen energies of the immobilized state into reassociated, purposeful actions and intentions. This will help the person both discharge the shock held in the system and reestablish the fight or flight resources. From here strong motions, movement, and emotions may be expressed as part of a discharge of the shock and of the process of completion.

Peter Levine has the patient slow the process down at this point. He has the patient sense himself or herself preparing to do whatever it is the body is moving towards expressing. This *preparing to do* phase is important not to miss. I have seen Maura Sills do a similar thing with patients. She has them stay with the *intention* to do something as a feeling sense in their body, before actually expressing it.

This staying with the *preparing to do* phase or the intentional phase lets the system begin to discharge the imploded energy in a very slow and resourced way. If it is missed, patients may jump to a physical or emotional expression of the imploded energy without actually processing and releasing it in a truly healing way. They miss the titration of the imploded energy and may explode into a dissociative reaction. Phrases like "Can you sense your body preparing to do that? Can you stay with the 'preparing to do' of that? Can you sense and stay with the intention of that in your body?" may be helpful. It's really about slowing things down and allowing things to resolve through the body with resources and appropriate pacing. The person may then move into more physical and cathartic expressions, but from a base of moving out of the shock response into an expression of power. Another thing to remember is that patients, as they move out of shock, may experience and express the fear or rage that may have also been cycling within the shock process. It is important that these are expressed within an associated and resourced state or the patient may just flip back into the shocked state.

Dissociation

In the last chapter we introduced the idea of *dissociation*. In this section, I would like to further explore the nature of dissociation as a stress response and place it more within the clinical context. Let's look at a scenario in which a person, holding some past shock and trauma in the system, meets stress at work, perhaps anger from their boss. Let's imagine that the boss is in a bad mood. Maybe he is stressed out and pressured by his own work, or his own boss. Imagine that he gets angry at our person. This might restimulate other instances of anger that were shocking or overwhelming for the person, or hook into personality processes relating to authority figures. Imagine that the person is cycling autonomic energies left over from past trauma. This cycling will lower his ability to appropriately meet new stresses

or potentially traumatic situations. As the boss expresses his anger, the person's system is overwhelmed by the experience. He doesn't have the resources, physical or psychological, to meet the anger. This may restimulate past traumatization, and he enters the shock response. One of the things that may occur is that the person will *dissociate*. Remember that an important shock response to an overwhelming experience is to dissociate, that is, to split off from the feelings and sensations of the body.

Dissociation is part of the natural defensive processes of the body. When a person's system is overwhelmed and the shock response is initiated, the parasympathetic nervous system surges and certain neurohormones flood the system. Under this influence a person will experience dissociative processes. The psyche may even dissociate from the soma. In other words, the person loses touch with current sensations and processes and may even become frozen and immobilized. The person may feel numb and immobilized or may inappropriately express emotions. Things will seem out of kilter. The person has entered the vortex of past traumatization. This is more likely to happen if he or she is cycling unresolved shock affects within the system. The person in the scenario above may freeze in response to the boss's anger; he may not be able to meet it in any skillful way. Alternately, he may express the cycling energies of his internalized trauma as terror or rage as his fight or flight mechanisms attempt to engage. He may thus express emotions that are inappropriate to the situation. The charge in the nervous system may be expressed in his own anger, or he may break down in a deluge of tears. Since this arises in a dissociative and unresourced state, the emotional expression is usually inappropriate and even retraumatizing to the system. Emotion is expressed in a dissociative state as an emotional affect and serves to reinforce the shock already held in the person's system. The person may be left retraumatized by the experience. A new layer of shock has been added to what is already held in the system. This is because he experienced the reactivation of the shock in a dissociated state and were not able to reassociate and process it.

The more traumatized the system, the more difficult it is to meet stressful situations, and the more difficult it is to process new experiences. Perhaps in this case, as the person's boss expresses anger, his defense mechanisms kick in. These are learned psychoemotional and psychic defenses that protect the person from confronting the shock and pain held in the system. As the boss expresses anger, the person will probably react in ways that are limited, familiar, and protective. Perhaps the person acts in a fawning and humble manner. This may placate the boss, but may also be an expression of low resources, which prevents him from dealing with the situation in a more forthright manner. Perhaps another person may run away and quit her job, or yet another may verbally attack the boss. The important thing is that these defensive reactions become automatic, and the person becomes locked into them. They are expressions of the traumatization held in the system. In other words, the effect of past traumatization is to reduce the range of possible responses available to the person in stressful situations. His options have become limited. Where there should be fluidity, there is fixity.

Dissociation: Clinical Discussion

In a clinical setting, a patient's system may express shock affects during a session. These may include hyperarousal states like emotional flooding and hypoarousal states like freezing and immobility. In these circumstances it is important that you, as practitioner, are aware of the possibility of dissociative states. This is important because, as mentioned above, one of the initial responses to trauma is to dissociate, that is, to split off from the feelings and sensations in the body. These sensations were originally experienced as overwhelming and their reactivation in sessions may also be experienced as overwhelming. As you pay attention to the process, you may notice some signs of dissociation. For instance, a patient's eyes may glaze over or he or she may seem distant and far away. What the person says may not be appropriate to the present circumstances. As you palpate the system, there may be a sense of distance, shut down, or very stagnant potencies. The system may seem to be shut down and tidal motions may not be evident. There may even be a sense of "vacancy" as though no one is home. The person may seem very distant and hard to contact.

If dissociative states arise in a session, it is important to engage the patient's process of inquiry in order to help him or her realign with present time. What is happening is that the system is accessing past traumatization as though it is happening now. What the person is really encountering are the cycling energies and hormones of the shock affect within their system. It is important to encourage the presence, or present awareness, of the patient so he or she remains in present time and doe not experience these affects as though the trauma is happening now. This is very much a factor of the practitioner's ability to maintain his or her presence and to encourage the patient's own presence or ability to be in the present. It is most important to help the patient stay in contact with the experience and in relationship with the practitioner. One way to do this is to maintain your verbal contact with the patient and to initiate an inquiry into what is being experienced.

Thus, if a patient experiences dissociation, one way of helping him or her to come into the present is to initiate an inquiry into the dissociative state. Initiating an inquiry into the state helps bring a person into present time. It helps to generate space by creating an inner witness who can begin to have a relationship to the experience. Questions like, "Where do you sense yourself to be just now? How far away are you? Can you describe that foggy state? What is the quality of that for you? What is happening just now? Can you sense that in your body?" may help bring the patient into a relationship to the felt sense of the dissociation. This is an open process in which the practitioner must offer suggestions slowly in relationship to the nature of the dissociative state being described.

Another important aspect of dissociative activation is a freezing and immobilization of the system. States of freezing and immobility may be activated, and a person may experience physical numbness, mental haziness, and confusion, even extremes of the immobilization and coldness. I have seen patients experience temporary paralysis as these states were activated within the system. The first step for the practitioner is to acknowledge the process and to reassure the patient that it is important, part of a healing and completion process. If a patient is expressing these kinds of shock affects, it is helpful to bring his or her awareness to the sensations and feeling tones of the experience in present time. If the person loses a sense of the present, it may feel as if the trauma is occurring again, and this can be very frightening. The experience in the treatment session may then just serve to reinforce the trauma or to send it deeper into the patient's system.

It is important to remember that the frozen, immobilized state that may accompany dissociation commonly has a huge amount of energy bound up within it. Encouraging present awareness in the body will also help the patient move from this frozen state to a state where the energy that has become bound up in the traumatized system can be accessed and discharged. Within the frozen state is the potential for its mobilization. If the energy bound up in the frozen state can be accessed by the patient, then the system may move to a more fluid and mobilized release of the affects. As we shall see, it is important to work slowly here and to help contain the patient's process by slowing things down. If your patient is aware of present sensations and feeling tones, and is resourced in himself or herself, the resolution of shock affect within the system becomes more likely. The practitioner's role here is to contain and support the process and to slow things down if the patient becomes overwhelmed by the experience.

Dissociation within the Cranial Context

The cranial practitioner may sense arising dissociative processes within the system in a number of ways. As you palpate a patient's system, there may be a sense of distance, as though the person has vacated or left the body. You may sense a vacancy and emptiness within the system. The person may seem very distant and hard to contact. The system may seem shut down, and tidal motions may not be evident. You may sense very stagnant potencies, as though the whole field of potency has become inertial. In overwhelmingly traumatic experiences, such as near fatal accidents, extremes of birth trauma, early childhood trauma, and the like, the whole field of potency may become inertial in order to center the shock within the system. Within the context of an arising process within a session, potency as a whole field of action may become inertial within the fluids in order to center and contain the arising experience. You may perceive that the fluid system is, or becomes, inertial and congested within the arising process. The potency that moves and permeates the fluids has become inertial in order to center the shock and shock affects within the system. These are common expressions of shock and shock affect within the system. You may even sense that the whole midline is congested or stagnant. Here the forces being centered are not necessarily localized fulcrums, but affect a whole area. The midline may seem dense, the vertebral column may express whole areas of compression, and natural fluid fluctuation may seem almost nonexistent. This is a common feature of birth trauma when the inertial forces involved are axial, powerful, and diffused throughout the midline.

I have also noted a very powerful dissociative process at work in some patients. In palpating their systems, the three functions of tissue, fluids, and potency seemed to be out of phase. The best way I can describe this is to remember an old black and white film I saw many years ago. The hero had been hit over the head and was knocked unconscious. As he came out of the unconscious state, the film director showed the room as though you were looking through the actor's eyes. Things were blurred and he had "double vision." The scene showed you a double image of everything. As the hero looked at a desk, there were at least two overlapping desks instead of one. In these patients' systems, the relationship between tissues, fluids, and potency felt something like that. They seemed shocked out of phase, like a "triple-vision." Potency, fluids, and tissues were centering around the shock affects, rather than the organizing principle of the Breath of Life. They seemed shocked and out of phase with each other. It was very difficult to help these systems access neutrals and states of balance. Tissues and fluids could not align to the midline, and the motion around the straight sinus was very slippery. The fluids and membranes would slip and slide around midline fulcrum,s, but could not orient to them. Work was very slow. Potencies within the midline were very inertial and fluctuation was restricted. Potencies had to be encouraged to manifest from the midline to begin to allow a realignment to occur. One classical process that can help this to occur is EV4. EV4 is very useful in dissociation. It helps potency to be expressed from the midline to the periphery and encourages the tidal motions. I worked with EV4 via the sacrum and tracked the manifestation of biodynamic potencies and inertial forces. Eventually these systems were able to express neutrals and states of balance. Shock affects could then be more safely processed within the resources of the system.

Another important phenomenon has to do with the ignition of the system at birth. As mentioned in Chapter Five, there is an ignition of the fluid system at birth. When the umbilical cord stops pulsing and the first breath is taken, there is a powerful welling up of potency through the cerebrospinal fluid within the dorsal midline. When this occurs, there is also an ignition of potency within the fluids of the third ventricle. You can sense this in patients as a dynamo-like action within the third ventricle. If this dynamo-like action is not present, then the system may not have fully ignited at birth. Shock may have a similar dampening down effect upon the system and upon the action within the third ventricle. This may occur due to birth trauma or anesthesia during the birth process. Anesthesia has a strong damping down effect on the system and, if unresolved, causes fluid stasis. The presence of anesthesia during birth may affect the ignition process as the potency acts to center the action of the anesthesia within the system. This is an aspect of anesthesia shock affect. If a patient accesses anesthesia shock affect during a session, you may perceive a systemwide stasis, global inertia within the whole tensile field of potency, and a general sense of vacancy. Resolution includes a process of reassociation and processing of the shock affects within the system. Again EV4 can be helpful here, as will the resolution of any inertial forces generated by birth trauma. A knowledge of cranial base patterns and of the birth process in general are essential here.

Summary: Processing Shock Affects within the Cranial Context

Overwhelming experiences, such as emotional flooding and freezing states, usually arise with the CRI level of process. Within the CRI level of experience, overwhelming emotional flooding, anxiety states, and frozen or numbed states may be activated. You might notice a shutting down of the system. The CRI will suddenly stop and a sense of shock will be felt. You may sense the fluids "locking up" as the shock affect is expressed within a CRI context. Within a cranial context, the most important intentions here are to help the patient's system shift from a cycling of affects to a deeper level of resource. It is imperative to help the system downshift to the mid-tide, or even to the Long Tide level of action if that is possible. I emphasize in courses that the CRI is a layer of affect and results. It is an expression of unresolved past experience. Autonomic cycling and set points affect its expression, and inertial issues of any kind will be expressed in its rate and quality. As noted above, in trauma counseling, if emotional flooding arises, the best initial clinical approach is to help slow things down. This is true within a cranial context also. If you are viewing the system from a CRI level, or if the system can only show you that level, there are some processes that help it to shift to the deeper tidal resources.

First of all, you can literally slow things down as you sense activation within the tissues and fluids. Slow the rate of expression down by subtly slowing the tissue motions down. This will help the system shift to stillness and to the mid-tide level of process. Along with this, make sure that you are viewing from a mid-tide perspective. Do not lose a sense of the whole. Let your hands float within fluids and hold the biosphere (the person's body and the field around it) within your field of awareness. See if you can help the system downshift to the mid-tide and the tidal potencies. The emotional process will then downshift too. It will shift from a cycling of emotional process to a process of completion. It feels different to both patient and practitioner. It becomes more spacious, and there is a sense of resource to it. Within your palpation sense, there will be subtler streamings of energy, perturbations of fluid, and a sense of a clearing of shock through the fluids throughout the body. Sensations of streaming of energy from the pelvis through the legs are common, as the sympathetic chain of ganglia discharge and clear their facilitation. (Much more on this in the next volume.) The patient will feel spacious within the process, and you will sense the action of potency within the fluids as the shock affects clear. From here, you can even go through the "eye of the needle" and shift to the Long Tide level of perception by deepening and widening your perceptual field. Within this level, potency at its most primal level of expression is accessed. It is basically essential to shift the system from a CRI level of expression to a level of action where resources are more easily accessed. Stillpoint processes, such as CV4, will also help to slow things down and help to access potency and resource within the process of discharge. This will again help the process shift from a cycling of energies to a completion of a process.

If your patient goes into a dissociative state, EV4s are a classical approach to a mobilization of potency and a reassociation of the psyche. You may notice dissociative state in a number of ways. There may be a perception of vacancy as you palpate. The patient may seem "far away." He or she may not be able to be in contact with you, or may seem dreamy and disconnected. Alternately, the patient may have dissociative experiences connected with what Peter Levine calls the "healing vortex" (see last chapter). As the system expresses its shock in an unresourced way, the person may be flooded with endorphins and dopamine. This will recapitulate the original trauma and the overwhelmed state. It is a tricky place. The patient may feel very comfortable here. Remember that dissociation is a defensive process. The patient may even experience what seem to be transpersonal or spiritual processes. These may actually be an expression of dissociation and ungroundedness. A truly spiritual process has a deep sense of ground and present time-ness to it. More commonly, dissociation within sessions is of the past; it is an expression of traumatization. See the discussion of this in the last chapter and above. In trauma counseling, the intention would be to explore the dissociative state within the present. Start an inquiry into its felt sense and the sensation of it. Remember, a lack of sensation *is* a sensation. EV4 can be very helpful here in the reassociation process.

To summarize, within the CRI level, emotional affects may arise in relationship to our particular conditioned state (e.g., our particular life experience). They are thus conditioned and conditioning. At CRI level, the activation of fight or flight emotions during treatment is more likely. Hyperarousal and hypoarousal states may manifest. These processes are the affects left over from unresolved past trauma. These may include a spectrum of emotion from fear to terror and from anger to rage. During a session, they may be expressed in a overwhelming and dissociated way. Emotions may flood, or the patient may experience freezing states. Then the person may reexperience overwhelm, dissociation, and traumatization. This is not necessarily therapeutic. The system may experience this as a reinforcement of the original traumatization. As these traumatic emotional states become inertial within the system, they will affect the expression of the CRI in some way.

Processes within the mid-tide level of expression are more about *present time*. During treatment, emotional affects of past trauma may be activated, but within the mid-tide they tend to be expressed in much milder forms within the resources of the person. Emotional processes are experienced as a completion of past experience and do not continue to cycle. Emotional affects complete; they are not reinforced. Emotional resolution may occur very quietly here and be experienced as a streaming of energy, warmth, and feeling. Within the Long Tide, shock affects are centered dynamically within the bioelectric matrix and can clear like a dropping away of something. The potency of the Breath of Life can be sensed to arise within the system as a field state, and something literally drops away. This is even more likely if the Dynamic Stillness is accessed by patient and practitioner. Then healing occurs within a kind of darkness under normal perceptual processes, with a deep sense of the vibrancy of life itself being reinstated. A simple process that helps to shift a system that cannot access its resources to a deeper relationship with its resources is outlined below.

Clinical Application: CV4 Process in the CRI

Sometimes a patient's system is so inertial, there is so much potency locked up centering the disturbances and shock affects within the system, that it is very difficult to initially get under the CRI level of action. All you may sense is activation and the CRI. Consider the CRI a level of results, affects, and autonomic activation. Find ways to get under it to

the deeper potencies that organize and center the system. A useful approach here may be to initiate a CV4 stillpoint within the CRI level of action, and to see if you can go through the "eye of the needle" to the deeper potencies and resources of the system. This was described in Chapter Sixteen.

Sometimes a person's system is so inertial that all you can sense is a CRI level of action. It may be very hard to make a perceptual shift to the mid-tide. There may be so much potency bound in centering traumatic conditions that the CRI is all that is obvious. If you begin to work within the CRI with an attitude of releasing or changing something, it is very likely that an activation of some kind will occur. This may take the form of increased symptoms, emotional flooding, freezing states, numbness, dissociation, reliving of a trauma in an unresourced manner, stress states and so on. What I recommend to practitioners is to find some way to help liberate potency beyond the conditions being centered. It is imperative to help the system access its own resources. When this occurs, the mid-tide will again become more available to your perceptual field. Stillpoints may help lead you and your patient there. Thus there are times when it is important to know how to initiate the stillpoint process within the CRI level of action. Previously, we have only described this from a mid-tide perspective. One way of approaching this is to work with the CV4 stillpoint process within the CRI, and within the stillpoint, to make a conscious shift to the mid-tide level of action. In essence, you will be following the system deeper into its tidal potencies because it can access them within stillness. It is a question of appreciating the qualities of deepening stillness as potency is initiated and accessed.

1. The patient is in the supine position. Use the CV4 hold as learned earlier. Place your perceptual field within the CRI. Let your hands float on tissues and narrow your perceptual field to bones and membranes. Get interested in the motion of the occiput. In inhalation-flexion the occiput will be perceived to widen and its

squama will rotate caudad as you sense a subtle pushing against your hands. In exhalation-extension, the occiput will be sensed to narrow and move cephalad.

2. As you become aware of the craniosacral motion of the occiput, listen to its exhalation-extension dynamic. The squama of the occiput will be sensed to narrow as its squama rotates cephalad. Follow this motion and notice the boundary of its excursion. At this boundary, suggest *wait* through your cupped hands. Don't force the stillpoint; simply suggest wait via a subtle intention in your hands. It is an offering of an option. *It must be negotiated.* You offer a suggestion as an inquiry, and you must hear the answer from the system. The system may not want to enter a stillpoint at that time. You must respect that. You can again suggest stillness, but it is an inquiry into the possibility of stillness, not a demand. As the system negotiates its entry into stillness, you may sense that the longitudinal fluctuation of the CSF begins to disorganize. You may notice various fluctuant phenomena arise within the fluids. Simply listen to this. On a tissue level, the system may go deeper into exhalation-extension. If it does, follow it in to the new boundary and again subtly suggest wait. As the system moves towards a stillpoint, you may sense a kind of deepening inward. It's like a deep settling down as the CRI stills. This is the initial expression of the stillpoint. It is important not to fight the system or to try to force a stillpoint on the system.

3. Now, as the stillpoint clarifies, synchronize your perceptual field within the mid-tide. Shift your perceptual field to the biosphere. Let your hands be immersed within fluid and widen your perceptual field to the biosphere. As you widen your perceptual field, you may sense the shift to the mid-tide and to deeper expressions of stillness. As this occurs, you are now in a more direct relationship to the potency and have

shifted the system to its resources under the CRI level of action. Wait within this stillness and notice how potency begins to manifest its healing intentions.

The intention here was to look at the stillpoint process within the context of a system that cannot access its deeper tidal potencies as a resource within session work. This is usually due to the presence of unresolved trauma-bound energies. This is simply a starting point for deeper perceptual shifts, for deeper forces to come into play, and for a healing process to be initiated from within.

Trauma Skills

In the following sections, I will outline and review some useful skills from trauma counseling work that are appropriate for any kind of practitioner to understand and become comfortable with. These are especially important if a patient shifts quickly to a CRI level of shock affect expression and the patient's process inappropriately speeds up. Also remember your cranial skills here.

Processing Shock Traumatization: The Zone of Activation

Peter Levine talks about a *Zone of Activation*, or a zone of the *warble*, in within which a patient is resourced and processes past traumatization. In this zone, the patient is in present time and the system moves to discharge trauma-bound energies and complete frozen defensive intentions. If the patient is not resourced and becomes overwhelmed by the process, he or she may go into dissociative states. In these, the patient may discharge too rapidly and move into hyperarousal states; or the patient may go into hypoarousal states of immobilization and numbness. The two poles of *overwhelm* are therefore (1) hyperarousal, in which the cycling fight or flight energies are rapidly expressed, and (2) freezing, in which the frozen and immobilized energy is experienced as stuckness, numbness, coldness, lack of sensation, and even as paralysis.

Within the scope of both states, powerful experiences of terror, fear, anger, rage, and anxiety may arise either in hyper- or hypoarousal processes. In hyperarousal states the patient may experience emotional flooding, rapid speeding up of process, physical states of trembling and shaking, heat and cold and sweating. These are all signs of autonomic discharge. In freezing states, the patient may experience states of immobilization, stuckness, numbness and coldness. Patients may lose contact with all or part of the body. This can be a scary and even terrifying experience. In both cases, they are experiencing the affect of previous traumatization and are being flooded by that affect. Dissociative states are common within this experience because dissociation is a most fundamental response to being overwhelmed by an experience. It is important to recognize when a patient is accessing shock traumatization. These states are commonly misinterpreted as emotional catharsis and emotional healing.

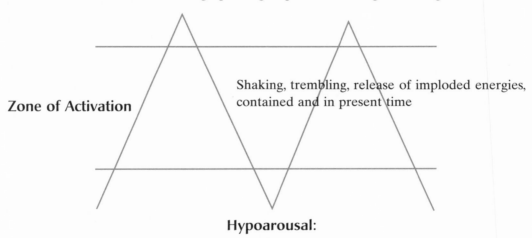

Hyperarousal:

Emotional flooding, speeding of process, shaking, trembling

Zone of Activation

Shaking, trembling, release of imploded energies, contained and in present time

Hypoarousal:

Freezing, immobilization, coldness, frozen defenses

Basic Therapeutic Intentions

Hyperarousal: Working with Speeding and Emotional Flooding

In states of hyperarousal it is important to slow the process down; help the patient reconnect to resources; and lower the hypertonicity of the system so that the patient settles into the *zone of activation*, a contained and resourced processing space. Helping to reestablish witness consciousness is impor-tant, as is helping the patient to ground in present time. If emotional flooding arises, the patient may totally identify with the state and will then be carried away by the flood and will lose sense of present time. At a time of emotional flooding it is important to maintain verbal contact and to gently slow the process down. It is not about stopping the process, but containing it within resources and ground. Phrases like, "Can you be with this?" and "Let that wave pass through" can be helpful. Slowing the process down by helping the patient to slow the breath down can also be helpful.

Summary: Basic Titrations in Emotional Flooding

1. Slow the process down and reestablish resources and space.

2. Bring attention to the body: "Where do you sense that _____ (naming the particular emotion they are experiencing) in your body?"

3. Bring attention to the sensation and felt sense of that in the body: "What sensations tell you that is _____" (naming the emotion they are experiencing).

4. Help patients track the sensations and felt sense of it in the body. The felt sense may also uncover deeper meanings and move the process along into a depth exploration of the traumatization.

5. Allow any processes of discharge such as trembling or autonomic discharge through the fluids to complete.

It is useful to ask patients where they sense the emotion in their body by using phrases like, "Where do you sense that (naming the particular emotion they are experiencing) in your body?" This helps to ground them in present time and enlists their curiosity. It initiates an inquiry. Help them track that with space and then shift their attention to sensations by using such phrases as, "What sensations tell you that is _____" (naming the emotion they are experiencing). This helps to uncouple the emotion from its sensations and allows the patient to stay with the sensation and felt sense of it, rather the emotional affect. It is less overwhelming to stay with the sensations and felt sense of the experience, rather than with the emotional state, and is potentially more transformative. Staying with the felt sense may also uncover deeper meanings and move the process along into a deeper exploration of the traumatization. The intention is to help the patient settle into the zone of activation where the shock affect is moving and discharging, the patient is resourced and is not overwhelmed by the experience. Remember our discussion about shuttling processes and the focusing work.

Freezing: Working with Frozen Defensive Energies

In states of freezing and immobilization, it is important to help the patient mobilize the imploded, frozen energies and to stimulate movement and activation. Here the intention is to help the patient to begin to discharge the frozen energy, to get things moving, and to rise up, so to speak, into the zone of activation. The patient may experience the frozen state of the shock affect within the system as numbness, coldness, stuckness, immobility, etc. Frozen or trauma-bound energy is simply the unresolved cycling energies of the fight or flight response as they were overlaid by a parasympathetic surge within the overwhelm response. As Peter Levine says, it is like having the accelerator and brake of a car on at the same time. The intention is to help the system express this energy in an appropriate and healing way. When there are trauma energies cycling, there is always an intention locked into the system. This may be to defend in some way. It commonly manifests within the joints, connective tissues, and muscles of the body, as tension and restriction. Let's look at some examples of working with these trauma-bound energies.

Basic Titrations

Scenario One

Let's say that the patient experiences a frozen sense in the body. It may be anywhere. Let's say that the patient experiences no sensation from the navel inferior, or a sense of numbness and coldness below the navel. One approach is to simply ask the patient to notice where there *is* movement. It might be a sense of warmth, tingling, or any sensation that is experienced as moving. Help the patient bring his or her attention to that part of the body. From there, see if the patient can gently bring his or her attention to the edge of the frozen area in the body. This commonly begins an activation of sensation from the frozen area, which the patient can then be encouraged to track as it moves in the system. This commonly moves the patient into the zone of activation and a discharge and clearing of the trauma-bound energy. Within a cranial context, a shift to the mid-tide or Long Tide level of action is essential here.

Scenario Two

Let's say that you notice that the patient's hand, arm, foot, or leg is moving. Perhaps it is jerking or shaking. This may indicate that a frozen defensive intention is beginning to be expressed. Simply bring the patient's attention to the area. He or she may begin to notice an intention being expressed. Help the patient track the sensations of the discharge and clearing. This may be expressed as a defensive movement such as blocking or hitting and/or by shaking and trembling. Slow the process down if it speeds up and help the patient stay in contact with resources. Help the patient to allow the physical discharge. If it is a true discharge of the trauma-bound energy from a resourced space, it will actually feel good.

Scenario Three

Let's say that a patient experiences a frozen quality in the shoulder. Perhaps it is a site of a chronic complaint. The first step is to be sure that the patient is resourced. Then simply bring attention to the shoulder involved. Ask if the patient senses an intention beginning to come through. Again this is commonly

some kind of defensive response. If it is the hands and arms, it may be about hitting, blocking, or pushing away; if it is the feet and legs, it may be about kicking or running. Let the patient explore the sensations and allow the intention to simply surface. When the intention begins to make itself known, you can use a simple process to help the patient titrate the experience and the discharge. The intention in all of these processes is to help mobilize the trauma-bound energy with the patient in present time, in a resourced and contained place. This titration process is described as four steps below.

1. Step one is to have the patient imagine that he or she is doing it (e.g., completing the intention). This is generally okay for even very traumatized patients. They can usually imagine doing something without going into overwhelm. Once they imagine doing it, say in this case it was pushing away, then have them relax and track the sensations that arise. Go slowly here.

2. If the patient's trauma-bound energy is still unresolved, then a second step is useful. In this step, ask the patient to prepare to do whatever it is that the shoulder seems to want to do. Here it was pushing. Ask him or her to engage all the muscles and joints necessary to *prepare to do* the pushing. The patient may be surprised at what parts of the body need to be engaged to help in the preparation. Have the patient *prepare to do* without actually doing it. Them have him or her relax and track the arising sensations. This may set off a cycle of discharge and clearing.

3. Again, if the patient's process is still unresolved, have him or her *prepare to do* by engaging all the joints and muscles that are needed in the preparation. Then ask the patient to slowly *do* the action, whatever it is. By first *preparing to do* and then slowly *doing,* no piece of the trauma-bound energy is left out of the process.

If the discharge occurs too rapidly, the energy may just recycle. Again, if emotional flooding occurs, or if the system goes into hyperarousal of any kind, slow the process down. Have the patient come into the breath and the resources. Then have the patient relax and track the arising sensations. This may set off a cycle of discharge and clearing.

4. A final step may be needed to complete the cycle of discharge and to help the trauma-bound energy find completion in its intention. Again have the patient *prepare to do*. Again ask him or her to slowly *do* it. This time, as the patient expresses the motion, give the patient's hand, arm, or shoulder a firm yet yielding resistance to push against. This generally helps to mobilize any energies still bound in the system. Go slowly and track the arising process.

Summary of Practical Considerations

When the system is expressing trauma and shock, it is important that you slow things down and help the patient be with the process with some space and with a clear witness consciousness. The safety of the therapeutic environment is essential, and the quality of the therapeutic relationship is the important foundation for healing to occur. The practitioner has to be able to hold the therapeutic space by being fully present and accepting what arises in the session with receptivity and without judgment. In a cranial context, you may sense the release of shock in the system by the perception of subtle tissue motions like vibration or trembling; or you may sense it in the central nervous system as an almost electric charge. Pay attention to this and bring the patient's attention to this too. See if the patient can be with the sensation of it in the body with a sense of space. See if the patient can be a witness to it and not become overwhelmed by it. This will greatly increase the likelihood of the release of the traumatic memory and decrease the likelihood of a retrauma-

tization of the system. Help the system downshift to deeper tidal and potency resources.

If your patient becomes overwhelmed by the experience, the system will experience the present release of shock as though a new trauma is happening in the present. The patient will thus dissociate from the reality of the present. Strong emotional charges may arise, which may overwhelm the patient. In this context, it is the role of the practitioner to help the patient contain the process and not be overwhelmed by it. If this occurs, it is important to bring the patient back to the present by slowing things down and encouraging an awareness of the sensations in the body. Sometimes, a simple thing like having the patient slow the breath down and remember the ability to be in the body with an awareness of sensation is all that is needed. Sometimes, simple phrases like, "Can you let that move through you?" or "Can you let that wave through you?" are helpful when strong emotions arise. The expression and release of strong emotional charge may be an essential part of the healing process, but containment within resources is essential if it is to be an empowering experience.

It is important that the patient have the inner resources to be with these strong emotions with space, with a clear sense of witness. Remind the patient of his or her resources and of the resourced sensations. It may take any number of sessions for the patient to begin to be able to be with the process with space. Once the patient can do this, it becomes a life skill that can be brought to everyday situations. The most important thing during the session is to work slowly and help the patient pace the work so that the tissue shock can be processed without retraumatizing the system. For a deeper and more complete discussion of trauma and its therapeutic repercussions, I refer you to the work *Waking the Tiger: How the Body Heals Trauma,* by Dr. Peter Levine. Peter Levine has worked with these issues for many years and has developed a language and a way of working with them that has consequences for every therapist in the healing arts.

I hope these last two chapters have been a useful introduction to trauma concepts. These skills are really essential to incorporate within your clinical practice and should be included in foundation courses in craniosacral biodynamics.

1. E. Gendlin, *Focusing* (Bantam Books).

23

Skills and the Tides

In this chapter, I will attempt to summarize and review the important perceptual and clinical aspects of work within the basic rhythms and tides associated with the primary organizing principle of the Breath of Life. I will also attempt to extend some of the concepts within a clinical context. A summary chart of this chapter is found in Appendix I of this volume. For each rhythm and tidal phenomenon, I will discuss how the healing process is perceived and the appropriate healing modalities involved. It is meant to be a rather dense review of many previ-

ous sections discussed in this volume. Please remember that this chapter is intended to be a summary and will not make much sense unless you have already spent time listening to these fields of action.

Prerequisite Skills

In the discussion below, certain prerequisite skills are assumed. These include the work discussed in previous chapters on accessing a practitioner neutral, centering and grounding the therapeutic relationship, establishing practitioner fulcrums, and negotiating appropriate distance and contact with the patient's system. Also assumed are the perceptual skills necessary for the work to have depth. These include the ability to access inner stillness, the development of listening skills, the ability to perceive the human system as it unfolds its information to you, the ability to synchronize with appropriate perceptual fields and to clinically relate to what is perceived, and the ability to perceive and relate clinically to the three functions of potency, fluids, and tissues within each of the three perceptual levels. All of these skills were introduced in previous chapters. The intention here is to gather together and augment the manifold intentions scattered throughout this volume and to present these within a clinical context.

In this chapter we will discuss:

- *Each rhythm and tidal unfoldment (the CRI, the mid-tide, the Long Tide) and the Dynamic Stillness and related perceptual experiences.*

- *The perception of inertial issues and forces within each unfoldment.*

- *The perception of organization.*

- *Healing processes and modes of clinical work at each level of process.*

- *The inherent treatment plan.*

CRI Level of Perception

Rate: 8–14 cycles/minute

Rhythmic Unfoldment

The CRI was called the *fast tide* by Dr. Rollin Becker. As earlier discussed, it is really not a tidal rhythm per se, but is an expression of added forces overlaid upon the deeper tidal forces and the Original bioelectric matrix. These added forces may include those of genetics, trauma, pathogens, toxins, and any other force added or overlaid upon the basic ordering matrix of the system. As the Breath of Life, through the potency it generates, acts to center these added forces, the CRI is generated. The CRI is thus not a direct expression of motility. It is an outer expression of motion conditioned by genetics and experiential processes. As we have seen, it is an expression of the results and affects of past experience and rests upon deeper forces at work within the system. It initially arises as genetic processes are centered by the action of the Breath of Life and is conditioned by all of the unresolved experiences of life. It is an expression of unresolved trauma and experience as they are held within the system as inertial forces. Again, the CRI is generated as the Breath of Life acts to center these conditions of our life. It is the wave form riding the Tide. It is variable and will change with changes within the system, such as traumatic activation and illness. Its rate and quality reflects autonomic activation and inertial affects, such as tissue compression and adhesion, fluid congestion, and neuroendocrine cycling and activation. It is a variable rate of motion whose rate of expression will change due to the nature of the unresolved forces of experience held within the system.

CRI Access

In previous chapters I have introduced a perceptual exercise that helps you gain clear access to various levels of organization within the human system. Let's review the entrée into the CRI here. Let your hands float on tissues. Establish your practitioner fulcrums and negotiate your contact with the patient's system as previously learned. Gently narrow your perceptual field to the bones, membranes, structural parts, tissue structures, and relationships being palpated. Do not grab onto the tissues as you do this. Remember to float on the tissues and let them show you their motions. Your mind is relatively active, analyzing, looking at relationships of parts and structures. As you stay with this intention the faster rhythm, usually described in terms of flexion and extension, will begin to become obvious. It must be remembered that this fast rhythm is a manifestation of the inertial issues being centered within the system by deeper tidal potencies at work.

CRI Perceptual Experience

The practitioner's perceptual field is focused on the structures being palpated as they hold the person's system within a relatively narrow field of awareness. The inhalation and exhalation phases of the underlying Tide are perceived as cycles of reciprocal tension tissue and fluid motion at this faster rate of expression. The practitioner commonly experiences tissue motion as the relationship of separate structures moving in cycles of reciprocal tension motion. Here craniosacral motion is perceived to be expressed as flexion and extension of separate parts. The relationship of separate parts and their external motions predominates in the practitioner's awareness. Motion is perceived to be organized around automatically shifting *tissue* fulcrums. The major fulcrum that organizes the reciprocal tension motion of tissues is perceived to be Sutherland's fulcrum located within the anteriormost aspect of the straight sinus.

CRI Level of Organization and the Perception of Inertia

Organization at the CRI level of action is generally perceived to be an expression of the relationship and motion of individual parts as they organize around a structural midline. The structural midline is the center line within the vertebral bodies and the cranial base defined by the axis of development of the notochord. Flexion and extension is sensed to be an expression of motion between individual tissue structures. Inherent motility, the inner cellular breath of these structures, is not as easily perceived within the CRI level of action. The reciprocal tension motion of flexion and extension is perceived to have its balance point around an automatically shifting fulcrum within the straight sinus known as Sutherland's fulcrum. Automatically shifting fulcrums are perceived to be sites within tissue relationships. Hence, reciprocal tension motion is perceived to be organized around embryologically derived *tissue* fulcrums, such as Sutherland's fulcrum.

Inertial organization is perceived through motion or fixation around lesion sites, tissue tension and tensile dynamics, and via tissue and fluid stasis. These are perceived as the results and affects of experience and suffering. Within the CRI, the perception of inertia and unresolved experience is via an awareness of results and affects. Expressions of inertial processes are perceived via tissue and fluid stasis and resistance. These are perceived as tissue and fluid affects, such as tissue resistance, adhesion, compression, stasis within fluids, tensile patterns within the tissue field, resistance between anatomical structures, and symptoms and pathology. Awareness of lesions predominates in the practitioner's perceptual field. A perception of activation and fragmentation predominates. These are commonly sensed as tissue compression, adhesion, changes in quality of tissues, strains, fluid fluctuations, and emotional processes. Perception tends to be about form and resistance. It is about how/where we hold unresolved trauma and resistance as CNS hyper- and hypo-states, as tissue and fluid inertia, as resistance between parts, as emotional affects, as psychological positions, and as pathological processes. The deeper centering potencies at work are not directly perceived within the CRI. Inertial fulcrums are perceived via tissue lesions, strain patterns, sites of tissue change, loss of

mobility, resistance, fluid congestion, and eccentric fluid fluctuation. Inertial fulcrums are located by the practitioner via motion testing, analysis and diagnosis, application of techniques, traction, fluid direction, and so on. The practitioner actively applies processes and techniques to locate and resolve inertial fulcrums, which are perceived as lesions needing to be fixed or released. Techniques applied may include exaggeration, direct techniques, traction, decompression, and points of balanced membranous tension, among others. Health, and its centering and healing functions, is not directly perceived here. The deeper forces at work are not as evident within this perceptual level.

CRI Level of Mental and Emotional Process

Again, the CRI is a level of affect and result. At the CRI level of manifestation, you are experiencing the conditioned mind. At this level the mind is busy. The practitioner's mind may be analyzing and seeking solutions. Therapeutic work tends to revolve around a linear, rational approach. There is a problem; here is a solution. The work is goal oriented and can be based on fixing whatever is found to be inertial and holding resistance. There is little sense that within the heart of this resistance Health is at work. Therapeutic interventions tend to be based on techniques and methods applied to release resistance and fix problems. Within the context of session work, conditioned states of mind arise within the patient's process. They are about images, memories, and thoughts linked to past experience and trauma. Like the activation within the brain stem and limbic system, they cycle and can become obsessive. Conditioned beliefs and life statements arise here, as does psychodynamic conditioning and confusion. The practitioner may find himself or herself exposed to transference issues, and his or her own transference issues may become stimulated. This is a realm of projection and psychological confusion.

Within the CRI, emotions are a manifestation of the nature of past experience and unresolved issues.

When shock affects arise within the context of the CRI level of action, emotional activation may also be generated within sessions. Emotions which arise within the context of the CRI are conditioned and a factor of the unresolved cycling of autonomic-limbic activity. They are very much about unresolved traumatization and neuroendocrine cycling. Here we are within the realm of the amygdala, the brain stem, and fight and flight issues. Emotional processes revolve around emotional affects, affects of trauma and past experience. There is emotional fixity. Thus, within the CRI, emotional affects may arise in relationship to our particular conditioned state (e.g., our particular life experience). They are thus conditioned and conditioning. During session work within the CRI, the activation of fight or flight emotions during treatment is thus more likely. Hyperarousal and hypoarousal states may manifest. These processes are the affects left over from unresolved past trauma. These may include a spectrum of emotion from fear to terror and from anger to rage. During a session, they may be expressed in an overwhelming and dissociated way. Emotions may flood, or the patient may experience freezing states. Then the person may reexperience overwhelm, dissociation, and traumatization. *This is not necessarily therapeutic.* The system may experience this as a reinforcement of the original traumatization. As these traumatic emotional states become inertial within the system, they will affect the expression of the CRI in some way. Within the CRI, emotional responses based on past conditioning and defended positions predominate.

CRI Level of Healing
Awareness and Process

Within the CRI level of action, healing processes are based on the acknowledgment of suffering, on a practitioner's relationship to the results and affects of suffering. Healing is perceived as a resolution of CNS activation, emotional affects, symptoms and pathologies and tissue and fluid congestion/resistance. The practitioner is very active. Work tends to be lesion, symptom, and activation oriented. However, even at this level of action, if suffering is truly acknowledged, a deepening into the underlying tidal potencies and forces at work can occur. Sometimes a patient needs you to know just how bad it has been. This can be an important step in the healing process. It may allow the patient to settle into deeper resources and tides where the potency centering their suffering is more accessible. Within the CRI level of work, the practitioner actively seeks neutrals, the point of balanced membranous, ligamentous, or fluid tension, within tissue, fluid, and emotional affects. The inherent neutral, relative to the inertial fulcrum sensed, is not easily perceived within this level of perception and action. The forces at work within the inertial fulcrums are not directly perceived. The *biodynamic potencies* centering the *biokinetic forces,* which maintain the inertial pattern, are not easily perceived here. The Health that centers the conditions present is not easily perceived here. The *inherent neutral* within the pattern being attended to, the state of balanced tension, a stillness, is not easily perceived here. Motion or lack of motion predominates in practitioner awareness. This might be the motion of tissues or of emotional and psychological affects. The Health centering these is not directly sensed here. The practitioner thus becomes very active in seeking the point of balanced membranous tension and other neutrals within the system. The relationship to tissues and fluids is *technique and method* based. Processes of decompression, traction, compression-decompression, fluid direction, lateral fluctuation of fluid, and soon may be applied to inertial tissue sites. Success is perceived to be a factor of the practitioner's intervention. Success is perceived to be achieved with the release of the tissue and structural lesion and, in some cases, with the release of coupled emotional affects. Disengagement is sensed to be a factor of practitioner intervention. Reorganization is perceived via the new balance of flexion and extension as reciprocal tension motions. *Within the CRI, healing is lesion and practitioner based.*

Mid-Tide Level of Perception

Rate: 2.5 cycles a minute

Rhythmic Unfoldment

Dr. William Garner Sutherland taught that the *cerebrospinal fluid tide* was driven by an invisible force, the potency of the Breath of Life. Potency acts like an Intelligence at work within the fluid and is the inherent force that drives its motions. This process occurs via transmutation. *Transmutation* is a shift in state. Potency, as a bioelectric field phenomenon, shifts in state within the fluids of the body and is then expressed as a physiologically active force. It is this force within the fluids that organized the original developmental motions of embryonic cells and which maintains order throughout life. As this force is expressed within the fluids, a tidal phenomenon of 2.5 cycles a minute, which I call the mid-tide, is generated. This tidal phenomenon, unlike the CRI, is relatively stable. The mid-tide is the realm of the transmutation of potency into a physiologically active ordering force within the fluids of the body. This force also acts to generate tissue motility and is the ordering factor within the cellular and tissue world. Within the mid-tide level of action, the three functions of potency, fluids, and tissues can be perceived as a unified dynamic. Potency is the organizing factor, fluid is the medium of exchange, and cells and tissues organize around its action. The mid-tide is a term I use to describe this whole level of action. Each function can be sensed to express motility at this rate of expression, and the wholeness of their dynamic can also be perceived. Each of the three functions acts as a tensile field that expresses reciprocal tension motion around automatically shifting fulcrums. In other words, potency, fluids, and tissues, as individual fields of action, express tensile motions around automatically shifting fulcrums. Within the mid-tide, potency, fluids, and tissues can also be perceived to be a unified tensile field expressing a tidal rhythm of 2.5 cycles a minute.

Mid-Tide Access

Within the mid-tide perceptual experience, the human system is sensed to be a whole, truly unified dynamic. Here I will repeat a simple process that helps practitioners gain access to the mid-tide level of perception. Negotiate your contact with the patient's system. Let your hands float on the tissues. While your hands float upon the tissues, sense that they are also immersed within fluid. Then widen your perceptual field to include the whole of person and the biosphere. (The biosphere includes the whole of the body, energy field, and area of environmental exchange around the patient's body.) Establish a relatively still field of listening. Let your mind still as it holds the whole of the patient within its field of listening. Your mind is relatively still and quiet, yet it is actively listening. The tendencies and conditioning of the mind still may arise here; let things settle. To help synchronize the mind with the mid-tide, allow your mind to settle, find a still inner neutral. Your mind is not interested in parts and relationships per se, but in whole units of function. Your awareness holds the whole of the person within its field of perception. Wait, listen, and the slower 2.5 cycles a minute tidal phenomena will clarify.

Mid-Tide Perceptual Experience

Within the mid-tide field of action, organization within the system is directly perceived to be a function of the action of potency within the fluids. The system is not perceived to be a mechanism, but a dynamic interplay of intrinsic forces at work. Potencies and forces at work are seen to be the organizing factors. Inherent motions are sensed to be generated by forces deeper than mechanical or hydraulic mechanisms. Organization is perceived to be based on a greater Intelligence manifesting within the fluids and tissues of the body. Tissues, fluids, and potency are experienced as interdependent and unified tensile fields of action. They mutual arise and are a true unit of function. Within this unified tensile field, each function, that of potency, fluids, and tissues, can be perceived as a tensile field of action in its own right. The fluids can be perceived to express a tidal motion which is commonly called the *fluid tide*. Perception of this phenomenon within the 2.5 cycles a minute mid-tide gives the practitioner information about how that system can manifest its resources.

Within the mid-tide, tissues are also perceived to express reciprocal tension motion as a unified tensile field of action. Tissue motility and motion are seen to be holistic. Although the craniosacral motion of individual structures is still discernible, their motion is perceived to be part of a much wider whole. Within this level of action, the craniosacral motions of tissues and their inner motility are perceived to be a unified phenomenon. Structures like the sphenoid bone can be sensed to express their inherent motions within the 2.5 cycles a minute rate and are sensed to be part of a much wider dynamic. The human body is thus perceived to be a true unit of function, a whole. For instance, within the mid-tide, the particular motion of the sphenoid bone is sensed to be part of a wider tissue field. Here the sphenoid and its particular dynamic is sensed to be part of a unified tensile tissue field, which expresses a unified reciprocal tension motion. Hence the unity of human organization is more directly perceived here. Tissue motion is perceived as a tensile surge and settling within the tissue field as a whole. This is perceived to be organized around automatically shifting fulcrums, which are sensed to be *points of potency* within a wider bioelectric matrix. These points of potency have the power to organize. They are a stillness within a greater field of action, which automatically shifts with the intentions of the Tide. This is an important perceptual shift from the CRI level of awareness, where automatically shifting fulcrums are perceived to be locations within the tissues. Automatically shifting fulcrums are here perceived to be coalescences of potency within a greater tensile field of action. A prominent organizing midline is perceived to be the dorsal or fluid midline, as it is expressed within the neural axis. The

fluid tide is perceived to be moved by the potency within the dorsal midline. The primal midline, within the notochord axis, may also be perceived here if the practitioner is maintaining a wide and still enough perceptual field.

Mid-Tide Level of Organization and the Perception of Inertia

Within the mid-tide level of action, individual tissue structures are directly perceived to be part of a unified motility throughout the body. The organization of flexion and extension dynamics are perceived to be a factor of deeper forces at work. An *inner breath* is perceptible within tissue motility. Flexion and extension of individual bones, of the reciprocal tension membrane, and of tissues generally is perceived to be part of a greater whole. Motion dynamics are perceived via awareness of unified tensile fields organized around automatically shifting fulcrums. Automatically shifting fulcrums are perceived to be loci or condensations of potency, which organize tensile fields of action. Thus, Sutherland's fulcrum is perceived to be a point of potency, ideally located within the anterior aspect of the straight sinus, which automatically shifts within the inhalation and exhalation cycles generated by the action of the Tide. The mid-tide is a relatively stable rhythm sensed as an inhalation surge and an exhalation settling within these tensile fields.

Within the mid-tide, inertial fulcrums are located via direct perceptual experience. Inertial fulcrums are directly perceived as sites of condensed potencies. They are sensed as condensations of inertial forces within tensile fields of action. The inertial patterns they generate are perceived as tensile distortions around these condensations. Within the mid-tide, there is a direct perception of biodynamic and biokinetic forces at work. The practitioner becomes aware of the biodynamic and biokinetic forces at work at the heart of organizing fulcrums. There is an experience of the coupling of biodynamic potencies with inertial forces in order to center and contain them. An acknowledgement of the

Health that centers disturbances within the system is possible here. As the practitioner listens within this field of action, the inherent treatment plan may begin to unfold. This occurs when the Intelligence of the ordering process begins to come through. The *exact* sequence of treatment will unfold within the practitioner's perception. This is a *precise* expression of what needs to happen for the healing of that particular person at that particular time. This is not something the practitioner can figure out or analyze. As the practitioner listens, with a still yet actively listening mind, the priorities set in motion by the Breath of Life will begin to make themselves known. These priorities must be respected. The inertial fulcrums within the system are being centered as a whole with precision. There is a precise order to this centering function, and a precise order of healing priorities will make themselves known, if the practitioner is still and patient enough and has the will to listen.

Potency, fluids, and tissues express their natural tensile motions around automatically shifting fulcrums. Inertial fulcrums are not automatically shifting fulcrums. They are sites of stasis that do not shift with the intentions of the Tide. These inertial sites will generate patterns of strained tension within the natural tensile fields of the body. Within the mid-tide, these inertial patterns are perceived as distortions within these natural tensile fields of action. The classic strain pattern results. These are sensed to be organized by condensations or concentrations of inertial potencies and forces. Expressions of inertial processes, such as conditioned tissue motion, and patterns of inertial motility and mobility, are perceived as distortions within whole tensile fields. The practitioner may perceive the whole tensile field distorting around an inertial fulcrum. For instance, while palpating the cranium via a vault hold, the practitioner may perceive a whole tensile distortion around a particular fulcrum. This is not a factor of analysis or motion testing, but a direct experience of organization. Tissue motility is perceived as a unified field, and inertial patterns are perceived as distortions within this field organized around inertial fulcrums. Information at this level of perception is more precise and encompassing than at the CRI level. There is no need to motion test in order to gain clinical information. The practitioner has a direct experience of inertial forces, shapes, and organizing fulcrums. The practitioner's mind is stiller and less active, and the work is less tiring.

Mid-Tide Level of Mental and Emotional Processes

Within the mid-tide, the mind is quieter. The practitioner's mind is still but may wander. The mind is taking in the *whole* and the details within the whole become clear. The practitioner learns to trust the *inherent treatment plan* and does not have to analyze or motion test to understand the dynamics at work. The practitioner can access and rely on his or her intuitive mind, and therapeutics is therefore less linear and more holistic. The practitioner appreciates the forces at work. Therapeutic interventions are perceived to truly be conversations with the three functions of potency, fluids, and tissue. In these therapeutic conversations the healing and inertial forces are more directly perceived. Work at this level is much less tiring and more clinically efficient.

Emotional process within the mid-tide level of expression is about *present time*. Emotions will arise appropriate to the circumstances being experienced and will then pass. Our emotional life is lived within the immediacy of our present experience and is a direct expression of the quality of the relationships within our life. Emotions within the mid-tide are more fluid and appropriate to the present experience. Emotional fixity is experienced more as energetic holding and density, rather than as activation. Within the mid-tide level of work, emotional affects and releases during sessions are generally expressed in more contained and resourced ways. Emotional affects and their resolution appropriately resolve in present time. Emotional activation has the quality of completion; the emotional state does not continue to cycle and is not reinforced. Thus work within the mid-tide tends to bring the patient more into relationship with his or her resources. There is a clear dynamic at work between the inherent healing potency of the Breath of Life and the inertial forces maintaining the pattern of disturbance. Session work within the mid-tide thus tends to be less activating and more contained. During treatment, emotional affects of past trauma may be activated, but they tend to be expressed in much milder forms within the resources of the person. Emotional processes are experienced as a completion of past experience and do not continue to cycle. Emotional affects complete; they are not reinforced. Emotional resolution may occur very quietly here and be experienced as a streaming of energy, warmth, and feeling. Work here helps to get under the results and affects of experience to the current organization of things. Emotional processing tends to be more about forces at work and their resolution than the activation that these forces may generate.

Mid-Tide Level of Healing Awareness and Processes

Within the mid-tide level of perception and action, healing is perceived as a function of transmutation. The activation of inertial potencies and forces, within the inertial fulcrums, is perceived to herald the beginning of a healing process. Healing is perceived as a resolution of the inertial forces that are maintaining the disturbances within the system. This occurs via the action of an inherent biodynamic potency within a larger field of action. Potency is perceived to be expressed as a whole tensile field of action within the fluids. A transmutation, or shift in state, of potency within this field can be experienced within the inertial fulcrum as the inertial forces are processed. *A change happens within the potencies involved*, and healing processes are initiated. When this occurs there is a reorganization of tissues, fluids, and potencies to the primal midline and natural fulcrums. The Original intention is reestablished.

Within the mid-tide, the treatment plan, which is inherent within the order of the system being pal-

pated, is perceived. As the practitioner listens, the treatment plan unfolds and is sensed to be inherent within the conditions present. The state of balanced tension is also perceived to be inherent within the inertial pattern and fulcrum being attended to. There is an inherent tendency for a state of balance, a *dynamic equilibrium*, to be accessed. At most, the practitioner facilitates the state of balance by slowing motions down. This can be facilitated within any or all of the three functions of potency, fluids, and tissues. Dr. Becker's three-stage healing awareness becomes obvious here.

Dr. Becker's Three-Stage Healing Awareness

1. Tissues, fluids, and potencies naturally seek a neutral. There is a natural movement towards a state of balance.

2. The state of balance is attained. A functional stillpoint arises. The state of balance is perceived to be the eye of a needle or the mysterious gateway, through which something can pass. Something happens within the state of balance. There is a *change in the potencies* involved within the inertial issue. There is a transmutation of potency within the inertial fulcrum being attended to. Biodynamic and biokinetic potencies are initiated. Expressions of Health are perceived. There is a permeation of potency, and inertial forces are ideally resolved.

3. Tissues, fluids, and potencies, the three functions discernible within the mid-tide, reorganize/realign to the primal midline and natural fulcrums.

The state of balance is a dynamic equilibrium within the conditions, potencies, and forces present. When accessed, this state is the gateway to the deeper organizing matrix generated by the Breath of Life. The bioelectric matrix is an expression of a dynamic equilibrium within the action of the Long Tide. A state of balance, a stillness within a dynamic equilibrium, takes you through the gateway to the deeper epigenetic potencies and ordering intentions generated by the intentions of the Breath of Life.

Within the context of the mid-tide, the practitioner may offer and engage in conversations about space and history via subtle negotiated intentions of disengagement, space, traction, direction of potencies, lateral fluctuations of potency, and so on. These are offered as conversations rather than as techniques or protocols. The key to healing at this level of work is based on a relationship in which the state of balance can be accessed. Here the inherent forces, not the intervention of the practitioner, are sensed to initiate healing. Disengagement is sensed to be a factor of transmutation and the potencies at work within the stillness. *Within the mid-tide, healing is perceived to be relationship and transmutation based.*

The Long Tide Level of Perception

*Rate: 50-second inhalation/
50-second exhalation*

Rhythmic Unfoldment

The Breath of Life is an *eternally creative intelligence*[1] at work within the infinite present. Through its action, past and future are enfolded within this present moment. The Breath of Life functions totally within present time. The creative intention of the Breath of Life generates the Long Tide, the great organizing wind[2] of the human system. Dr Rollin Becker coined the term Long Tide. The Long Tide is a manifestation of the Original motion that Victor Schauberger discusses. We reviewed some of his concepts in Chapter Five. As we have seen in earlier chapters, the Long Tide is the Original motion generated by the Breath of Life. This Original motion lays down the bioelectric field, or Original

matrix, the organizing field for human form. This is Originality made manifest. The Long Tide seems to arise out of "somewhere" and return to "somewhere." It is a local phenomenon, which is expressed within a huge field of action. This field takes in the whole of the universe we inhabit. In David Bohm's terms, the Long Tide is an explicate expression of a deeper implicate creativity. It is generated by the deeper creative intentions of the Breath of Life. As the Long Tide functions to generate a particular form, the whole universe is enfolded in its action.

Long Tide Access

Here again, I will review a simple exercise that helps practitioners resonate with this field of action. From your perception of the biosphere and the mid-tide, you will shift your imagery and perceptual field so that a synchronization with the Long Tide field of action is more likely. To do this, while your hands float on the tissues, let them be immersed within the field of potency surrounding the patient. Let them lighten and see if a sense of being supported by a wider field of bioenergy comes to you. Once you have a sense of this, widen your perceptual field from the biosphere towards the horizon. Do this slowly and carefully. Do not go beyond your comfort level. If you sense yourself getting lost in the field, or losing contact with the patient, gently narrow your field to a more grounded sense of relationship. Allow your mind to settle. A balance between its outgoing motor field and its incoming sensory field will naturally arise. In other words, your mind rests within a state of dynamic equilibrium. As you extend your perceptual field out from your practitioner neutral, your mind may settle into a state of balance. In this state, your sensory and motor fields, that is, the extension of your field of awareness and the sensory information returning, may settle into a state of balanced listening. You may have the sense that your mind, indeed your very being, is being breathed by the Breath of Life. Your perceptual field is very wide and deep. Listen within this widened perceptual field. Do not look for anything. Let information come to you.

Long Tide Perceptual Experience

The Long Tide is the grand organizing wind of the human system. It may be perceived like a great wind that arises out of "somewhere and returns to somewhere." Again, it is a local phenomenon that is part of a huge field of action. In its centripetal and centrifugal expression, it lays down a stable bioelectric matrix, the ordering field for the human body. The Original matrix is a stable form. It is generated by a dynamic equilibrium in the centripetal and centrifugal action of the Long Tide. A dynamic and stable field of action results. Practitioners may tend to be more aware of this stable field than of the centripetal and centrifugal motion that generates it. When practitioners synchronize their field of awareness with the Long Tide, various phenomena may be perceived. Within this perceptual field, the potency of Breath of Life is more directly perceived. There may be an airy yet powerful experience of radiance. The practitioner may sense potency as a radiance permeating everything. The experience of radiance passes through the practitioner's hands. There may even be a perception of cellular permeation as this radiance passes through everything. This is a perception of potency as a unified field phenomenon. The Original bioelectric matrix may be directly perceived as an ordering and organizing field. There may also be a sense of vibrancy within this field, an alive stillness, which underlies the expression of the human form. The practitioner may also sense a very slow, deep rhythm generated by the action of the Long Tide within space. This will be expressed in cycles of 50-second inhalations and exhalations (100 seconds for both inhalation and exhalation). The practitioner may also sense very slow, wavelike cycles of expansion around the body. This has the quality of a pebble being dropped into a pond every 20 minutes. It is as if the Breath of Life drops a creative intention into the pond of life and motion is generated. Here the practitioner is sensing the Long Tide as a wider field of action. This is the organizing wind of life. The practitioner may also perceive the primal midline as an uprising force within a wider bioelectric field. The notochord within the embryonic disc organizes in relationship to this midline. This awareness can give excellent clinical information about the organization of form and structure within that particular person's system.

Long Tide Level of Organization and the Perception of Inertia

The Long Tide is a manifestation of the creative intentions of the Breath of Life. As this intention unfolds, a Tide of creativity is generated. The Long Tide is thus the Tide per se. The Long Tide can be perceived as a direct ordering and organizing intention within and around the patient. A bioelectric field is generated via centripetal and centrifugal spiraling forces as the Long Tide, like a great wind, lays down the Original matrix of a human being. Bioelectric potency is seen to be an unfoldment of a particular intention to incarnate which carries the universal form of a human being. Organization within this field of action is perceived as a factor of the radiance of the Breath of Life and the Original matrix it generates. The primal midline is more obvious within this field of action. Within the perceptual field of the Long Tide, the geometric precision of the Original matrix is perceived. "God geometizes, man cognises."[3] Within this field of action, the organizing axis is perceived via the primal midline as an emergent reality. The primal midline may be experienced as an uprising force within the center of the field. This becomes the main organizing axis for the development and maintenance of the form of the human body. The notochord of the embryo and the structural axis of the body organize in relationship to its action. Inertial fulcrums are perceived as density and distortion within an energetic field. Inertia patterns are not perceived via fulcrums or inertial motion patterns per se. Instead, inertial patterns are perceived as coalescences and distortions within a matrix, like Einstein's concept of mass bending the space-time continuum. The bioelectric matrix is perceived to distort as the centering intentions of the Breath of Life are expressed. Inertia is perceived as density and distortion within a wider bioelectric matrix. This is similar to how mass is said to bend space-time in the theory of relativity.

Long Tide Level of Mental and Emotional Process

Within this perceptual field the mind is very still. A balance has been attained between its outgoing motor field and its incoming sensory field. In other words, the mind is in a state of dynamic equilibrium. Its perceptual field is very wide. Local phenomena like the Long Tide are sensed to arise in a vast field of action. It is a humbling experience. There may be a sense of being breathed by the Breath of Life here. The mind deepens and stills, breathes with the Breath of Life within a wide perceptual field. There is radiance. Within this perceptual field, there is still the experience of an observer, although very subtle and still. Expansive emotional tones predominate. Joy, warmth, a sense of connection, and humbleness are the predominant emotional forms. There is a direct experience of what the Buddhists call *maitri,* an inner warmth, gratitude, and appreciation for all manifest things. There is an experience of the interconnectedness of all things. The practitioner and patient are not separate, but are perceived to be interdependent and mutually arising. They are discrete, yet totally connected, a true unit of function. Here the life of patient and practitioner are sensed to mutually arise, and the forces that support both are not separate. The same Breath of Life and the same Long Tide support and order both. Humility naturally arises here.

Long Tide Level of Healing Awareness and Processes

Within this field of action, there is a direct experience of the potencies of the Breath of Life doing the healing. Potency shimmers like sunlight on the sea as inertial issues are addressed. Inertial fulcrums vibrate and inertial forces resolve via permeation, transmutation, and a reconnection to the Original matrix. Healing is perceived as a shift or resolution within the bioelectric matrix. The practitioner's mind is still and balanced. Healing is perceived to arise "from the without to the within" via transmutation and reconnection to the Original matrix. The practitioner is a humble observer holding space and relationship. Here the practitioner keenly listens to processes of reconnection and transmutation. Disengagement is sensed to arise from within. *Within the Long Field of action, healing is perceived to be resonance and reconnection based.*

The Dynamic Stillness
Perceptual Experience within the Dynamic Stillness

Within this state there is perception without a perceiver. There are no tides, only an alive, dynamic Stillness. Vibrancy predominates. There is a state of vibrancy, an aliveness that permeates everything. You don't know it; you are it. You sense it in the depths of your being. Within the Dynamic Stillness, order is seen to be an expression of the intentions of the divine. All potential rests within its stillness. It is a Stillness that is both vibrant and alive. As you come out of the state of unknowing, a sense of the divine remains. You simply know it as a fact. There is an intermediary perceptual experience in which the vibrancy of the Stillness is directly perceived in space. It is like having a foot in two worlds. You sense a dynamic aliveness, a vibrancy, within the body and within the space you inhabit. You may directly sense an exchange between the stillness and the form you are palpating. You may perceive a rhythmic interchange between stillness and form. This may have an electric-like sense to it, like a vibrancy that seems to arise out of nowhere and to infuse the conditions present. This is a direct perception of healing intentions at work. More on this in the next chapter.

Access into the Dynamic Stillness

The practitioner's mind stills, settles, deepens, and expands, letting go of self-view. Access into the Dynamic Stillness is about truly letting go of the known. It cannot be accessed within the context of what the mind knows. It is about letting go of knowing, trying, and even of self-view, that is, what and who I think I am. There is never a question of how to enter it, only a process of letting go. This is very challenging for most practitioners, who are trained to know and do a lot. It is also challenging on a deeper level, where our sense of selfhood may be challenged. By this I mean the challenge to let go of what we know, of our needs, and of any desire for outcome or knowledge. It is like entering a darkness.

State of Mind/Consciousness and Emotion within the Dynamic Stillness

The state of mind is unified, still, expanded. No-self, no self-constructs, no subject-object relationship. No knowing. Unity consciousness. The practitioner enters a darkness. This is not the darkness of light and dark. It is the darkness of unknowing. Boundaries melt away as the state of unknowing is allowed, yet there is no merging. This has nothing to do with doing. It is about letting go. This is a deep relaxation into the present moment and a relinquishing of all that one knows. It is humbling because what we know commonly defines our sense of who we are. We are much more than that.

Within the Dynamic Stillness there is no self-other perception. There is only a unified field of compassion. Equanimity and compassion are directly sensed as an illimitable and unified natural state of grace. As the Buddhists say, compassion is the archetypal energy that holds the whole universe together and is the only origin for its manifestation. In the Christian tradition, it is said that love is the force that molds the universe and upon which it rests. This state is not personal, but a universal. It is not known by the ego, but only within a state of unknowing. What's more, it is natural. The Dynamic Stillness permeates and supports everything.

Healing Processes within the Dynamic Stillness

Healing processes within the Dynamic Stillness are mysterious. Both patient and practitioner know that something has happened, but it will be difficult to describe. Whatever happened occurred within Stillness. We may try to figure it out, but all we may notice are the changes that arose after we came out of the depths of the Stillness. Within the Stillness, healing occurs via direct resonance with a deeper creative source. Space-time is irrelevant. Healing can be instantaneous. Even if healing does not occur on the physical level, an appreciation of life and a deep sense of peace can arise. This can be extremely beneficial for terminally ill patients. It allows a much wider perspective about what our life rests within. Wholeness has been touched and we are forever part of that wholeness.

1. See Callum Coates, *Living Energies* (Gateway Books), for a discussion of the eternally creative intelligence.

2. This level of manifestation is called the "wind of the vital forces" in the Tibetan system. It is considered to be a nonconditioned organizing field of action for the unfoldment of the human form.

3. A saying coined by Dr. Randolph Stone, D.O.

24

The Treatment Plan, Rhythmic Balanced Interchange, and the Empty Vessel

This is the last chapter of the first volume of *Craniosacral Biodynamics*. This chapter is meant to bring some aspects of this volume into a wider clinical context. It is also meant to introduce some important clinical experiences and possibilities. I would like to start this inquiry with a more detailed exploration of what Dr. Becker called the *inherent treatment plan*. I would also like to discuss another term he used, *rhythmic balanced interchange*. Finally, I would like to explore some thoughts about being an *empty vessel*. It seems to me that it is only when we can truly empty ourselves of ourselves that something else beyond our narrow perspective begins to show itself. A *presence* arises beyond my narrow human intelligence, which takes over and leads me to much deeper potentials within our human experience. Perhaps this is what Dr. Sutherland pointed to when he spoke of *Intelligence*. Perhaps I can call this presence the Breath of Life; however, to be truthful, it brings me to a loss for words.

In this chapter we will:

- *Discuss the inherent treatment plan.*
- *Discuss rhythmic balanced interchange.*
- *Discuss the empty vessel.*

I would like to give some of my own comments on these ideas, which come from my clinical and teaching experience. They are given in all humility as starting points, not as places of completion. Each and every day of our life, indeed each moment, is another opportunity for inquiry. Please take these musings within that frame of reference.

Prerequisites

Dr. Rollin Becker coined the term *inherent treatment plan*. I have also used this term various times in this volume. I would like to tease this concept out here and to offer some of my ideas about it. For me the inherent treatment plan has to do with the deep Intelligence present within the human system. There is an Intelligence within, which is orchestrating the work we do. I think that all experienced practitioners come to this awareness. The Intelligence holds everything together. It centers all of the conditions of life within a unified whole. As we have seen, this Intelligence works to center any added forces within the mind-body physiology in precise ways. These added forces may be traumatic, pathogenic, genetic, and so on. The bioelectric matrix, the energetic blueprint of the human system, is a precise expression of this Intelligence and of the creative intentions of the divine. Its centering function is also precise. Inertial fulcra within the system are centered in precise ways within this matrix as a whole and the healing process necessary for that person will also unfold in a precise way. By this I mean that the sequence of what has to happen within any given healing process is precise and is a function of that Intelligence, not of my clinical analysis. I, as practitioner, can never figure this out. That is why treatment protocols are not appropriate at deeper levels of the work. They just get in the way. The treatment plan is inherent within the conditions already being centered by the potency of the Breath of Life. The treatment plan will precisely unfold in the exact sequence appropriate to the conditions being centered within the system as a whole. I heard Dr. Becker, on a recorded tape, say, "Trust the Tide and get out of the way!" That certainly sums it up. As one listens to the human system with a wide and still perceptual field, needing and expecting nothing, something begins to emerge. A clarification of intention begins to happen. It is not my intention or your intention as practitioner, it is the healing and centering intention of the Breath of Life in action. It is simply a matter of listening to it as it unfolds.

Some questions may arise here: "How does one recognize the inherent treatment plan? How can one interface with it in appropriate ways?" Let's look at some possibilities here. First of all, you must be able to access the deeper tidal rhythms with consistency and clarity. You must also have the ability to generate practitioner fulcrums from which the healing process can be initiated. Your practitioner fulcrums allow the patient's system to have a neutral ground from which to explore its patterns and its relationship to the Health which is never lost. Your fulcrums are the ground from which the patient's system is held safely within the healing process. They are an external neutral, which holds the whole process with safety and containment. They generate a relationship in which the patient's process can be reflected in a resourced way so that overwhelm is less likely. The ability to negotiate an appropriate viewing distance from the patient's system, and to hold a relatively wide perceptual field, is also crucial here. A wide and still field of listening is essential. This must be a listening without the need to know or find anything. The patient's system must be held within a field of curiosity and inquiry. It is about discovery and mystery, not about assumptions and analysis. Let's look at these ideas within a few different contexts.

The Inherent Treatment Plan: A Mid-Tide Perspective

Let's say you are viewing a system within the mid-tide level of action. You are holding the whole person and the field of energetic interchange around him or her, within your perceptual field. Once appropriate fulcrums are established and an appropriate contact is made, you may perceive a huge amount of information. It is like meeting a friend after a long period of time and everything spills out all at once. It is not a matter of sorting it out. It is a matter of listening. Over time, the action of potency, fluids, and tissues begins to clarify. As you hold the system within your wide perceptual field in stillness, things will gradually settle and something else will begin to emerge. A pattern, a particular within the system, will begin to express itself. Remember that you are holding whole tensile fields of action within your perceptual field. You perceive not just individual structures and their motions, but the whole tensile field they are part of. The whole will begin to speak to you. The intentions of the Breath of Life, in its precise ordering and centering function, will begin to clarify. It simply takes patience. The inertial patterns, with their traumatic and pathological origins, are all being centered in a precise way all at once within the system. This precision is found within the heart of every fulcrum perceived. Each inertial fulcrum is already a manifestation of this treatment plan. Every inertial force and fulcrum within the system is being centered within the whole all at once.

As you listen to this whole, a particular inertial fulcrum may begin to manifest. The tensile field begins to precisely organize around a particular fulcrum. Something seems to engage from within, and the whole tensile field begins to distort around one particular fulcrum. Everything begins to organize around it at every level of action. This is a precise expression of what needs to happen for that system at that particular time. The precision of the organization around it may then be perceived by the practitioner. This fulcrum may have many layers and may be coupled with other fulcrums, but the system begins to organize around it in a precise way. The system focuses its healing intentions on one particular issue. The bioenergy field of potency, the fluid field, and the entire tissue field organize around this particular fulcrum all at once. Everything is now organized around this one particular. All of the resources of the system can be focused here. This inertial fulcrum is essentially uncoupled from all the others within the system. This is crucial to understand. There is a deep precision at work here. You didn't have to figure this out. You couldn't have. You can't motion test for this, nor can you analyze to discover it. You have to hold a particular kind of awareness and be patient in your listening. You have to be unobtrusive and be open to the Intelligence within the system. This is a great gift, which makes clinical work much less tiring and much more efficient.

The inherent treatment plan may also manifest through the action, or drive, of the potency within the fluids. As you settle into a listening within the mid-tide, you may begin to sense the inhalation surge of potency through the fluids. As you follow this surge of potency over a number of cycles, you may sense a powerful phenomenon. While listening, with special attention within the inhalation surge, you may sense that the potency begins to shift within the fluids. A drive of potency through the fluids may be sensed, which begins to focus on a specific fulcrum. You can follow this drive of potency towards the fulcrum with your awareness. Potency begins to build within the inertial area. You may follow it deeper into that area. You may sense a settling into a state of balance and a building of potency, or the process may seem so fast that the potency builds and something seems to be directly processed. The tissues involved then seem to expand and reorganize to their suspended automatically shifting fulcrums and the primal midline. The key to this seems to be the practitioner's ability to track the inhalation phase of the Tide and the expression of potency within the fluids during this phase of action. It is almost as if you become a surfer on the inhalation surge of the Tide, and it takes you into its intentions.

Once the treatment plan unfolds and a particular fulcrum shows itself to you, then the issue is about supporting this intention appropriately and humbly. Remember that healing happens within stillness. The state of balance is essential to comprehend here. This is the gateway into the depth of the healing process. Previously, we discussed clinical approaches and the state of balanced tension. Dr. Becker's three-step healing awareness is important to comprehend here. In previous chapters, we also discussed ways to facilitate space and to initiate the action of potency in deeply inertial conditions. We introduced clinical skills such as direction of fluid, use of lateral fluctuation, disengagement processes, and others. We also discussed the synchronization and shifting of your perceptual field to initiate relationships with deeper forces at work. All of these clinical skills have to become internalized and spontaneous, arising in relationship to the conditions present.

The Inherent Treatment Plan: A Long Tide Perspective

From a mid-tide perspective, you may sense a particular pattern arising within a whole tensile field of action. You may sense a settling around the fulcrum that organizes it. As you listen, a state of balance may be attained. You may facilitate this in various ways. Once the state of balance is attained, a change may be perceived within the potencies involved. Expressions of Health may be sensed. You may then shift your perceptual field to the wider Long Tide field of action. This has more depth and breadth to it. As you do this, it is like moving through a mysterious gateway to the deeper forces at work. It brings you more directly to the Original matrix, its ordering potencies, and the organizing winds of the Long Tide. A deeper perception of the treatment plan then unfolds. It is seen to be not just a factor of inertial potencies within a fulcrum, but to be a function of the Long tide and of the Original matrix itself.

The Long Tide, as a most primal potency, may be sensed to rise like a great wind within the midline of the bioelectric field. There is then a permeation and transmutation of potency within the fulcrum being attended to, and the whole bioelectric matrix shifts as inertial forces are resolved. The treatment plan is seen to be held as a whole within space and within the wider bioelectric field as its potency precisely centers the conditions present. As the forces within an inertial fulcrum resolve, there will be expansion within the tissue elements and a reorganization process will occur. Potencies, fluids, and tissues will realign to the primal midline and suspended automatically shifting fulcrums. You may then perceive that the fluid tide is strongly expressed with a different quality than at the beginning of the session. A new pattern may then arise as the next step in the treatment process, or that may be a point of completion for that session. Over a number of sessions, the treatment plan will unfold its precise order and intentions to you. It is a matter of listening with a wide and still perceptual field, which needs and expects nothing. It becomes a matter of supporting the process and truly being a servant to the Breath of Life and the mystery of life.

Alternately, as you hold a wide perceptual field, you may sense the treatment plan unfolding from the "outside-in" and the "inside-out." The Long Tide enters your perceptual field. Its huge field of action and the bioelectric field it generates may come into your awareness. An Intelligence seems to enter the field. This is a humbling experience. You sense field phenomena here. A larger field of action is sensed beyond the physical confines of the body. You may sense how the whole bioelectric matrix may be organized around unresolved issues, similar to how, in Einstein's theory of relativity, mass bends space-time. (See Figure 24.1.)

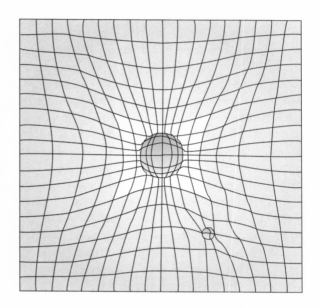

24.1 The bioelectric matrix distorts
to center inertial forces
similar to how mass bends space-time

The healing intentions of the Breath of Life clarify here. Motion and potency may seem to come from "somewhere else" and rise up the midline, through the tensile fields of the body, right through an appropriate fulcrum. It works from the outside-in and the inside-out. This fulcrum is chosen by the centering function of the Breath of Life and the precision of its intentions. Here the state of balance is not a factor of shape or form, or even of a stillness being accessed, but is truly sensed to be inherent within the conditions present. Here it is a not a matter of accessing a stillness and a state of balance. It is perceived that the Stillness is already present within the conditions being centered. There is a shimmering within the system as inertial forces are engaged within the fluids. Something happens beyond the conditions being centered and the compensations held. It can be lightning fast. There will be a change in the potencies within the fluids as a transmutation of potency occurs. There will also be a change in the potencies within the inertial fulcrum being attended to. A transmutation of potency occurs within the inertial potencies and forces present. Inertial forces are processed, and there is then a shift within the fluids and tissues as a reorganization to suspended automatically shifting fulcrums and the midline becomes possible.

Some Ways into the Treatment Plan

In this section, I would like to share some of the ways we introduce students to the inherent treatment plan. We do this in the second year of the training when students have already begun to sense some of these dynamics. Over five seminars we introduce different aspects of listening. I will share three of these processes here.

First Session

In the first session, we work with a quality of listening within the mid-tide, which students have already begun to develop:

1. Negotiate your contact via the vault hold. Maintain an appropriate viewing distance from the patient's system. Settle into the biosphere and mid-tide level of action. Let the fluid tide come to you and include an awareness of the whole tissue field.

2. Notice the quality of information that comes. Simply listen. Do not follow or go to anything. Wait. Be patient. As you listen, wait for something to seem to engage from within. Wait for something to clarify as a manifestation of the whole. You may sense a drive of potency towards a particular fulcrum and the whole tissue field will seem to distort around it. The distortion will have an "organic" feel to it. The *whole* tensile field will respond. An inertial shape will be expressed throughout the field as a distortion in its entire dynamic. It may seem as if the whole tissue field distorts around a particular fulcrum. You are directly sensing the actual inertial dynamics of the field around that particular fulcrum.

3. Notice what organizes this field of action and facilitate the healing intentions as appropriate. Listen for Dr. Becker's three-step awareness. Use any of your skills to help facilitate space, initiate potency, and access the state of balance. This may include any of the skills you have at your command. The important thing here is to respond appropriately and to not get in the way of the intentions of the treatment plan. You are a servant of the Breath of Life here. You must follow the conductor of the symphony and not get in the way. It is a question of supporting the process already in play.

Second Session

In a second session we add another listening factor:

1. As you settle into the relationship as described above, become especially aware of the action of the potency in the inhalation phase of the mid-tide. As you sense inhalation, it is as if you are riding the fluid tide as the potency surges within it.

2. Follow the surge of potency for as many cycles as necessary. You may notice a moment when the potency begins to shift within the fluids. It may seem to surge towards a particular fulcrum or area within the body. Follow this surge to the fulcrum being attended to. You may again sense the tissue field distorting around the fulcrum towards which the potency is surging.

Third Session

In a third session, we open the process up to a much wider field of listening:

1. Again settle into your relationship to the system. Gently let your perceptual field open and move towards the horizon. Settle into a wide field of listening as you do this. Simply listen without any need to know anything or to find anything. Let your needs settle into a stillness. Simply listen within this wide field.

2. As you do this, you may become aware of a larger field of action around the person's body. You may sense a stable bioelectric phenomenon. It may seem like a living field of energy. You may have a felt sense of bioenergy and of a bioelectric matrix. It may be sensed as a vibrancy, almost electric, but softer and more dynamic. It may seem like a field within which the person is organized.

3. This bioelectric field is not separate from the wider space it rests in. Space and form are one dynamic. You may sense a movement of an intention from an even wider field of action. It may seem as if a great yet subtle wind enters the space. This wind is like a focused presence. It may seem to arise out of nothing, or to come from "somewhere else." It enters the space and rises within the system.

4. Again, something seems to engage from within. The whole bioelectric field seems to distort around a particular. It has the quality of space being bent or distorted. The potency, fluids, and tissues respond to this intention. A healing process is engaged. You are a still and present observer to these phenomena. The treatment plan seems to engage from the outside-in and the inside-out. It is a factor of the deeper centering and healing intentions arising from within. It is not about coupled forces or inertial potencies. There is a more direct sense to the treatment plan truly being inherent within the conditions present as an Intelligence at work.

The Dynamic Stillness

Stillness permeates the world. It is an expression of wholeness and of the divine creative intention. It is the ground of emergence for all form. This Stillness is not void; it is dynamic and vibrant. As the practitioner grows in awareness, it may be sensed that healing is a factor of Stillness, not of motion or form. This Stillness is accessible. Words are difficult here for me. It is very hard to describe something that is unformed, imminent. It is about essence rather than form. Yet is also about the relationship of that essence to form. Again, from the Heart Sutra, emptiness *is* form and form *is* emptiness. They co-arise. There are, for me, a number of experiences that relate to the presence of this sacred ground. In one, an immersion into Stillness seems to occur. If your consciousness deeply settles into the Dynamic Stillness, a depth of unknowing is accessed. It is like a darkness, a freedom from the known. It is a space of vast potential. Here the treatment plan is an expression of mystery. It is not really about a *plan* per se, it is not linear or even about particulars. It is more as if past and future enter the present moment and what arises is totally appropriate. Something happens within this darkness and then, when you come out of it, you *know* something has happened, but may not be able to describe it. There may then be a process like that described above, where, upon leaving the darkness, there is a Long Tide field of action, organizing winds are perceived, and then a shift to the mid-tide is sensed. Potencies at each level are initiated in the healing process, inertial forces resolve, and potency, fluids, and tissues realign to suspended automatically shifting fulcrums and the midline. There has been a reconnection to the deeper intentions of the Breath of Life and the Original matrix it generates.

There is also another experience in which the Dynamic Stillness seems to be a ground of emergence for the ordering intentions of the Breath of Life. This experience is like having your feet in two worlds, the world of Stillness and the world of form. A rhythmic balanced interchange between the Stillness and the world of form can be perceived. A literal exchange between Stillness, potency, and form is experienced directly. This is described in the next section in much more detail. It has vast clinical significance.

Again, as the practitioner listens to the system with an open awareness, this process is seen to unfold in a very precise way. One thing needs to happen before another. It is a matter of following this inherent treatment plan as it unfolds and supporting it as appropriate. As you listen to a patient's system over a number of sessions, the particular fulcrums which need to be addressed will be expressed in a precise order and precise way. Again, it is then a matter of supporting the process in any way that is clinically appropriate and does not get in the way of the forces acting to resolve the issue. This whole process is humbling, and a great gratitude to the Intelligence inherent within all conditions, the Health that is never lost, will surely arise.

Rhythmic Balanced Interchange

When I first came across the term *rhythmic balanced interchange*, I was very touched. Tears came to my eyes, because it resonated with much of my clinical experience. For discussions of this concept and much more, please see, *The Stillness of Life,* edited transcripts of Dr. Becker's papers and letters.[1] I would like to give my thoughts on this concept with an acknowledgment that these are not Dr. Becker's interpretations, but my own. The organization of the human system is founded upon rhythmic balanced interchange. There is an interchange between the Dynamic Stillness and space. The Breath of Life mediates this exchange. Within this process, organizing winds are generated by the action of the Breath of Life, and its creative intention is set into motion. There is a rhythmic balanced interchange between space, movement, and form. The Breath of

Life organizes space and form follows. The Long Tide is the great organizing wind set into play by the intentions of the Breath of Life. The bioelectric matrix is laid down as the centripetal and centrifugal motions of the Long Tide express a dynamic equilibrium. The dynamic equilibrium is again a factor of rhythmic balanced interchange. It is an interchange between the formless and the formed.

There is then a rhythmic balanced interchange within the potency, fluids, and tissues of the body. The rhythmic order, expressed via the inhalation and exhalation cycles of the Tide, manifest within the fluids, cells, and tissues of the body as a rhythmic exchange between potency and fluids. The transmutation of potency within the fluids is a factor of this rhythmic balanced interchange, and the cellular and tissue world follows. In essence, there is a rhythmic balanced interchange between our deepest spiritual Source and the world of form. This exchange organizes order out of chaos. Indeed, order and chaos are simply the two poles of this interchange. It is a constant and ever going process. It holds things together in their interactions within the arms of the eternal present.

Rhythmic Balanced Interchange

The Dynamic Stillness

⇓⇑

The Breath of Life

⇓⇑

The Long Tide

⇓⇑

The Bioelectric Matrix

⇓⇑

The Potency

⇓⇑

The Fluid, Cellular and Tissue world

Within the world of experience and form, there is also a constant rhythmic balanced interchange at work. There is a constant interchange between the biodynamic potencies that order the human system, the Stillness that manifests that potency, the mind-body physiology, and all of the genetic, environmental, and stress factors we must meet in life. Health centers it all. As we have seen in previous chapters, the biodynamic potency of the Breath of Life acts to center the biokinetic force factors within the system, and this too is a rhythmic balanced interchange of potency to force factor, be it genetic, environmental, or traumatic. All of this is held within a dynamic equilibrium by the ordering intentions of the Breath of Life. It is the precision of this balance that centers all of our conditions and allows the inherent treatment plan to manifest. It is a function of the Stillness, the ground of emergence from whence it all arises.

Rhythmic Balanced Interchange:

Stillness–to Biodynamic Potency–to Mind-Body Physiology–to biokinetic forces present

The Stillness

Biodynamic Potency

Mind-Body Physiology

Unresolved Biokinetic Forces: Genetic, Traumatic, and Environmental Forces Present

---

Rhythmic Balanced Interchange within the Treatment Process

This has become an important perceptual awareness for me. I have described this process in a num-ber of ways in this volume. Here I would like to expand upon some ideas and again bring this concept of rhythmic balanced interchange into the equation. One of the first things we discussed in this volume was the creation of practitioner fulcrums. The creation of these fulcrums gives the practitioner a ground to come from and a fulcrum for the patient's system to relate to. It helps generate a relational field of action within which a healing process can be initiated and held. Within this relationship field, there is a rhythmic balanced interchange between the practitioner and the patient. This is a living relationship, which has its ebb and flow. There is an exchange of life process, of consciousness, and of intentions. So much moves and resonates within the co-joined fields of practitioner and patient. There is a rhythmic balanced interchange between the universal aspects of both. The same primary breath enlivens both, and the same ordering field is at work. The same Long Tide organizes and generates the Original matrix, and this matrix is the same in both. Mind states are exchanged within this field and thought forms resonate. Warmth and compassion, a universal acknowledgment of love, is rhythmically exchanged, especially when a depth of balance and stillness is attained within the relationship.

There is a rhythmic balanced interchange within all treatment processes. This concept sums up all of the work presented in this book. When we discussed Dr. Becker's three-step healing awareness, we were discussing this rhythmic balanced interchange. Within the state of balance, a state of dynamic equilibrium is attained. Within the state of balance, a rhythmic balanced interchange among Stillness, potency, and the forces that maintain the disturbance is initiated. Within the stillness of the state of balance, rhythmic balanced interchange is occurring. Biodynamic potencies are initiated, and there is an exchange between these ordering potencies and the genetic, environmental, or traumatic forces present. Within the stillness of the state of balance, a transmutation of potency occurs within the fulcrum being attended to. Transmutation is an expression of a rhythmic balanced interchange between potency as a bioenergy field and the fluids within the body. There is a change in the potency as this occurs, and *something happens* within the inertial fulcrum beyond the conditions being centered.

There is an even deeper aspect to this. This rhythmic balanced interchange has depth. It is not horizontal; it goes deep. Within the state of balance, the practitioner is focused not just on the resistance or forces present, but on the dynamic nature of the Stillness, which is not separate from it all. As the practitioner resonates with this Stillness, he or she may sense a rhythmic balanced interchange between the potencies and forces at work and the stillness that centers the whole. A sense of aliveness, a rhythmic exchange between all of the factors present may be appreciated. As seen earlier, the Dynamic Stillness is the ground of emergence for the organization of form. As the practitioner deeply enters the Dynamic Stillness, a darkness of knowing occurs. *But there is an intermediate experience.* It is like being within the doorway of the Stillness and not completely entering. Or it is like having a foot in both worlds. The practitioner becomes aware of an interchange among Stillness, space, and form. A vibrancy is sensed, which underlies and permeates everything. There is a direct perception of the Dynamic Stillness as a ground of emergence for all form and organization. It is alive, vibrant, and dynamic in its creative processes. Stillness is in constant rhythmic balanced interchange with all of the form within the universe, all at once, as a whole. It is vast, yet it is contained within the head of a pin, the eye of the needle. Form is not separate from that Stillness. Remember the Heart Sutra discussed in an earlier chapter: form is emptiness and emptiness is form.

There is a constant rhythmic balanced interchange among the Dynamic Stillness, space, and form. Stillness permeates form and orders its dynamics. It is like a dynamic spiral, which takes you ever deeper into the present. In this, nothing is separate. This truth is accessible within the state of balance. As I hold the patient's system within my hands, I am aware of a Stillness that centers the

forces and potencies at work. This is a vibrancy, an aliveness that pervades everything. As a depth of relationship is accessed, as we move through the eye of the needle, a rhythmic balanced interchange among the Stillness and the potencies and forces within the fulcrum occurs. It is a vibrancy, an infusion of light. Something arises from a depth of Stillness and a rhythmic balanced interchange occurs. As you palpate the patient's system, it may seem that there is a vacuum between your hands within which there is an exchange or interchange of potencies and forces. It is vibrant and alive and you perceive this within your hands and within all of your senses at once. Potency seems to arise from a "nowhere" and return to that nowhere. This is truly the treatment plan in action! Thus we can see that there is a rhythmic balanced interchange among the Stillness, the potencies, the inertial forces present, and the mind-body physiology. All of this attains a dynamic equilibrium within the state of balance, and a rhythmic balanced interchange is initiated beyond the conditions being centered. It is constantly and always a humbling experience. I give you may thoughts on these ideas as pointers, as words that cannot describe this adequately or clearly. I can only speak from my own limited perspective, but hopefully a dialogue has been initiated.

The Rhythmic Balanced Interchange within States of Balance

The Stillness

⇓⇑

The Biodynamic Potency

⇓⇑

The Biokinetic, Inertial Forces

⇓⇑

The Mind-Body Physiology

Clinical Application: Stillness and the Rhythmic Balanced Interchange

In the following short application, the intention will be to initiate a relationship to the Stillness within the potencies and forces centering and maintaining disturbances within the system. It is meant to initiate an exploration into the possibility of sensing the Stillness at work within the state of balance and all healing processes. In the exploration, you will help access a state of balance within the mid-tide and work to sense the stillness at work within the midst of the conditions being centered.

1. Start with a vault hold and synchronize your perceptual field with the mid-tide. Hold the whole biosphere within your perceptual field, yet do not lose a sense of the tissues being palpated. Let the mid-tide field of action come into your awareness. First be aware of the fluid tide, then include the tissue elements.

2. Settle into this field of action. Do not follow anything, do not grab onto any of the three functions of potency, fluids, or tissues. Let things clarify. Wait for the inherent treatment plan to unfold. You may sense something engaging from within. The whole tensile field of action may begin to distort around an inertial fulcrum or, during the inhalation phase, you may sense a surge of potency within the fluids towards an inertial fulcrum.

3. Listen for the settling of this field into a state of balanced tension. It may be sensed that the potencies, fluids, and tissues are working their way towards a state of balance. Assist this if needed. Simply slow things down. Do not grab onto any of the three functions as you intend this. Listen for the state of balance, a dynamic equilibrium within the potencies and forces present, to be accessed.

4. Now, let's try something here. Within the state of balance, as you become aware of any motion, even if it is the action of potency at some level, settle into the space that supports the motion. Do not disengage from the system or the form of things; simply settle into the *space* between the motion and the form of things. Be more aware of the *space* within and between motion and form. Slowly go back and forth from an awareness of motion to a settling into space. Sense the space that supports the form. Do this slowly. First listen to motion and then settle into space and stillness. Spend a few minutes with each awareness as it comes to you.

5. After a while, you may begin to sense something extraordinary. Space and Stillness begin to come to the foreground. As you settle into this space, without a loss of awareness, you may then sense a vibrancy within the heart of the motion of potencies and forces at work. You may sense a rhythmic balanced interchange between Dynamic Stillness and form. Something like a vacuum, or a void, may seem to open up between your hands. You may perceive a vibrant exchange among Stillness, space, and form. Stillness to potency, to the conditioned form of things and back. Something will happen here beyond the forces and conditions present. A vibrancy occurs. You will discover that this rhythmic balanced interchange *is* the treatment process, and what is needed for that day has occurred.

The Empty Vessel

There is a further perceptual experience that I would like to talk about here. It is difficult to describe and really pushes me to the extreme of language. It has to do with an experience of emptying wherein something fills the space created, which I can only term Presence. This emptying I am talking about is an emptying of self. As we go through our ritual of generating practitioner fulcrums and negotiating our contact with the patient's system, we can settle into the stillness of listening. As we hold a wide perceptual field with the patient in the center of this field, our sense of separate self may temporarily be suspended. Within this state, this emptiness of self, I have humbly witnessed something I can only surmise is the Breath of Life in action. Perhaps it is an expression of a divine intention deeper and much more Intelligent than my limited mental and intuitive processes. In my own words, it is a sense of a Presence, which is huge yet can move through the most diminutive spaces.

The first time I sensed this was at a time of clinical crisis. Over a number of sessions, I had been struggling to help a patient and was at the end of my clinical tether. Nothing would help. I was helpless and hapless. I was empty of all clinical possibility. I stopped trying to do anything and literally gave in to the present moment. It was not an intentional act. I had no choice. It was a letting go of any machinations and any sense of doing anything. My patient's suffering was mine, and I was humbled by the moment. I said a prayer, to whom or what I still have no idea, but something happened that was beyond my limited experience. I sensed a Presence. As this occurred my heart opened, I was pushed out of the way, and something else took over. It was a mutual experience for me and my patient. We were truly fellow travelers here. It was as if this Presence was saying to me, "Step aside sonny, there is work to do." There was a sense of vibrancy and permeation everywhere at once. Multiple fulcrums were safely attended to, light filled the spaces, and form was transformed. I still don't know how long this took. It seemed to happen in an instant. Both of us knew we had been in the presence of something special. A gift was bestowed.

Over the years this Presence sometimes makes itself known to me during sessions, other times when I am simply sitting in meditation. I have no control over this. It seems to be a factor of my interior state, a letting go in all humility to something "other." It also seems to be a matter of the heart. The heart resonates where my brain cannot. It is an openness to

the present moment, while still maintaining a humble awareness that waits in all humility. It is, to me, about an emptying of my self-sense. In the Zen tradition there is a saying, "one must become like an empty vessel." Something may come to fill this empty vessel with its Presence. There is the possibility of a resonance with Big Mind, or Bodhicitta, the brilliant sanity that underlies all of manifestation. There is the possibility of a relationship to a Presence that seems to be orchestrating what needs to happen next. There is an availability to "something other" than our narrow conditioned state. It seems to me that this Presence is discovered only in the eternal present and completes its creative intention in every moment of our lives. We are eternally and ever presently being created and nurtured in its womb-like presence. What I sense as the presence of something much greater than my limited viewpoint is perhaps best summed up in a beautiful stanza from a book by Haven Trevino:

The Breath of Life inspires
The eternal womb of the
Divine Mother
Who conceives and gives birth to the promise
of God in every being.

Thus our well is eternal
The Breath of Life fills us
Again and again.[2]

In the Daoist tradition the Dao is likened to an empty vessel, which may be drawn from without ever needing to be filled. It fills us again and again. In its emptiness, it is full of all potential. In becoming like an empty vessel, there is the potential to be filled. There is the possibility that in all humility the Intelligence that permeates the universe may make its Presence known and something may occur beyond the conditions present. Enough said. In the *Dao De Jing* Laozi states that the best teachings occur in silence, so I will quiet myself here.

Completions

This is the last chapter in this volume. There are also a number of appendices, which may be of use to you. One summarizes the unfoldments of the tidal phenomena within the context of clinical skills. This was dealt with in more detail in the previous chapter. There are also a number of transcribed talks of mine, which may be of interest to you. They are meant to summarize some important ideas in a less formal way than my written words.

The second volume of this work is about the relationships and patterns of the human system. It goes deeper into structure and function and covers the motility and motion of the major tissue relationships of the body. It is about how to create an appropriate clinical relationship to the structures and systems of the human body, given the perceptual and clinical skills developed so far. We start with an awareness of the primal midline, and the rest of the volume organizes around that perceptual skill. A chapter on the nervous system is crucial to appreciate.

I hope this first volume will be of some help to you all.

Best wishes.
    —Franklyn Sills

1. See R. E. Becker, *The Stillness of Life*, ed. Rachel E. Brooks (Stillness Press, 2000).

2. Haven Trevino, *The Tao of Healing* (New World Library).

* *Looking Glass Universe, The Emerging Science of Wholeness*, by John P. Briggs, Ph.D., & F. David Peet, Ph.D., Simon & Schuster (Touchstone), New York, 1984, p.66.

Appendix I: Perceptual Levels and Skills

Prerequisite Skills:

- Accessing a practitioner neutral, centering, establishing practitioner fulcrums, grounding.

- Negotiating distance and appropriate contact.

- Perceptual skills, inner stillness, listening skills, maintaining and synchronizing with appropriate perceptual fields, the ability to perceive the human system as it unfolds its information to you.

- The ability to perceive and relate clinically to the three functions of potency, fluids, and tissues at each of the three perceptual levels.

CRI Level of Perception

Rate: 8–14 cycles/minute

Palpation: Hands float on tissues, perceptual field narrows to bones, membranes, structural parts, tissue structures, and relationships.

Mind: Relatively active, analyzing, looking at relationship of parts and structures.

Emotion: Emotional affects, affects of trauma and experience, emotional fixity. Activation may arise in sessions. Emotional responses based on past conditioning and defended positions.

Perceptual Experience: Inhalation and exhalation phases perceived as cycles of reciprocal tension motion. Tissue and fluid motion experienced via reciprocal tension motions. Practitioner commonly experiences tissue motion as relationship of separate structures in reciprocal tension. Craniosacral motion, flexion and extension of separate parts, predominates awareness. Motion is perceived to be organized around automatically shifting tissue fulcrums.

Tidal Unfoldment: The CRI is not a direct expression of motility. The CRI is an outer expression of motion conditioned by genetics and experiential processes. The CRI level of motion is generated as an expression of the relationship of parts and structures as these are effected by the experiences of life. It initially arises as genetic processes are centered by the action of the Breath of Life. The CRI is also an expression of unresolved trauma and experience as they are held within the system as inertial forces. The CRI is generated as the Breath of Life acts to center these conditions of our life. The quality of the CRI is directly effected by the state of the autonomic nervous system. Autonomic set points affect CRI expression. It is the wave form of our experience; it is not a direct expression of the Tide. The CRI ha a variable rate of 8–14 cycles a minute, which is an expression of conditioned processes. Its rate of expression will change due the forces of unresolved inertia and the nature of the unresolved experiences held within the system.

Inertial Perception: Within the CRI level of perception, the perception of inertia and unresolved experience is via an awareness of results and affects. Expressions of inertial processes are perceived via tissue and fluid affects, resistance between anatomical structures, and via symptoms and pathology. The deeper forces at work are not directly perceived. Awareness of lesions predominates the practitioner's perceptual field. These are perceived as tissue and fluid affects, such as tissue resistance, adhesion, compression, pathology, stasis within fluids, and resistance between tissue structures. A perception of activation and fragmentation predominates. These are commonly perceived as tissue compression, adhesion, changes in quality of tissues, strains and fluid fluctuations. Perception is about form and resistance, about how/where we hold unresolved trauma and resistance as CNS hyper- and hypo-states, as tissue and fluid inertia, as resistance between parts, as emotional affects, psychological positions, and as pathological processes.

Inertial Fulcrums: Inertial fulcrums are perceived via tissue lesions, strain patterns, sites of tissue change, loss of mobility, resistance; as fluid congestion and eccentric fluid fluctuation. Inertial fulcrums are located via motion testing, analysis and diagnosis, application of techniques, traction, fluid direction, etc. Practitioner actively applies processes to locate and resolve inertial fulcrums perceived as lesions.

Organization Perceived: Organization perceived to be an expression of the relationship and motion of parts. Inertial organization is perceived through motion or fixation around lesion sites, and via tissue and fluid stasis. These are perceived as the results and affects of experience and suffering. The organizing midline is perceived to be a structural axis through the vertebral bodies and cranial base. Automatically shifting fulcrums are perceived to be sites within tissue relationships. Hence, reciprocal tension motion is perceived to be organized around embryologically derived tissue fulcrums, such as Sutherland's fulcrum.

Healing Perceived: Healing processes are based on the acknowledgment of suffering, on a practitioner's relationship to the results and affects of suffering. Healing is perceived as a resolution of CNS activation, emotional affects, symptoms and pathologies, and tissue and fluid congestion/resistance. Disengagement is perceived to be a factor of practitioner intervention.

Healing Modes: Practitioner is active. Work is lesion, symptom, and activation oriented. The practitioner actively seeks neutrals within tissue, fluid, and emotional affects. The practitioner is more active in seeking the point of balanced membranous tension. Conversations with tissues and fluids are technique and method based. Processes of decompression, traction, compression, fluid direction, lateral fluctuation of fluid, may be applied to inertial tissue site. *Healing processes are lesion and practitioner oriented.*

Mid-Tide Level of Perception

Rate: 2.5 cycles a minute Palpation:

Hands immersed/floats within fluid. The practitioner widens the perceptual field to include the whole of person and his or her biosphere. (The biosphere includes the whole of the body, energy field, and area of environmental exchange around the patient's body.)

Mind: The mind is relatively still/quiet. The tendencies and conditioning of the mind still may arise. To help synchronize the mind with the mid-tide, allow the mind to settle, find a still inner neutral. The practitioner's mind is not interested in parts and relationships per se, but in whole units of function.

Emotion: Emotions are fluid and appropriate to the present experience. Emotional responses and resolutions appropriately arise in present time. Emotional affects and releases are expressed in contained and resourced ways. Emotional activation has the quality of completion. The emotional state does not continue to cycle and is not reinforced.

Perceptual Experience: Potency, fluids, and tissues are perceived by the practitioner as a unified field of action. At this level of perception, the practitioner is aware of potency as a transmutation within the fluids. Potency is experienced as a physiological ordering factor within the fluid system. The practitioner is aware of each function of potency, fluid, and tissue as a unified and whole tensile field of action. Tissue motility and motion is perceived as a unified tensile field. Individual structures are directly perceived to be part of a unified motility throughout the body. Flexion and extension dynamics are perceived to be a factor of deeper forces at work. An inner breath is perceptible within tissue motility. Flexion and extension of individual bones, of the reciprocal tension membrane, and of tissues generally is perceived to be part of a greater whole. Inhalation and exhalation cycles are perceived as a surge and settling within tensile fields. Motion dynamics are perceived via awareness of unified tensile fields organized around automatically shifting fulcrums. Automatically shifting fulcrums are perceived to be loci or condensations of potency, which organize tensile fields of action.

Tidal Unfoldment: The mid-tide is an expression of the transmutation of potency within the fluids of the body. Here we have a direct experience of potency within fluids. Potency is the organizing factor, fluid is the medium of exchange, and cells and tissues organize around its action. Potency, fluids, and tissues are perceived to be a unified tensile field expressing a tidal rhythm of 2.5 cycles a minute. Tissues, fluids, and potency are experienced as whole tensile fields of action. The mid-tide is a relatively stable rhythm sensed as an inhalation surge and an exhalation settling within tensile fields.

Inertial Perception: Expressions of inertial processes such as conditioned tissue motion and patterns of inertial motility and mobility are perceived as distortions within whole tensile fields. The practitioner perceives the whole tensile field distorting around inertial fulcrums. Tissue motility is

perceived as a unified field, inertial patterns are perceived as distortions of this field organized around inertial fulcrums. Information at this level of perception is more precise and encompassing than at the CRI level. There is no need to motion test in order to gain clinical information. Practitioner has a direct experience of inertial forces, shapes, and organizing fulcrums. The practitioner's mind is stiller, less active, and the work is less tiring.

Inertial Fulcrums: Inertial fulcrums are directly perceived as sites of inertial potencies. Inertial fulcrums are perceived as condensations of inertial forces within tensile fields of action. There is a direct perception of biodynamic and biokinetic forces at work. Within the mid-tide level of perception, inertial fulcrums are located via direct perceptual experience. The practitioner is aware of the biodynamic and biokinetic forces at work at the heart of organizing fulcrums. There is an experience of the coupling of biodynamic potencies with inertial forces in order to center and contain them. Inertial fulcrums are not automatically shifting fulcrums. They are sites of stasis that do not shift with the intentions of the Tide. Inertial patterns are perceived via distortions within tensile fields of action organized by condensations or concentrations of inertial forces.

Organization Perceived: Organization directly perceived to be a factor of the potency within the fluids. Inertial organization perceived as tensile distortions around the condensation of inertial potencies. Forces at work are seen to be the organizing factors. The organizing midline is perceived to be the dorsal or fluid midline, as it is expressed along the neural axis. The fluid tide is perceived to be a function of the dorsal midline.

Healing Perceived: Healing perceived as a factor of transmutation. Healing perceived as resolution of inertial forces and via the reorganization of tissues, fluids, and potencies to the primal midline and natural fulcrums. Original intention is reestablished.

Healing Modes: State of balanced tension seen to be inherent within the inertial pattern. The treatment plan inherent within the disturbance is perceived. There is an inherent tendency for a neutral to be accessed. At most, practitioner facilitates state of balance by slowing motion down. Dr. Becker's three-stage healing awareness becomes obvious:

1. Tissues, fluids, and potencies naturally seek a neutral. There is a movement towards a state of balance.

2. The state of balance is accessed. A functional stillpoint arises. The state of balance is perceived to be the "eye of a needle through which something can pass." Something happens within the state of balance. Biodynamic and biokinetic potencies are initiated. Expressions of Health are perceived. There is a permeation of potency and inertial forces are resolved.

3. Tissues, fluids, and potencies reorganize/realign to the primal midline and natural fulcrums.

Practitioner may offer and engage in conversations about space and history via subtle negotiated intentions of disengagement, space, traction, direction of potencies, lateral fluctuations of potency, etc., offered as conversations rather than as techniques or protocols. Healing is perceived to be transmutation and potency based.

Long Tide Level of Perception

Rate: 50 second cycles of inhalation and exhalation (100 seconds in all)

Palpation: Hands immersed/floats within potency. The practitioner widens the perceptual field towards the horizon. Wide perceptual field is maintained.

Mind: Mind deepens and is still, breathes with the Breath of Life within a wide perceptual field. There is still an experience of an observer, although very subtle and still.

Emotion: Expansive emotions predominate. Joy, warmth, sense of connection and humbleness.

Perceptual Experience: Long tide is the potency of the Breath of Life per se. Potency of Breath of Life is more directly perceived. The practitioner senses potency as a radiance permeating everything. The experience of radiance passes through the practitioner's hands. There is a light, airy, yet powerful experience of radiance. There is a perception of cellular permeation. There is a perception of potency as a field phenomenon. The Original or primal bioelectric ordering matrix is directly perceived. The primal midline is perceived as an uprising force within the bioelectric field.

Tidal Unfoldment: The Long Tide is an expression of the intention of the Breath of Life to create a human being. It is the "Original motion" that Victor Schauberger wrote of. This is the Tide per se. The Long Tide is perceived as a direct organizing intention within and around the patient. The bioelectric matrix is generated via centrifugal and centripetal spiraling forces as the Long Tide, like a great wind, lays down the stable bioelectric form of a human being. The Long Tide can be perceived within the biosphere to generate deep, airy, powerful tidal motions in 100-second cycles (50 seconds inhalation, 50 seconds exhalation). Its intention may be experienced in a wider field in very slow cycles of expansion (15–20 minute cycles). The Long Tide generates the most fundamental ordering matrix, a bioelectric form, as a field phenomenon. The Original matrix of a human being is laid down. Bioelectric potency is seen to be an unfoldment of a particular intention to incarnate, which carries the universal matrix of a human being. The primal midline coalesces within the bioelectric ordering field generated by the action of the Long Tide. The primal midline may be experienced as an uprising force within the center of the organism. This becomes the main organizing axis for the development and maintenance of the form of the human body. The notochord of the embryo and the structural axis of the body organize in relationship to its action.

Inertial Perception: Inertia is not perceived via fulcrums or inertial motion patterns. Inertial issues perceived as coalescence and distortions within a matrix like Einstein's concept of mass bending the space-time continuum. Inertia is perceived as density and distortion within a wider matrix. This is similar to how mass is said to bend space-time in the theory of relativity.

Inertial Fulcrums: Inertial fulcrums are perceived as a density and distortion within an energetic matrix.

Organization Perceived: Organization is perceived as a factor of the radiance of the potency of the Breath of Life and its Original matrix. The primal midline is more obvious. The geometric precision of the original matrix is perceived. "God geometizes, man cognises" (Dr. Randolph Stone, D.O.) The organizing axis is perceived via the primal midline as an emergent reality.

Healing Perceived: Direct experience of the potencies of the Breath of Life doing the healing. Potency shimmers like sunlight on the sea, inertial fulcrums vibrate, inertial forces resolve via permeation, transmutation, and a reconnection to the Original matrix. Healing perceived as a shift or resolution within the bioelectric matrix.

Healing Modes: The practitioner's mind is still, potency is directly perceived. Healing is perceived to arise "from the without to the within" via transmutation and reconnection to the Original matrix. The practitioner is a humble observer holding space and relationship. Practitioner keenly listens to processes of reconnection and transmutation. *Healing is resonance and reconnection based.*

The Dynamic Stillness

Entry: The practitioner's mind stills, settles, deepens, and expands, letting go of self-view.

Mind/Consciousness: State of mind is unified, still, expanded. No-self, no self-constructs, no subject-object relationship. Unity consciousness.

Emotion: Within the Stillness there is no self-other perception. There is only a unified field of compassion. Equanimity, compassion directly sensed as an illimitable and unified natural state of grace. This state is not personal, but a universal.

Perceptual Experience: Within this state there is perception without a perceiver. There are no tides, only an alive, dynamic Stillness. Vibrancy predominates.

Organization Perceived: Organization is an expression of the intention of the divine.

Healing: Healing via direct resonance. Space-time irrelevant. Healing is instantaneous. *Healing occurs within the darkness of unknowing and is mysterious.*

419

Appendix II: The Mysterious Gateway

The intention of this appendix is simply to bring together some of the sections of this volume that relate directly to the awareness of and the accessing of deeper healing processes. This will include the exercise about shifting perceptual fields and the discussions of the mysterious gateway, or the eye of the needle from sections on the state of balanced tension, stillpoint, and disengagement. The ability to shift perceptual fields and to appreciate deeper healing processes as they arise is an important clinical skill whose depths continually deepen.

A. Shifting Perceptual Fields

Let me introduce a perceptual exercise that will become the foundation for many future clinical explorations. We will return to it over and over again. In this process, you will use different modes of intention and a widening perceptual field to help gain access to the different tidal unfoldments. We will work within the three basic levels of the CRI, the potency tide, and the Long Tide. The CRI tends to express itself anywhere from 8 to 10 cycles a minute. The potency tide expresses itself at a more stable 2.5 cycles a minute, and the Long Tide in 100-second cycles (50-second inhalation and 50-second exhalation). Refer back to Chapter Five for a more detailed discussion of each layer of unfoldment. Later, we will develop the means to consciously access the Dynamic Stillness.

1. With the patient in the supine position, place your hands in the vault hold. Access your inner neutral, negotiate your contact, and let your hands float on the tissues as though they are corks on the water. Do not place any pressure or force on the tissues. Simply float and let yourself be moved by the tissues and fluids being palpated.

2. In the first perceptual process, you will shift, or synchronize, your attention to the *CRI level of perception*. To do this, maintain the image of your hands floating on the tissues like corks on the water. Narrow your perceptual field to tissues, bones, and membranes. Get interested in how these tissues are moving. Let your hands float on the tissues, and let them show you their motions. Listen, don't look for anything, and don't expect anything. Let it come to you. See if the faster rhythm, the CRI, comes into your field of awareness. Stay with this for a number of minutes until you are clear about its expression.

3. Now shift your intentions to the *mid-tide level of perception*. To do this, you will shift your imagery and will widen your perceptual field. In the CRI level of perception, your hands were floating on the tissues. In this shift, let your hands instead *float within fluids*. Imagine/sense that your hands are floating in a wider field of

fluid as they palpate the tissues. Your hands are immersed within this fluid field.

4. Now widen your perceptual field to hold the whole of the person and the field around him or her. Dr. Rollin Becker, D.O., called this the *biosphere*. The biosphere is a useful concept. It denotes the whole of the person, the body, and the field of potency and environmental exchange around their body. In this process, you widen your field of awareness from the individual tissues and structures palpated above to include the whole of the person and the wider field of potency around the body. Within this field you are sensing the fluids and tissues of the body *as a whole*.

5. As you do this, allow your mind to settle and be relatively still. Your quality of awareness is wide and soft, yet you also maintain a keen precision within your listening. You are now holding the *whole* of the person within your field of attention. You may sense a deepening and slowing of the rhythmic unfoldment. See if the slower rhythm of the potency tide, 2.5 cycles a minute, begins to unfold its presence. Stay with this for a number of minutes.

6. Now shift your perceptual field to the Long Tide. To do this, you will again shift your intentions and widen your perceptual field. Above you imagined/sensed that your hands were immersed within fluid. Now see if you can imagine/sense that your hands are floating within potency. Imagine a field of potency within which the patient is centered and your hands are immersed. It is like being within a subtle yet palpable bioelectric field.

7. With this sense, slowly widen your perceptual field towards the horizon. Move out towards the horizon while holding the patient within the center of your field of attention. Do not extend your awareness beyond what feels safe and contained for now. Simply let your mind hold a wider sense of the whole. Let it still, and see if you have the sense that your intention to move towards the horizon is at balance with the sensory information returning. It may seem as if your mind is literally being breathed by the Breath of Life in total balance. The patient is in the centre of this widened field of perception.

8. See if the deeper, slower Long Tide unfolds within your perceptual field. This may seem as if the Breath of Life is radiating from the core of the person and permeating everything. It may also seem as if you are immersed within the ocean and the tidal forces are moving through you. Simply listen within this wider field. You may be surprised at the nature of communication within this widened field of attention. Stay with this awareness for a number of minutes, then gently and slowly shift your perceptual field back to the biosphere and the potency tide level of perception. After anchoring your perceptual field within the potency tide, slowly negotiate a disengagement of your physical contact.

After the sessions, spend some time with your tutor exploring the experience and come together in the large group to share the essential insights gained with the whole class. This exercise can also be explored in threes with two people sharing the practitioner role. You will repeat this process many times as we unfold the different intentions of the work and the different relationships of the system. A summary of this process is outlined opposite.

B. The State of Balance as the Eye of the Needle

The state of balanced tension is also the eye of the needle into the deeper forces at work within the system. The state of balance can be the "eye" into the intentions of the Breath of Life and the Dynamic Stillness itself. In this last exploration you will again access the state of balanced tension and work to explore this state as a mysterious gateway to even deeper forces at work. You will do this by shifting

---

Summary of Access to Perceptual Levels

CRI
8–14 Cycles a Minute
- **Hands** float on tissues like corks on water.
- **Perceptual field** narrows to tissue, bone, membrane.
- **Mind** is interested in individual structures and relationships of structures/parts.

Mid-Tide
2.5 cycles a minute
- **Hands** are immersed/float within fluid.
- **Perceptual field** widens to hold the whole of the person and the biosphere. (The biosphere is the body and the field of potency and environmental exchange around it.)
- **Mind** is relatively quiet, holds a wider field, and is in relationship to whole of person.

Long Tide
100-second cycles
- **Hands** are immersed/float within potency (the fluid within the fluid).
- **Perceptual field** widens to the horizon.
- **Mind** is expansive and still, breathes with the Breath of Life.

---

your perceptual fields within the stillness accessed in the state of balance. You shift your perceptual field to the different unfoldments of the Breath of Life while maintaining an awareness of the state of balance. In this exercise, you will again start within the mid-tide level of perception. This process calls for a quality of listening in which you are open to the unknown and do not bring any preconceptions or judgments to a unique clinical encounter. You will first facilitate the state of balance within the mid-tide level of perception and then widen your perceptual field towards the horizon. This may open your perceptual field to the Long Tide level of perception and even to an experience of the Original matrix, which underlies the organization of form. As you widen your perceptual field, you will listen for any phenomena that arise within the state of balance.

The first step is to establish a safe and trustworthy space. Review concepts presented in Chapter Six. Gently negotiate your relationship and be open to listening within a context of unknowing. It is really important here to establish a still clinical space. It contains, initiates, and holds the process. It is a call to the deeper forces and Intentions at work within the human system. It is a call towards a relationship with the Breath of Life itself. Remember your practitioner fulcrums, come into breath and sensation, let your mind still and hold a wide and natural field of listening. This establishes a safe therapeutic space and is a call to the deeper healing resources within and beyond the conditional forces being centered. Much more important, it is a humbling entrée into a healing process, which is a mutual journey for both therapist and patient.

1. Start at the vault hold and negotiate your contact with the patient's system. In this position,

synchronize your perceptual field with the mid-tide, 2.5 cycles a minute. Do this by allowing your hands to float in fluid as they float on the tissues. Then widen your perceptual field to the biosphere as previously learned.

2. Within the biosphere, notice reciprocal tension motion as a unified motion dynamic within tissues, fluids, and potency. Listen to this as the cycles of primary respiration are expressed. Notice the tissue field as it expresses its tensile motion. Notice any distortions or inertial patterns within that field. Notice what organizes that motion. Notice Dr. Becker's three-step process. Listen to the tissues as they seek a neutral. Subtly slow their motions down until a state of balanced tension is obtained as learned earlier. Do not grab any function (tissues, fluids of potency) as you explore *reciprocal tension balance* within tissues, fluids, and potency.

3. Maintain an awareness of the inertial fulcrums and state of balanced tension within the biosphere. *Do not narrow your perceptual field as you listen.* Listen within this wider field of awareness. Include the tissues, fluids, and potency as a unified tensile field. Notice the three function of tissues, fluids, and potency accessing the state of balance. Listen for forces and potencies at work. Listen for expressions of Health.

4. Now, within the state of balance, gently shift your perceptual field towards the horizon. Let your hands float in potency and widen your perceptual field towards the horizon. Widen your field to wherever it is sensed to be safe and tolerable. Do not lose awareness of the state of balance and fulcrums being palpated as you do this. It is like holding a dual awareness, a wide perceptual field *and* an awareness of the particulars within it.

5. As you do this, you may sense the deeper, slower tidal phenomenon of the Long Tide. The midline imperative of the Breath of Life may also become more obvious here. Listen within the stillness of the state of balance to the inherent biodynamic forces as they begin to express their healing intentions. You may actually have an experience of the Breath of Life moving into the midline, arising through the tensile fields of the body, right through the inertial fulcrums being attended to. Like a mysterious gateway, the shift in your perceptual fields can bring you to the most formative organizing forces at work. The state of balance can bring you, like the eye of a needle, to the Original matrix itself. Biodynamic, epigenetic forces are perceived more directly here. The permeation of the potency of the Breath of Life through the inertial fulcrums is most clearly experienced here. Experiences of radiance, luminescence, and field phenomena are common here. The practitioner may have a sense of being in the ocean, in the midst of huge tidal forces at work. This is directly perceived to be part of a greater whole, a universal process of Original motion coming into play.

6. As your mind synchronizes with a depth of stillness and accesses a state of balance in which it is neither coming nor going, another gateway may open for you. You may enter a depth of Stillness from which all things arise. In Taoism it is called the Subtle Essence. It is entered in unknowing, a darkness. The mind is totally at balance and peace. It is wide and deep. Here the Dynamic Stillness, the ground of emergence of the human system, may be appreciated. It is truly a humbling experience. It is a stillness that permeates everything, that is alive with potential. It underpins the unfoldment of life. It is the ground of vibrancy from which particular forms arise. Here healing processes are directly a function of a greater plan and organization beyond the local inertial forces being centered. Perhaps it is like a subtle ground matrix in which all potential is unfolded. Within this state, what is appropriate to unfold will unfold.

7. As the tissues, fluids, and potencies again express motion, slowly shift your perceptual field

back to the biosphere. Allow the reorganization process to unfold. Do not rush this. Wait for a sense of tissue reorganization relative to Sutherland's fulcrum and for a clear expression of the fluid tide to come through. You may literally have the experience of the Breath of Life moving through the inertial fulcrum like light through the eye of a needle.

The Mysterious Gateway: Summary of the Process

1. Synchronize your perceptual field with the mid-tide (the 2.5 cycles a minute tide) Widen your perceptual field to the biosphere and listen to the unit of function of tissues, fluids, and potency as a whole unified tensile field of action. Facilitate the state of balanced tension. Listen for expression of forces at work.

2. Within the state of balance, again widen your perceptual field towards the horizon. See if the Long Tide and the midline function of the Breath of Life become more obvious. Settle into the stillness and allow your mind to still. Listen for healing to occur truly from the inside out as the Original intention of the Breath of Life clarifies within the system. You may literally have the experience of the potency of the Breath of Life moving through the inertial fulcrum like light through the eye of a needle. Biodynamic, epigenetic forces are perceived more directly here.

3. In this process a neutral may be entered in which your mind is neither coming nor going. Mind itself totally settles and enters a state of balance where the Dynamic Stillness is accessed. Another mysterious gateway may open here, a timeless state from which the most formative healing processes may arise.

C. Stillpoint as the Mysterious Gateway

In the next clinical application, we are going to further explore the stillpoint process as the mysterious gateway into deeper stillness and to the Dynamic Stillness itself. In this application, you will consciously be shifting your perceptual fields as the way into deeper depths of stillness. We started to do this above, but here we will move from the mid-tide, to the Long Tide, into deepening stillness. To paraphrase Dr. Jim Jealous, think of the stillpoint process as the *eye of the needle* into deeper and deeper experiences of stillness and inherent Health.

You will discover that as each unfoldment stills, different qualities of stillness will be perceived. The stillness accessed within each unfoldment has depth. If you are palpating within the CRI level, you may perceive a stilling of the CRI and different aspects of work being done physiologically. You may perceive fluid fluctuations, tissue reorganization, relaxation of tensions, and so on. Within the mid-tide level, you may perceive a deepening potency, a greater availability of resources, a welling up of the potency within the system and a clarity of healing forces at work. The inherent treatment plan may clarify as the forces of potency are expressed within the system. You may perceive a subtle processing of shock affect as fluid perturbations, tissue trembling, and resolution of autonomic affects. Within the Long Tide you may perceive a deepening relationship to the potency of the Breath of Life itself. A sense of the aliveness of the bioelectric field and its potency, a sense of its vibrancy, and a sense of radiance may arise.

The inherent treatment plan may become obvious as the potency of the Breath of Life moves to resolve inertial issues. Within the stillness here, patients may even connect to archetypal forms and energies as the Original matrix unfolds. This can be a very integrative experience. An inherent interconnection to life *as a whole* may be sensed and acknowledged here.

Within the Dynamic Stillness, we are talking about a depth experience that is difficult to describe.

It is about perception without a perceiver, or more correctly, it is a state of "neither perception nor non-perception." I am afraid that words seem to elude me here. It is a depth of Stillness in which self-view is truly dropped, even for an instant. A state without subject-object relationship, a Whole. Healing can be instantaneous here, as can a spiritual resonance. It is, in essence, a state of grace within a clinical context. The practitioner and patient are totally within the depth of present time and something happens. It may even be said that they are beyond time, even for an instant. The practitioner may not realize the repercussions of the session work until returning to the world of form and relationship. Even in the most desperate situations, with impending death obvious, fear can be dropped, and life and death can be seen as an expression of the Whole.

Application: Stillpoint as the Mysterious Gateway

In this section you will use the stillpoint process as the "mysterious gateway" into deeper and deeper depths of stillness. We introduced this idea in the chapter on the state of balanced tension. You may have perceived that, within a state of balanced tension, as you widen your perceptual field towards the horizon, a shift in both perception and healing process may occur. As you synchronize your perceptual field with the deeper unfoldments of the Breath of Life, deeper healing processes and forces become more evident. In this section we will begin again within the mid-tide level of perception and action. You will initiate a CV4 process within the mid-tide as above and will then broaden and deepen your perceptual field using each tidal unfoldment as the mysterious gateway into a deepening stillness. This process can also be initiated from the CRI, but I find it more direct to begin this process within the mid-tide and then widen your perceptual field towards the horizon into a deepening stillness. The spectrum traveled will include the mid-tide, the Long Tide, and the possibility of entry into the Dynamic Stillness itself. This is not to be taken lightly. Have patience. Do not expect anything and do not be disappointed, as everything is perfect in its own right. All of this has its own timing, its own tone and tempo.

The most important thing here is the quality of the space you are holding for entrée into deeper healing processes. It is based upon your negotiated contact and the nature of the perceptual field you are holding. The nature of your stillness and listening is a call to the deeper forces at work within the human system. It is about resonance and humility. It is again really important here to establish a still clinical space. The quality of this space contains, initiates, and holds the process. It is a call, in the darkness of unknowing, for a relationship to the Breath of Life itself as its mysterious intentions unfold. Remember your practitioner fulcrums, come into breath and sensation, let your mind still and hold a wide and natural field of listening. Let this deepen. Again, this is a call to the deeper healing intentions within and beyond the conditional forces being centered. Much more important, it is a humbling entrée into a healing process, which is a mutual journey for both therapist and patient.

1. With the patient in the supine position, place your hands in the CV4 hold. Synchronize your perceptual field to the mid-tide. Let your hands float within fluid and widen your perceptual field to the biosphere. Let the mid-tide rhythm come into your field of awareness.

2. Notice the boundary of excursion of the exhalation-extension motion. At this boundary, suggest "wait" through the occiput and the tissue field as a whole. If you are aware of the fluid tide, notice the unified dynamic between tissues and fluids and suggest a back pressure via your hand contact within the occiput and the fluids at the same time. This is a subtle suggestion, an inquiry into stillness. As you do this, you may sense a natural deepening of the stillpoint. A deeper quality of stillness may be perceived.

The tidal potencies and fluid tide will still. Again, this is a negotiated intention, an exploration into the possibility of deepening the stillpoint. Listen within the stillness for a sense of deepening.

3. When stillness is perceived to deepen, again widen your perceptual field, this time towards the horizon. Let your hands float within potency and widen your perceptual field towards the horizon. Do this very slowly and gently. Do not widen past your sense of safety and containment. With this intention, you are welcoming the Long Tide level of perception. You may again perceive a natural deepening of the stillness. At this level, it is not a matter of intending stillness or even of suggesting it. It is simply a matter of accessing that depth within yourself and of recognizing it within the patient. You are both within the Tide and even may have an experience of being the Tide. This level of stillness can be a gateway into the Dynamic Stillness itself. The wide perceptual field, and a mind that is neither coming nor going, are the keys to this gateway. There is a further stilling, a further deepening, then unknowing, a darkness. At the level of the Dynamic Stillness, there is truly perception without a perceiver. Here the Originality opens itself to itself as subject and object fade away. It is in essence a state of unity consciousness. At this level there is deep interconnection and mutuality as life heals itself. There may be a merging into a silence. Within the darkness, even time recedes.

4. As you come out of this darkness, or as you notice tidal phenomena again being generated, narrow your perceptual field to the biosphere and the embodied nature of the potencies and forces within the human system. This allows for integration and reentry into the embodied nature of experience. Give this process time. You are now back within space-time and embodied forces are at work. Let a process of realignment and reorientation occur. Wait for a clear sense of the fluid tide and for the tissue to complete any reorganization process occurring.

This section was meant to be a further exploration of the stillpoint process. In this there is a pointing to the depths of Stillness itself. It is up to each of us to journey into possibility and to know this territory for ourselves. In essence it cannot be taught. I can only give contexts and guidelines. It is a self-taught process.

D. Disengagement as the Mysterious Gateway

As we have seen, sometimes traumatic forces are so strong and the resulting compression is so deep that the inertial potencies involved do not have enough space to be expressed within states of balanced tension. The state of balanced tension may have a flat or dull quality to it. The tissues, fluids, and potencies involved may be deeply and intransigently inertial. Tissue and fluid changes may have occurred as a result. The *history* of the trauma may be deeply entrenched. There may be so much impaction between the structures involved that even within a state of balanced tension, the compressive forces are so intense that potencies within the fulcrum cannot be accessed. There is simply too much inertia to overcome. In these situations the skill of *disengagement* can help access the space needed to allow inertial potencies to be expressed. It is most commonly used in relationship to compression within sutures and joints. You will learn to use this skill within the context of a conversation with the potencies, forces, fluids, and tissues involved in the relationship. In other words, you will be conversing with the Health and with the history around which the system is organized.

Disengagement is a truly profound concept to grasp. It is really about the deeper intentions of the Breath of Life manifesting as the Original matrix is reestablished. It is about the intentions of the Breath of Life, which initially manifest in the development of the fetus, disengaging inertial forces from within. In some respects, if you understand disengagement, you have an entrée into developmental forces as they organize form throughout our lives. As you work with the intentions of disengagement and widen your perceptual field more and more, you will discover that disengagement truly comes from within. It is not a factor of your intervention, but is about a reconnection to the most primal organizing forces within the human body. We have discussed the state of balance and stillpoint as entrées into the epigenetic forces and the Original matrix itself. Here we will discuss disengagement in this same light.

Within the CRI level of perception, disengagement can be perceived to be a factor of practitioner intervention. "There is compression, I will decompress it." Disengagement can seem to be a factor of practitioner intention as resistance is perceived to be a problem to solve. At a mid-tide level of perception, disengagement may seem to be a factor of the potencies and forces at work within the system. The interplay between universal and conditional forces is perceived, and within the state of balance, the potency, as it acts within the fluids, is perceived to do the work. Within the Long Tide perceptual level, something else happens. There is a perception of potencies acting from the outside in and the inside out. There can literally be an experience of the potency of the Breath of Life coming from space, entering the midline, and moving right through the inertial fulcrum being explored. It is as if something gathers from the outside, wells up within the system, and moves right through the specific inertial fulcrum like wind through the eye of a hurricane. An actual sense of the permeation of the Breath of Life is appreciated. Then the experience is truly one of disengagement from within. Here there is a natural realignment to the Original intention of fluid, cellular, and tissue organization. The inherent potencies, within the depth of a stillness, bring you to the Original matrix itself as it unfolds its ordering function. It is about the nature of your presence, the stillness of your mind, and the natural balance of the sensory and motor functions of your awareness.

Application: Disengagement as the Mysterious Gateway

In the following process, you will use perceptual shifts to use the intentions of disengagement, the mysterious gateway or the eye of the needle, as an entrée into the deeper healing and ordering intentions of the Breath of Life. You will start from a perception of the biosphere and then shift to a much wider perceptual field. As you do this, the Long Tide may express itself. You may sense a much wider field of action, as if both you and the patient are within the same ocean or greater field of organization. We will use the frontozygomatic suture as an example.

Fundamentals Reviewed

It is really important here to establish a still clinical space. It contains, initiates, and holds the process. Remember your practitioner fulcrums, come into breath and sensation, let your mind still and hold a wide and natural field of listening. This establishes a safe therapeutic space and is a call to the deeper healing resources within and beyond the conditional forces being centered. Much more important, it is a humbling entrée into a healing process, which is a mutual journey for both therapist and patient.

1. Make contact with each bone on either side of the suture. In this exercise you will start at a mid-tide level of perception. Let your hands float on the bones and shift your perceptual field to the biosphere and the mid-tide. Let your hands be immersed within fluid and widen your perceptual field to the biosphere. Hold the whole body and the field around it within your field of awareness. Let the fluid tide come to you, then include the tissues as a tensile field.

2. As you hold this whole within your perceptual field, you may sense the tissues as a unified tensile field of action. Notice the suture as a particular within that field. You may sense the whole tensile tissue field distort around the inertial forces held within the suture. Very subtly intend space across the suture. This is given in the sense of an offering. It is an inquiry into pos-

sibility and space. It is not a demand. Do not grab the tissues as your explore this. If you do, you will lock the tissues up and may unconsciously shift to the CRI.

3. As space is accessed, you may sense the inertial forces at work within the suture. Biodynamic and biokinetic forces have become coupled and an inertial fulcrum has resulted. In this process, biodynamic forces will attempt to center the inertial forces that are maintaining the disturbance in the system. Facilitate a state of balanced tension as outlined above. At most you may have to simply and subtly slow down the tissue, fluid, or potency elements involved. At this level of perception, you may experience that the state of balance is inherent within the inertial fulcrum being palpated.

4. Once the state of balance is obtained, widen your perceptual field towards the horizon. Let your hands float within potency and shift your perceptual field towards the horizon. Widen your perceptual field to where it still feels safe and contained. As you do this, you may sense the deeper, slower tidal phenomenon of the Long Tide. The midline imperative generated by the Breath of Life may also become more obvious here.

5. Listen with an awareness of the intention of disengagement within the state of balance. The inherent biodynamic forces may begin to express their healing intentions. You may actually have an experience of the potency of the Breath of Life coming from "somewhere else," moving through the midline, through the tensile fields of the body, through the heart of the inertial fulcrum being attended to. As this occurs, you may have a direct perception of the biodynamic forces disengaging the sutural tissue. The biokinetic forces resolve, and disengagement is perceived to truly occur from the inside out.

6. It may feel as if intrinsic forces from within coming through a mysterious gateway to disengage the sutural compression. Like the eye of the needle, the shift in your perceptual fields can bring you to the most formative organizing forces at work. The intention of disengagement and the state of balance can bring you, like the eye of a needle, to the Original matrix itself. The motion of the potency of the Breath of Life through the inertial fulcrum, like a fountain spray of life, is most clearly experienced here as the force that disengages and resolves the inertial issue. Even deeper, within this context as, you settle into an even deeper stillness, one in which your mind is truly neither coming nor going, the Dynamic Stillness may unfold. This ground of emergence is one where a mystery truly unfolds and healing processes are impersonal, natural, and not about the centering of conditional forces. Here the question truly unfolds into its own answer.

I hope the processes outlined above give you a way into the "mysterious gateway." You will find that this will deepen your work and enhance its efficiency. It is about a deepening appreciation of the forces at work and the treatment plan generated by the centering intentions of the Breath of Life. Explore this over and over again in your practice sessions until the intentions and responses of the system become clear to you. This learning process is truly part of your developing ability to hear and respond. You are in the privileged position of appreciating the Health at the heart of the healing process.

Appendix III: Listen, It Is All About Perception

[This is an edited talk, which was given by Franklyn Sills in 1997 to a group of skilled practitioners at the end of an advanced course. It was meant to summarize some important ideas. The concepts were already familiar to the participants.][1]

I would like to give a summary of some of the things we have been talking about so far. It is all about perception. Perceptual skills are the *ground* of this work. Presence, contact, grounding, and the quality of space you hold are essential for success. Listen, don't look. Listening expands, looking narrows. The purpose of this work is not to release resistance or to process issues, but to liberate the health inherent within the resistance. This can be instantaneous. The treatment plan is inherent within the disturbance. The potency of the Breath of Life is always centering the disturbance, is always found within the heart of the inertial fulcrum. The state of balance allows it to be expressed beyond the compensation. Health is never lost; it centers our experience. Truth is found in the depths of our listening. Find the stillness that takes you beyond the form. It is from an intrinsic stillness, which is both still and yet dynamic, that this truth is found. The Breath of Life arises from stillness and returns to that stillness. The Dao is neutral and still. Yet within it are images, the blueprint of eternity. From it all motion arises and to it all returns. It is a dynamic process of generation and creation. It is always in present time. Past and future are holographically enfolded within the present. Healing occurs in this eternal present. Attention and intention are of key importance in the therapeutic relationship. The purpose of this work is not about tissue resistance per se; it is not to release something. Our intention is not to come from this place or that place, not to process issues, though issues will come up and be processed. Our intention is to be present for, and to relate to, the Health that is never lost. The purpose of the work is to access the Health that has centered the disturbance. The purpose is to liberate the health inherent within the resistance or the disturbance. We help the system to liberate potency so something else can happen beyond the compensations that we normally maintain. Sometimes the system will reestablish compensation as the first step when it has been exhausted. Sometimes the person's system is ready to shift. Sometimes it is not, and that's okay. It can take ten to fifteen minutes just to settle in and relate to that health. Suddenly there is relationship, and then things start to happen.

Listen, listen, listen. Let images come, but don't narrow the looking down. Have a spacious sense of listening (spaciousness and patience). As we get closer to the original reference beam it means acknowledging and connecting with the health within. Even if the physical body is collapsing, that doesn't mean all is lost. Death can be a transition and a transmutation. Relate to the health in the system.

Listen for it, listen to it. Especially when there is exhaustion at the end of a day in clinical work, shift to acknowledge health. Get out of the way and hold the field. Listen for the expression of health at many levels. Listen for potency and cellular pulsation. Then, when resistances come up, you have a different relationship from the viewpoint of the health in the system. Work from the mid-tide and the Long Tide. This is where the healing forces are expressed. This is much less tiring. This work is a joint practice of inquiry by practitioner and patient. Come into your fulcrums. Come into a receptive perceptual field. There is vast Intelligence in this process. If order was not inherent, we would fall to pieces and fragment. This is what keeps us together in the midst of our conditions. In the midst of all the shapes and forms generated, there is something that holds them and us. This is the Breath of Life and its potency. Centering it all is this health. All the compensatory shapes and relationships are also intelligent. Listen for the Intelligence centering them. Densification happens in what would naturally be fluid. Within the density, look for what is still fluid. Health is always expressed. Instead of seeing patterns of resistance to get rid of, perceive the Intelligence. Move beyond that other view. Open your perceptual field. Get out of the way.

Learn to negotiate your boundaries. Listen for space, not just the form of things. Do not invade; there is no need to. Do not grab any of the three functions (potency, fluids, and tissues). Do not lock up the structure and function of the system. Your *attention* can lock up the system if it is not negotiated or inappropriate. This is very subtle. It is easy to miss this. It is easy to fool yourself here. The system will then react to your presence, and you will end up chasing shadows.

Potency, fluids, and tissues will speak to you if you hold respectful and negotiated space. Listen; do not look for anything. Remember—no expectations— not for yourself, not for the work, not for any results. Let go of the need to do anything, to have anything happen, and listen. Listen, please, it *is* about perception. What is the patient's system saying to you? Can you allow the inherent treatment plan to arise in its own time? Let your hands be buoyant and go beyond the bounds of palpation to truly listen. Listen with a caring interest and space, not with need.

All tensions are reciprocal in nature. Even fluids express reciprocal tension motion, both longitudinal and lateral. Even potency is a tensile field of action. Potency is a tensile field of action, fluid is a tensile field of action, and tissues are a tensile field of action. All three express reciprocal tension motion around suspended automatically shifting fulcrums. Fulcrums are energetic in nature. They are points of potency—a stillness within a larger field of action. Listen—all three functions are organized around automatically shifting fulcrums, and all three functions will speak to you. They will show you their story with precision as the Breath of Life centers everything with precision. Individual tissue structures express reciprocal tension motion as part of a unified dynamic—as part of a whole tensile field of action. Do not get lost in the parts; always hold an awareness of the whole. The parts will speak to you more precisely then. When you palpate/sense the whole of someone, that whole will speak to you. The treatment plan will clarify over time and the whole tensile field will express it. You may sense the whole tensile tissue field distort around a fulcrum as the potency expresses the treatment plan from within. You do not need to do anything to find what needs to happen. You do not need to motion test, to analyze, to figure it out— this only gets in the way. Listen within a wide field of awareness and it will clarify.

Bone, membrane, tissues, fluids, and potency are a unit of function. They are a unified dynamic. They are whole. Potency is the motive force, fluids are the medium of exchange, and the cellular and tissue world organizes around its action. Motility is generated by the action of the potency within the fluids and this is all one thing, a unit of function. Units of function are whole and are organized by fulcrums. A fulcrum is a still place, a point of potency that has the power to organize and move. Listen for its action within the heart of the form. All reciprocal tension motions are organized around fulcrums, both inertial and natural. Automatically shifting fulcrums shift with the intentions of the Tide. Remember that inertial fulcrums are not automatically shifting fulcrums. They do not shift with the intentions of the Tide. The whole tensile field will lead you to its action.

A fulcrum is a still place, in essence—a point of condensed potency around which organization is generated. Natural fulcrums, like Sutherland's fulcrum, are distinct points of potency that organize the reciprocal tension motion of fluids and tissues, and which shift with the intentions of the Tide. They are suspended automatically shifting fulcrums. They are suspended, so to speak, within the whole tensile field of action, be it potency, fluid, or tissue, and organize and move that field. Inertial fulcrums are expressions of unresolved experience, even of genetics if they overlay and distort the organizing field of potency. Inertial fulcrums are centered within the whole field of action. As this occurs, suspended automatically shifting fulcrums will shift in their action in order to center the conditions present. The whole field distorts to accommodate this. The inertial fulcrum then becomes an organizing factor within the whole tensile field. Distortions occur at every level: tissue and structural distortion, fluid distortions, and distortions in the unified field of potency, the bioenergy field. The osteopathic lesions result. It is an affect, not a cause or origin. All are organized around inertial fulcrums, which are sites of inertial potency. These inertial sites have the potency, or power, to organize. Stasis, inertia, and loss of motion results—this is the first movement to disease states. Inertial forces generate inertial fluids and tissues, and vitality is lost, disorder sets in.

But remember—within the heart of every inertial fulcrum there is Health at work, centering the unresolved forces that generate the disturbance within the system. Remember Dr. Becker's concept here. At the heart of every inertial fulcrum there is potency, the biodynamic potency of the Breath of Life, centering the inertial, or added, forces present.

This is crucial to understand. Potency becomes inertial in order to center and contain the unresolvable forces present. There is biodynamic potency at work centering the unresolved forces of experience, trauma and disease states. The inertial forces within the system are centered in precise ways. They will also be attended to by the Breath of Life in precise ways and in a precise order. Dr. Becker said that the *treatment plan* is inherent within the conditions present. The treatment plan lies hidden within the very fulcrum organizing the disturbance within the system. If you are silent and maintain a wide field of listening, this treatment plan will begin to express itself. It is inherent within the conditions being centered within the body as a whole. The treatment plan arises within the field of potency from ever deeper sources. It moves *through* the fulcrum. Listen and you will sense things clarifying—a particular fulcrum and a particular shape of altered reciprocal tension motion will clarify, and the Tide will focus its intentions precisely within the fulcrum at the heart of it all. Please recognize the precision of all this. You must listen for this treatment plan, for this precision, and clinical work becomes much less tiring and more efficient.

All reciprocal tension motion expresses a precise proportionality of form. Dr. Randolph Stone used to say, "God geometizes, man cognizes." We cannot approach this precision by thinking—only by listening within a wide and neutral field of awareness. All reciprocal tension expresses boundaries. It is the fulcrum that organizes these motions that establishes the boundary. Palpate the limits and then let them go. Sense the fulcrum that organizes the shape, sense the heart of the motion, not the poles of its expression. Remember that all tension is reciprocal, even altered tensions due to the presence of inertial forces. States of balance occur within reciprocal tension fields. These are states of dynamic equilibrium. The state of dynamic equilibrium reorients the potencies and inertial forces present to natural automatically shifting fulcrums and to the primal midline. Fulcrums reorient to the midline. Midlines are expressions of the organizing inten-

433

tions of the Breath of Life in action. Look for re-orientation to midline phenomena and naturally suspended automatically shifting fulcrums. This gives you much clinical information. The Breath of Life is the Tide within this midline. It is eternally primal and primary. It acts to center our existence.

The state of balance initiates a process of easing into receptivity. It is a receptivity to Originality, to origin. The state of balance is like a mysterious gateway into something beyond the conditions being centered. The state of balance, a dynamic equilibrium, resonates with the Stillness at the heart of all form and all natural organization. Appreciate this. It is the heart of clinical practice. Wait for this neutral to appear, listen for it, don't miss it. It is a settling within all of the potencies and forces present. It is a settling of the conditions present. It is a gateway to the deeper organizing forces within the human system.

Listen for expressions of Health. It is relatively easy to palpate resistance and disorder. But can you sense the Health that centers it all? This is your challenge. Can you sense the potency centering the inertial forces present? Can you sense the bioelectric, epigenetic matrix, the blueprint of form? Can you sense the action of the Long Tide, the ordering winds of the human system? Can you sense the Stillness at the heart of it all? All are at work, always acting in the eternal present. Don't be led by conditions, only by expressions of Health. Center on the deeper healing resources of the system, not just on the results and affects of suffering. Stillness is at the heart of the fulcrum. Deepen into Stillness. Don't get lost in stillpoints. As Dr. Becker mentioned, there are thousands of stillpoints, but only one Stillness. Let the stillpoint be a gateway to the deeper experience of Stillness. The Dynamic Stillness is a ground of emergence and is known only in silence and *unknowing*.

Do not try to change the disturbance; leave it be. Let suffering be. Attend to the health, which centers it always. It wants to tell its story without interruption or intervention. Listen to the story and access the health. Do not worry about results and affects. Lesions will take care of themselves once the potency is accessed. The Breath of Life and its potency is at the heart of the healing process. It is unconditional health in action. It is self-correcting and self-balancing. The Breath of Life arises from the Dynamic Stillness. This is only known in unknowing. Your mind cannot grasp this, only your heart. Settle into the Stillness and the Health will take over. Originality will emerge. Listen within the silence.

Remember that all of your classical skills are conversations, not demands. They are skills, not techniques. Learn the primary relationships. Let them lead you to the heart of things. Osseous to membrane, membrane to fluid, fluid to potency, potency to the Breath of Life, and Breath of Life to the Dynamic Stillness. Discrete phenomena, yet totally interconnected, all mutually arise and are interdependently originated. All lead back to Origin and Source, not to causes. All are mysterious gateways to the truth of things, but only if you listen. Simply listen; it is all about perception. Be still and present and the essence of Originality will emerge.

1. Some additional material has been added to this talk from another talk.

Appendix IV: Space and Form[1]

Let's take a breath together. Settle into stillness. Let the silence take you. Simply let your mind settle. There is nothing to do in that. . . . Now feel the space for a minute, in the room. Just take a minute, come into your center and let your awareness extend out and sense the *space* in the room that we inhabit. As you sense that space, notice that it is the space which allows your awareness to move. Notice how we inhabit space. . . .

Now coming into your midline, the center of yourself, almost sense that you're a coalescence within the space. Something that has coalesced, that has condensed, that has intended to inhabit this space. Just feel yourself, in the very present moment, coalescing and inhabiting this space. And just notice that it's the space which allows things to unfold. And just bring your awareness to the whole of the space you're in and sense now the other people in the room inhabiting that space, coalescing, condensing, intending to be here together in this space. Extend your awareness out so you're holding everyone, your perceptual field is holding the whole building. Just sense us all for a moment inhabiting this space together. . . . Now take another minute staying within this space and very slowly open your eyes and see if you can maintain an awareness of co-inhabiting this space together. . . . So let's come into relationship within this space we are inhabiting just now.

Know that the work we do is about space more than about form. It is space which allows things to move, to change, to grow. The natural world is based on space. The Breath of Life organizes space in order to organize form. And we're part of that, literally, as a coalescence in space. . . . If you just work with the form of things—and in this work the tendency might be to just work with the resistance, the pain, the results of experience; then you've lost the opportunity of reconnecting to what allows that to unfold, which is space. The significance of the room we're in is in its space. Isn't it? It's nice to look at the walls and the things hanging on them, but the usefulness of the room is in its space. What allows us to use the room is its space and its doors and windows. Doors and windows are functions of space, they open to space. What would this room be without doors and windows? It would be hard to inhabit, wouldn't it? So there is something about the permeability of the space and the ability to move through space which allows form to unfold.

So the work we do is really about space and the space between things; what inhabits that space. And what inhabits the space between things is very much about intention. We are here as a direct intention to be a human being. And that intention is a movement through space. The spaces in our body are full of fluids. Dr. Sutherland gave a talk in which he said there is an ocean of cerebrospinal fluid in this very room. And it's the fluids within the spaces that support that intention to be here as a human being. And that's the heart of the work, reestablishing that connection. From the space to what supports that intention to be here. And what allows that, what really inhabits space and is perhaps the essence of space, is what Dr. Sutherland called the Breath of Life. It is this Breath of Life which organizes order out of chaos, form out of space.

Space in essence is emptiness. And it is emptiness which supports the unfoldment of all form. Stillness imbues emptiness with meaning and potential. Within the space, if you're all tuned into it, there is this palpable quality of Stillness. Stillness is the ground of emergence from which the Breath of Life acts. Stillness connects, it maintains integrity. It's a universal. Life is whole, it is not separate.

When we look at each other, we look like very separate beings, and there is that aspect. I have a particular form, and I've become conditioned to believe I'm a "Franklyn." (I don't quite believe that but . . . —[laughter] It's very easy to see each other through the separateness, through the differences. And we all get very involved in our lives and it's very easy to feel, within that, disconnected from the whole. We get caught up in the particulars of our life. But they are like the waves on the ocean. You see separate waves. But they're all part of the Tide and they rise and they pass just as we will. Just as this body will arise and pass. But there is something else there also. So being a discrete person is sort of like being a wave that has become rigid for a period of time. Like we're kind of frozen in time, and then all we see are the waves and we relate to each other like separate wave forms. We lose touch with the whole, with the Tide we are all part of. We lose touch with the fluidity of what's possible and the mutual arising and passing of the waves. We're all mutually arising from the same tide. That's how the natural world is. It is whole. Things are totally interconnected and co-arise. And when you're there holding or palpating someone's system you're both separate waves and yet you're part of the same Tide. So in the relationship of the waves, there is

clarity of boundaries, there is clarity of form, there are roles and all of that, but at the level of the Tide there is the wholeness, there is the mutual arising nature of two human beings. There is interconnectedness.

And when you're there, these things that we're teaching aren't arbitrary. When you're there, holding someone's head, or their big toe, or any body part, and you're holding this wide perceptual field that we encourage you to hold, within that field, within the holding of that field, there is a possibility to sense the universality of your relationship to the whole. And within that universality, within that possibility of wholeness there is a conversation that starts, in a way, tide to tide. And in that conversation, as you're holding your attention, your perceptual field in relationship to that person, that "seemingly other," if you like, something else can happen beyond the form, beyond the suffering within that spaciousness that you're holding. It's almost like a reminder: there is space here. And within the space, moment to moment, there is the possibility of something else beyond our conditioning to reestablish itself. That which holds everything together. When you go down to the depths of this work there is a highly spiritual quality to it. Without calling it anything. Without having to make it into a thing. Spiritual by the very fact we're here in relationship. Without having to call it a religion or anything. So the early practitioners of this work, and many current ones, have an incredible reverence for the work. Which really means they have a reverence for our relationship as human beings together. That there is something within that possibility of contact and relationship which can reestablish the whole. That calls upon the potential beyond the conditioned forms we hold.

What we usually do in our relationships is come from our conditioning and our particulars. But in having a relationship here, with another human being, holding spaciousness and presence, something else becomes possible. When I'm in the still center, where I'm appreciating space, this allows some other conversation to take place, beyond "I'm a Franklyn." Beyond you're a Jim or a Jane, or whatever. Something deeper which is quite magical. And no matter how much you want to rationalize and analyze the work you do—this lesion pattern does that and this pathology shifts, these emotions are expressed, and CV4s do this, and all that—no matter how we want to rationalize or understand whatever kind of healing work we do, whether you give pills, whether you stick needles in people, whether you do adjustments, it doesn't matter; what heals is something which is very mysterious. No matter how much we understand the immune system, the neuroendocrine immune system and all that, underlying it all, there is something which is beautifully mysterious. And as healers if we forget that, if we lose touch with that, if we got lost in the form, then we have lost a lot.

And within all that, it's also really important to have the particular knowledge you need to help the person in their suffering. You need to know how to be in relationship to suffering in specific ways that are helpful. And that's the other side of what we learn, the other side of the coin, so to speak. We learn how to be very precise and specific and efficient in meeting suffering. In meeting places that have become frozen, distressed, abandoned. And that's about an awareness of clinical issues, of anatomy and physiology, so you can work within any level that's appropriate, where that person's system needs to work as a reflection of the inherent treatment plan and of the Breath of Life and its intentions. And to be able to reflect the Health within all of that. Not just to reflect the pain and the resistance. Not just to release the symptoms, but to touch the Health which is never lost again. Many people learn this work in ways that just reflect resistance. And you can get a certain level of change in that. But what I encourage you all to do, no matter what form your work takes, is to learn how to reflect the Health.

And in order to do that you have to be in relationship to it in some way. You have to learn how to sense it, to palpate it, to feel it. It has to be a perceptual experience, a felt sense. Not just in your mind, but in your body, a felt experience. And when you can reflect Health to that person's system, it is one of the most powerful things anyone can do. I am not saying this is the only way to do it, but I find this a very powerful way to work. And that's really where I want to start from. That this work is about the perception and reflection of Health. And within that is the ability to reflect how we're holding our suffering to acknowledge, "Oh, this is what it's like. This is how bad it's been." In the acknowledgment of a pattern, of inertia and pain, there can be a deep recognition. An acknowledgment of suffering. So we must hold both the Health *and* the suffering. Carl Jung wrote elegantly towards the end of his life about what he called the *transcendent function*. He said that it is the role of the therapist to hold both the universal and the conditional. As the therapist does this, the possibility for a balance between these poles arises and it is in this balance that the transcendent function naturally arises. Then something else can happen beyond the conditions present. Sound familiar?

So in that there can be a deep acknowledgment of suffering as you meet another's process, as a practitioner in that reflective process. There is something here about acknowledging, "Ah, this is how it has been for you." And in that there may be an "Ah, someone can see how it's been." It is heard. Then, "You've done really well, you're really holding this together. As desperate as the situation may be, you're still here. You're still holding it together in some way. How do you do that?" That's the next level of conversation. "How does your Health center this disturbance? And can that Health be expressed in another way, beyond the conditions and compensations that we have to hold right now?" So the conversation shifts from "Aha, so this is how it is," to "Wow! So this is how it can be!" "What centers this? What is holding this together? What allows yourself to remain an integrated human being? What is whole and never lost? How do you express this Health to center this disturbance, this distortion in your system?"

In many ways we're not really working with the

distortion. We're relating to the Health that's centering it. We go under the distortion. And that's the beauty of this work. And that has to do, coming back to where I started, with space and spaciousness. That is what maintains life. The forms we create are important because that is how we generate our sense of self and our sense of joy and suffering. All those forms are important to acknowledge and to meet, but the essence of the work is what holds that, what integrates that, what is whole within that? Where is the Health? How is that expressed?

And that is a really good lead-in to what I want to talk about, which is how Health is expressed from the moment of conception. How we actually organize ourselves around Health. It may not seem like that. And our minds do a lot of funny things with our lives, don't they? I can only speak for myself. I'm sorry, my mind does funny things! [laughter]

But you know, the body never lies. When you're meeting a person and palpating in this way, truth is naturally communicated. The body will tell you, "This is how it's been and this is how it is now." The body will show you how it's compensated, its defensive strategies, its suffering. The body never lies. The mind does all sorts of funny things with it. So as we're learning to palpate in deeper and deeper ways, we're meeting truth. We're meeting that person's truth. This is so important to understand.

I have this wonderful little sign on my roll-top desk that says, "Truth is truth, wherever you find it." It may be in all sorts of guises and shapes and forms, and when you meet that person's system, and you're meeting it through the anatomy and physiology, through the subtle physiology of that system, through its energies, you're meeting the truth of that person. Their history, their life, how it's been. Their joys, their sorrows. Their neutral places. Their hopes, their fears. You're meeting that directly. The shape and form of the truth of who that person is. And that's a very privileged thing to be able to do. And we must hold that quality of respect. We learn to be very deep listeners to a person, their story, and it's totally nonverbal. It doesn't have to have any words attached to it. The body holds the story

and it tells it. The mind may do all sorts of funny things with the story and distort it. And within that, in that clinical relationship, we're also holding the truth of what organizes all that. The Health that allows that to unfold.

As compensated and shaped as I am, there is still that which is allowing all that to unfold and holding things together. And that's the essence that we work with. It starts from the moment of conception. It becomes a midline phenomenon. Initially within the embryo, which we'll see. That truth, that Breath of Life, that neuter essence, that blueprint energy. And the cellular and tissue world unfolds as it needs to in order to maintain an intention of being a human being.

So that one cell at conception starts dividing and dividing and dividing and dividing, and it's driven to complete an intention. The intention of being a human being. And that may mean that a certain number of those cells complete in the intention of becoming a liver. Certain other number of cells complete in becoming an intention of lungs. But that intention is still whole. The intention of the human being as a whole. The particular has to be there. So that functions can arise, so we can be here. But those functions which we tend to separate out—this is the digestive system, this is the cardiovascular system, this is the musculoskeletal system—they're all still that one cell carried through an intention to be particular functions. The are all still whole and never truly separate. Even when there are billions of cells, there is the whole human being, never fragmented, never lost. So we're still always whole at any particular time. It takes a still and wide perceptual field to begin to appreciate that. And that's another thing in our work—holding that wide perceptual field. Holding the whole allows that awareness of the whole to actually be there. So that when particulars arise, whether they're particular structures or places of inertia or functions, those particulars can be seen by the practitioner in the context of the whole. Indeed, the system can see itself in that context.

So we kind of work with a split attention in many

ways. Our attention is on the whole and yet we can also be aware of the particular. But if you lose the whole and you narrow down to just the particular, you lose the potential of allowing that Health to start to show itself because you have narrowed down just to the particular condition in that system. So holding the whole allows us to hold more than just that particular condition and allows the Health to start to express itself through that condition, that strain, that compression, that pathology, it doesn't matter. So what I'd like to do—I can talk about this for hours, let's be careful. I want to focus this a bit in terms of what happens in the early embryo and how the midline is established around which the vertebrae condense. This is our seminar for this time. The vertebrae—which is a particular and the centerline of our body—which become the vertebral axis, coalesce around the initial midline laid down by the Breath of Life within the embryo, and we're continually coalescing, if you like, in relationship to that midline throughout our lives. So I'd

like to talk about that. Remember that the cellular and tissue world is organized by potency and the natural world is organized by the great Breath of Life. A tree is part of the whole just as we are part of the whole. The mouse that escaped my cat's clutches last night and is now inhabiting my house is part of the whole. I have to respect that. I may have lots of feelings about that mouse at the moment. No, it's the cat, that's the one whom I have feelings about, actually [laughter]. But we're all part of the whole, and it's a great cosmic universal play unfolding, of all sorts of things. . . . Let's take a break now and after the break, let's look at some embryology together. From these, we will introduce some clinical work in relationship to vertebral dynamics.

1. Talk by Franklyn Sills, February 1998, ©Karuna Institute. Thanks to Sarah Delphont for transcribing this talk.

Some Recommended Books In the Cranial Field

Becker, Rollin. *Life in Motion.* Rudra Press.

Becker, Rollin. *The Stillness of Life.* Stillness Press.

Kern, Michael. *The Craniosacral Approach to Essential Health.* Thorsons/Harper Collins.

Magoun, H. *Osteopathy in the Cranial Field.* Sutherland Cranial Teaching Foundation.

Milne, H. *The Heart of Listening.* North Atlantic Books.

Sutherland, W. G. *Contributions of Thought.* Rudra Press.

Sutherland, W. G. *Teachings in the Science of Osteopathy.* Rudra Press.

Upledger, John. *Craniosacral Therapy,* 2 vols. Eastland Press.

Other Recommended Books

Bloom, Sandra. *Creating Sanctuary.* Routledge. An excellent exploration into trauma from a societal and developmental perspective.

Bohm, David. *Wholeness and the Implicate Order.* Ark Paperbacks. The seminal work which explores the physics of the holographic universe.

Briggs and Peat. *Looking Glass Universe.* Simon and Schuster. An introduction into new physics.

Briggs and Peat. *Turbulent Mirror.* Harper & Row. An introduction into chaos theory and the science of wholeness.

Coates, Callum. *Living Energies.* Gateway Books. An exploration into the work of Victor Schauberger.

Herman, Judith. *Trauma and Recovery.* Pandora. An excellent journey into the psychology and healing of trauma.

Ho, Mae-Wan. *The Rainbow and the Worm, the Physics of Organisms.* World Scientific. An extraordinary enquiry into physics and living organisms.

Juhan, Deane. *Job's Body.* Station Hill. A classic exploration into the nature of tissues written for bodyworkers.

Ledoux, Joseph. *The Emotional Brain.* Phoenix Press. An exceptional inquiry into the nature of the brain and its stress responses.

Levine, Peter. *Waking the Tiger*. North Atlantic Books. An essential introduction to trauma in the human system.

Oschman, James. *Energy Medicine*. Churchill Livingstone. An excellent exploration into the science of energy medicine.

Pert, Candace. *Molecules of Emotion*. Scriber Press. An excellent introduction into the Biochemical links among consciousness, mind, and body.

Rothschild, Babette. *The Body Remembers: the Psychophysiology of Trauma and Trauma Treatment*. (Norton & Co.)

Schwenk, Theodor. *Sensitive Chaos*. Rudolph Steiner Press. An extraordinary inquiry into the nature of water, flow and living organisms.

This book list is by no means meant to be exhaustive. It highlights some important contributions to the cranial field and points to some other important areas of inquiry.

For Training information about a craniosacral biodynamic approach to work within the cranial field, contact:

The Karuna Institute
Natsworthy Manor
Widecombe in the Moor
Devon, United Kingdom
TQ13 7TR
Karuna@eurobell.co.uk
www.karuna-institute.co.uk

Index

About the Author

· ·

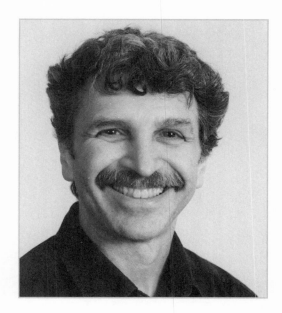

Franklyn Sills is Co-director of the Karuna Institute, a respected post-graduate Institute for Craniosacral Biodynamics and Core Process Psychotherapy. Throughout his career, he has been in the forefront of pioneering a biodynamic approach to work within the cranial field. His training includes medical research, Osteopathic work, and an in-depth study of the work of Dr. Randolph Stone. His main focus has been placed within the context of craniosacral teaching and clinical practice. He is the author of the award-winning book *The Polarity Process*.